NUTRITION
IN THE COMMUNITY
The Art of Delivering Services

NUTRITION IN THE COMMUNITY
The Art of Delivering Services

ANITA YANOCHIK OWEN, M.A., R.D.

President, Owen Associates, Inc., Consultants in Health Care and
Nutrition Education; Adjunct Assistant Professor,
Department of Home Economics and Nutrition,
New York University, New York, New York;
Adjunct Associate Professor, Graduate School of Health
Sciences, New York Medical College, Valhalla, New York;
President, The American Dietetic Association (1985-1986)

REVA T. FRANKLE, M.S., Ed. D., R.D.

Director of Nutrition, Weight Watchers International, Inc.,
Manhasset, New York; Adjunct Associate Professor,
Graduate School of Health Sciences, New York
Medical College, Valhalla, New York; President,
Frankle Associates, Nutrition Consultants

Second Edition

with 94 *illustrations*

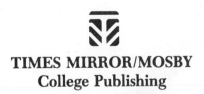

TIMES MIRROR/MOSBY
College Publishing

ST. LOUIS • TORONTO • SANTA CLARA   1986

Editor: Nancy K. Roberson
Assistant editor: Kathy Sedovic
Project editor: Connie Povilat
Manuscript editor: Linda Duncan
Cover designer: John R. Rokusek
Production: Susan Trail, Teresa Breckwoldt

SECOND EDITION

Library of Congress Cataloging-in-Publication Data

Frankle, Reva T.
   Nutrition in the community.

   Authors' names in reverse order in previous ed.
   Bibliography: p.
   Includes index.
   1. Nutrition policy—United States. 2. Community
health services—United States. I. Owen, Anita
Yanochik, 1937–   . II. Title. [DNLM: 1. Community
Health Services—United States. 2. Nutrition.
QU 145 F831n]
TX360.U6F73   1986   363.8'83   85-24495
ISBN 0-8016-1678-6

F/VH/VH   9 8 7 6 5 4 3 2   02/D/291

To
George, Gregory,
and my parents,
Louis and Evelyn Vangarelli

Anita Yanochik Owen

To
George, Joyce, Jon, and Joshua
and my parents,
Belle and Hick Treelisky

Reva T. Frankle

Preface

Occasionally a book so accurately captures the essence of its time that it becomes a classic for that decade. In the 1950s it was *The Organization Man*; in the 1970s it was *Future Shock*; and in the 1980s it was *Megatrends*. The second edition of *Nutrition in the Community: The Art of Delivering Services* captures the tumultuous times in which health and nutrition professionals live and work. This book presents a new plan to aid dietitians/nutritionists in serving the community. The second edition is more than a revision—it is a new book in message, content, and style. With only Chapters 3 and 8 retained from the first edition, this 15-chapter textbook can be considered a primer and a "survival kit" for undergraduates, graduate students, teachers, and practitioners because of its strong emphasis on managing both the internal and external environment to achieve health outcomes.

Health care has changed considerably since the publication of the first edition in 1978. Because of the emphasis on cost containment and the limits on the amount that will be paid for performance of health care, it is predicted that hospitals will become tertiary care centers. Many of the traditional services now offered by hospitals will be delivered in community settings. Growth of alternate health care delivery systems, such as outpatient facilities, community models, and home health care, are envisioned.

In addition, there is a great deal of consumer interest in nutrition and healthy life-styles, as evidenced by the growing national enthusiasm for exercise and the number of persons who have decreased consumption of calories, fat, and sodium.

This national preoccupation with healthy life-styles is evidenced by the nation's new set of major health goals. For the first time a set of major goals for improving the health of Americans over the coming decades was introduced by the Department of Health and Human Services with the publication in 1979 of *Healthy People: The Surgeon General's Report on Health Promotion and Disease Prevention*. *Promoting Health/Preventing Disease*, which described specific health objectives for the nation to be achieved by 1990 was published in 1980. A 1983 document detailed an implementation plan to accomplish these objectives.

Because they set forth health goals for the nation, these documents helped shed light on the second public health revolution in the United States. The first revolution came with the dramatic shift in the leading causes of death and disability in the United States. Coronary heart disease, cancer, stroke, and accidents have replaced infectious diseases as the leading causes of death for Americans. Controllable risk factors such as smoking, diet, alcohol use, and lack of exercise are now associated with the leading causes of death. Action based on new understanding of how Americans can respond to the challenge posed by chronic disease and behavior-related health problems comprises the second public health revolution. Knowledge about the relationship between health and behavior continues to expand, and strategies for preventing disease and promoting healthy life-styles help ensure major strides in attainment of better health.

This book addresses the major health initiatives for the 1980s and 1990s. It provides student, faculty member, and practitioner with guidelines for management and delivery of nutrition services.

THE PURPOSE OF THIS NEW EDITION AND WHY A MAJOR CHANGE

The purpose of this edition is to present a new and stimulating approach to community nutrition by fully developing the skills needed by community dietitians/nutritionists and health professionals for the 1980s and 1990s. It covers a broad range of topics, yet it offers sufficient depth to provide significant information for the undergraduate, graduate, teacher, and practitioner.

The new agenda for community dietitians/nutritionists discussed in the text is based on several documents that describe the changing role of the nutrition professional. The most comprehensive and recent document is *A New Look at the Profession of Dietetics*, a 1984 report by the Study Commission on Dietetics (Chapter 1). This study recommended future courses of action for the profession based on a changing health care delivery system. The study commission recommended a broader base of education for dietitians/nutritionists, particularly in behavioral sciences, greater emphasis on management and communication, use of new technology, and greater scientific knowledge of nutrition.

This edition of *Nutrition in the Community* covers each of these topics in depth. In Part I, Managing Community Nutrition Services, seven chapters are devoted to management, business, and communications. In Part II, Delivering Quality Nutrition Services, emphasis is on scientific knowledge of nutrition throughout the life cycle. Part III, Tools for Developing Effective Community Nutrition Services, contains chapters on developing analytical, behavioral change, grantsmanship, and public policy skills.

NEW IN THIS EDITION

Substantial changes have been made in the development and organization of the second edition.

Part I, Managing Community Nutrition Services, provides a comprehensive treatment of the subject matter. Six of the seven chapters in this section are new.

"Community Nutrition: An Essential Component of Health and Health Care" (Chapter 1) sets the tone for the learning experience by identifying the unique role of the community dietitian/nutritionist and other nutrition personnel in health care. Each of the subsequent chapters provides detailed descriptions for developing the skills needed to become an effective practitioner. A discussion of the major trends in our society and their effect on consumers assists the dietetic and nutrition student and practitioner in understanding the world in which nutrition services must be delivered.

With its multitude of topics and issues, a systematic approach to management can easily become an overwhelming subject for the reader. Abundant material is presented within a systematic framework so that the student can progress in an orderly manner. The cornerstone of the foundation is Chapter 2, "Managing and Managers: Their Role in Community Nutrition." In this chapter, the concept of management and its four basic functions is defined. The nutrition manager's role in planning, organizing, leading, and controlling to obtain organizational effectiveness is described.

In "Planning and Decision Making in Community Nutrition to Produce Outcomes" (Chapter 3) there is a detailed discussion of strategic planning and the role that values play in formulating plans. The case study of a community (Everywheresville) brings to life the baseline data and needs assessment required to understand a community. It prepares the reader to use information provided in succeeding chapters.

A social marketing plan is developed for Everywheresville in Chapter 4 to demonstrate the use of marketing strategies for nutrition services. Contemporary management strategies are described in "Organizing and Developing Action Plans for Nutrition," such as the successful use of power in an organization, the changing views of conflict, and how to stimulate and encourage creativity in a changing organization.

What is your leadership style? How well do you communicate and listen? How do you motivate people? These are the elements that are developed in Chapter 5, "Leading to Achieve Individual and Organizational Goals." After reading this chapter, the student will be able to determine a leadership style and to understand effective and ineffective methods of communication.

Sound management requires effective control. Chapter 6, "Controlling Nutrition Services for Productivity," describes the essential steps in program evaluation. With the use of a case study, the basic processes of evaluation are clearly delineated. These include what to evaluate, the measures used in evaluation, and what can go wrong in evaluating a program.

The important steps in and potential use of cost-effectiveness and cost-benefit analysis in nutritional care are addressed in Chapter 7, along with a method for developing a quality assurance program.

Part II, Delivering Quality Nutrition Services, is greatly expanded from the first edition. "The Elements of Quality Nutrition Services for Prevention of Disease and Promotion of Health" (Chapter 8) includes nutrition assessment, intervention, and referral systems. General information is provided for each element. In Chapters 9 through 11 guidelines for nutrition services throughout the life cycle are specified, including nutrition and nutrition services for pregnant women, infants, children, adolescents, adults, and the elderly. Strategies at the local level are depicted in each chapter, and innovative action programs throughout the life cycle are described. For example, Massachusetts Nutrition Resource Center, where consumers receive nutrition information through a hot line and mail service, is described. The health promotion worksite program at Southern New England Telephone is discussed, and the nutrition component of the community-based Minnesota Heart Health Program is described.

Part III, Tools for Developing Effective Community Nutrition Services, has two new chapters. These chapters were included to present the student with a total picture of the skills needed to be an effective practitioner. In Chapter 12, "Tools for Developing Effective Community Nutrition Services," both statistics and epidemi-ology are reviewed. Because effective use of computers is a challenge for dietitians, Chapter 12 includes their basic uses in nutrition services.

Becoming a more effective change agent for patients and clients requires knowledge of the behavioral sciences. Methods for changing behavior, elements in nutrition counseling, and assessment of intervention outcomes are some of the strategies and techniques discussed in Chapter 13. Updated information in "Grants and Grantsmanship" (Chapter 14) and "Developing Public Policy Skills and Legislation" (Chapter 15) provides a set of tools that every student, faculty member, and practitioner requires to meet consumer needs.

PEDAGOGICAL AIDS

Various learning aids are employed to enhance the usefulness of this text by students and faculty.

Applications and Case Studies. Our extensive experience in the field has helped us provide many applications of community nutrition throughout the text. A case study is presented in Chapter 3 and is then further developed throughout the management chapters. With one case study, used as consistent thread throughout these chapters, the student's learning will be enhanced. In Chapter 6 a case study is built into the entire chapter for ease in understanding of how to control nutrition services for productivity.

General Concept. Each chapter begins with a brief opening paragraph that provides an overview of the chapter.

Objectives. The major learning objectives for each chapter are stated to reinforce their significance for the student.

Chapter Opening Illustrations. All new illustrations open each chapter to help identify and reinforce the concepts covered in the chapter.

Figures and Tables. Strong visual materials are used in each chapter to illustrate important points. The theme of management process is carried through Chapters 2 to 7 by the use of figures that highlight the planning, organizing, leading, and controlling processes.

Chapter Summaries. Each chapter ends with a brief summary that is particularly valuable for quick review of the subjects discussed in that chapter.

References. Each chapter provides current references to allow the reader to gain further information.

Glossary. A glossary at the end of the text covers a wide range of terms used throughout the book.

Recommended Resources. In addition to the references, additional readings and resources are provided to enhance the reader's knowledge of the subjects covered.

Common Abbreviations. A list of common abbreviations is included on the endpapers to aid the student in understanding the various organizations involved in health care.

ACKNOWLEDGMENTS

Numerous persons have made significant contributions to this edition. Without their experience, guidance, and advice, this book would not have been completed. Receiving continual feedback from colleagues, practitioners, and students helped us create a truly teachable textbook. A special thanks and public acknowledgment should be made to the contributing authors, who provided materials, consultations, and their precious time:

Judith Brown, M.P.H., Ph.D., R.D., Director and Associate Professor, Program in Public Health Nutrition, School of Public Health, University of Minnesota, Minneapolis, Minnesota

Jean Hankin, M.S., M.P.H., Dr. P.H., R.D., Professor of Public Health, Director, Public Health Nutrition Program, and Nutritionist, Epidemiology Program, Cancer Research Center, University of Hawaii, Honolulu, Hawaii

Sheryl Lee, M.P.H., R.D., Chief, Bureau of Nutrition Services, Arizona Department of Health Services, Phoenix, Arizona

George M. Owen, M.D., Vice President and Medical Director, Nutritional Research and Development, Bristol-Myers International Group, New York, New York

Patricia L. Simonis, M.S., R.D., Instructor and Doctoral Candidate, Department of Dietetics, Restaurant and Institutional Management, Kansas State University, Manhattan, Kansas

Allene G. Vaden, Ph.D., R.D., Dean, School of Home Economics, and Professor, Department of Institutional Management, University of Southern Mississippi, Hattiesburg, Mississippi

Faye Wong, M.P.H., R.D., Public Health Nutritionist, Centers for Disease Control, Atlanta, Georgia

Times Mirror/Mosby College Publishing obtained an experienced group of excellent reviewers. We appreciate their many suggestions and criticisms, which have had an influence on various aspects of this text. Our special thanks go to the following persons:

Judith Brown, M.P.H., Ph.D., R.D., University of Minnesota

Maurine Hegsted, M.S., University of Utah

Shiriki Kumanyika, Ph.D., Cornell University

Edward Sheehan, Ph.D., R.D., University of Arizona

Diana Spillman, Ph.D., R.D., Florida State University

Dale Terry, Ph.D., Iowa State University

Mary Nelle Traylor, R.D., University of Tennessee

Linda Vaughan, Ph.D., R.D., Arizona State University

Jane Wentworth, Ph.D., Virginia Polytechnic Institute and State University

The stimulating, new, and effective community nutrition models described in the text were provided by several leaders in our profession: Angelica Cantlon, R.D.; Paul Deigman, R.D.; Johanna Dwyer, D. Sc., R.D.; Kathy King Helm, R.D.; Mary Abbott Hess, R.D.; Ann Hunt, R.D.; Barbara Ann Hughes, R.D.; Roseann Ippolito, R.D.; Elvira Johnson, R.D.; Maria Mueseler, R.D.; Rebecca Mullis, Ph.D., R.D.; Lynn Parker from FRAC; Caroline Patacchiola-

Roy, R.D.; and Catherine Wotecki, Ph.D., R.D. (NHANES data).

A work of this kind involves the assistance and expertise of many persons who contributed in various ways to its completion. They include several dietitians/nutritionists from federal agencies who provided a wealth of materials and consultations on various aspects of this text: Elizabeth Brannon, R.D., Mary Egan, R.D., Marilyn Farrand, R.D., and Lenora Moragne, Ph.D., R.D., from the U.S. Department of Health and Human Services and Edith Thomas, R.D., from the U.S. Department of Agriculture.

Judith Gilbride, Ph.D., R.D., and her student Lisa Stollman assisted with the tedious job of literature review and research.

Our heartfelt thanks to the secretaries who assisted with the preparation of the manuscript, especially Cheryl Zeranti, Dorothy Kamil, Pam Papay, Bobbie Lane, and Suzie Owen.

How fortunate we are to be part of the health community and the very exciting field of community nutrition. Futurists tell us that a seed of change planted today can become a mighty force in the years ahead. May the seeds from this text bear many fruits for our clients, the American public.

Anita Yanochik Owen
Reva T. Frankle

Contents

PART I
Managing Community Nutrition Services

1 **Community Nutrition: An Essential Component of Health and Health Care,** 3

Unique opportunity for community dietitians/nutritionists in providing nutrition services, 4
Who performs community nutrition services? 5
Where are community dietitians/nutritionists employed? 8
What are the significant nutrition problems to address in the 1980s and 1990s? 10
Consumer views on the importance of nutrition, 11
What are the societal trends that will affect community nutrition programs? 11
Health promotion: new frontiers for community nutrition, 15
The future for community dietitians/nutritionists, 17
Future educational needs for community dietitians/nutritionists, 18
Summary, 19

2 **Managing and Managers: Their Role in Community Nutrition,** 21

Defining management, 22
Managerial functions and coordination, 26
Performance in the organization, 28
The evolution of management theory, 33
Management and change for the twenty-first century, 33
The external environment, 34
Summary, 35

3 **Planning and Decision Making in Community Nutrition to Produce Outcomes,** 37

Strategic planning, 38
Community assessment: diagnosing the community's health and nutrition needs, 43
Decision making, 60
Summary, 64

4 **Organizing and Developing Action Plans for Nutrition Services,** 67

Basic elements of organizing, 68
Authority, delegation, and decentralization, 70
Organizing for changing environments, 74
Managing organizational change, 75
Managing organizational conflict and creativity, 76
Organizing for action in nutrition services, 82
Summary, 91

5 **Leading to Achieve Individual and Organizational Goals,** 93

The importance of motivation, 94
Motivation theories, 94
Leadership, 98
Communications, 104
The vitamins of human relations, 111
Summary, 112

6 **Controlling Nutrition Services for Productivity,** 113

The control process, 114
Evaluation: how to measure outcomes, 114
Evaluation design, 117
Evaluation in action settings (service programs), 119
What are the essential steps in program evaluation? 120
What to evaluate, 125
What is being measured: the characteristics of measures, 126
What can go wrong: threats to internal validity, 127
Use of evaluation results: implication for program administrators, 128
Summary, 130

7   **Quality Assurance, Financial Control, and Cost-Effectiveness/Benefit Measures,** 133

Quality assurance, 134
Financial control, 153
Cost-effectiveness/benefit, 157
Reimbursement for nutrition services, 163
Summary, 164
Appendix 7-1: State programs, 165

PART II
Delivering Quality Nutrition Services

8   **The Elements of Quality Nutrition Services for Prevention of Disease and Promotion of Health,** 173

Delivering quality nutrition services, 174
Nutrition surveillance, 180
Elements of quality nutrition services, 183
Summary, 214
Appendix 8-1: Guidelines for criteria of nutritional status for laboratory evaluation, 216
Appendix 8-2: 1985 edition of the Recommended Dietary Allowances, 218

9   **Maternal Nutrition,** 219

Nutrition-related health problems of pregnant women, 220
Identifying problems in the community: pregnancy nutrition surveillance system, 220
Physiological changes in pregnancy, 221
Nutritional needs of pregnant women, 222
Weight gain during pregnancy, 222
Nutritional risk factors during pregnancy, 225
Lactation, 227
Guidelines for patient management, 231
Nutrition counseling for pregnant women, 237
Nutrition guidelines for lactation, 243
Referral for additional services, 243
Examples of strategies at the local level, 247
Summary, 247

10   **Guidelines for Nutrition Services for Infants, Children, and Adolescents,** 249

Nutrition-related health problems of infants, children, and adolescents, 250
Identifying problems in the community: pediatric nutrition surveillance system, 250
Infants, 252
Children, 278
Adolescents, 284
Referral for additional services, 294
Examples of strategies at the local level, 295
Summary, 296
Appendix 10-1: Neuromuscular and psychosocial development in infants, 297

11   **Adults and the Elderly,** 303

Nutrition-related health problems of adults and the elderly, 304
The aging process: physiological changes, 308
Nutritional needs of adults and the elderly, 308
Supplementation and faddism, 311
Diet-drug interactions, 312
Poverty and other sociological concerns, 314
Guidelines for prevention of nutrition-related diseases, 316
Assessment of nutritional status, 327
Assuring quality of health care for adults and elderly, 333
Nutrition services at the community level, 334
Summary, 343

PART III
Tools for Developing Effective Community Nutrition Services

12   **Analytical Skills: Tools of Nutrition Science,** 347

Nutrition-related disciplines in the delivery of nutrition services, 348
Computers and computer science, 349
Epidemiology, 356
Statistics, 362
Summary, 371

13 Developing Behavioral Change Skills, 373

Life-style behavior, 374

Learning theories: how is behavior changed? 374

How to change behavior: nutrition counseling, 376

Practical application: behavior change at the community level, 384

Summary, 387

14 Grants and Grantsmanship, 389

History of grants and grant legislation, 391

Grant versus contract, 393

Types of grants, 394

Sources of funding, 395

The proposal, 407

Shortcomings found in disapproved grant applications, 411

Summary, 412

15 Developing Public Policy Skills and Legislation, 413

Public policy, 414

Nutrition policy, 414

Federal legislation supporting nutrition services, 415

Current public policy and legislative issues that relate to nutrition, 416

Lobbying: why and how nutritionists should be involved, 419

What it takes to pass legislation, 421

The federal budget, 422

Summary, 424

Appendix 15-1: A nutritionist's guide to Washington, 425

Glossary, G-1

Recommended Resources, R-1

P·A·R·T I

Managing Community Nutrition Services

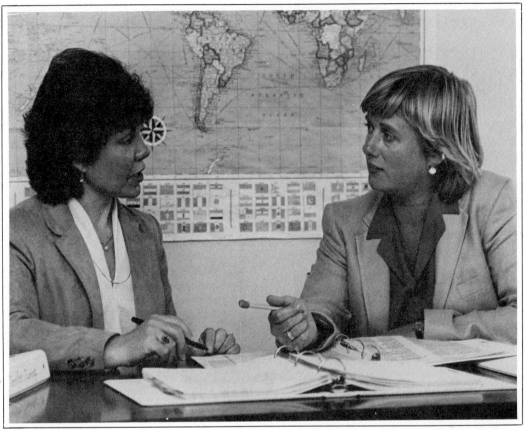

H. Armstrong Roberts

Community Nutrition: An Essential Component of Health and Health Care

GENERAL CONCEPT

In our rapidly changing environment, with major transformations taking place, community dietitians/nutritionists need to "stay ahead" to meet challenges. If community dietitians/ nutritionists are to gain full support and legitimacy in this era of convulsive change, they will need a rich mix of creativity, experimentation, and change. Community dietitians/ nutritionists have a unique contribution to make to society with their knowledge of the interrelationships of food, nutrition, and health.

Today the American public is interested in nutrition. Consumers are more aware of the actions they can take to maintain health through their daily eating patterns and have initiated changes in their nutritional practices. Such changes include the lower consumption of total fat, saturated fat, and cholesterol. An aware public understands that appropriate nutrition is necessary for optimum growth and development, physical activity, reproduction, lactation, recovery from illness and injury, and maintenance of health throughout the life cycle (USDHHS, 1983).

A variety of health problems can occur when persons have deficits of essential nutrients or consume excessive or inappropriate amounts of some nutrients.

Along with the benefits of consumer interest about nutrition come the risks of entrepreneurs who capitalize on this interest with a lot of misinformation. In this fitness-conscious era nutrition advice has become an extensive and highly lucrative business. Unfortunately the advice many people are getting is often useless and sometimes dangerous. Typically it is based on inappropriate tests of nutritional needs and is characterized by irrational dietary restrictions and generous doses of costly supplements often sold by the purveyors of the advice. At no other time in history have the services of the community dietitian/nutritionist been so important to consumers.

Greater emphasis is being placed on the role of community dietitians/nutritionists and other health care providers in preventive medicine. In fact, numerous reports document that prevention is one of the most cost-effective and best scientific approaches in the conquest of nutrition-related diseases (Levy, 1977; Davidson, Delcher, and England, 1979). In this text public health nutritionists and community dietitians will be referred to as community dietitians/nutritionists.

UNIQUE OPPORTUNITY FOR COMMUNITY DIETITIANS/NUTRITIONISTS IN PROVIDING NUTRITION SERVICES

Community dietitians/nutritionists have the unique opportunity and responsibility of improving the nutritional status of the population they serve. There is a need for including nutrition in preventive, diagnostic, curative, and restorative services. Nutrition services should be integrated with medical and social services and should be included at all levels of the health care delivery system (Owen, Lanna, and Owen, 1979). The primary level of care focuses on the welfare of the whole person and provides an assessment of that person's needs. At the secondary and tertiary levels, health care becomes increasingly specialized, but nutrition services may constitute a major part of the treatment plan.

The academic discipline that deals with the identification and solution of health and nutrition problems within communities is called *community nutrition*. As the physician plays a major role in the medical aspects of preventive medicine, the community dietitian/nutritionist delivers nutrition care services with a focus on community health in order to promote and maintain health, prevent disease, and continue rehabilitative efforts (Baird and Sylvester, 1983).

WHO PERFORMS COMMUNITY NUTRITION SERVICES?
Public Health Nutritionists and Community Dietitians

Public health nutritionists are the members of the public health agency staff with advanced training who manage the nutrition services for the agency. Their role is to assess community nutrition needs and to plan, organize, direct, coordinate, and evaluate the nutrition component of the health agency's services (Baird and Sylvester, 1983). Public health nutritionists establish links with related community nutrition programs, nutrition education, food assistance, social or welfare services, child care, services to the elderly, other human services, and community-based research (Kaufman, 1982). The roles and functions of public health nutrition personnel include planner/evaluator, coordinator, educator, consultant, standard setter, manager (fiscal), counselor, advocate, supervisor, manager (personnel), researcher/investigator, teacher, and outreach worker. Table 1-1 summarizes the recommended roles for the various classifications and indicates the chapter in this text that relates to the identified role.

The educational qualifications of the public health nutritionist include a master's degree in public health nutrition; or a master's degree in nutrition, with emphasis in public or community health, or in applied human nutrition, with course work in public health. The range of experience required is 3 to 5 years of full-time professional employment in the field of nutrition or dietetics, at least 2 to 3 years as a nutritionist in a public health or community nutrition program. Persons employed for this position must be registered dietitians (RDs) and maintain this status (Kaufman, 1982).

The Community Dietitians

Community dietitians provide direct nutrition care and nutrition education to patients or clients and to the public. This is the entry-level position for professional public health nutrition personnel. Roles of the community dietitian include counselor, educator, coordinator, standard setter, advocate, and supervisor (Table 1-1). Since this is an entry-level position, the community dietitian is not expected to perform the roles of planner/evaluator, consultant, manager, or researcher/investigator that were identified for the public health nutritionist.

Educational requirements for the community dietitian include a bachelor's degree in community nutrition or dietetics, in food and nutrition, or in dietetics from an accredited college or university. Courses must meet the current minimum academic requirements for dietetic registration established by the American Dietetic Association (ADA). Academic course work should include emphasis in the area of community dietetics. The individual must be a registered dietitian and maintain this status (Baird and Sylvester, 1983).

The roles of the community dietitian were arrived at by the Role Delineation and Verification Study conducted by the ADA (Baird and Sylvester, 1983). This study describes statements of major and specific performance responsibilities for each level of practice. In addition, the relationships between the public health nutritionist, the community dietitian, and the community dietetic technician are deliberated. Table 1-2 describes the major performance responsibility statements of the community dietitian and the community dietetic technician. For example, the public health nutritionist has advanced training and is responsible for the overall nutrition program of a health service agency. The community dietitian works under the supervision of the public health nutritionist, whereas the community dietetic technician works under the supervision of the community dietitian.

The Community Dietetic Technicians

Dietetic technicians in the community assist the public health nutritionist and the community dietitian in the areas of nutrition screening, delivery of direct nutrition care services, and outreach. The roles they perform include teacher

Table 1-1. Roles of public health nutrition personnel*

Role	Chapters in Text Relating to Role	Public Health Nutritionist — Sole	Public Health Nutritionist — Supervisor	Public Health Nutritionist — Consultant	Public Health Nutrition Director/Administrator	Nutrition Care Provider — Community Nutritionist/Dietitian	Nutrition Care Provider — Dietetic Technician in Nutrition Care	Researcher in Public Health Nutrition	Educator of Public Health Nutrition Personnel
Planner/evaluator	3 to 7, 12	◯	◯	◯	◯				
Coordinator	8 to 11	◯	◯	◯	◯	∘			
Educator	13	◯	○	◯	◯	◯		○	◯
Consultant	Text	◯	◯	◯	∘	◯		○	○
Standard setter	6, 7	∘	∘	∘	◯	○			∘
Manager	2 to 7	∘	∘		◯				
Manager (fiscal)	6, 7	∘	∘		∘				
Counselor	13	∘				◯			
Advocate	15	∘	∘	∘	∘	∘			∘
Supervisor	3 to 7		◯		∘	□			
Manager (personnel)	3, 4, 5		∘		∘				
Researcher/investigator	1, 12, 13		□	□	□			◯	◯
Teacher	8 to 11, 13						○		
Outreach worker	13						○		

From Kaufman, M., editor: Personnel in public health nutrition for the 1980's, McLean, Va., 1982, Association of State and Territorial Health Officials Foundation.

*Key: ◯, Major role (limited to 4 per position); ○, intermediate role; ∘, minor role; □, optional role.

Table 1-2. Role delineation and verification for entry-level positions in community dietetics: major performance responsibility statements

Focus	Community Dietitian	Community Dietetic Technician
Client	1.0* Provides community nutrition program services	1.0 Implements selected community nutrition program services (i.e., client care, group education, training) for the *not*-at-risk client population
	2.0 Provides comprehensive nutrition care in a variety of settings to individual clients	2.0 Provides nutrition care in a variety of settings to individual clients *not* at nutrition risk
	3.0 Provides nutrition education to selected groups for health promotion, health maintenance, and rehabilitation	3.0 Provides nutrition education to selected groups for health promotion, health maintenance, and rehabilitation, as specified by a protocol
Intraprofessional	4.0 Advances competence as a practitioner in community dietetics	4.0 Advances competence as a practitioner in community dietetics
	5.0 Applies current research information and methods to nutrition practice	
Interprofessional	6.0 Interacts with other community service providers	5.0 Interacts with other community service providers, as specified by a protocol
Intraorganizational	7.0* Manages community nutrition support personnel	6.0 Implements components of training program for community nutrition support personnel, as specified by a protocol
	8.0* Provides nutrition-related in-service education to dietetics students and other providers within the organization	
Interorganizational	9.0* Provides nutrition-related technical assistance to consumer groups and community organizations	
	10.0 Advocates action to meet nutrition-related needs of consumers	

From Baird, S.C., and Sylvester, J.: Role delineation and verification for entry-level positions in community dietetics, Chicago, 1983, The American Dietetic Association. Copyright The American Dietetic Association. Reprinted by permission.
*The verification study indicates that these responsibilities are performed *independently* substantially more often by entry-level master's trained personnel than by entry-level bachelor's trained personnel.

and outreach worker. Their educational requirements include successful completion of a 2-year dietetic technician program approved by the ADA.

Other Health Care Providers

In health care, other team members deliver quality nutrition services to patients and clients. *Physicians* provide medical direction and participate in establishing standards and policies for nutrition services. They reinforce and support the need for the patient's attention to nutrition advice offered by other health care team members (USDHHS, 1978). *Nursing personnel* can assist with nutritional assessment and provide some education and counseling to patients with uncomplicated nutrition problems. *Social workers* can contribute by assisting with community resources and social services needed to support adequate nutrition care. *Physical therapists, occupational therapists, dentists, dental hygienists, pharmacists,* and other health care workers can be helpful in counseling persons who have physical conditions that interfere with adequate nutrition (e.g., neurological impairment affecting chewing and swallowing). *Health educators* and *behavioral scientists* can assist in implementing educational programs in nutrition for patients, clients, and staff.

WHERE ARE COMMUNITY DIETITIANS/ NUTRITIONISTS EMPLOYED?

The public health nutritionist may be employed at the international, federal, state, county, city, or neighborhood level. Depending on the program's organization, the public health nutritionist may be employed either as an administrator who develops all nutrition services or as a specialist who serves in a specific program or population group. For example, health programs designed for different population groups may be organized to meet specific needs: special high-risk groups such as pregnant women, infants, children, and the elderly; populations with special needs for care as a result of socioeconomic status

or life-style, such as the elderly who live alone or in groups and migrant workers; or various health problems, such as cardiovascular disease, diabetes, or obesity.

International Level

Community dietitians/nutritionists employed at the international level can be found in such international agencies as the World Health Organization (WHO), Pan American Health Organization (PAHO), Food and Agriculture Organization (FAO), and United Nations Children's Emergency Fund (UNICEF). One of the roles of the international community dietitian/nutritionist is to consult the planner and give technical advice on nutrition. For nutrition personnel working in the international area, it is important, for example, in their training to study political science, the techniques of decision making and policy making, and modern managerial methods. With these skills, nutrition personnel will be more aware of the financial and social burden of malnutrition.

National Level

At the federal (national) level most nutrition programs and services are sanctioned by the U.S. Department of Health and Human Services and the U.S. Department of Agriculture. Nutritionists in these agencies provide technical assistance and professional consultation to their respective regional, state, and local health programs. They are program planners; they can assist grantees, project officers, and program administrators to develop and implement an appropriate nutrition program.

State and Local Levels

Before 1935, little existed in the way of nutrition services in state health departments or other community agencies. However, from 1933 to 1935, during the Depression years, hundreds of workers trained in nutrition were employed by state and local emergency relief administrations to give advisory service to directors concerned with the responsibility for preserving the health of unemployed families and individuals.

Title V of the 1935 Social Security Act gave the first national impetus for employment of public health nutritionists or consultants in maternal and child health programs. These consultants provided consultation and training to physicians, nurses, health educators, and teachers, attempting to extend nutrition services through other health care providers (Kaufman, 1982).

The directors of nutrition in the state and territorial health departments organized in 1952 (Association of State and Territorial Public Health Nutrition Directors) as an affiliate of the Association of State and Territorial Health Officials. This action gave national recognition to public health nutrition by developing a separate area for nutrition.

Problems of dietary overabundance, such as obesity, diabetes, hypertension, heart disease, and dental caries, were identified as emerging public health problems in the 1950s and early 1960s. In addition, the proliferation of nursing homes to serve the growing aging population stimulated the role of institutional nutrition consultants who were employed by state and local health agencies that were responsible for the licensing of nursing homes. As public health agencies developed programs in chronic disease control, adult health, and health services for the aging, public health nutritionists were employed in these programs (Kaufman, 1982).

Title V of the Social Security Act was amended in the mid-1960s to include special project funding for maternity and infant care projects and health service projects for children and youth and special programs for prevention of mental retardation and handicapping conditions. These amendments were included because of the identification of special problems in the community by public health workers.

With the passage of the Social Security Act amendments, Title XVIII (Medicare) and Title XIX (Medicaid), participating health professionals were required to have a formal credentialing system. In 1969 the ADA instituted dietetic registration to meet this criterion.* It was recommended that nutritionists employed in public health agencies qualify as registered dietitians, since it was important to have a mimimum entry level competence and an emphasis on continuing education. Dietetic registration is currently the formal credentialing for nutrition and dietetic personnel.

Nutrition became a public policy issue in the United States with the publication of *Hunger U.S.A.* in 1968 and the CBS television documentary, "Hunger in America."

As an outgrowth of the hunger issue, the 1969 White House Conference on Food, Nutrition and Health was held, and the 1968–1970 Ten-State Nutrition Survey and the Preschool Nutrition Surveys were conducted (USDHHS, 1968; Owen, 1974). After data were released from these surveys, a proliferation of food and nutrition programs occurred. The most significant of these was the 1972 Child Nutrition Act, which provided funding to implement the Special Supplemental Food Program for Women, Infants and Children (WIC). WIC began as a $20 million pilot program for fiscal year 1973, and by 1984 it had grown to over $1 billion. The WIC program is administered by the U.S. Department of Agriculture through state public health agencies. A significant number of nutrition personnel are employed in the WIC program. Its unique features include a voucher system for food, plus medical and nutritional assessment and counseling.

During the 1970s the Food Stamp Act was revised and expanded. The Older Americans Act, Title VII (now incorporated into Title III), provides congregate meals and home delivered meals for the elderly through the area or local agencies on aging. Public health nutritionists are employed in this program also.

*Dietitians who meet the standards and qualification established by the Commission on Dietetic Registration (CDR), an autonomous certifying component of the ADA, may be registered and may use the professional designation registered dietitian, or RD.

An expansion of nutrition education for school-children, parents, and school food service personnel occurred with the authorization of the Nutrition Education and Training Program (NET) by an amendment to the Child Nutrition Act of 1977.

During the 1970s the focus on nutrition changed from problems of undernutrition to those of overnutrition. Interest soared on the role of nutrition and diet in preventing certain chronic degenerative diseases. Programs were initiated for prevention and control of cardiovascular disease, hypertension, and diabetes. Nutritionists were included as part of the interdisciplinary team providing services to these programs.

In the 1980s *Dietary Guidelines for Americans* was published by the U.S. Department of Health and Human Services and U.S. Department of Agriculture (USDHHS-USDA, 1980) (see Chapter 8). Also in the 1980s, *Guidelines for Diet, Nutrition and Cancer* was published by the National Academy of Sciences (Chapter 8).

In 1982 block grant funding was instituted for major public health and nutrition programs, providing states with an opportunity to plan for their own needs (see Chapter 15).

The field of health promotion and disease prevention is an exciting area and presents a great challenge for community dietitians/nutritionists in the development of nutrition programs in the 1980s and 1990s.

WHAT ARE THE SIGNIFICANT NUTRITION PROBLEMS TO ADDRESS IN THE 1980s AND 1990s?

In the United States, nutrition problems include undernutrition and overnutrition; the availability, quality, and safety of the food supply; the links between foods eaten and the development of disease, and the patient's treatment and rehabilitation. The most significant nutrition problem seen in national nutrition surveys conducted in the 1960s and 1970s, regardless of socioeconomic status, was iron deficiency anemia. The prevalence of obesity was high, particularly among women, of whom nearly one third were obese. Evidence of retarded growth was apparent in children of families living in poverty (USDHHS, 1968, 1971-1972).

The nutrition problems of the 1980s and 1990s can best be described as either overnutrition and overconsumption of energy and nutrients or undernutrition, which is prevalent in certain high-risk groups. The following nutrition problems have been identified (USDHHS, 1980):

1. *Obesity.* Mean body weight of American men and women ages 18 to 74 increased by an average of 2.7 kg (6 lb) and 1.3 kg (3 lb) respectively, from 1963 to 1973. Some subsets of the population are more prone to obesity than others: for people ages 20 to 74, about 14% of men and 24% of women meet the criterion for obesity (120% of "ideal weight").

2. *Cardiovascular disease risk factors.* Average blood cholesterol levels in the United States among men of all age groups declined slightly between surveys conducted in 1960 to 1962 and 1971 to 1974; among women, blood cholesterol levels declined as much as 9% in the age group 55 to 64 and 6% in the age group 65 to 74. Some persons consume excessive amounts of sodium; in 1979 estimates ranged between averages of 4 and 10 gm of sodium ingested per person per day.

3. *Deficiencies in pregnant women.* Iron and folic acid deficiencies are particularly common among pregnant or lactating women. In 1978, 7.7% of pregnant women were iron deficient as estimated by hemoglobin concentrations early in pregnancy.

4. *Deficiencies and growth retardation in infants and children.* Among migratory workers and certain poor rural populations, approximately 10% to 15% of infants and children suffer growth retardation as a result of dietary inadequacies. Iron deficiency is a nutrition problem in approximately 10% of the low-income pediatric population (CDC, 1980).

5. *Dental problems.* Dental caries affects

98% of the U.S. population. By 17 years of age 94% of children have cavities in their permanent teeth. Low-income children have about four times as many untreated decayed teeth as do higher-income children. About 31 million adults ages 18 to 74 have lost all of their upper or lower teeth.

CONSUMER VIEWS ON THE IMPORTANCE OF NUTRITION

As we review the significant nutrition problems in our society, it is important to understand how consumers view these developments. Consumers often find it difficult to make informed choices about food and nutrition. They are bombarded with confusing and even conflicting information from many sources, thus making wise food choices and the selection of health practices even more complex. The lack of knowledge about nutrition has, in some instances, led to susceptibility to nutritional quackery. Limited information about nutrition provides an excellent medium for the wide dissemination of misinformation about foods and their roles in health and disease (Alfin-Slater and Aftergood, 1983). This lack of knowledge is exemplified by the recent trend in the number of health food stores in the United States. In 1968, 1200 health food stores were in existence; by 1981, 8300. Health food sales rose from $170 million in 1970 to $2 billion in 1981 (Naisbitt, 1982).

A study by Yankelovich, Skelley, and White (1979) on consumers' views of health and nutrition provides some useful insights for the health care provider. They concluded that the majority of American families are ready to accept in principle a new and more active approach to nutrition and health care—one that would require supplementing traditional means of health care with new approaches aimed primarily at preventing health problems before they arise. This trend is demonstrated by the following statistics (USDHHS, 1979):

1. At least 100 million Americans, almost half the population, are now exercising in some way.

This figure is up from only about one fourth of the population in 1960.

2. Fat intake has been reduced considerably; butter consumption is down 28% and milk and cream consumption down 21% since 1965.

3. Between 1978 and 1982, there was a 37% increase in the number of consumers who are on a sodium-controlled diet.

4. Smoking is down substantially, 28% among adult men and 13% among women since 1965.

Despite the many positive steps toward a healthier population, there are several obstacles to overcome before people are prepared to make the lifestyle changes necessary to improve their health. For example, American families are cutting back in some essential health areas, such as visits to physicians on a consistent basis, to cope with inflation. Despite all of the materials released by the government and media on health, only one in four families feels well informed about good nutrition and health practices (Yankelovich, Skelley, and White, 1979).

WHAT ARE THE SOCIETAL TRENDS THAT WILL AFFECT COMMUNITY NUTRITION PROGRAMS?

In our society, the coming decades will represent a period of great change and transition. The forecast is optimistic. A renaissance for the United States can occur in political prestige and technological power. In the next 50 years people will live to a healthy old age of 100 or more as medical advances find cures for diseases such as cancer and disorders such as senility (What the Next 50 Years Will Bring, 1983). Genetic techniques may expand food production and curb pollution, robots will do household and factory chores, and cars will be programmed to avoid accidents.

The Family

In the last two decades the American woman has redefined herself and her role in society. Breaking old forms and releasing new energies, she has grown and changed in ways not dreamed of in

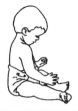

AMERICANS IN 2033
LIFE EXPECTANCY AT BIRTH

Men	1983	70.8 years
	2033	74.4 years
Women	1983	78.2 years
	2033	82.7 years

Figure 1-1. Life expectancy at birth, 2033.
Redrawn from U.S. Public Health Service, Department of Health and Human Services: State of America's health, Washington, D.C., 1984, U.S. Government Printing Office.

the early 1960s, in turn forcing growth and change in the world around her, leaving virtually no institution or individual untouched as a result. These changes have been positive in terms of achievements. However, there are some trouble spots.

There was a 69% increase in single-parent families in the last decade. Only 13% of the nation's families have a working father, a nonworking mother, and one or more children. Ninety percent of one-parent families are maintained by mothers, as compared to 85% in 1978, and 16% of these mothers are unwed. Whereas men's income improves by 42% after divorce, women show a 73% loss of income. In 1981 53% of families headed by white females and 70% of families headed by black females lived in poverty (U.S. Bureau of Census, 1982-1983).

Over the next five decades, experts say, society will redefine its concept of the family. Through the pattern of divorce and remarriage, a whole new network of kinship will arise. There will be double sets of grandparents, brothers, and sisters. This kinship is called the new divorce–extended family. Although these families will be larger, natural families will be smaller as couples decide to have fewer and fewer children or no children at all. The U.S. birthrate is currently 1.8 children per woman. Projections are that the United States will achieve zero population growth by the mid-twenty-first century. However, any unit with a husband, wife, and children present will be considered a nuclear family, no matter how it was formed (What the Next 50 Years Will Bring, 1983).

Elderly Population

As a result of better health, more money, and increased political power, tomorrow's elderly will be a dominant force in the United States. In the next century those 65 and over will account for more than one of every five persons and will alter the way the U.S. population lives and works. The elderly will be active much longer as medical advances reduce illness and disability. By 2033 the Census Bureau anticipates life expectancy to increase by about 4 years to 74.4 for men and 82.7 for women (Figure 1-1).

Over the next 50 years the Census Bureau projects that the number of Americans 65 and over will more than double from 27 million today to 66 million in 2033. As a result, programs designed for senior citizens could comprise as much as 65% of the federal health budget, compared with almost 28% today.

Key issues for the elderly will involve housing and health care. Even with medical advances, a segment of the population, especially those over 85, will likely have disabling diseases that will require costly medical care. Not only is spending in medical care expected to increase dramatically, but also health officials worry who will care for the chronically ill aged. For a significant number of elderly people whose chronic ailments do not require institutional care, sociologists anticipate the growth of *congregate housing*, apartment complexes offering a range of health and social services.

Health

Early in 1984 the Public Health Service issued its annual report on the state of American health. It was concluded that America's health was "better than ever" but that the seemingly intractable disparities between blacks and whites continued. The 1982 life expectancy for blacks, 69.3 years, was 6 years less than the 75-year life expectancy for whites. The mortality rate for black infants is

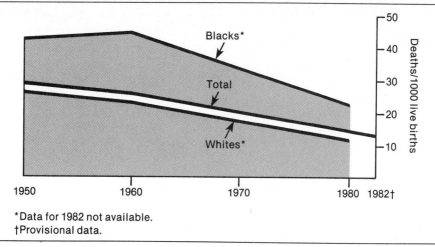

*Data for 1982 not available.
†Provisional data.

Figure 1-2. Deaths per 1000 live births. Infant mortality rates: black and white, 1950-1982.
Redrawn from U.S. Public Health Service, Department of Health and Human Services: State of America's health, Washington, D.C., 1984, U.S. Government Printing Office.

almost twice as high as for white infants (Figure 1-2). This rate has remained constant for over a decade.

The nation's increased awareness of health, reflected in exercise and careful attention to diet, seems to be paying off. Heart disease remains the number one killer, but the death rate has decreased 25% since 1970, when heart disease caused 254 deaths for every 100,000 people (Figure 1-3). In 1982 the rate fell to 191/100,000. The decline in the death rate for strokes and other cerebrovascular diseases was even more dramatic, from 66 deaths per 100,000 in 1970 to 36 in 1982 (Figure 1-3).

Consumers' concern about healthy life-styles have played a role in these decreased statistics. What will be important in the next few decades will be the rise of systematic research and development activities to further clarify the role of positive life-styles in maintaining health.

The challenge for all health care workers will be to address the question of appropriate care at an appropriate cost, while continuing to reach out to the medically indigent and the elderly.

	1950	1960	1970	1980	1982
Total	841.5	760.9	714.3	585.8	556.4
Selected causes					
Diseases of heart	307.6	286.2	253.6	202.0	190.8
Stroke	88.8	79.7	66.3	40.8	36.1
Cancer	125.4	125.8	129.9	132.8	133.3
Accidents	57.5	49.9	53.7	42.3	37.1
Homicide and legal intervention	5.4	5.2	9.1	10.8	9.7

Figure 1-3. Age-adjusted death rates per 100,000 population, 1950-1982.
Redrawn from U.S. Public Health Service, Department of Health and Human Services: State of America's health, Washington, D.C., 1984, U.S. Government Printing Office.

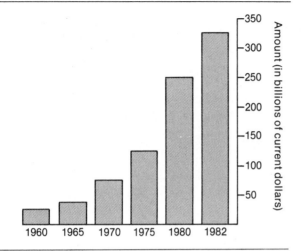

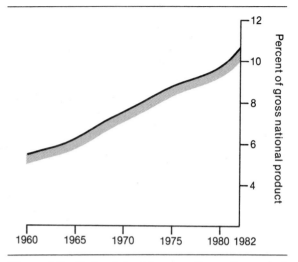

Figure 1-4. National health expenditures (public and personal spending), 1960-1982. Amount in billions of current dollars.
Redrawn from Office of Management and Budget (OMB): U.S. Budget, 1984, Washington, D.C., 1984, U.S. Government Printing Office.

Figure 1-5. National health expenditure. Percent of gross national product, 1960-1982.
Redrawn from Office of Management and Budget (OMB): U.S. Budget, 1984, Washington, D.C., 1984, U.S. Government Printing Office.

Health Care Costs

During the last 20 years or so the average cost of a day in the hospital has increased over 700%. National health expenditures rose from $42 billion, or 6% of the gross national product, in 1965 to $322 billion, or 10.5% of the gross national product in 1982. Translated into individual costs, this amounted to $1350 per capita (Figures 1-4 and 1-5).

By 1982 health care cost containment had become a national preoccupation with everyone, from state legislators to insurance companies to employers. According to a Chrysler Corporation executive, the single largest supplier for the Big Three auto makers is not a steel company or a rubber company or a glass company; it is Blue Cross and Blue Shield. He states that $600 of the price of an average American car goes for health care for auto industry employees, compared with $80 in the average Japanese auto (What the Next Fifty Years Will Bring, 1983). Business and industry are totally immersed in the health care picture.

In 1983 the emphasis on cost containment shifted from controlling health care delivery expenses to putting limits on the amount that would be paid for the performance of health care services. Consequently, the business environment for health care providers is becoming one of increasingly stringent control on patient charges. Third-party payers—insurers, federal and state governments through Medicare and Medicaid—are now specifying the amount providers must charge, rather than simply paying part or all of the bills, determined solely by the providers. Limiting the amount that will be paid for health care has already engendered dramatic changes in the way health care services are delivered and how they are paid for. Today's preferred payment organizations (PPOs) have become a mainstay of the health care delivery network (PL 98-21, 1982). PPOs provide a channel through which health care deliverers can bid for the right to serve the health needs of a particular group or organization. PPOs and their first cousins, health maintenance organizations

(HMOs), are considered successful; as a result, they may become the means by which the great majority of people will receive their health care in the future.

As the drive to limit the dollars spent on health care gathers steam, concern is growing in this country that a two-tier health care system is being created—one for those who can pay and another for those who cannot. The ability to pay for health care has already become a significant factor for people with little or no ability to pay.

• • •

These trends in the population, in health, and in the family have far-reaching implications for the role of community dietitians/nutritionists, their work, and their benchmarks for the future. Can they, as professionals, prosper in an era of rapid technological change? Community dietitians/nutritionists will need to look at the present and do sound planning to meet consumers' needs, particularly with their new-found interest in healthy life-styles.

HEALTH PROMOTION: NEW FRONTIERS FOR COMMUNITY NUTRITION

Among the more significant developments of the 1970s was the growth in knowledge and awareness of how important health promotion and disease prevention could be to realizing further reductions in unnecessary death and disability in the United States. The challenge for the 1980s and 1990s is to apply that knowledge in a productive and timely manner.

Why has health promotion and disease prevention become a national preoccupation? A brief historical account will put the health promotion movement into perspective. This nation's first public health revolution was the struggle against infectious diseases that spanned the late nineteenth and twentieth centuries. That revolution has successfully run its course, at least in the United States and the major industrial nations. Its strategies included major sanitation measures, the development of effective vaccines, and mass immunization. So successful was this first revolu-

tion that today only 1% of people who die before age 75 in the United States die from infectious disease.

Remarkable gains in life expectancy and declines in infant mortality have occurred since 1900. They were achieved not only by treatment and by curative medicine but also by preventive and health-promoting measures such as improved sanitation, better nutrition, pasteurization of milk, and control of infectious disease.

The success of that first revolution means that today the pattern of fatal and disabling diseases has shifted drastically. While the number of deaths from major acute infectious diseases plummeted between 1900 and 1970, the proportion of mortality from major chronic diseases such as heart disease, cancer, and stroke increased more than 250%. Today, cardiovascular disease, including both heart disease and stroke, accounts for roughly half of all deaths. Cancer accounts for another 20%. Accidents, such as automobile and home, exact a fearsome toll of death and disability, particularly among young people.

The Next Public Health Revolution

The next public health revolution must be aimed at these new killers and cripplers (heart disease, cancer, and accidents), with emphasis on preventing these afflictions rather than treating them after they have already struck.

For many years, lack of knowledge about the origins of these chronic diseases barred the development of preventive strategies. Today, however, new knowledge from research is steadily increasing the capacity for prevention.

Redefinition of Health

What has actually emerged in our society is a redefinition of health in the last decade: from the mere absence of disease to the existence of a positive state of health in the whole person. This definition has gained wide acceptance from health professionals, the private and public sectors, and consumers (USDHHS, 1979).

What is health promotion? Unlike traditional curative medicine, health promotion begins with people who are basically healthy and fosters the development of life-styles to monitor and enhance the state of health and well-being. Actions to stop smoking, reduce misuse of alcohol and drugs, improve diet and nutrition, manage stress, exercise, adhere to medical regimens, and appropriately use preventive services can reduce the risk of illness and premature death. The specific areas of health relevant to health promotion include personal habits in nutrition, exercise, smoking and alcohol use, and stress management. Therefore health promotion activities, whether they consist of programs and policies to facilitate life-style changes or educational interventions to increase public and professional awareness, seek to reduce risk factors that affect health status. For example, specific risk factors are identifiable for the major health problems confronting Americans:

Problem	Risk Factors
Heart disease	Smoking, high blood pressure, elevated serum cholesterol, diabetes, obesity, lack of exercise
Cancer	Smoking, diet, alcohol, solar radiation, ionizing radiation, worksite hazards, environmental contaminants, infectious agents, certain medications
Accidents	Alcohol, smoking (fires), product design, home hazards

Two recent publications give credence to the basic and applied research that is being completed to bring the health promotion message to the American public.

Dietary Guidelines for Americans

In 1980 the U.S. Department of Health and Human Services and the Department of Agriculture recommended dietary guidelines for Americans in a publication entitled *Nutrition and Your Health—Dietary Guidelines for Americans* (USDHHS-USDA, 1980) (see Chapter 8). These

recommendations were based on the assumption that Americans need to make some prudent changes in their diets, based on the best available knowledge. For instance, it has been established that people need to eat a wide range of nutrients to maintain good health. In addition, there is a relationship between obesity and eating more calories than needed and between hypertension and eating a lot of salt. Many experts believe there is a relationship between heart attacks and eating too much of foods high in fat, saturated fat, and cholesterol.

Community dietitians/nutritionists also recognize that people do not eat for nutritional benefit alone. Food must be appealing and enjoyable or no one will eat it. Another assumption made in the publication is that moderation is the best guide in eating to maintain health.

The guidelines (USDHHS-USDA, 1980) recommend that people:

- Eat a variety of foods
- Maintain ideal weight
- Avoid too much fat, saturated fat, and cholesterol
- Eat foods with adequate starch and fiber
- Avoid too much sugar
- Avoid too much sodium
- Avoid excessive alcohol consumption

The object of the guidelines is to ensure the right balance of vitamins, minerals, and fiber without overdoing the salt or the calories, especially the calories from fat and sugar.

Guidelines for Diet, Nutrition, and Cancer

Diet, Nutrition and Cancer describes the relationship between diet and the incidence of cancer (National Academy of Sciences, 1982). It summarizes what is known about the nature of cancer and reviews the basis for suspecting a relationship between cancer and diet. Basing its recommendations on careful assessment of current scientific evidence, interim dietary guidelines are provided that are both consistent with general nutritional practice and likely to reduce the risk of cancer (National Academy of Sciences, 1983):

1. Reduce the consumption of both saturated and unsaturated fats.
2. Include fruits (especially citrus fruits), vegetables (particularly carotene-rich and cruciferous vegetables), and whole-grain products in the daily diet.
3. Minimize consumption of foods preserved by salt-curing, salt-pickling, or smoking.
4. Minimize contamination of foods with carcinogens from any source and continue to evaluate food additives for carcinogenic activity.
5. Reduce the concentration of mutagens in foods when feasible to do so.
6. Consume only moderate amounts of alcohol, if any.

Personal choice is a factor in the leading causes of death. As understanding deepens about the influences personal behavior can have on health status, a significant effort is developing to help Americans achieve greater gains in the maintenance and improvement of their health. More emphasis on strategies for prevention of disease is required by both the private and the public sector if these gains are to be made.

Objectives for the Nation

The many issues surrounding the area of prevention, including the role of health promotion, have been discussed in the Surgeon General's report "Healthy People in 1979" (USDHHS, 1979). This report led to the publication of *Promoting Health, Preventing Disease: Objectives for the Nation* in 1980. (USDHHS, 1980). In this document 15 targeted primary action areas are listed, including Preventive Health Services, Health Protection, and an area called Health Promotion, which includes nutrition and physical fitness as two of the major components. The following objectives in the area of nutrition are to be accomplished by 1990 (USDHHS, 1980). There are some clear approaches to be taken by community nutrition professionals.

1. By 1990 the prevalence of significant overweight among the U.S. adult population should be decreased to 10% of men and 17% of women, without nutritional impairment.

2. By 1990 the mean serum cholesterol level in the adult population aged 18 to 74 should be at or below 200 mg/dl.
3. By 1990 the average daily salt ingestion by adults should be reduced at least to the 3 to 6 gm range. (In 1979 estimates ranged between averages of 4 and 10 gm salt.)
4. By 1990 all states should include nutrition education as part of required comprehensive school health education at elementary and secondary levels.
5. By 1990 virtually all routine health contacts with health professionals should include some elements of nutrition education and nutrition counseling.

Although the objectives for health promotion were developed through the efforts of federal agencies, they do not necessarily reflect a federal agency's perspective only. Approximately 167 experts representing public service organizations and the private sector prepared these quantifiable objectives. These objectives actually represent the development of a consensus about this nation's health goals and about some means of attaining them. Setting the objectives is only a starting point. This process also reveals the need for a commitment by individuals and organizations in both private and public sectors to realign some activities and resources to address these pressing health needs.

•   •   •

Community dietitians/nutritionists can assist Americans to make substantial gains in their health status by using health promotion strategies. If a commitment is made at every level, the objectives to be attained by 1990 can be realized and Americans who might otherwise have suffered disease and disability will instead be healthy people.

THE FUTURE FOR COMMUNITY DIETITIANS/NUTRITIONISTS

A recent study of the dietetics profession explored its relationship to a changing health care delivery system. The 1984 Study Commission on Dietetics was established by the boards of directors of the ADA and the ADA Foundation (Study Commission on Dietetics, 1984).

The study findings indicate that there has been rapid growth in knowledge of foods and nutrition in recent years and that the domain of dietetics has increased substantially. In addition, the American public has greater understanding of foods and nutrition and their importance to a full and happy life. However, dietitians are not widely recognized by the public as those qualified by education and training to provide the necessary expertise in the field.

The largest number of dietitians continues to be employed as clinical dietitians in health care institutions. The most recent ADA membership census (1981) found respondents classifying themselves as clinical dietitians, 39%; food service, 26%; community nutritionists, 10%; general, 9%; educators, 4%; counselors, 4%; and other, 8%. The typical dietitian is young, white, and female. The membership census showed that 97% were females, 87% were white, 7% were Asian, 4% were black, 1% were Hispanic, and very few were native Americans. It is interesting to note that over 50% were between the ages of 26 and 40. About 55% had been in practice less than 10 years and 35% less than 5 years.

One of the major study commission recommendations addresses the issue of the present practice areas of dietetics and the need for new areas of practice. Hospitals are predicted to become tertiary care centers with much health care being provided in the community setting. As a result of this change, community dietitian/nutritionists will have new markets for their services requiring a different set of skills to provide these services.

Over 25 recommendations were made in this study of the dietetics profession. The following recommendations have great implications for the community dietitian/nutritionist:

- Major changes [should] be made to revitalize the profession and enable it to make its maximum

contribution to society. The profession must become more dynamic and assertive but in order to do so it must increase its depth of knowledge and expertise. This will require changes in the education of dietitians at undergraduate, graduate, and continuing levels. It will also require changes in the patterns of dietetic practice and in the activities of the American Dietetic Association.

- ADA [should] give greater consideration to its statement of purpose "to promote optimal health and nutritional status of the population" and specific plans be drawn for its implementation.

FUTURE EDUCATIONAL NEEDS FOR COMMUNITY DIETITIANS/NUTRITIONISTS

The study commission identified several areas where the education of dietitians should be strengthened to increase depth of knowledge and expertise:

- A broader base, particularly in the arts, humanities, and behavioral sciences.
- Greater emphasis on management and business
- Greater emphasis on communications and networking
- Greater emphasis on new technology, especially the computer
- Greater depth in scientific knowledge of nutrition

Major emphasis in this text has been placed on management and marketing skills for community dietitian/nutritionist services. Community dietitians/nutritionists of the future will need to upgrade their management skills to a more rigorous level to compete effectively for diminishing levels of funds. New funding sources and new markets must be pursued vigorously. A marketing strategy provides great promise for community nutrition. This strategy includes defining the market segments that will be serviced, identifying the needs of each segment, developing a plan to obtain and monitor the desired market share of each segment, and finally evaluating outcomes.

Community dietitians/nutritionists must carefully monitor the trends in our tumultuous society. Using these trends as a barometer, their future is bright to become the "executives in nutrition systems" of the future if they develop competencies as:

1. Marketers of nutrition services with a bias for action
2. Conceptual managers who can provide quality services that are cost-effective in a competitive environment under considerable economic pressure
3. Basic and applied researchers to learn new information about the efficacy of their services

Moving forward in community nutrition will require much more than keeping pace; it will mean staying ahead, exploring technology and new markets aggressively and imaginatively, and applying this knowledge experimentally to new ideas. The health promotion movement is one example of a new, blossoming area where the time is right for experimenting with and creating new models for nutrition services.

SUMMARY

The unique skills that community dietitians/nutritionists possess are becoming better understood by the public as they address the issues of healthy life-styles. The public health nutritionist takes the lead in developing community programs, and the community dietitian occupies the entry-level position and performs several of the direct services to clients.

There are many challenges for the community dietitian/nutritionist in the next decade as one looks at the health problems of the population. Cardiovascular disease, obesity, and cancer are some of the leading problem areas where a great deal of resources, both human and financial, need to be expended to manage death and/or disability from these diseases.

Keeping people healthy will be the major impetus for health workers in the next decade. How to sustain consumer interest in healthy life-styles and obtain lasting behavioral change in the population will be part of the next health revolution.

The future is bright for the community dietitian/nutritionist if new skills are developed to meet the needs of the population with creativity, experimentation, and change.

REFERENCES

Alfin-Slater, R.B., and Aftergood, L.L.: Food fads. In Schneider, H.A., Anderson, C.E., and Coursin, D.B., editors: Nutritional support of medical practice, ed. 2, New York, 1983, Harper & Row Publishers, Inc.

Baird, S.C., and Sylvester, J.: Role delineation and verification for entry-level positions in community dietetics, Chicago, 1983, ADA.

Centers for Disease Control: Nutrition surveillance bulletin, Atlanta, 1980, CDC.

Davidson, J.K., Delcher, H.K., and England, A.: Spin-off cost benefits of expanded nutritional care, J. Am. Diet. Assoc. 75:250, 1979.

Kaufman, M., editor: Personnel in public health nutrition for the 1980's, McLean, Va., 1982, Association of State and Territorial Health Officials Foundation.

Levy, R.: Testimony on diet and cardiovascular diseases, Select Committee on Nutrition and Human Needs, U.S. Senate, Dietary Goals for the U.S., Rev. Pub. no. N0052-072-04376-8, Washington, D.C., 1977, U.S. Government Printing Office.

Naisbitt, J.: Megatrends: the new directions transforming our lives, New York, 1982, Warner Books, Inc.

National Academy of Sciences, Committee on Diet, Nutrition and Cancer: Diet, nutrition and cancer, Washington, D.C., 1982, National Academy Press.

Owen, A.L., Lanna, G., and Owen, G.M.: Counseling patients about diet, Nurs. Clin. North Am. 14:2, June 1979.

Owen, G.M., et al.: A study of nutritional status of pre-school children in the U.S., 1968-1970, Pediatrics 53:597, 1974.

Public Law 98-21, Tax equity and fiscal responsibility act of 1982, Social security amendment of 1983, U.S. Congress, Washington, D.C., 1982, TEFRA.

Study Commission on Dietetics: A new look at the profession of dietetics, Chicago, 1984, ADA and W.K. Kellogg Foundation.

U.S. Bureau of Census, Division of Marriage and Families: Bureau of Census Income Division, Washington, D.C., 1982-1983.

U.S. Department of Health and Human Services: Ten-state nutrition survey, DHEW Pub. no. (HSM) 72-81-30-8234, Washington, D.C., 1968, U.S. Government Printing Office.

U.S. Department of Health and Human Services: Preliminary findings of the first Health and Nutrition Examination Survey, DHEW Pub. no. (HRA) 74-1219-1, Washington, D.C., 1971-1972, U.S. Government Printing Office.

U.S. Department of Health and Human Services: Guide for developing nutrition services in community health programs, HSA Bureau of Community Health Services, Rockville, Md., 1978.

U.S. Department of Health and Human Services: Healthy people: the Surgeon General's report on health promotion and disease prevention, Washington, D.C., 1979, U.S. Government Printing Office.

U.S. Department of Health and Human Services: Promoting health, preventing disease: objectives for the nation, Washington, D.C., 1980, U.S. Government Printing Office.

U.S. Department of Health and Human Services: Public health reports: promoting health/preventing disease, PHS implementation for attaining the objectives for the nation (Suppl.), Washington, D.C., Sept./Oct. 1983, U.S. Government Printing Office.

U.S. Department of Health and Human Services and U.S. Department of Agriculture: Nutrition and your health: dietary guidelines for Americans, Washington, D.C., 1980, U.S. Government Printing Office.

What the next 50 years will bring, U.S. News and World Report 94:18, May 9, 1983.

Yankelovich, Skelley, and White: Our family health in an era of stress, Minneapolis, 1979, General Mills, Inc.

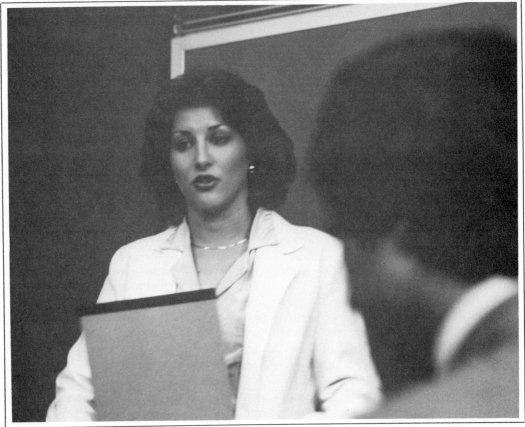

H. Armstrong Roberts

Managing and Managers: Their Role in Community Nutrition

GENERAL CONCEPT

Today the community dietitian/nutritionist must possess managerial skills to be seen by others as capable of assuming high-level positions. Since management is the art of getting things done through people, managers can best help the organization by having the ability to design and achieve their goals. Getting things done is accomplished by arranging for others to perform whatever tasks may be necessary to achieve these goals.

Enhancing the managerial effectiveness of the community dietitian/nutritionist may be the greatest challenge facing the profession in the 1980s and 1990s. In these difficult economic times dietitians/nutritionists in leadership positions are being evaluated in terms of their managerial effectiveness. Technical expertise is not enough; one must have managerial skills. Much more emphasis must be placed on mastering resource management and managerial skills if dietitians/nutritionists are to be recognized as effective professionals and chosen to assume leadership positions (Hoover, 1983). The real challenge will be to provide a high level of services, cost-effectively, in a competitive environment, and under considerable economic pressure. Governmental pressures have forced the curbing of cost increases in health care, and regulatory influences are demanding financial accountability (PL 93-641, 1974; PL 96-79, 1979).

Skillful management of resources results in desired output targeted to meet the goals of an organization. What abilities are needed by the community dietitian/nutritionist to keep efforts moving in the right direction? Why are many dietetic practitioners stereotyped as deficient in managerial skills? What is the result of emphasis on technical and clinical skills at the expense of managerial competency? What is to be done about the employment opportunities lost because of inadequate management skills?

Institutional administrators expect cost-effective decisions relative to range of service, organization environment, quality assurance, risk management, productivity, energy accountability, and technology adoption (Hoover, 1983). Being cost-effective requires creative problem solving, risk taking, and highly effective planning, resulting from a blend of operations management techniques, financial expertise, leadership and marketing orientation, and systems design skills. In health care institutions cost-effectiveness has become a password, or one used by administrators to discuss the "bottom line" before any other issue can be covered. With limited funds for community health services, the fiscal situation is usually placed first above all other considerations.

In this section emphasis will be placed on the community dietitian/nutritionist as manager. The management process will be discussed in detail in subsequent chapters. Figure 2-1 describes the management process that will be used as the basis for each of the sections on management.

DEFINING MANAGEMENT

Management has been called "the art of getting things done through people." This definition calls attention to the fact that managers achieve organization goals by arranging for others to perform whatever tasks may be necessary—not by performing the tasks themselves (Stoner, 1982). Bennett (1979) suggested that certain qualities of an artist are essential for effective management: (1) global consciousness, (2) vision of newness, (3) desire for qualitative results, (4) positive attitude, (5) humanism, and (6) growth orientation. We will attempt to apply these qualities to community nutrition.

Community dietitians/nutritionists need a global view of the community they serve and the

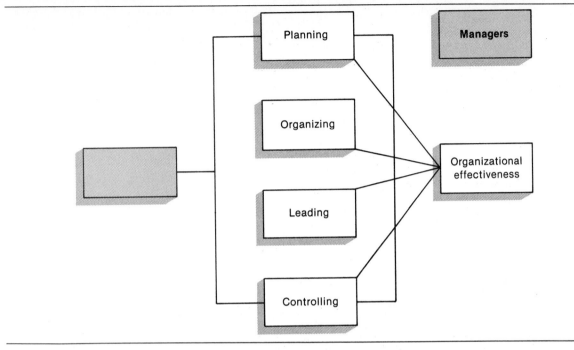

Figure 2-1. The management process.

organization where they are employed. Looking at these areas together will provide a better perspective of how to deliver community nutrition services because nutritionists will understand community needs, particular health problems, and which ones are amenable to nutrition services. In an organization there is nothing more damaging than to have an insular view of one's job and department. One is doomed to failure if the total organization is not considered in the planning and implementing of services.

A vision of newness refers to new models and methods to do a job more effectively. Continuing education for the community dietitian/nutritionist will help to spark new ideas and teach new methods.

Obtaining qualitative results requires a system that includes data collection methods, with specific objectives and retrievable information to use to quantify the results. The Centers for Disease Control (CDC) Surveillance System provides some of the quantitative aspects that are needed in a health department.

Learning to work with people and having a positive attitude can make a difference in job satisfaction. A county health department nutrition staff undertaking a problem and using good problem-solving techniques to arrive at a solution can be a rewarding experience. This is a win-win situation; clients get better service, and the nutrition staff feel good about themselves.

A growth orientation is necessary, whether it be to expand the nutrition staff to serve a larger segment of the population or to reorganize personnel to achieve a greater growth in services. This aspect must be dynamic to keep up to date with new services and new ways of giving more services with less money and personnel.

Management includes all of these qualities and more. Our discussion will start with a more complex definition so that we may call attention to other important aspects of managing.

Management is the process of planning, organizing, leading, and controlling the efforts of organization members and of using all other organizational resources to achieve stated organizational goals (Stoner, 1982) (Figure 2-1). A process is a systematic way of doing things. Community dietitians/nutritionists' training should reflect an ability to plan, organize, lead, and control. This is not only an activity of the manager of all services; people at every level must be prepared to understand and implement the process. We define management as a process because all managers, regardless of their particular aptitudes or skills, engage in certain interrelated activities to achieve their desired goals. The tasks that make up the process are many and varied. By and large, writers in the field agree with the following aspects of management.

Planning

Planning is making the strategic decisions from which objectives, policies, programs, and procedures logically follow. Planning is the primary function: nothing can be accomplished without a plan. However, planning is also a continuing function. Planning implies that managers think through their goals and actions in advance. Their actions are usually based on some method, plan, or logic, rather than on a hunch. Plans are revised and adjusted throughout the process (Pekar, 1982). Community dietitians/nutritionists are expected to develop a precise plan for their portion of the services.

Organizing

Organizing is the development of a work structure—a framework in which the necessary tasks are carried out to reach the organization's objectives. The effectiveness of an organization depends on its ability to marshal its resources to attain its goals. Organizing includes assigning activities, dividing work into particular jobs, and defining the relationship among them. It also involves delegation of authority necessary to com-

plete the tasks. Authority is the key to the manager's job; its delegation, the key to organizing. Community dietitians/nutritionists are often involved in the organizing aspects; however, the total planning can be left to someone else. Knowledge of only one piece of the plan can lead to disillusionment and negative attitudes. It is important for the community dietitian/nutritionist to review the organizational chart of the health agency and determine where the nutrition staff fits into the overall plan of operation.

Leading

Leading describes how managers direct and influence subordinates, getting others to perform essential tasks. Motivation is an integral part of this process, and it has many dimensions: morale, employee satisfaction and productivity, communication, and leadership. Leadership is the creation of a work environment that both satisfies employees and promotes the organization's objectives. For the community dietitian/nutritionist the professional organization is often one way to learn how to lead.* Leadership skills can then be used in the workplace.

Controlling

Controlling is the process through which there is insurance that plans are being followed. Although it can be a corrective function—adjustments are made as necessary—it is also a means of foreseeing and offsetting events, both within and outside the organization, that could have a negative effect on the plans. Controlling services and resources is an area where community dietitians/nutritionists need additional skills, since this area is rapidly changing; the use of computer technology demands that dietitians/nutritionists keep pace.

The success with which managers carry out managerial functions determines how effectively the organization operates. The organization is an

---

*The professional organization provides a training ground for ideas without total response for every action. Work with peers can stimulate new ideas and options.

instrument, developed to perform a set of tasks; it is the manager's job to wield that instrument as effectively as possible. Managers use all the resources of the organization—its finances, equipment, and information, as well as its people—to attain their goals. Community dietitians/nutritionists use the entire organization to foster the goals of the department of nutrition. People are the most important resource of any organization, but managers would be limiting their achievements if they did not also rely on the other available organizational resources, such as fiscal and personnel departments. The definition of management also involves achieving the organization's "stated goals." This means that managers of any organization—a public health agency, a university, or a professional football team—try to attain specific ends. These ends are, of course, unique to each organization. The stated goal of the public health agency is to deliver quality health care to high-risk populations. At the university the goal might be to give students a well-rounded education in an academic community. The stated goal of a football team might be to win every game in a season. Whatever the stated goals of a particular organization, management is the process by which goals are achieved.

Coordination: The Essence of Management

Many authorities consider coordination as a function of the manager that is separate from other managerial activities. It seems more accurate, however, to regard coordination as the essence of managership, for the achievement of harmony of individual efforts toward the accomplishment of group goals is the purpose of management. Each of the managerial functions is an exercise in coordination. This is so true in public health, since no one agency has the total capability to deliver all of the services. By coordinating with other groups such as Expanded Food and Nutrition Education Program (EFNEP) and Nutrition Education and Training (NET), for example, more services can be rendered to a larger group of clients.

Need for Coordination

The necessity for synchronizing individual action arises out of differences in opinion as to how group goals can be reached or how individual and group objectives can be harmonized. Thus the central task of the manager is to reconcile differences in approach, timing, effort, or interest and to harmonize cooperative and individual goals.

The best coordination occurs when individuals see how their jobs contribute to the dominant goals of the enterprise. Understanding of the enterprise implies knowledge and understanding of the organization's objectives, not just on the part of a few at the top but by everyone throughout the organization. If, for example, managers are not aware that the basic goal of their institution is quality, profit, advanced techniques, or patient service, they cannot coordinate their efforts to achieve the true objective. Each would be guided by his or her own ideas of what is in the interest of the agency or, without any such conviction, would work for self-aggrandizement. To avoid such splintering efforts, the dominant goal of the enterprise should be clearly defined and communicated to everyone concerned. Naturally, goals of all departments must be designed to contribute to the enterprise's goals.

Principles of Coordination

The principle of direct contact states that coordination must be achieved through interpersonal, vertical, and horizontal relationships of people in an organization. People exchange ideas, ideals, prejudices, and purposes through direct personal communication much more efficiently than by any other method, and, with the understanding gained in this way, they find means to achieve both common and personal goals. This recognized identity of ultimate interests then tends to bring agreement on methods and actions. For instance, rivalry and consequent criticism, which all too frequently mar the relationships of employees in different departments, are evidences of poor coordination. In community nutrition the use of nutrition councils, composed of several agencies with common goals, can foster good communication and coordination among agencies.

A second principle stresses the importance of achieving coordination in the early stages of planning and policy making. It is clear that after departmental plans are put into operation, it becomes more difficult to unify and time them properly. The cry "Why doesn't someone tell me about this?" thus becomes a common refrain.

A third principle states that all factors in a situation are reciprocally related. When A works with B, for instance, each influences the other, and both are influenced by all persons in the organization. If, for example, through the Nutrition Council community dietitians/nutritionists know that the Dairy Council has a large program to educate elementary students about nutrition, they will support this effort and spend precious resources on a high-risk group rather than go into elementary schools.

These principles indicate, finally, that the method of achieving coordination is largely horizontal rather than vertical. People cooperate as a result of understanding one another's tasks; thus the administrator's dictum "Coordinate!" is both unrealistic and uninforceable.

MANAGERIAL FUNCTIONS AND COORDINATION

What the manager does to accomplish a synchronized effort of subordinates is to carry out managerial functions, that is, to plan, organize, staff, direct, and control. Coordination is achieved in two ways. First, one assures that the environment facilitates coordination by creating an appropriate organization structure, selecting skillful subordinates and training and supervising them effectively, providing and explaining the integrated plans and programs that subordinates will carry out, and establishing means to determine whether plans are being carried out properly and programs are on schedule. Second, managers make clear that subordinates understand the principles of coordination and the importance of acting on them. In community nutrition the nutrition manager must work with other programs, such as the hypertension or smoking programs, as

a way of demonstrating intraorganization coordination. Joint planning with other agencies is a sound way to facilitate coordination.

What Do Managers Actually Do?

Our working definition describes managers as organization planners, organizers, leaders, controllers, and coordinators. Actually, every manager, from the hospital administrator to the director of food service and nutrition, takes on a much wider range of roles to move the organization toward its stated objectives (Files, 1981). *Managers work with and through other people.* The term *people* includes not only subordinates and supervisors but also other managers in the organization and individuals outside the organization, such as clients, community leaders, suppliers, and union representatives. Managers, then, work with anyone at any level within or outside their organizations who can help achieve unity or organizational goals. In community nutrition dietitians/nutritionists work with many levels of employees and community representatives to get the job done. In addition, managers in any organization work with each other to establish the organization's long-range goals and to plan how to achieve them. They also work together to provide one another with accurate information needed to perform tasks. Thus managers act as channels of communication within the organization. Peters and Waterman (1982), in addressing corporate excellence, identified several attributes that distinguish excellent innovative companies. These attributes all emphasize work with and through other people and consider people as the most important asset.

A Bias for Action

Even though these companies may be analytical in their approach to decision making, they are not paralyzed by that fact. In many of these companies the standard operating procedure is "Do it, fix it, try it"; instead of allowing 250 engineers and marketers to work on a new product in isolation for 15 months, bands of 5 to 25 form and test ideas out.

An application to community nutrition would be a group of community dietitians/nutritionists who have had several committee meetings to develop standards for maternal nutrition services. Since there are conflicting reports in the literature and strong personal opinions about the appropriate weight gain for obese pregnant women, the committee met four more times than was planned because of lack of resolution of this issue. If the leader had a bias for action and used problem-solving techniques such as the nominal group process, this issue could have been resolved at the first meeting. Precious time is wasted if there is not a bias for action and knowledge of how to proceed to achieve appropriate action.

Close to the Customer

"These companies learn from the people they serve. They provide unparalleled quality service and reliability—things that work and last. Many of the innovative companies got their product ideas from customers. That comes from listening intently and regularly" (Andreasen, 1982).

In developing the Supplemental Feeding Program for Women, Infants and Children (WIC), a combination of health professionals and the community listening to one another to minimize the problems of infant mortality and undernutrition was the motivating force for people to work together for an understood goal. Community leaders were aware of the health problems in these age groups and worked with the health and public policy committees to facilitate this program. Being close to the customer made this program a reality. Community dietitians/nutritionists have a unique opportunity to be close to their consumers.

Autonomy and Entrepreneurship

The innovative companies foster many leaders and many innovators throughout the organization. They encourage practical risk taking and support good efforts (Peters and Waterman, 1982).

Community dietitians/nutritionists are now beginning to become entrepreneurs through the use of marketing strategies in new areas, such as work site nutrition programs, computer-generated dietary information for clients, work with athletes, and a host of other markets involving consumers.

Productivity Through People

The excellent companies treat the rank and file as the source of quality and productivity gain. They do not foster "we/they" labor attitudes or regard capital investment as the fundamental source of efficiency improvement. Respect for the individual permeates throughout the organization.

Managers of community nutrition have used participatory management as a major style. Since community nutrition is a people-oriented profession, this area is one that has potential in fostering productivity through people. Pursuing continuing education programs that address productivity is an excellent way to develop and refine skills to obtain results.

Hands-On Value Drives

Thomas Watson, Jr., of IBM said that "the basic philosophy of an organization has far more to do with its achievements than do technological or economic resources, organizational structure, innovation and timing." Values are the underpinning of any organization.

The value system in community nutrition indicates that nutritionists wish to serve people through the use of skills in the area of food, nutrition, and health.

Managers Are Responsible and Accountable

Managers are in charge of seeing that specific tasks are done successfully. They are usually evaluated on how well they arrange for these tasks to be accomplished. All members of an organization, including those who are not managers, are responsible for their particular tasks. The difference is that managers are held responsible or accountable, not only for their own work but also for the work of others. The chief nutritionist or nutrition manager is held responsible and accountable for community nutrition programs.

Managers Balance Competing Goals and Set Priorities

At any given time every manager faces a number of organizational goals, problems, and needs, all of which compete for the manager's time and resources (both human and material). Because such resources are always limited, each manager must strike a balance between the various goals and needs. Many managers, for example, arrange each day's tasks in order of priority: the most important things are done right away, and the less important tasks are looked at later. In this way managerial time is used more effectively. Managers are often caught between conflicting human and organizational needs and must identify priorities. In recruiting staff for public health nutritionist positions, we would always make an attempt to determine the amount of flexibility a potential applicant was able to handle. This is necessary in community nutrition, since each day brings myriad problems, both diverse and time consuming. Setting priorities and being flexible are essential. For example, the nutrition administrator of the Arizona Department of Health Services recently was in a position to develop a new data system for all programs. To do this, she had to review the present system but also think toward the future in terms of numbers of clients, disease entities, and high-risk groups. Doing so required analytical skills.

Managers Are Mediators

Disputes within a unit or organization can lower morale and productivity. Such occurrences hinder work toward unit or organization goals; therefore managers must at times take on the role of mediator and iron out disputes before they get out of hand. Settling quarrels requires skill and tact.

Managers Are Politicians

Managers must build relationships, use persuasion, and compromise in order to promote organizational goals, just as politicians do to move their programs forward. Managers should develop other political skills, also. All effective managers "play politics" by developing networks of

mutual obligations with other managers in the organization. They may also have to build or join alliances and coalitions (Kanter, 1979). In nutrition, knowledge of the political arena, whether formal or informal, is essential, since agencies and departments are often competing for some of the same funds.

Managers Are Diplomats

Managers may represent the entire organization, as well as a particular unit, in dealing with clients, customers, contractors, government officials, and personnel of other organizations. Managers' image in the community is a vital part of the external environment of a company or agency. Therefore tact and diplomacy are necessary attributes.

Managers Are Decision Makers

No organization runs smoothly all the time. Many types of problems can occur, including financial difficulties, problems with employees, or differences of opinion in interpreting organization policy or with the medical staff over nutritional therapy. Managers are expected to come up with solutions to difficult problems and to follow through on their decisions, even when doing so may be unpopular. The brief description of these roles shows that managers must be flexible, "change hats" frequently, and be alert to the particular role needed at a given time. A mark of an effective manager is the ability to recognize the appropriate role to be played and to change roles readily (Stoner, 1982). The public health nutritionist has had to make many difficult decisions in the past few years related to serious budget cuts. Appropriate data to make good decisions are essential.

PERFORMANCE IN THE ORGANIZATION

How successful an organization is in achieving its objectives and in meeting society's needs depends on how well the organization's managers do their jobs. Just as managers function within the organization, organizations function within the larger society. How well managers do their jobs, or managerial "performance," is the subject of much debate, analysis, and confusion in the United States and other countries (Lohr, 1981). How well the organizations of a society do their "jobs," or organizational performance, gives fuel to an equally lively debate (Connolly, Conlon, and Deutsch, 1980; Drucker, 1981). Underlying many of these debates are two concepts suggested by Drucker (1964). He has indicated that a manager's performance can be measured in terms of efficiency and effectiveness. Efficiency, according to Drucker, means "doing things right," and effectiveness means "doing the right thing." Efficiency—that is, the ability to get things done correctly—is an input/output concept. An efficient manager is one who achieves outputs, or results that measure up to the inputs (labor, materials, and time) used to achieve them. Managers who minimize the cost of the resources they use to attain their goals are acting efficiently.

However, it is not enough to measure efficiency of a manager's use of employees only in terms of keeping costs low. Effectiveness, on the other hand, is the ability to choose appropriate objectives. An effective manager is one who selects the right things to get done. A community nutritionist must do a complete needs assessment in order to make decisions. A manager who selects an inappropriate objective is an ineffective manager. Such a manager would be ineffective even if this objective were completed with great efficiency. No amount of efficiency can compensate for lack of effectiveness. The greatest temptation, says Drucker, is to work on doing better and better what should not be done at all. A manager's responsibilities require performance that is both efficient and effective; although efficiency is important, effectiveness is critical. Drucker implies that effectiveness, rather than efficiency, is essential to business. The pertinent question is not how to do things right, but how to find the right things to do and to concentrate resources and efforts on them.

Managerial Skills and Time Allocation

All managers need to plan, organize, lead, and control. There are differences among managers in the amount of time they devote to each of these activities. A dietitian manager who supervises a group of community health workers will use her time differently from the community dietitian/nutritionist manager of a large public health nutrition department whose subordinates are a cadre of dietitians/nutritionists who cover specific regions of the state.

The assumption that there is an executive type is widely accepted, either openly or implicitly. However, any executive presumably knows that a company or agency needs all kinds of managers for different levels of jobs. The literature of executive development is replete with efforts to define the qualities needed by executives, and by themselves these sound quite rational. Few, for instance, would dispute the fact that a top nutrition manager needs good judgment, the ability to make decisions, the ability to win the respect of others, and all the other well-worn phrases any management person could mention. One has only to look at successful managers in any company or agency to see how broadly their particular qualities vary from any ideal list of executive virtues.

Robert L. Katz (1974), an educator and business executive, has identified three basic types of skills that he thinks are needed by all managers: technical, human, and conceptual.

Technical Skill

Technical skill implies an understanding of and proficiency in a specific kind of activity, particularly one involving methods, processes, procedures, or techniques. For example, a surgeon, community dietitian/nutritionist, accountant, and engineer all have technical skills when they are performing their own special function. Technical skills involve specialized knowledge, analytical ability within that specialty, and facility in the use of the tools and techniques of the specific discipline. Managers need enough technical skills "to accomplish the mechanics of the particular job" they are responsible for.

Human Skill

Human skill is the executive's ability to work effectively as a group member and to build cooper-

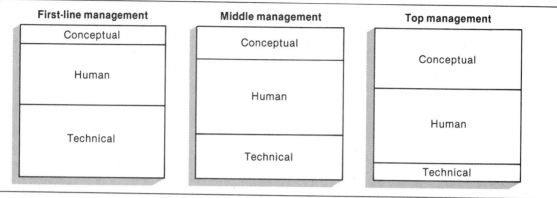

Figure 2-2. Relative skills needed for effective performance at different levels of management.

ative efforts within the team. As technical skill is primarily concerned with working with "things" (processes or physical objects), so human skill is primarily concerned with working with people. This skill is demonstrated in the way a person perceives and recognizes the perceptions of his or her superior, equals, and subordinates and in the way one behaves subsequently.

Persons with highly developed human skill are aware of their own attitudes, assumptions, and beliefs about other individuals and groups; they are able to see the usefulness and limitations of these feelings. Such persons work to create an atmosphere of approval and security in which subordinates feel free to express themselves without fear of censure or ridicule; they do so by encouraging subordinates to participate in planning and carrying out those things which directly affect them. Persons with human skill are sufficiently sensitive to the needs and motivations of others in the organization so that they can judge the possible reactions to and outcomes of various courses of action that may be undertaken. Skill in working with others must become a natural, continuous activity, since it involves sensitivity not only at times of decision making but also in the day-by-day behavior of the individual. Human

skill cannot be a "sometime" thing. Consistency in behavior is necessary because everything that a manager says or does has an effect on associates.

Conceptual Skill

Conceptual skill involves the ability to see the enterprise (organization) as a whole; it includes recognizing how the various functions of the organization depend on one another and how changes in one part affect all others; and it extends to visualizing the relationship of the individual business to the industry, other areas such as the community, and political, social, and economic forces. A manager needs enough conceptual skill to recognize how the various factors in a given situation are interrelated so that the actions that are taken will be in the best interest of the total organization. Katz (1974) suggests that although technical, human, and conceptual skills are all essential to effective management, their relative importance to a specific manager depends on his or her rank in the organization (Figure 2-2). Technical skill is most important at the lower levels of management; it becomes less important higher in the chain of command. A dietitian assigned to a diabetic patient service, for example, is likely to need more technical skills than the chief dietitian for the entire hospital, because the manager will have to deal with the day-to-day problems that arise. Similarly, although human skill is important at every level of organization, it is imperative at the lowest level where the greatest number of manager-subordinate interactions are likely to take place.

On the other hand, the importance of conceptual skill increases higher in the ranks of management. The higher the manager is in the hierarchy, the more he or she will be involved in the broad, long-term decisions that affect large parts of the organization. For top management, which is responsible for the entire organization, conceptual skill is probably the most important skill of all.

• • •

In a recent study by Rinke, David, and Bjoraker (1982) Katz's skill model was applied to the four routes used to train dietitians: internship, coordinated undergraduate, traineeship, and advanced degrees. They considered that the four routes to professional preparation in dietetics appeared to provide more adequate preparation in technical than in either human or conceptual skill. This observation is significant because it implies that dietitians are prepared for their specialist roles but are falling short of the human and conceptual skills needed to advance to higher level positions in an organization.

Another approach to determine how managers spent their time was taken by Mahoney, Jerdee, and Carroll (1965). They measured management behavior in terms of the amount of time managers estimated that they devoted to various activities. Their study involved 452 managers, representing all levels of management from first-line supervisors to the president. The managers were employed in 13 companies and represented a typical cross section of business and industry. The managers in the study received questionnaires instructing them to estimate how much time they usually spent on each of eight manage-

Table 2-1. Percentage of workday spent by managers on various tasks

Function	Percentage of Workday
Supervising	28.4
Planning	19.5
Coordinating	15.0
Evaluating	12.7
Investigating	12.6
Negotiating	6.0
Staffing	4.1
Representing	1.8

From Thomas A. Mahoney, Thomas H. Jerdee, and Stephen J. Carroll, "The Job(s) of Management," *Industrial Relations*, 4, no. 2 (February 1965), 103. Used by permission. In James A.F. Stoner, Management, ed. 2, © 1982, pp. 408, 593. Reprinted by permission of Prentice-Hall, Inc., Englewood Cliffs, N.J.

ment tasks: planning, investigating, coordinating, evaluating, supervising, staffing, negotiating, and representing. As a group, the managers reported that they spent more of their workday performing supervisory activities (28.4%) than any other function. The planning function came next, taking up 19.5% of their average workday (Table 2-1).

Mintzberg (1975) made an extensive survey of existing research on the manager's role and integrated those findings with the results of his own study of the activities of five chief executive officers. The combined survey covered all kinds and levels of managers: factory foremen, sales managers, administrators, presidents, and even some street gang leaders. Mintzberg concluded that there is considerable similarity in the behavior of managers at all levels. All managers, he concluded, have formal authority over their own organizational units, and they derive status from authority. This status causes all managers to be involved in interpersonal relations with subordinates, peers, and superiors, who in turn provide managers with the information they need to make decisions. These different aspects of the job cause managers at all levels to be involved in a series of interpersonal, informational, and decisional roles, which Mintzberg defined as organized sets of behavior (Figure 2-3).

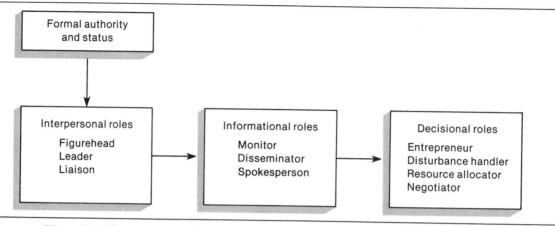

Figure 2-3. The manager's roles.
Reprinted by permission of the Harvard Business Review. An exhibit from "The Manager's Job: Folklore and Fact" by Henry Mintzberg (July/August 1975). Copyright © 1975 by the President and Fellows of Harvard College; all rights reserved. Redrawn from James A.F. Stoner, Management, ed. 2, © 1982, pp. 408, 593. Reprinted by permission of Prentice-Hall, Inc., Englewood Cliffs, N.J.

The Manager's Negotiator Roles

Managers spend much of their time as negotiators, because only they have the information and authority that negotiators require. There are three informational roles in which managers gather and disseminate information. The first is the *monitor* role. As monitor, the manager constantly looks for information that can be used to advantage, for example, statistics on the lower rate of anemia in preschool children over the 3-year period that the program has been working with this population. Second is the *disseminator* role. The manager distributes to subordinates important information that would otherwise be inaccessible to them—data showing the rate of anemia decreasing since the program started. Finally, as a *spokesperson*, the manager transmits some of the information he or she has collected to persons outside the unit or even outside the organization. For example, the administrator of the health department is presented with data on decreasing rates of anemia at the appropriate time to receive good coverage with the press and legislature or the director of the agency, since this represents the results of the nutrition program.

The Manager's Decisional Roles

Information is the basic input to decision making for managers. In the role of the entrepreneur the manager has a leader role—hiring, training, motivating, and encouraging employees. Finally, the manager must play the interpersonal role of liaison, by dealing with people other than subordinates or supervisors, such as peers within the organization and allied health groups outside of it.

The Manager's Informational Roles

Mintzberg (1975) suggests that receiving and communicating information are perhaps the most important aspects of a manager's job. A manager needs information to make the right decisions, and others in the manager's unit or organization depend on the information they receive from and transmit through the manager. Ideal information for community dietitians/nutritionists would be CDC surveillance data on the population they are serving over time. Mintzberg's work is particularly interesting because it calls attention to the uncertain, turbulent environment in which the manager operates. Real-life events and situations, he stresses, are only partially predictable and controllable—the manager often must deal with them as they come. In his view managers have neither the time nor the inclination to be reflective thinkers; they are, above all, doers, coping with a dynamic parade of challenges and surprises. Thus Mintzberg's concept of the manager's job offers a useful reminder that our definition of management as a series of functions, planning, and organizing is a somewhat idealized but useful overview of what managers try to do. In fact, managers operate in a constantly changing environment. Although they attempt to follow systematic and rational procedures, they are often interrupted in their work. Community dietitians/nutritionists reflect Mintzberg's concept, since a vast number of activities are handled on a daily basis, which could be viewed as outside the manager's strict definition.

THE EVOLUTION OF MANAGEMENT THEORY

Three well-established schools of management thought—classical, behavioral, and quantitative—have contributed to managers' understanding of organizations and their ability to manage them. Each offers a different perspective for defining management problems and opportunities and for developing ways to deal with them (Wren, 1979).

Frederick W. Taylor (1911) created the scientific management movement—the application of scientific and analytical theory to management practice. That movement evolved in the late 1920s and 1930s into three areas: the management process (classical), human relations (behavioral), and organization theory (quantitative). He looked at management through its functions, distinguishing those functions from the policies that form and guide them. Human relations entered the science when the Hawthorne studies showed the relationships between productivity and morale. These experiments led to an important discovery: special attention, such as being selected as participants in a study backed by top management, frequently causes people to in-

crease their efforts. This phenomenon is known as the Hawthorne effect (Mayo, 1953).

Organization theory, in a sense, combined both classical and behavioral movements. By the 1930s, management theory was in transition. Chester Barnard and James Burnham, two researchers in organizational theory, accurately predicted the power managers would have to influence, even to shape, the society we live in. Barnard and Burnham set the stage for the decades to follow (Stoner, 1982).

MANAGEMENT AND CHANGE FOR THE TWENTY-FIRST CENTURY

Management has become the dominant social, economic, and political force of the twentieth century. This rise to power took place against a backdrop of changes in technology, work force, and organizational structure. To cope with the new methods and products, better educated workers, and larger, more complex organizations, management has been forced to change. The early emphasis on the principles of management has given way to the concepts of systems and contingencies.

Technological Change

Technological change has had the greatest impact on the nature of management today and community nutrition, with the use of computers to generate and store data. New applications of science have forced managers to adapt, not only to revolutionary products and methods of production but also to the effects these products and methods have had on the work force and organizational structure. Technology comprises two areas: the application of organized science to practical tasks and a division of labor that focuses scientific knowledge on specific segments of work. Technological change, then, is the progressive use of applied science specialization. Galbraith (1978) has pointed out six specific effects of technological change on the operation of an organization:

1. Longer production cycles
2. An increase in the capital needed to run an enterprise

3. A tendency toward inflexibility in task performance (Longer production cycles and greater capital needs slow the speed with which a technology can be altered for any particular job.)
4. A growth of specialists in the labor force
5. Increased intensity of organization
6. The growing importance of planning for the most effective use of time, capital, and labor

Organizational Change

Technological change has been responsible for organizations becoming larger and more complex. One aspect of this change is specialization. As people specialize and thus limit each area of expertise, they increase the overall number of areas and their interaction. To cope with the size and complexity of today's organizations, modern managers have had to restructure them. There are times when the vertical chain of command, the traditional line organization, does not work. In its place managers are using project organization structures that work laterally, as well as vertically.

THE EXTERNAL ENVIRONMENT

The external environment consists of those elements outside an organization relevant to its operation, whereas the internal environment deals with elements inside the organization. As the size and complexity of the organization itself increase, so do those of the elements in the organization's task environment. Modern managers and community dietitians/nutritionists must deal with an external system far more complex than their own organization—a system that includes government regulatory agencies, labor unions, consumer groups, and a large number of other independent but related organizations.

Managers today must establish some method or approach that will enable them to maintain and improve their performance in a changing environment. For example, as the social and technological environment has changed, hospital managers have faced rapidly rising costs and var-

ious pressures from government. Obviously, an approach to management must take the external environment into account so that an organization can function effectively.

In responding effectively to the external environment, both "systems" and "contingency" approaches come into their own. Both take explicit account of the total environment within which an organization operates, and both specifically emphasize the adjustments needed as managers attempt to dominate, control, neutralize, or adapt to that environment.

Systems Theory

Systems theory is one of the most important concepts in modern management because it deals with change and interrelationships in complex organizations (Haimann, Scott, and Connor, 1982). A critical aspect of the theory is interdependency. A change in one part of the system must affect other parts of that system. A managerial decision to increase outpatient care in a hospital affects nursing, nutrition, and treatment resources as the nature of patients' needs changes. The systems approach sees the organization as more than an economic unit that makes rational use of people, machines, and materials to increase efficiency and profits. It sees the organization as a fusion of parts, processes, and goals that makes a living, changing human enterprise. The *parts* are people and material resources. The *processes* that tie them together are planning, organizing, leading, and controlling—the managerial function. These processes link the parts and aim them squarely at organizational goals.

The systems concept frees management from the narrow, efficiency-oriented view of the organization; it incorporates many variables that affect the system and influence managers' actions. The concept gives dietitians and nutritionists more leverage for adjusting the system and a more realistic picture of their impact on it.

Contingency Approach

The contingency approach was developed by managers, consultants, and researchers who tried to apply the concept of the major schools to real-life situations. They often found that methods that were highly effective in one situation would not work in other situations. They then sought an explanation for these experiences. Why, for example, did an organizational development program work brilliantly in one situation and fail miserably in another? The contingency approach had a single, logical answer to such questions. Results differ because situations differ. A technique that works in one case will not necessarily work in all cases.

According to the contingency approach, the task of managers is to identify which techniques will, in a particular situation, under particular circumstances, and at a particular time, best contribute to the attainment of management goals.

SUMMARY

The classic managerial functions of planning, organizing, leading, controlling, and coordinating are important elements for the community dietitian/nutritionist in today's health care system with cost constraints as a major focus of all care. Since managing implies getting things done through people, the community dietitian/nutritionist takes on an additional set of functions beyond scientific information. For example, the roles of a goal and priority setter are critical to this process. In addition, analytical skills are needed, plus a whole array of others, such as mediator, politician, developer, and above all, decision maker.

Applying Katz's managerial skill model of technical, human, and conceptual skills to the community dietitian/nutritionist, the strengths and weaknesses of the dietitian's training and where continuing education is needed to meet the needs of clients in these difficult economic times are identified.

Management theory provides a framework to look at where an organization has been and to help give a sense of direction, both technological and organizational, to prepare for management of health care systems in the twenty-first century.

REFERENCES

Andreasen, A.R.: Nonprofits: check your attention to customers, Harvard Bus. Rev. **60**:105, May/June 1982.

Bennett, A.C.: Managers apply artistic attributes to reach beyond job fundamentals, Mod. Health Care **9**:72, 1979.

Connolly, T., Conlon, E., and Deutsch, S.J.: Organizational effectiveness: a multiple constituency approach, Acad. Management Rev. **2**:211, 1980.

Drucker, P.F.: Managing for results, New York, 1964, Harper & Row Publishers, Inc.

Drucker, P.F.: Behind Japan's success, Harvard Bus. Rev. **59**:83, 1981.

Files, L.A.: The human services management task: a time allocation study, Public Administration Rev. **41**:686, 1981.

Galbraith, J.K.: The new industrial state, ed. 3, Boston, 1978, Houghton Mifflin Co.

Haimann, T., Scott, W.G., and Connor, P.E.: Management, ed. 4, Boston, 1982, Houghton Mifflin Co.

Hoover, L.W.: Enhancing managerial effectiveness in dietetics, J. Am. Diet. Assoc. **82**:58, 1983.

Kanter, R.M.: Power failure in management circuits, Harvard Bus. Rev. **57**:65, 1979.

Katz, L.R.: Skills of an effective administrator, Harvard Bus. Rev. **52**:23, Sept./Oct. 1974.

Lohr, S.: Overhauling America's business management, New York Times Magazine, Jan. 1981.

Mahoney, T.A., Jerdee, T.H., and Carroll, S.J.: The job(s) of management, Industrial Relations **4**(2):103, 1965.

Mayo, E.: The human problems of an industrial civilization, New York, 1953, Macmillan.

Mintzberg, H.: The manager's job: folklore and fact, Harvard Bus. Rev. **57**(4):55, July/Aug. 1975.

Pekar, P.P.: Setting goals in the non-profit environment, Managerial Planning **30**:43, March/April 1982.

Peters, T.J., and Waterman, R.H.: In search of excellence, New York, 1982, Harper & Row Publishers, Inc.

PL 93-641, National Health Planning and Resources Act of 1974, Washington, D.C., Superintendent of Documents.

PL 96-79, National Health Planning—Resource Development Act Amendments of 1979, Washington, D.C., Superintendent of Documents.

Rinke, W.J., David, B.D., and Bjoraker, W.T.: The entry-level generalist dietitian. II. Employers' perceptions of the adequacy of preparation for specific administrative competencies, J. Am. Diet. Assoc. **80**:139, 1982.

Stoner, J.A.F.: Management, ed. 2, Englewood Cliffs, N.J., 1982, Prentice-Hall, Inc.

Taylor, F.W.: The principles of scientific management, New York, 1911, Harper & Row Publishers, Inc.

Wren, D.A.: The evolution of management thought, ed. 2, New York, 1979, John Wiley & Sons, Inc.

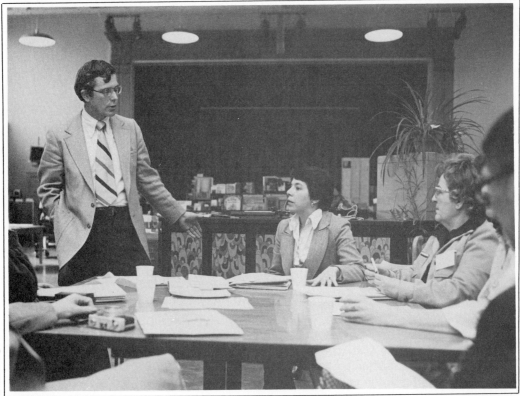

H. Armstrong Roberts

Planning and Decision Making in Community Nutrition to Produce Outcomes

GENERAL CONCEPT

Planning is a primary managerial function that involves decision making. Planning entails developing a course of action to achieve predetermined objectives within a framework of implementation and then assessing effects (evaluation). Objectives are the focal point around which managers place their energies and mobilize their resources. Setting priorities and determining a course of action are important steps in defining the specific objective that will be implemented.

When you finish this chapter, you should be able to

- Explain why it is important to understand strategic and operational (program) planning
- Describe how managers can devise a correct strategy for their organization or agency
- Define the elements of the strategic planning process, including value formation, problem/need, goals and objectives, setting priorities, and choosing alternative courses of action
- Define the elements required to identify the problem/need for a community
- Define goals and objectives and identify the difference between outcome and process objectives
- Describe the decision-making process and the essential steps necessary to arrive at a sound decision

Planning is the primary managerial function, whether one is discussing individual health planning or planning for an organization or agency. It precedes and is the framework for organizing, leading, and controlling (Figure 3-1). It begins with decision making—the process of selecting from among alternatives. Through that process emerge organizational strategies, objectives, policies, and procedures—the standards against which performance is measured. The modern organization or agency operates in an environment that is always changing in ways it can neither control nor predict. This changing environment does not do away with the need for planning; it heightens it. The only way that the organization or agency can survive is through rational anticipation of and preparation for new developments.

STRATEGIC PLANNING
The Concept of Strategy

The concept of strategic planning is vital to the dietitian/nutritionist who is attempting to be eff

zation. What is strategic planning? Strategic planning is the formalized, long-range planning process used to define and achieve organizational goals. Strategic planning is also called *comprehensive planning* and *long-range planning* in some literature (Steiner, 1979). There are three reasons why strategic planning is important. First, the need for strategic planning has increasingly become a fact of organizational life. The strategic plan—or lack of one—is often the starting point for understanding and evaluating the actions of managers and their organizations. Second, strategic planning provides the basic framework within which all other forms of planning should take place (Heroux, 1981). Because all activities of an organization ultimately depend on its strategy, strategic planning is the most important type of planning. Third, an understanding of strategic planning—potentially the most complex and sophisticated type—makes it easier to understand the other forms of planning.

Characteristics of Strategic Planning

Stoner (1982) describes the characteristics of strategic planning:

1. It deals with fundamental or basic questions. It provides answers to questions such as Who are our customers? Who should they be? and How can we meet their needs?
2. It provides a framework for more detailed planning and for day-to-day managerial decisions.
3. It involves a longer time frame than other types of planning.
4. It lends a sense of coherence and momentum to an organization's actions and decisions over time.
5. It is a top-level activity in the sense that top management must be actively involved. Only top management has access to the information necessary to consider all aspects of the organization. Commitment from top management is necessary to generate commitment at lower levels.

Strategic Versus Operational Planning

Strategic planning is not the only planning activity of an organization; however, it is the one in

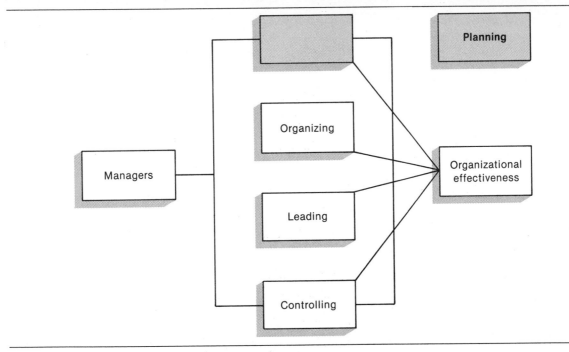

Figure 3-1. The management process.

Planning done at lower levels is called *operational (program) planning* (Connors and Spaulding, 1982). Its focus is on present operations, and its prime concern is efficiency (doing things right) rather than effectiveness (doing the right things).

In a sense, strategic planning provides guidance and boundaries for operational management; the two types of planning overlap, and both are necessary. Effective management must have a strategy and must operate the day-to-day level to achieve its goals (Tucker and Burr, 1982). Table 3-1 summarizes the main differences between strategic and operational planning.

Strategic Planning in Not-for-Profit Organizations

Wortman (1981) reviewed the research on strategy formulation and implementation in not-for-profit organizations and concluded that "not-for-profit organizations are in the initial stage of using the strategic management concept." He classified not-for-profit organizations into three categories: public (health departments), third sector (food co-ops), and institutional organizations (universities). Despite their diversity, many not-for-profit organizations share characteristics that distinguish them from profit-oriented firms. Newman and Wallender (1978) have listed six characteristics that are fairly common in not-for-profit organizations:

1. The service they provide is intangible and hard to measure.
2. Customer influence may be weak.
3. Strong employee commitment to professions or to a cause may weaken their allegiance to the organization.
4. Resource contributors may intrude into internal management.
5. Restraints on the use of rewards and punishments result from 1, 3, and 4 above.

Table 3-1. Operational planning versus strategic planning

	Operational Planning	Strategic Planning
Focus	Operating problems	Longer-term survival and development
Objective	Present accomplishments	Future accomplishments
Constraints	Present resources environment	Future resources environment
Rewards	Efficiency, stability	Development of future potential
Information	Present business	Future opportunities
Organization	Bureaucratic/stable	Entrepreneurial/flexible
Leadership	Conservative	Inspires radical change
Problem solving	Reacts, relies on past experience	Anticipates, finds new approaches
	Low risk	Higher risk

Modified with permission from *Long Range Planning*, Vol. 9, B. Taylor, Strategies for planning, © 1975, Pergamon Press, Ltd. In James A.F. Stoner, Management, ed. 2, © 1982, pp. 408, 593. Reprinted by permission of Prentice-Hall, Inc., Englewood Cliffs, N.J.

Table 3-2. Steps in the planning process

Planning Steps	Planning Questions
Defining the problem	What is the present situation? Who says it is a problem? What will happen if nothing is done?
Setting the objective	What do I want the situation to be in the future? How will I know when I have achieved it?
Choosing among alternate strategies	What are all the possible ways to solve the problem? What resources would be needed to do each alternative? Which alternatives are most feasible? Who needs to be involved in choosing which way is best?
Preparing for implementation	What arrangements need to be made with other organizations and people to carry out the plan? How will we get everything done on schedule? How will the needed resources be found?
Designing the evaluation	How will I know when I have reached my objective? How well did the strategies and activities work out? How efficiently were the resources used?
Using evaluative information	What will I do with this information? Who needs to receive it? How can I make it possible for others to use this information?
Organizational effectiveness (initiating change)	What is the organization's capacity for change? How do organizations change? What problems will I face in introducing my plan? How can I get my plan accepted?

From Craig, D.P.: HIP pocket guide to planning and evaluation, Learning Concepts, Inc. Distributed by University Associates, San Diego, Calif.

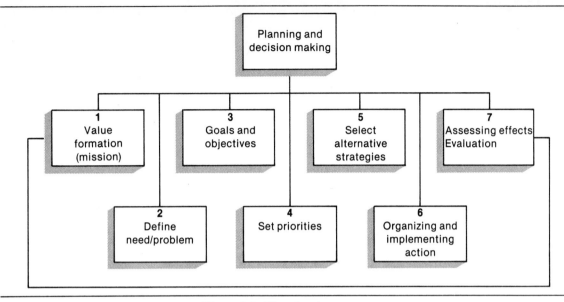

Figure 3-2. The planning process.

6. Charismatic leaders and/or the "mystique" of the enterprise may be important means of resolving conflict in objectives and overcoming restraints.

Wortman (1981) found that not-for-profit organizations tended to be "managed much more in a short-term operation sense than in a strategic sense." There is evidence that some of these organizations have no strategy at all (Belohlav and Waggener, 1980). Rather, they seem motivated more by short-term budget cycles and personal goals than by any interest in reexamining their purpose or mission in light of altered environmental circumstances.

In spite of the barriers, strategic planning efforts appear to be increasing in not-for-profit organizations, as they have been in business firms. The same rapid changes in environmental factors that have led business organizations to undertake strategic planning have similarly had direct impact on not-for-profit organizations. For these and other reasons, reports of strategic planning efforts in health departments, colleges, hospitals, and local and state governments are now starting to appear regularly in such professional journals as *Long Range Planning* (Hawkins and Tarr, 1980).

The Process of Strategic Planning

The importance of strategic planning for managers (community dietitians/nutritionists) and organizations has grown in recent years. Managers found that by describing the organization's value system and by defining the organization's mission in specific terms, they were better able to give their organization direction and purpose. Organizations function better as a result and become more responsive to a changing environment. Organization values and mission will be described in this chapter as part of the strategic planning process along with the other elements of planning, including defining needs, describing goals and objectives, setting priorities, and selecting alternative courses of action. Organizing and implementing action and assessing effectiveness (evaluation) will be described in detail in Chapters 4 and 6 (Figure 3-2 and Table 3-2).

Value Formation

What are values? Values provide a general "guidance system" for a person's behavior. They are different from attitudes in that they transcend specific objects, events, or people. Values may be defined as beliefs about what is "good" (freedom, justice, charity) and what is "bad" (war, poverty, disease). A common observation made about values today is that they are changing.

Managers need to be aware of their own values and the values of those who influence their accountability for performance (Albanese, 1978). Furthermore, it is significant to managers not only that values are changing but also that multiple and sometimes conflicting scales of values characterize work environments. (For practical help in understanding the process of value formation and techniques of value clarification, see Maury Smith, *A Practical Guide to Values Clarification* [1977]).

Peters and Waterman (1982), in their research on America's best-run companies, were impressed by the explicit attention that these companies pay to values. They state that the foundation of an institution is marked by the formation of value commitments. These values fix the assumptions of policymakers as to the nature of the enterprise, its distinctive aims, methods, and roles. Excellent company beliefs are usually narrow in scope and include just a few basic values:

1. A belief in being the best
2. A belief in the importance of the details of execution, the nuts and bolts of doing the job well
3. A belief in the importance of people as individuals
4. A belief in superior quality and service
5. A belief that most members of the organization should be innovators; however, there should be a willingness to support failure
6. A belief in the importance of informality to enhance communication
7. Explicit belief in and recognition of the importance of economic growth and profits

Values for health practitioners. The recognition of values helps health practitioners to establish priorities and hierarchies of importance among needs and goals (Haimann, Scott, and Connor, 1982). Such value orientation occurs in all public services. Value determination on the part of the professional and public creates the objectives and often the destiny of public service programs.

The relationship between values that are inherently conceived and those which are actually operative vary greatly in different circumstances and may be determined only through empirical investigation. For example, any program designed to reduce the incidence of cardiovascular disease by changing the risk factors of individuals must first establish the inherent value of the risk factors as a cause of cardiovascular disease; then it must identify those who have these risk factors. This discovery must then be translated into the operative value of removing the risk factors of elevated serum cholesterol, smoking, obesity, and stress.

Organizational Purpose and Mission

Once the value system has been formulated for an organization or agency, then a discussion of purpose and mission is the next logical step in the strategic planning process. The purpose is a broad aim that applies not only to a given organization but to all organizations of its type in that society. For example, a hospital's purpose is to provide health care to the community, whereas a community nutrition program's purpose is to provide nutrition services to people in the community.

The *mission* of an organization is the unique aim that sets the organization apart from others of its type. Narrower than purpose, the mission is the broadest aim that a particular organization chooses for itself. Within the broad limits of an organization's purpose, each organization chooses its own mission, which can be described in terms of the clients served, such as infants and children.

In strategic planning the first step is to define an organization's mission. Drucker (1974) calls this step determining the "common thread" for the organization's activities. Often, managers have to explore several possibilities and even make false starts before defining the right mission. Exploration of choices is particularly true in not-for-profit areas such as hospitals and health departments. Many managers find the common thread of their organization by asking themselves some of the following questions:

1. *What is our business, and what should it be?* This question is not simple. For instance, if an organization's business or purpose is defined too broadly, the organization may lack a sense of direction; if purpose is too narrowly defined, the organization may overlook atractive opportunities.

2. *Who are our clients or customers, and who should they be?* An examination of the needs and characteristics of clients and customers may point the direction for an organization to take.

3. *Where are we heading?* This question is relevant even if an organization produces unrelated goods or services.

4. *What major competitive advantage do we enjoy?* Managers can identify and isolate those factors which give the institution a strong competitive edge, such as unique services or a favorable location. A hospital interested in developing a health promotion program may be unique in the community by offering such services.

5. *In what areas of competence do we excel?* Boundaries may be ill-defined or changing. In this case special capabilities of the organization, such as an outstanding staff of dietitians/nutritionists who may attract clients to the health promotion program, could be the common thread for a new venture.

COMMUNITY ASSESSMENT: DIAGNOSING THE COMMUNITY'S HEALTH AND NUTRITION NEEDS

Nutrition problems originate from complex interrelationships between environmental and social factors and the individuals in a community. Therefore to look at a community only in terms of medical assessment of nutritional status (clinical, dietary, and biochemical) is of limited practical value if the different factors from which problems result are ignored.

Community assessment relies primarily on existing sources of information. It is a relatively simple technique for which cost and manpower requirements are relatively small. Some existing sources of information may include statistics from U.S. Census studies, vital statistics, hospital records, public assistance records, private and public health agencies, and social welfare agencies.

What Is a Community and How Can One Diagnose It?

Because the major emphasis of this text is on delivering nutrition services in the community, the community will be diagnosed and assessed as one example of defining the need/problem.

A *community*, as the term is used here, is defined as a group of individuals or families living together in a defined geographical area, usually comprising a village, town, or city; it may represent only a few families in a rural area or may include heavily populated cities; it may range in size from less than a hundred to a few thousand people. Members of a community live and work together, feel a sense of loyalty to the community, and share a limited number of common interests.

Accepting the definition of a community, what, then, is community nutrition? A definition that allows for flexibility and scope in both teaching and practice is that community nutrition is the academic discipline that deals with the identification and solution of health problems with nutritional implications within communities or human population groups.

This description of the community includes its background, history, and geographical determinants. The people must be characterized—not just their demography, but their culture and their ethnic differences. In addition, other major factors that contribute to the color and texture of the community map are the people's religion, taboos, education, interests and concerns, socioeconomic status, housing, schools, and other institutions. Too often in the past the knowledge, attitudes, and practices as related to values have been overlooked.

Gathering existing data on these and other factors will help to determine whether the community's nutritional resources are adequate, what groups are potentially at high nutrition risk, and how well the community's nutritional and related health needs are being met by existing curative and preventive health programs.

There are existing sources of information on which community assessment relies. What is known about the community from its health, vital statistics, morbidity, and mortality records? What is known about health services, number of professionals, and number of health-related facilities? In addition to U.S. Census data, which give the characteristics of the population group—sex, age, race, marital status, education, income, and housing—what is known from hospital records, public assistance records, and private, public, and social welfare agency statistics? The community assessment paints a picture of the health of the community, its ecology, and the factors influencing the way its people live (Christakis, 1973).

CASE STUDY OF A COMMUNITY

The hypothetical community presented here is the county of Everywheresville, U.S.A. Although this community may resemble other communities throughout the United States, its differences are in actuality marked. Population structure, family characteristics, employment and economic situation, educational profile, transportation system, programs available for specific population groups, available health services, the community health and nutrition problems are all factors that will vary nationwide. However, basic elements of effective program planning can be applied to any Everywheresville in the United States. Pertinent data concerning the community should be gathered and collated, as in this profile of Everywheresville.

Location

Everywheresville is located in the Southwest

Population Characteristics

Population—500,000
Urban setting, with many shopping malls
Population mix—white, 60%; black, 20%; Hispanic, 15%; other, 5%

Age Distribution of Population

Large percentage of population is 30 years of age and under 15% of population elderly
High birthrate

Employment and Economic Situation

Industry—marketing of area for tourists, sunshine and good weather all year; light manufacturing consisting of leather factories and some clothing factories that make men's sports apparel
Average—$10,000 to $12,000 per year for a family of four persons (after taxes)
Poverty level—20% of population below poverty level
Unemployment rate—10%

Family Characteristics

Family size
  Average—4 persons
  Low-income average—5 persons
  One-parent households—22%
Working mothers—60% employed; children taken care of in day-care centers, and some neighbors take care of two or three children

Educational Level

High school graduates—75%
College and above—10%
Noneducated—15%

Educational Resources

Elementary schools
High schools
Community colleges (2)
Vocational schools (3)
No mandatory health education in schools
School Lunch Program available in most schools, with free or reduced-price lunches available; cost of lunch daily is 95¢ per meal
School Breakfast Program available in selected areas only

Transportation Characteristics

No mass transportation; private automobiles provide transportation

Programs Available for Specific Population Groups

Day-care facilities available for 50% of children of working mothers and 50% of children cared for in private homes

Food and nutrition programs (other than schools)

Food stamps—serving only 25% of those eligible

Women, Infants, and Children (WIC) Supplemental Feeding Program for pregnant and lactating women, infants, children—case load of 1000 clients representing approximately 10% utilization by those in need*

Title III—several congregate feeding sites for the elderly throughout major population centers with transportation available to all sites

Health Services Available (Other Than Private Providers)—County Health Department

Personnel

Health director (MD)—1

Pediatric nurse assistants—2

Sanitarians—3

Nurses—15

Health educator—1

Nutritionist—1

Services for behavioral health

Services for planning environmental health

Social workers—2

Health workers—2 per clinic setting

Health worker trainees—2

Services available

General community hospital

Family planning clinics

Limited prenatal clinics for population (clinics staffed primarily by pediatric nurse assistants)

Equipment available for nutritional assessment, such as calibrated scales and steel measuring tapes and baby boards (wooden to measure length of infants)

Outdated or inappropriate equipment available for measuring heights and weights

Limited facilities for biochemical determinations, which include hemoglobin and hematocrit values; no clinical laboratory available

Computer services at health department very limited

Health and Nutrition Problems in Community

Cardiovascular disease in adult population—40% — and has increased by 25% with decreasing age in the last 10 years

Cancer

Accidents

Diabetes

Anemia in 17% of 1- to 2-year-old indigent population, determined by medical staff and laboratory tests to be iron deficiency anemia

Overweight in 19% of child population—2 to 18 years old

Obesity in 40% of total population

High incidence of women with complications in pregnancy

Short stature in 18% of indigent population (preschool children and schoolchildren)

Elevated serum cholesterol levels in large percentage of population 18 years and under; of these, a large number had two or more additional cardiovascular risk factors

Poorly nourished elderly population: 10% undernutrition, 5% anemic

Widespread dental disease—dental caries

Areas for Community Assessment

The purposes of collecting data are to obtain factual knowledge about the problem, to permit an accurate diagnosis of its causes and systematic approaches to its solutions, and to help assess or evaluate changes that follow. Types of data that may be collected include the following:

1. Anthropometric studies
2. Clinical nutrition surveys
3. Biochemical studies
4. Vital and health statistics
5. Studies on local foods, the marketplace, and food economics
6. Cutural and sociological data, including material on food habits and food preference, "power structure in local communities, the decision-making process, and leadership patterns
7. Role of family members

If the need or want is not clearly identified and described, what to do about it cannot be considered. Problems arise in describing the need when the statement is one of the solution rather than a clear expression of the need. For example, "We need to supply iron supplements to children"

---

*500,000 total population; 20% poor = 100,000 persons; 10% women, infants, and children = 8000 to 10,000 eligible for WIC program but not covered.

Table 3-3. Some sources of information for nutrition needs/problems in the community

Need/Problem	Source of Information
Population	Census Bureau (most recent data)
	Health departments
	Social service departments
	Universities and colleges—programs in nutrition, medicine, urban health, allied health, community health, nursing
	Offices of congressional, state, and local representatives
	Federal, state, and local bureaus of labor, statistics, or commerce
	Department of Aging
	Board of Education
	City/county government offices
Housing	Same as above and in addition:
	Department of Housing and Urban Development
Food marketing facilities	Local offices for supermarket chains
	Local office of consumer affairs or markets
	Local association of food stores or farmers' markets
	Local newspapers and advertisements
Health statistics	Regional, state, and municipal health/hospital departments
	State and local health agencies
	State health planning agencies
	State and local universities and colleges, community medicine, population studies, health planning
	Health systems agencies
	Data from National Center for Health Statistics and Health and Nutrition Examination Survey
	Data from Centers for Disease Control Nutrition Surveillance System
Community and mental health care programs	Local hospitals, nursing homes, home health care agencies
	Local health and social services departments
	Local prepaid health care groups
	Local programs for the elderly, handicapped, and special groups
	Community health centers
	Migrant health centers
	Indian health clinics
	School health services for data on pregnant teenagers
Community agencies	Local United Fund or equivalent
	Local telephone directory
	Local health, social services department and education agencies
	Local March of Dimes
	Local community action and/or legal services organizations
	Local Agricultural Extension Service
	Local community colleges, universities, and professional schools
	Local home health care agencies
	Local heart, cancer, and similar associations

From Simko, M.D., Cowell, C., and Gilbride, J.A.: Nutrition assessment: a comprehensive guide for planning intervention, Rockville, Md., 1984, Aspen Systems Corp. Reprinted with permission of Aspen Systems Corporation.

Table 3-3. Some sources of information for nutrition needs/problems in the community—cont'd

Need/Problem	Source of Information
Food and nutrition programs	State and local health departments, social services State or local Board of Education Local community action groups
Nutrition education programs	County, city health departments Board of Education Social services departments Local Extension or Farm Bureau Office Local office of Dairy Council and of similar interest groups
Educational facilities	Local Board of Education State Commissioner of Education
Nutrition training programs	Local educational institutions, universities, and colleges Community colleges and vocational (trade) schools National, state, and local organizations of dietitians and nutritionists Local school food service office

is really a solution, whereas the need may be to reduce iron deficiency anemia among 1 to 5 year olds.

The sixteen areas of information that pertain to community assessment are described in detail in this chapter (Christakis, 1973). Table 3-3 summarizes some sources of information that should be helpful for the community assessment profile (Simko, Cowell, and Gilbride, 1984).

Demographic Information

Demography is the statistical study of human populations, especially with reference to size and density, distribution, and vital statistics. Age, ethnicity, sex, population density, birthrates, and death rates are all important aspects of demographic data. The U.S. Census tabulations are good source documents for such data. In Everywheresville the population mix is 60% white, 20% black, and 15% Hispanic. Places to obtain information for small areas where problems exist include the local health systems agency; local city planning; health, welfare, and social service agencies; school boards; chambers of commerce; local banks; and local newspapers. In the community

diagnosis of Everywheresville population characteristics are given along with the age distribution of the population.

Socioeconomic Stratification

One of the fundamental tools of community nutrition analyses is determining socioeconomic stratification. The two main devices for social stratification include (1) socioeconomic profile of geographical areas, which is useful to define and locate poverty pockets; and (2) evaluation of individuals, for which levels of income are relevant because income may be directly related to the adequacy of nutritional status. In Everywheresville 20% of the population is below the poverty level.

Census data are useful in stratifying areas, since they contain information about socioeconomic indicators such as crowding, racial composition, and housing characteristics.

Housing adequacy and the health environment correlate closely with socioeconomic status and are indicators of potential nutrition problems. Local health departments usually have these data.

Health Statistics Resources: Morbidity and Mortality

The vital statistics department of any health agency has a wealth of information derived from local and state data on health problems in the community. The vital statistics department usually has records on the actual numbers of births and crude birthrates. This information is especially important if comparisons are made over periods of years. Additional data that are significant in nutritional assessment are the numbers of illegitimate births, births of less than 2500 gm (5½ lb), the number of home births, and births to mothers under 18 or over 40 years of age. These data may indicate community health problems. High neonatal, postnatal, and infant mortality is a gross indicator of the need for better health and nutrition services.

For the community as a whole, compiling the causes of deaths and the number of deaths attributed to each cause can be useful. However, the common practice of examining the 10 leading causes of death provides inadequate information for community nutritional assessment. Nutritional factors are often a highly important component of morbidity and mortality resulting from coronary heart disease, hypertension, diabetes, and alcoholism. These disease indices should all be examined in terms of their nutritional implications.

Statistics on the prevalence of incidence of diseases that may be poverty related—for example, tuberculosis or other nutritionally related diseases such as coronary heart disease, hypertension, diabetes, and alcoholism—are often available from public health sources or voluntary health organizations that are concerned with these specific diseases. Family planning clinics also have data on diet histories that can be made available to the assessment team.

Data available in the Early Periodic Screening, Diagnosis, and Treatment (EPSDT) portion of the Medicaid program are also a valuable source of health information, particularly for children from birth to 18 years of age. The Supplemental Feeding Program for Pregnant and Lactating Women, Infants, and Children (WIC Program) is another source of data for specific indices such as height, weight, hemoglobin, or hematocrit. In addition, data from several health problems are identified in Everywheresville, including cardiovascular disease in 40% of the adult population, anemia in 17% of the 1- to 2-year-old indigent population, overweight in 19% of children, and poorly nourished elderly.

Local Health Resources

Some of the questions that might be asked of agencies working in the area of community health and nutrition services follow:

- Are dietitians/nutritionists available to agencies' staff?
- Is a health educator available?
- Are effective child health programs in operation? Do these have adequate nutrition evaluation? Is parent education adequate?
- Are maternity clinics adequate, and do they have credible nutrition programs?
- Is nutrition a significant part of local health units or public education program?
- Are public programs available for coronary heart disease, diabetes, and hypertension? Is the nutrition component an effective and significant one?
- Are there work site life-style programs being conducted at any of the industrial plants, where employees are encouraged to exercise and practice nutrition and stress management?
- Does an exercise program exist?
- Does an effective alcoholism program exist? Does it have an effective nutrition component?
- Do drug addiction and rehabilitation programs have a nutrition component?
- Do child feeding and school lunch programs exist and under whose supervision? Are there qualified people to run them?

Hospitals, extended care facilities, and nursing homes also should be identified and their bed capacity and occupancy rates evaluated in terms of the community's health needs. Within these institutions the number of qualified dietitians employed and adequacy of food service facilities should be measured. Also, public health agencies should be viewed in terms of their nutrition component.

In a particular area the number of available health personnel such as physicians, dentists, public health nutritionists, public health nurses, school nurses, health educators, social service workers, nurse practitioners, and other health workers should be determined, including osteopaths and other licensed practitioners. This information can be obtained from local licensing agencies, professional societies, and social service agencies. It may be wise to explore other influences on community health, such as the extent to which a population uses faith and spiritual healers or other quasimedical practitioners. Fortunately, in Everywheresville, the county health department provides basic public health services to the population.

Dental Health

The availability of dental care for all members of the community regardless of income or age should be investigated, since nutrition is an important factor in dental health. If dental health programs do exist, the amount and number of patients being seen in various economic categories should be determined.

Cultural Factors

Knowledge of cultural factors in a community, such as differences in life-style and ethnic eating patterns, are crucial to community nutritional assessment. Although some of these cultural factors are difficult to define and isolate, community assessment should summarize the identifiable cultural traditions and goals of the community and its subgroups, particularly with reference to food preferences and eating habits. An evaluation should be made of the shopping area where produce and meat are purchased and of shopping patterns as well.

These data may only be available from local

nutritionists, dietitians, home economists, school lunch supervisors, public health nurses, and social service workers, who are generally good sources of information.

Community Political Organizations

A program for a given community should never be conceived exclusively by health professionals without any input from the community. This type of approach can ensure failure from the very beginning. Also, it is necessary to determine who the community leaders are and where the power structure lies. Interviews with various government officials, community coordinators, and people in administrative positions can provide clues as to who is in charge. Interviews can be made of the public officials and community leaders in the following way:

1. Determine whether nutritional problems exist in the community. Is the community aware of them?
2. Determine whether an educational program is necessary to increase awareness of the local government and community groups to the need for health action programs.
3. Determine how to locate and use available resources for developing programs in this area.

Housing

Housing data are important in community and nutrition assessment for two reasons: (1) they are an excellent indicator of social and environmental deprivation, and (2) the family's ability to utilize foodstuffs is directly related to the adequacy of kitchen facilities.

Since these data again can be a useful source of selected housing characteristics, they can be used to measure crowding, that is, the number of persons per room, and sanitation facilities.

Data on kitchen facilities might be supplemented by information from local utility companies, which may have records of household appliances such as stoves, refrigerators, freezers, and dishwashers. A direct household survey that has been completed in the area is certainly even more informative. Specific information on housing may be obtained from local housing authorities, the local health department, and urban planning groups.

Food Programs/Resources

Assessments of the local marketplaces, supermarkets, small grocery stores, food cooperatives, delicatessens, health food stores, organic food stores, and other food outlets are necessary for a complete community diagnosis. The number of small corner vendors, snack stands, and other popular chains and the extent to which they are used by the population are also relevant.

Food consumption studies on a national basis are available from the U.S. Department of Agriculture in regional and national offices. Other factors should be considered.

Food costs. The determination of relative food costs for a community, indicating whether an adequate food supply can be purchased, is important. Local departments of welfare, community service agencies, and consumer groups often compile food costs on a weekly and monthly basis. Department of Agriculture publications, issued on a regular basis, indicate costs of food in various parts of the United States. A yearly survey is done on food costs and is often reported in local newspapers. Another consideration is credit purchases as opposed to cash purchases of food, which may also indicate variances in cost.

Food standards. It is desirable to determine the presence or absence of compliance with local or state food standards, including fortification requirements, and also if the state has an enrichment law for breads and cereals. It should be determined whether a consumer protection agency is available and how strong its role is in local government.

Nutrition resources. A survey of the numbers of dietitians/nutritionists, home economists, and nutrition aides within the community, their level of training and certification, their functions, and a definition and assessment of the population they serve is desirable. The amount of in-service training of these various personnel groups should be known, as well as the kinds of institutions and universities that provide their training. There are several programs available for the indigent population in Everywheresville: food stamps, WIC, and Title III. (See Chapters 8 to 11 for a description of these programs.)

School Nutrition Programs

The number of school breakfast and school lunch programs requires evaluation. The amount of federal funds compared with local funds for school lunch and school breakfast programs is also a consideration.

The extent of nutrition education in the school systems and also at the preschool level should be defined. Further possibilities for nutrition education programs for teachers in the primary and secondary schools, their students, and food service personnel became a reality with the passage of the Child Nutrition Act (H.R. 1139 Amendments to the National School Lunch Act and Child Nutrition Act of 1966) called the Nutrition Education and Training (NET) Program. Feeding programs such as the WIC Program, which has a strong medical and nutrition component, should be identified if they are available. Fortunately, a school lunch is available in Everywheresville; however, school breakfasts are limited.

Social Welfare Programs

National figures and percentages of the population receiving public assistance may be obtained from local welfare departments and social service agency records. Eligibility standards may need careful review, particularly since many barriers stand in the way of people obtaining social services. Although public assistance and Aid to Dependent Children figures are not presented in the Everywheresville community statistics, they will provide additional information for the assessment of (1) income levels, (2) poverty levels, and (3) unemployment rate. It is useful to determine the eligibility standards for Medicaid. The use of food stamps, donated foods, and supplemental food programs all require documentation, as well as description and evaluation of the quality of the diets provided. The accessibility of these feeding programs to clients should be investigated.

Food and social services for senior citizens (Title III programs) and children should be explored. For example, are there day-care programs for senior citizens? Does the program provide nutrition education and meal services? In children's programs, such as Head Start, are the meals adequately prepared and is there an adequate nutrition component including food service and nutrition education?

Transportation

Transportation is important to nutritional patterns for the following reasons:
1. It provides accessability to food supplies.
2. Mobility of persons has a direct bearing on their ability to obtain nutritional counseling and to visit health and educational facilities.
3. Freeways may present problems that limit social or commercial contacts between segments of the community.

No mass transit system is available in Everywheresville.

Education

An understanding of the literacy and the extent to which the English language is understood and spoken must be considered in the evaluation of health and nutrition programs. If the program is to be oriented toward an English-speaking population and the nutritionist is dealing with a primarily Spanish-speaking population, obviously the program is doomed to failure. Unfortunately, detailed data in this area are difficult to acquire, but public and parochial schools can often provide useful facts concerning education levels, illiteracy, and whether or not English is understood. Often, community leaders can provide this kind of information. Everywheresville's statistics on educational characteristics are available.

Occupational Data

Data on occupations, unemployment, and industrial health practices may not be essential to nutritional assessment but may be helpful in providing a profile of the whole community. Marketing and manufacturing are the major industries in Everywheresville.

Geography and Environment

In rural and underdeveloped areas particular attention should be given to soil type and other factors related to agricultural production. The level of food supply can be a direct function of whether and in what conditions the land affects production.

Human-induced environmental changes are significant considerations as well. Polluted animal-feeding areas, creation of land subsidies, and crop or livestock loss from air or water contamination are all factors in determining food availability and, consequently, nutritional status.

Surveys and Surveillance

There are two sources of data for nutrition statistics that will be very useful in determining need. First, nutrition surveys examine a population group at a particular point in time. The National Health and Nutrition Examination Survey (NHANES) is an excellent data base that describes a large sample of the population. Caution must be taken not to extrapolate data specifically to a select community; however, these data can reveal national trends and present a good picture and some clues as to what dietitians/nutritionists should be looking for in the community.

Second, nutrition surveillance data can be invaluable in describing problems at the local level. The Nutrition Surveillance program developed at the Centers for Disease Control has provided useful data on children and pregnant women since the early 1970s. Data are collected and used by state and local health departments. A complete description of survey and surveillance data is found in Chapter 8.

In addition to services delivered in the community, the community dietitian/nutritionist serves a variety of institutions and clients. A complete guide to assessing facilities and clients is developed in *Nutrition Assessment: A Comprehensive Guide for Planning Intervention* (Simko, Cowell, and Gilbride, 1984).

• • •

Knowledge about the preceding 16 factors can provide enough information to make sound judgments on community assessment. A word of caution is necessary in community assessment: Specific cutoff points in the collection of data must be made. It is self-defeating if the gathering of data becomes the main objective and the true purpose of alleviating the nutrition problems in a given area is missed.

Defining the Need/Problem: The Process

Defining the need/problem in strategic planning is critical; however, it is the most difficult and often the most neglected step. Table 3-2 describes the steps in the planning process and the planning questions needed at each step. *The terms*

STEPS TO DEFINE THE NEED/PROBLEM

---

1. Develop a rough narrative description of the problem situation and underline key words.
2. Write a more concise (one paragraph) statement of the problem.
3. Determine who has the problem.
4. Determine what would happen if nothing is done about this problem.
5. Consider whether it is appropriate for your organization to be doing something about this problem.
6. Determine the appropriateness of the problem in terms of your and your agency's value system.
7. Analyze the cause of the problem.
8. Rewrite the final problem statement based on your complete understanding of problem and refine it.
9. Review the checklist to be sure the problem statement is complete (p. 54).

---

need *and* problem *(need/problem) are used interchangeably for our purposes.* If this step is overlooked or done carelessly, the rest of the process may end up being completely off base. This result may not surface until a lot of time, energy, and money has been wasted. In describing the problem, several questions should be asked: What are the specific health problems with a nutrition component? What are the patterns of health and illness? This step often consists of a straightforward collection of already available and easily obtainable data.

Before any program is conceived, a clear description is necessary of the need/problem and the condition the program is going to solve is extremely important. The term *need/problem* may be defined as:
1. a situation or condition
2. of people or the organization
3. that will exist in the future and
4. that is considered undesirable
5. by the members of the organization

In this definition one should think of the problem as something that will happen in the future if action is not taken (Craig, 1978). The final achievement of all planning, strategic and operational (program), is to meet a need, satisfy a want, or alleviate an existing condition.

There are several steps that should be followed in order to clearly and concisely state the problem (see box on left).

Step 1: Develop a Rough Narrative Description of the Problem Situation and Underline Key Words

In Everywheresville several areas of need are identified. For example, there is a problem of anemia in children: 17% of 1 to 2 year olds from the indigent population have iron deficiency anemia and are at nutritional risk. There is a need to reduce iron deficiency anemia in children.

Another example is the prevalence of cardiovascular disease. The rate of cardiovascular disease in Everywheresville is 40% and has increased by 25% with decreasing age in the last 10 years. There is a need to design a program to reduce cardiovascular disease risk.

Thus, in the process of need determination or problem identification, the planner pinpoints the exact area where problems are seen. For example, there are two specific nutrition problems in Everywheresville: iron deficiency anemia in children and a prevalence of cardiovascular disease in an increasingly youthful population.

Step 2: Write a More Concise (One Paragraph) Statement of the Problem

Everywheresville faces two specific health problems: (1) 17% of the 1 to 2 year olds in the indigent population have been diagnosed as having anemia, and (2) the prevalence of cardiovascular disease is 40% and has increased by 25% with decreasing age in the last 10 years.

Step 3: Determine Who Has the Problem

Anemia
- Indigent children ages 1 to 2 years old
- Parents of children—they may not have an ample food supply and medical care to prevent and alleviate problems
- Siblings of these children—parents may not understand the process of disease; anemia may occur in other children in the family
- Health workers—county health department staff, nutritionists, physicians, nurses—who see this as a public health problem
- Community and family—anemic children may be lethargic and have difficulty learning in school

Cardiovascular disease
- Male population over 45
- Male and female population who are predisposed to one or more cardiovascular disease risks, such as elevated serum cholesterol, obesity, and smoking
- Employers who realize the importance of keeping people well and productive throughout their lives
- Health workers who see this as a public health problem
- Community and family with cardiovascular disease—life span may be short; service to the community may be hampered because of debilitating disease

Step 4: Determine What Would Happen if Nothing Is Done About This Problem

Anemia
- Children may have a lower resistance to infection
- Children may not be able to learn well in school
- Increased medical costs to family and community

Cardiovascular disease
- Debilitating disease for all segments of the population
- Fewer years of productivity because of disease
- Decrease in productivity within society
- Quality of life may be lessened
- Early retirement
- Early mortality
- Increased medical costs to family and community

Step 5: Consider Whether It Is Appropriate for Your Organization to Be Doing Something About This Problem

- What is the purpose of your organization? Its purpose is to provide health care to indigent populations in the community of Everywheresville.
- Does the problem fit the purpose?

  Yes (X)   No ( )   Useless ( )

- How is the problem related to the organization's purpose? The two problems identified are health problems that have been found in the community. It is important for the Public Health Department to deal with these problems as soon as possible.

Step 6: Determine the Appropriateness of the Problem in Terms of You and Your Agency's Value System

- It is the job of the public health worker and department to reduce the prevalence of disease in the population.
- We obtain satisfaction by helping children and adults achieve better health status.

- The Public Health Department may lose funding and credibility if the problems are not resolved.
- We believe it is the right of all people to have good health care.

Step 7: Analyze the Cause of the Problem

Anemia

- Recent layoffs in Everywheresville have led to a limited food supply for the indigent population.
- Parents are not taking children to the health clinics because there is some question of their eligibility for services at the time of layoff.
- This is a proud community, and many people feel the stigma of taking food stamps or other help.
- WIC has just started a study; no results are available to date.

Cardiovascular disease

- Sedentary life-style of factory workers
- Limited recreational facilities in the town for exercise programs
- Stress from factory work and from unemployment
- Large numbers of smokers
- High alcohol consumption
- Obesity is a major problem—some cultural groups find obesity attractive in women
- Cultural groups represented eat a diet high in saturated fat and salt

Step 8: Rewrite the Final Problem Statement Based on Your More Complete Understanding of Problem and Refine It

Final problem statement

The following five basic elements should be contained in the problem statement:

1. Future point in time that you are concerned about
2. Geographical area or parts of the organization that the problem affects
3. Nature of the problem
4. Estimate of size of problem
5. Individuals or group of people the problem affects

Refined problem statement

Anemia

1. If health and food services are not provided within 3 months, a larger number of
2. the indigent children in the community of Everywheresville
3. will have iron deficiency anemia.
4/5. Now 17% of the 1 to 2 year olds have anemia.

Cardiovascular disease

1. If a cardiovascular disease risk factor program is not initiated within the next 6 months
2. the adult population (over 40 years old) of Everywheresville
3. will manifest a greater number of cardiovascular disease risk factors.
4/5. Now the rate of cardiovascular disease in Everywheresville is 40% and has increased by 25% with decreasing age in the last 10 years.

Step 9: Checklist for Problem Statement

The following checklist is important to review as you finalize your problem statement:

- Relates to purposes and goals of organization
- Is of reasonable dimensions
- Is supported by statements from authorities
- Is stated in terms of clients or beneficiaries
- Does not make assumptions
- Does not use jargon
- Is interesting to read

With an adequate description of the scope, nature, and victims of the nutritional problems of a community in hand, the next step is to begin to develop a precise plan. Here, the manager (community dietitian/nutritionist) determines what the program will accomplish, states the goal of the program, and develops specific objectives in precise terms.

Developing Goals and Objectives
Differences Between Goals and Objectives

An arbitrary differentiation has been made by many people between goals and objectives, even though both imply a "results orientation" or what will be accomplished. However, to differentiate between the two terms, a goal, mission, or purpose is usually a statement of broad direction, general purpose, or interest. It may be somewhat unreachable, and it is seldom quantifiable. One example of a statement of a goal follows: "To increase the health status and the quality of life for the citizens of the state."

Goals tend to be broad, all-encompassing ideals because they are derived from values. The formulation of abstract goals is essential because many of the most important human goals can be adequately or meaningfully stated only in general terms.

Objectives often explain behavior better than any other contributing factor in a managerial situation, and the understanding and control of objectives is more vital than other factors, since they provide the main energizing and directive force for managerial action. Objectives are the focal point around which managers concentrate their efforts and mobilize their resources.

This discussion of objectives can apply to organization and management of a public health system, since the same factors of money, manpower, resources and accomplishment, and results orientation are the ones that must be utilized, coordinated, and evaluated.

Writing Objectives

Guidelines. The definition of an objective is very similar to the definition of a problem. This fact should not be surprising, since the objective is basically to reduce or eliminate the problem. Objectives are specific measurable statements of what one wants to accomplish by a given point in time (Craig, 1978).

There are several ways of distinguishing among types of objectives. Objectives may aim to solve a problem external to the organization, usually a problem of the community and/or target population, or they may aim to solve problems internal to the organization, such as employee training or motivation. Also, objectives may be directed to changing the skills, knowledge, or attitudes of people, for example, patients, clients, customers, and staff. These types of objectives are often referred to as behavioral objectives (Chapter 13). Whether an objective is a specific program or is behavioral, the basic elements are the same.

The following general guidelines apply to formulating objectives for a person, unit, section, or department:

- State objectives in terms of expected results, not in terms of activities or processes.
- Specify results that will be tangible and recognizable so that all involved in planning, including advisory board and other agencies or special interest groups, will also recognize the objectives.
- State objectives so that expected results are very specific, not general.
- State objectives in terms of results to be accomplished this month or this year (if the program is continued next year and the years thereafter, include specific time limitations).
- Show how the objectives of a specific program help further the objectives of the organization, or department or unit, and the mission and purposes of the statewide or national structure.

Steps. Developing meaningful written objectives of program statements is the basis of program management. In writing objectives, these steps should be followed:

1. Translate your problem statement into an objective.
2. Check your objective to see if it is clear and complete.
3. Establish your criteria for success.

Two specific formulas for writing sound objectives follow:

1. To/action verb/desired result/time frame/resource required.
   Example from Everywheresville:
   To reduce/anemia by 40% in the 1 to 2 year olds/in 1 year/utilizing the nutrition staff from Everywheresville's health department.
2. By ____(date)____ , the following results will have been accomplished.

Example from Everywheresville:

By March 1987, a 40% reduction in the prevalence of anemia will occur in the 1 to 2 year olds by using the existing nutrition team.

Using the basic formula to develop objectives as applied to Everywheresville, it is possible to develop sound objectives.

Earlier, two specific needs/problems were identified in Everywheresville:

1. Seventeen percent of children ages 1 to 2 years from the indigent population have iron deficiency anemia and are at nutritional risk.

Example:

To deal with the incidence of anemia, the following objectives could be completed:

To reduce the prevalence of anemia in 1 to 2 years olds by 40% in those identified at risk in 1 year by utilizing the nutrition team in each of the 14 counties.

2. The prevalence of cardiovascular disease in Everywheresville is 40% and has increased by 25% with decreasing age in the last 10 years.

Example:

To design an objective for the need in the cardiovascular disease area, the following objective could be completed:

To reduce the prevalence of cardiovascular disease risk factors (hypercholesterolemia, obesity, hypertension, smoking, and inactivity) by 40% and obesity by 30% in the 10,000 people screened, utilizing personnel and funds from the state appropriations and county health department nutrition staffs, within 1 year.

Process and outcome objectives. A differentiation should be made between process and outcome objectives for the purpose of writing clear, concise objectives that will have a results orientation. Outcome objectives are those which state the ultimate result and *not* steps, processes, or actions to achieve that result. In the medical area outcome objectives are intended to achieve the ultimate health outcome. For example, reducing anemia is a health outcome and thus an outcome objective. However, if the objective states that you are going to develop a pediatric program in Everywheresville, it is a process objective because it is a step in reaching the outcome (health) objective. The difference between process and outcome objectives is a very important concept in the health arena, since the quality assurance program (described in detail in Chapter 7) stresses outcome and process criteria as major elements of the program. If writing outcome objectives is neglected, community dietitians/nutritionists may never see the forest for the trees and may never get to the objective they are striving for—better health care for clients.

An illustration of an outcome and process objective follows:

Outcome objective: To reduce anemia by 40% in the 1 to 2 year olds in 1 year utilizing the nutrition staff from Everywheresville's health department (note the health outcome to reduce anemia).

Process objective: To develop a system of pediatric clinics including nutrition services to meet the health needs of children in a 1-year period, utilizing resources from Everywheresville's health department. This process objective is one step in obtaining the outcome objective of reducing anemia. There may be several process objectives to achieve the outcome objective over time.

Both process and outcome objectives are necessary, since merely stating an outcome objective with no steps to achieve it will be frustrating to employees and will not be achievable on an incremental basis.

Benefits from writing sound objectives. Some of the benefits resulting from writing sound objectives are summarized by Drucker (1974):

Objectives identify the basic ideas, principles, and fundamental concepts of the organization and what it is trying to achieve. They give meaning and direction to the work of the people associated with the organization.

Objectives provide the basis for guiding, leading, and directing the organization.

Objectives provide standards of performance that are essential to the control of human effort in an organization. Evaluation of individual performance is based on the extent to which mutually agreed on objectives are being achieved.

Objectives motivate people. They help provide a sense of unity, harmony, cooperation, and concern for achievements that are essential for all organized endeavors.

Objectives help program planners to:

Organize and explain the whole range of organizational phenomena in a few general statements

Test these statements in actual practice

Predict behavior

Appraise the soundness of decisions

Analyze their own experiences and, as a result, improve their performance.

Checklist. The following checklist should be reviewed before finalizing objectives:

- Describes problem-related outcomes of the program
- Does not describe methods
- Defines the population served
- States the time when the objectives will be met
- Describes the objectives in quantifiable terms, if possible.

Setting Priorities

The relationship of possible goals and objectives to each other is of particular interest and concern to health managers. It necessitates the development of some means of determining the relative importance of various health problems and hence various health activities. Today, because of limited funds and resources it is important to prioritize the objectives for any organizational unit.

At any given moment or place there are many public health problems, many more than can be treated adequately with the resources that are available. Some problems obviously must take precedence over others. As previously indicated, the decisions too frequently are made on the basis of personal whims or interests or because of some political or public pressure groups rather than as a result of careful study and analysis.

In determining program priorities, there are certain fundamental factors that should be considered. For example, generally a problem that affects a large number of people should take precedence over one that affects relatively few people, but not if the former is the common cold and the latter a smallpox epidemic. A disease that kills or disables should take precedence over one that does not, but only if an effective method of treatment is available. Similar factors should also be considered, particularly the existence of scientific knowledge and techniques, the availability of suitable personnel and funding, the propriety and legality of the contemplated action, and its acceptance by the community. Several techniques are available to assist the evaluator with simplicity in prioritizing objectives. Table 3-4 provides a review of the solutions to the problems of too many objectives (Morris and Fitz-Gibbon, 1978).

A Matrix for Priorities

Another method that has been used to determine priorities is the use of a priority matrix. The purpose of the matrix is to measure each objective against all other objectives. This method has been used successfully in setting priorities for a nutrition program at the Arizona Department of Health Services. The 22 objectives developed for a particular program (A to V) are inserted on the vertical and horizontal axes of the priority matrix (Figure 3-3).

A. Complete screening

B. Make and record referrals

C. Write patient care plan; include behavioral objectives

D. Intervene on underweight

E. Intervene on obesity

F. Intervene on high-risk pregnancy

G. Intervene on anemia

H. Intervene on cardiovascular disease risk

I. Intervene on short stature

Table 3-4. Solutions to the problem of too many objectives

Method	Quick Summary	Advantages	Disadvantages	Recommendations
Sampling objectives	Randomly select objectives from the total set.	Can be done by the evaluator alone—without cooperation from others. The quickest, simplest method. Treats all program objectives —on the test or not—as instructionally important.	The risk exists of missing objectives or items that might be important, thus reducing the credibility of the evaluation.	Highly recommended when all objectives are of about equal importance.
Sampling the important objectives	Two or three raters select the few objectives they think are most important. From this pool, objectives are then randomly chosen, if necessary.	Fairly fast method. Gives people (the raters) a say in the evaluation. Makes it unlikely that important objectives will be missed.	Focuses evaluation on a small number of objectives. Depends on cooperation of raters. Raters' choices may not represent opinions of other concerned persons.	Highly recommended when you have credible raters available and objectives which are not all of equal importance and feel you will be able to narrow down to as few as 10 objectives measured by 50 items.
Matrix sampling	All objectives are used. They are assigned to parts of a test, and each part is given to a randomly selected group of students.	Can be done by the evaluator alone—without cooperation from others. All objectives are tested, albeit with samples of students rather than all students.	Somewhat involved procedure. Data not entirely appropriate for use with some statistical tests.	The only method by which you can assess all objectives. Due to the procedure's complexity, however, use it only when you cannot avoid testing all objectives or items.
Assigning priorities to all objectives through ratings (retrospective needs assessment)	A group of approximately 15 raters rate all objectives according to a 5-point scale. Mean ratings determine priorities.	Yields accurate assessment of the priorities of interest groups represented by the raters. Involves raters in the evaluation and is therefore likely to increase credibility.	Focuses evaluation on a small number of objectives. Depends on cooperation of raters. Time-consuming for evaluators and raters.	A good procedure to use, if you have time for it and can gain cooperation from enough raters. Especially recommended when the acceptance of the evaluation by various groups is a major concern.
Assigning priorities through objectives hierarchies	Objectives grouped into content areas, then charted from simple to complex. The more complex or "terminal" ones receive highest priority.	Can be done by the evaluator alone—without cooperation from others. Assigns priority to the most logically complex objectives, avoiding attention to too simple ones.	Relatively time-consuming, depending on the number of objectives. It may not be desirable to test only terminal, difficult objectives.	Probably should be used only when you, as evaluator, must narrow down the number of objectives yourself, without assistance, and when the subject matter lends itself to logical hierarchies.

From Morris, L.L., and Fitz-Gibbon, C.T.: How to deal with goals and objectives, Center for the Study of Evaluation, 1978, University of California, Los Angeles.

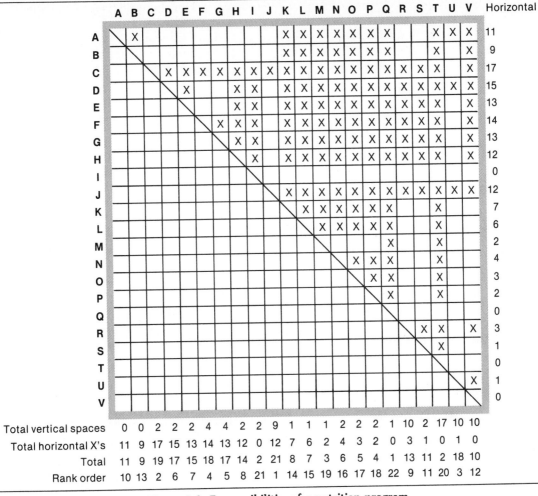

	A	B	C	D	E	F	G	H	I	J	K	L	M	N	O	P	Q	R	S	T	U	V	Horizontal
Total vertical spaces	0	0	2	2	2	4	4	2	2	9	1	1	1	2	2	2	1	10	2	17	10	10	
Total horizontal X's	11	9	17	15	13	14	13	12	0	12	7	6	2	4	3	2	0	3	1	0	1	0	
Total	11	9	19	17	15	18	17	14	2	21	8	7	3	6	5	4	1	13	11	2	18	10	
Rank order	10	13	2	6	7	4	5	8	21	1	14	15	19	16	17	18	22	9	11	20	3	12	

Figure 3-3. Responsibilities of a nutrition program.

J. Community nutrition worker routine training

K. Community nutrition worker modular training

L. In-service for other health personnel

M. Training for nutritionists

N. Training for personnel in aged, group care, and educational facilities

O. Training for the public by use of media

P. Training for the public by group presentations

Q. Training for the public by individual sessions (telephone or office)

R. Submitting monthly, quarterly, and annual reports

S. Identify nutrition needs and resources to community and governmental agencies

T. Develop materials and evaluate existing materials

U. Complete voucher issuance and records

V. Monitor grocer relations

A priority list of these 22 objectives can be established in the following manner:

1. If the objective in the left column is more important than the objective across the top, put an X in the box. If not, leave blank.
2. Work only to the right of the diagonal line.
3. Sum the Xs on each horizontal line, and transfer these sums to the bottom of the page where it says "Total Horizontal Xs."
4. Sum the blank spaces above the diagonal line in each vertical column.
5. Total the vertical spaces and horizontal Xs for each objective.
6. Assign rank order to the objectives, with the first priority being the objective with the highest total.

Using this matrix, the following priority listing occurred:

1. Community nutrition worker routine training
2. Write patient care plan; include behavioral objectives
3. Complete voucher issuance and records
4. Intervene on high-risk pregnancy
5. Intervene on anemia
6. Intervene on underweight
7. Intervene on obesity
8. Intervene on cardiovascular disease risk
9. Submit monthly, quarterly, and annual reports
10. Complete screening
11. Identify nutrition needs and resources to community and governmental agencies
12. Monitor grocer relations
13. Make and record referrals
14. Community nutrition worker modular training
15. In-service training for other health personnel
16. Training for personnel in aged, group care, and educational facilities
17. Training for the public by use of media
18. Training for the public by group presentation
19. Training for nutritionists
20. Develop materials and evaluate existing materials
21. Intervene on short stature
22. Training for the public by individual sessions (telephone or office)

DECISION MAKING

Effective managing demands the efficient use of resources. Optimum use of an organization's resources is the cornerstone of the management process. All managers, whether they are hospital administrators, directors of dietary departments, government officials, or business executives, are responsible for the property of others. Because resources are limited, managers cannot possibly take advantage of every opportunity.

Before a manager can act to use or withhold resources then, opportunities must be looked at. *Decision making* is the choice process—the deliberation about alternative ways to use resources (Haimann, Scott, and Connor, 1982). Only after a single alternative (objective) is chosen, can planning begin.

The Value of Forecasting Information in Decision Making

Forecasting is the difference in accuracy between a predicted outcome that is based on sound information and one that is not. Most daily actions people take, as individuals or managers, are based on some type of forecast. Forecasts are necessary. Without them, individuals, as well as organizations, are at the mercy of future events. The most important use of forecasts is as premises for planning. When managers assess the alternatives available to them, they try to forecast how events within and outside the organization will be. These forecasts are the premises or basic assumptions on which managers' planning and decision making are based (Balachandra, 1980).

The Process of Decision Making

Decision making is a basic human activity. It begins in early childhood and it continues until death. The process used to make everyday decisions—What shall I prepare for dinner tonight?

Which movie should I see?—is much the same as the one used to make managerial decisions.

The decision process involves four steps (Huber, 1980):

1. Identify the problem and then the objective.
2. Determine the alternative course of action.
3. Predict the outcome of each alternative.
4. Select the alternative that best meets the need.

Identify the Problem

The process begins with a problem: "Something isn't right and we've got to do something about it to make it right" such as the anemia problem in Everywheresville (pp. 60 and 61).

Determine the Alternative Course of Action

After the problem is identified and the objectives set, then activities designed to achieve these objectives must be developed. If there were only one possible action that would result in the desired objective, we could end the discussion here. But there is always more than one way to get from point A to point B. When domestic car makers were faced with declining market shares, they had several options open to them. They could advertise heavily, pushing the safety aspects of large cars. They could lobby for increased tariffs on foreign imports, raising the price of those imports above what the average consumer could afford. Or they could compete by reducing the size of their product to match the foreign machines. All of these courses of action—and there were many more—could have led Detroit's manufacturers to their objective. When nutrition programs were threatened by budget cuts, there were several options to pursue, including (1) serve only high-risk clients, (2) seek funds from clients on a fee-for-service basis; and (3) determine if another community agency could pick up some of the case load.

Where do these ideas come from? There are as many sources as there are alternative actions. Some are even outside of the organization. Whatever the source, each reasonable alternative must be considered as a possible means for reaching the objective.

Now that the problem has been defined and the objectives set, figuring out how to solve the problem is undertaken. As a first effort, list all possible ways of reaching the stated goal (Craig, 1978).

This task may be the most enjoyable part of planning. Now is the time to be creative and to pretend that money and resources are unlimited. At this stage, as many ideas as possible are listed; the more ideas listed, the better chance there will be of having a good plan.

The purpose of this phase is to break away from the standard solutions, to generate new ideas and new approaches to old ideas. The brainstorming process is one way to generate a lot of ideas in a hurry. In 15 minutes a small group can often generate 50 to 100 ideas. Presented with an idea, the group thinks of as many courses of action as possible for reaching the objective. There are three basic ground rules in this process:

1. No criticism or evaluation of ideas is allowed.
2. Far-out ideas are encouraged. They may trigger some practical ideas for someone else.
3. Do not hold back. Quantity is the main objective. If you cannot think of something, try a variance on someone else's ideas.

Once a group has brainstormed a list of options, it may be possible to combine several of these ideas into one course of action.

The objective for Everywheresville was to reduce anemia by 40% in the 1 to 2 year olds in 1 year utilizing the existing nutrition staff from the health department. A sample list of alternate courses of action for this objective follow:

1. Survey clinics to determine if the present staff can handle the project.
2. Seek funds from maternal and child health grants or other areas of the federal government.
3. Ask community leaders for suggestions for sites to hold clinics, if new clinics are a possibility.
4. Seek supplies for the project, such as iron

Sample objective

To reduce anemia by 40% in the 1 to 2 year olds in 1 year utilizing the existing nutrition staff.

Sample course of action

Form a task force composed of community leaders and health department personnel to develop a plan to get the children at risk into the health care system.

Helping forces ⟶

Interest in this health problem has recently been expressed by advocate groups in the community.

The health team is anxious to work with the community leaders, since they have ideas on funding sources.

⟵ **Hindering forces**

We have never involved the community in solving internal problems.

The board of supervisors, who oversee the health department health team, feel that they are the community leaders and need no help from additional groups.

Figure 3-4. Force field analysis.

supplements, from pharmaceutical companies.

5. Expand the WIC program to be sure that families are obtaining an additional food supply.
6. Ask parent groups to help volunteer in clinics.
7. Get the nutrition council or another health agency to cite problems of children with anemia in the community.
8. Form a task force composed of community leaders and health personnel to review alternative courses of action.
9. Seek local funds and assistance.

Predict the Outcome of Each Alternative

Now that you have generated different options, let's look at some possible ways to analyze alternate courses of action. At this point, you will look at each alternative from different perspectives. Think about how desirable each one may be without making a final decision about which one is best. Most often, this part of the process if done

somewhat intuitively. Certain strategies are rejected because they are too expensive or they will not work. The intent of the exercise is to slow the process down, to allow a careful consideration of all the possibilities.

The suggested techniques follow:

1. A "force field" analysis of forces in the environment that may help or hinder you in carrying out the strategy
2. A review of resources that would be needed for this strategy—resources you have and those you can get
3. A check against a number of criteria you will use later in evaluating success

Force field analysis. In force field analysis there are helping forces and hindering forces. Once these helping and hindering forces have been identified, a number of additional questions can be asked:

1. Do we have some influence over any of these forces? Which ones?
2. Can the effects of any helping forces be increased? How?

GUIDE FOR RESOURCES

Resource	Needed Resource Is this resource needed for this strategy? Yes/No	Resources Available Is it possible to direct resources to this strategy? Yes/No	Resources Not Available Is it possible to acquire this resource elsewhere? Yes/No
Personnel			
Money			
Equipment			
Facilities			
Time			
Knowledge			
Skill			
Political influence			
Prestige (reputation)			
Legitimacy			
Energy			
Control of information			

From Craig, F.P.: HIP pocket guide to planning and evaluation, Learning Concepts, Inc. Distributed by University Associates, San Diego, Calif.

3. Can the effects of some hindering forces be reduced?
4. What new forces might be generated to help out the strategy?

Figure 3-4 is a force field analysis from the Everywheresville case study.

Review of resources. The second technique for considering the feasibility of each alternative is to look at the resources that would be needed to carry out the strategy and to think about which of these resources are available and which would need to be acquired in order to implement the strategy.

Resources are tangible things (such as personnel, money, equipment, facilities) or intangible things (such as time, knowledge, skill, political influence prestige, legitimacy, control over information and energy) used by an organization's personnel to carry out a strategy or activity that is designed to reach desired objectives.

The box above provides a guide for considering what resources will be needed to carry out each strategy.

Select Alternative That Best Meets Needs

You have now listed all decisions and completed an analysis of possible alternate ways to meet your objective. You have analyzed each alternative and made comparisons based on helping or hindering forces and resources needed.

With all this information available, the manager should now be able to come to some reasonable decision. Who will make the decision? How will the decision be made? The answers depend on the decision-making structure of the organization and the type of decision to be made (Craig, 1978).

Who Makes the Decision?

In some organizations and in some situations the decisions will be made unilaterally by the supervisor, nutrition director, manager, or president.

The manager may decide without staff input, without explaining the problem or asking for opinions about how to solve it: "Here's what I want you to do." Or, the manager may make the decision after asking for others' opinions: "I'm thinking about doing it this way. What's your reaction?" The manager may or may not consider these opinions in making the decision.

Each of these decision-making styles is appropriate at various times and for various kinds of decisions. Probably the best time to use group decision making is when a high level of involvement and commitment by group members will be needed to implement the decision being made (Fink, 1984).

Decision-Making Styles of Dietitians

Mobley et al. (1984) studied the decision-making styles of 61 dietitians and 55 dietetic students by using the Myers-Briggs Type Indicator (MBTI). The four decision-making styles that are used include the technician, planner, teacher, and artist.

The technician style (impersonal, matter-of-fact analysis expressed in technical skills) was preferred to other styles by the greatest percentage of subjects studied. Subgroups of clinical dietitians, those 40 years or older, and dietetic internship graduates preferred the technical style that is related to academic achievement in applied and physical sciences.

Dietitians in administration, consulting, education, and community/public health indicated a preference for the artistic style, an insightful approach to possibilities expressed as an ability to communicate well with others.

Coordinated undergraduate program graduates indicated the most diversity in style preferences. The planner style identified with researchers was preferred to the artistic by students. Identification of individual decision-making styles and the theory of adaptation to various situations are important parts of continuing education programs for dietitians.

How Is the Decision to Be Made?

Within a group setting, there are many ways to make a decision, some more common than others (Welsh, 1981):

1. "Plop" decision—Various suggestions are bypassed without response. One proposal is finally agreed on, but most members believe their ideas have not been considered.

2. Decision by authority rule—The group discusses an issue, but the group leader or someone else in authority makes the decision.
3. Decision by minority—One or several people railroad a proposal through without giving opponents an opportunity to be heard.
4. Decision by majority rule—A poll or vote is taken. The majority go away satisfied, but some are dissatisfied and may not cooperate in implementing the proposal.
5. Consensus decision—Discussion continues until a decision is reached that everyone can accept and support.
6. Unanimous decision—Everyone agrees on the action to be taken.

Again, each of these techniques may be appropriate for some situations. Some are more efficient and less time-consuming. Others take more time, but when high commitment and involvement are needed, the extra time may be well spent.

Most people have a lot of experience with group decision by "plop," authority and minority and majority rule. That is why community dietitians/nutritionists should practice using the consensus approach in their organization when they work through the process of listing alternate strategies, analyzing them, and choosing the one to be used.

Now that the decision is made about how to proceed with the objectives and the strategies selected, the next step is organization and implementation (Chapter 4).

SUMMARY

Strategic planning is a primary function of the community dietitian/nutritionist. In strategic planning a description of the organization's value system and definition of the organization's mission provide a framework for clear direction and purpose. Diagnosing a community and its nutritional needs provides the necessary data to begin the development of specific objectives to deal with nutrition problems.

Decision making requires that the problem be identified and objectives set and that alternative courses of action be considered. Finally, decision making requires the selection of alternatives that best meet the needs of the community.

REFERENCES

Albanese, R.: Managing toward accountability for performance, Homewood, Ill., 1978, Richard D. Irwin, Inc.

Balachandra, R.: Perceived usefulness of technological forecasting techniques, Technological Forecasting and Social Change 16:2, Feb. 1980.

Belohlav, J.A., and Waggener, H.A.: Keeping the strategic in your strategic planning, Managerial Planning 28:23, March/April 1980.

Christakis, G., editor: Nutritional assessment in health programs, Am. J. Public Health 63 (suppl.):1, 1973.

Connors, E.J., and Spaulding, P.W.: Strategic planning: multiinstitutional systems present pros and cons to planning process, Hospitals 56:64, June 1982.

Craig, F.P.: HIP pocket guide to planning and evaluation, Austin, Tex., 1978, Learning Concepts.

Drucker, P.F.: Management: tasks, responsibilities, practices, New York, 1974, Harper & Row Publishers, Inc.

Fink, A., et al.: Consensus methods: characteristics and guidelines for use, Am. J. Public Health 74:979, 1984.

Haimann, T., Scott, W.G., and Connor, P.E.: Management, ed. 4, Boston, 1982, Houghton Mifflin Co.

Hawkins, K., and Tarr, R.J.: Corporate planning and local government: a case study, Long Range Planning 13:2, April 1980.

Heroux, R.L.: How effective is your planning? Managerial Planning 30:3, Sept./Oct. 1981.

Huber, G.P.: Managerial decision making, Glenview, Ill., 1980, Scott, Foresman & Co.

Mobley, C., et al.: Decision making styles of dietitians, J. Am. Diet. Assoc. 84:1013, 1984.

Morris, L.L., and Fitz-Gibbon, C.T.: How to deal with goals and objectives, Center for the Study of Evaluation, University of California-Los Angeles, Los Angeles, 1978, Sage Publications, Inc.

Newman, W.H., and Wallender, H.W., III: Managing not for profit enterprises, Acad. Management Rev. 3(1):28, Jan. 1978.

Peters, T.J., and Waterman, R.H., Jr.: In search of excellence, New York, 1982, Harper & Row Publishers, Inc.

Simko, M.D., Cowell, C., and Gilbride, J.A.: Nutrition assessment: a comprehensive guide for planning intervention, Rockville, Md., 1984, Aspen Systems Corp.

Smith, M.O.: A practical guide to values classification, San Diego, 1977, University Associates, Inc.

Steiner, G.A.: Strategic planning: what every manager must know, New York, 1979, The Free Press.

Stoner, J.A.F.: Management, ed. 2, Englewood Cliffs, N.J., 1982, Prentice-Hall, Inc.

Tucker, S.L., and Burr, R.M.: Strategic planning: analysis must precede adoption of competitive strategies, Long Range Planning 56:80, June 1982.

Welsh, A.N.: The skills of management, New York, 1981, AMACOM.

Wortman, M.S., Jr.: Strategic management: not for profit organizations. In Schnendel, D.E., and Hofer, C., editors: Strategic management, New York, 1981, Columbia University Press.

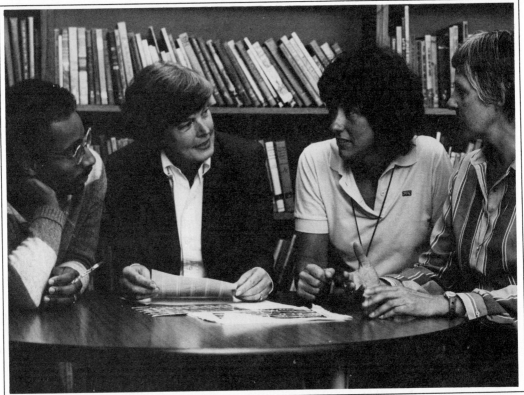

H. Armstrong Roberts

Organizing and Developing Action Plans for Nutrition Services

GENERAL CONCEPT

Organizing includes a functional group or institution that is involved in the process of determining the way in which work is arranged and allocated among members of the institution so that the goals of the organization can be efficiently achieved. Without orgnization, goals and objectives cannot be accomplished and action plans cannot be completed. Because the environment plays a major role in organizations, it is important to understand how organizations can be designed to fit with the environment in which they are involved.

When you finish this chapter, you should be able to
- Describe the organizing process and explain why it is important for organizations
- Define the elements of organizational structure and describe how they fit together for effective organization
- Define the five types of conflict possible in organizational life
- Explain how creativity can be stimulated and encouraged in organizations
- Define marketing and its role in not-for-profit organizations
- Develop an action plan including marketing strategies for one project in which you would like to be involved

BASIC ELEMENTS OF ORGANIZING

Organizing is based on planning; planning defines expectations and organizes the activities needed to reach them (Figure 4-1). Organizing, then, is setting up a formal structure of activities. It is the *division of work* to make that structure efficient, it is a measurable *span of management* to make the structure effective, and it is *coordination* to make the structure functional (Haimann, Scott, and Connor, 1982).

The design of the structure—what it looks like and how it works—rests on the organization's objectives, size, technology, values, and culture. In addition to the basic elements, the issue of organizing in a changing environment will be discussed. Organizing to formulate action plans will be stressed along with a marketing approach to action in nutrition services.

The Importance of Organizing

Organizing is a multistep process that includes the following:
- Detailing all the work that must be done to attain the organization's goals

- Dividing the total work load into activities that can be logically and comfortably performed by one person or by a group
- Setting up a mechanism to coordinate the work of organization members into a unified, harmonious whole
- Monitoring the effectiveness of the organization and making adjustments to maintain or increase effectiveness

There is no one optimum way for all organizations to be designed. The most desirable structure is an individual matter that will vary from one organization to the next and within one organization over time. There are two major aspects of organizational structure: division of work and span of management (Miles, 1980).

Division of Work

Division of work is the breakdown of a work task so that each individual in the organization is responsible for and performs a limited set of activities rather than the entire task. In a nutrition department, in addition to the director, there may be regional nutritionists who cover segments of the state and local community dietitians/nutritionists who deliver the services; they perform all specific activities.

Hackman and Lawler (1971) described five core job characteristics: skill variety, task identity, task significance, autonomy, and feedback. Jobs of broad scope (number of different operations such as coverage of five or six major departments) are likely to require greater skill variety and perhaps will encompass more task identity. Job depth (the extent to which a person can control work) is directly related to autonomy and may encompass skill variety, task identity, and feedback. The job of nutrition director has all of these characteristics, but the job of the community dietitian has less depth since this position limits skill variety and autonomy. Hackman and Lawler observed that responsibility and an understanding of the results of work contribute to motivation and job satisfaction. Persons whose jobs involve high levels of skill variety, task identity, and task significance experience work as

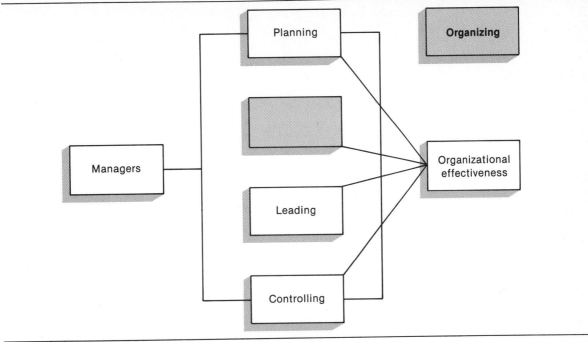

Figure 4-1. Management process.

highly meaningful. A high level of autonomy leads to a greater sense of responsibility and accountability. Where feedback is provided, workers develop a useful understanding of their specific roles and functions. Thus the greater the extent of all five task characteristics in a job, the more likely it is that the job holder will be highly motivated and experience job satisfaction (Figure 4-2).

Departmentalization. In the division of work departmentalization is the grouping together of similar or logically related work activities. Efficiency of work flow depends on the successful integration of various units within the organization (Litterer, 1980). Division of work and logical combinations of tasks should lead to logical department and subunit structures. In nutrition a typical organization chart would show the nutrition department under the Assistant Director for Health Services or as a unit in Personal Health

Services or as a part of Preventive Health Services.

To show the organization's structure, managers customarily draw up an organization chart that diagrams the functions, departments, or positions of an organization and shows how they are related. The separate units of the organization usually appear in boxes, which are connected to each other by solid lines that indicate the chain of command and official channels of communication.

Coordination. Division of work and departmentalization in organizations make coordination an important managerial activity. Through coordination, the activities and objectives of an organization's subunits are harmoniously integrated so that the organization's goals can be efficiently achieved. The need for coordination varies according to the type of interdependence that exists between organization units (Chapter 3).

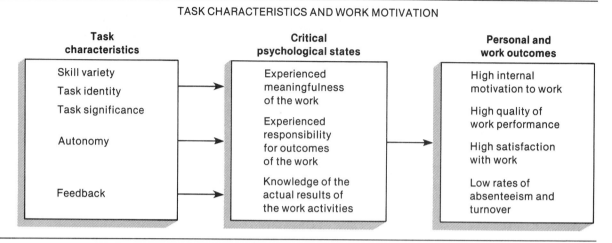

Figure 4-2. Task characteristics and work motivation.
From J.R. Hackman, *Work Redesign*, © 1980, Addison-Wesley, Reading, Mass. Adapted material.
Reprinted with permission.

Span of Management

Span of management can be simply defined as the number of subordinates who report directly to a given manager (Ouchi and Dowling, 1974). Span of management and coordination are closely related. There are two reasons why the choice of an appropriate span of management is important. First, span of management affects the efficient utilization of managers and the effective performance of their subordinates. Too broad a span may mean that managers are overextending themselves and that their subordinates are receiving too little guidance or control. Too narrow a span may mean that managers are underutilized. For example, one community dietitian giving direct services may be able to supervise four to six community dietetic technicians. Any larger numbers may sacrifice appropriate supervision and jeopardize good patient care. Second, there is a relationship between span of management throughout the organization and organizational structure. A narrow span of management results in an organizational structure with many supervisory levels between top management and the lowest level. A broad span, for the same number of employees,

means fewer management levels between the top and bottom. Either structure may influence the effectiveness of managers at any level. Ouchi suggested the concept of an optimum span, which indicates that spans could be too broad or too narrow in specific instances, resulting in inefficiency (Ouchi and Dowling, 1974).

AUTHORITY, DELEGATION, AND DECENTRALIZATION
Authority

For an organization to function efficiently, a formal authority system must be supplemented by informal bases of power and influence. Unless managers have authority themselves and can give authority to subordinates to carry out work responsibilities, the structure has no meaning. The delegation of authority is the process by which managers receive and give out authority; decentralization is the degree to which the authority is delegated throughout the organization. Managers use more than their official authority to obtain the cooperation of their subordinates. They also rely on their knowledge, experience, and leadership abilities (Scanlon and Atherton, 1981).

Influence

We will define influence or actions or examples that, either directly or indirectly, cause a change in behavior or attitude of another person or group. For example, a hard-working community dietitian/nutritionist may, by setting an example, influence others to increase their productivity. This definition also takes into account those types of influence which do not lead to more direct changes in behavior. For example, managers may use their influence to improve morale. This influence would not necessarily change behavior; it might simply bring about a change in attitude.

Power

Power may be defined as the ability to exert influence. To have power is to be able to change the behavior and attitudes of other individuals. Hard-working community dietitians/nutritionists would be more likely to have power to influence the work group if they were popular than if they were disliked.

Formal authority is one type of power. It is based on the recognition of the legitimacy or lawfulness of the attempt to exert influence. The individuals or groups attempting to exert influence are seen as having the right to do so within recognized boundaries. This right arises from their formal position in an organization.

The sources of power. Power does not simply derive from an individual's level in the organization hierarchy. Five sources or bases of power have been identified, and each may occur at all levels:

1. *Reward power* is based on one person (the influencer) having the ability to reward another person (the influencee) for carrying out orders or meeting other requirements.
2. *Coercive power*, based on the influencer's ability to punish the influencee for not meeting requirements, is the negative side of reward power. Coercive power is used to maintain a minimum standard of performance or conformity among subordinates.

3. *Legitimate power*, which corresponds to our term *authority*, exists when a subordinate or influencee acknowledges that the influencer has a "right" or is lawfully entitled to exert influence—within certain bounds. For example, the nutrition director has legitimate power to expect outcomes from staff in terms of patient care. The right of a manager to establish reasonable work schedules is an example of "downward" legitimate power. A hospital guard may have the "upward" authority to require even the chairman of the hospital board to present an identification card before being allowed to enter the surgery suite.
4. *Expert power* is based on the perception or belief that the influencer has some relevant expertise or special knowledge that the influencee does not. When people accept advice from the community dietitian/nutritionist, they acknowledge his or her expert power. Expert power is usually applied to a specific, limited subject area.
5. *Referent power*, which may be held by a person or a group, is based on the influencee's desire to identify with or imitate the influencer. For example, a community dietitian/nutritionist manager will have referent power if subordinates are motivated to emulate his or her work habits.

Characteristics of successful power users. What do managers do with their power? What specific techniques and styles are most effective? The following characteristics are common in managers who use their power successfully:

1. Effective managers are sensitive to the source of their power and are careful to keep their actions consistent with people's expectations.
2. Good managers understand—at least intuitively—the five bases of power and recognize which to draw on in different situations and with different people. They are aware of the costs, risks, and benefits of using each kind of power.
3. Effective managers recognize that all bases

of power have merit in certain circumstances. They try to develop their skills and credibility so they can use whatever method is needed.

4. Successful managers have career goals that allow them to develop and use power.
5. Effective managers temper power with maturity and self-control.
6. Successful managers know that power is necessary to get things done. They feel comfortable in their use of power and accept the fact that they must be able to influence the behavior of others to achieve goals. The power of a department of nutrition is evident when the nutritionist is called to give expert testimony before a legislative committee on a nutrition issue such as food quackery. The nutritionist has power because of his or her knowledge and position in the health department.

Power, then, is an important part of organizational life; it cannot be ignored. Managers must not only accept and understand power as an integral part of their jobs, but also they must learn how to use and not abuse it to further their and the organization's goals.

Delegation

We define delegation as the assignment to another person of formal authority and responsibility for carrying out specific activities. The delegation of authority by supervisor to subordinates is obviously necessary for the efficient functioning of any organization, since no supervisor can personally accomplish or completely supervise all the organization's tasks.

The extent to which managers delegate authority is influenced by such factors as the type of the organization, the specific situation involved, and the relationships, personalities, and capabilities of the people in that situation.

How to Delegate

The first step in the delegation process requires that the manager has a clear understanding of what he or she wants done. The manager must

establish the scope, depth, and framework of the responsibility and work demanded (Lagges, 1979).

For successful delegation, instructions must be specified clearly; the manager should explain the context of the assignment and define the expected output. After precisely defining the task, the manager must establish the framework for the work to be accomplished by:

- Soliciting the views of subordinates about suggested approaches, expected schedules, and necessary resources
- Ensuring that subordinates have the authority, time, and resources (finances, people, equipment) to accomplish this assignment
- Knowing the capabilities of his or her staff; if the skills are not equal to the task, lost time, morale problems, and failure to meet deadlines will occur
- Establishing a clear understanding as to the time required for task completion

It is imperative that supervisors and subordinates work together and that communication between them be clear and consistent. The manager must be available to clarify issues and to help solve problems. Montana and Nash (1981) have compiled a list of delegation do's and dont's (p. 73).

Effective Delegation

When used properly, delegation has several important advantages. The first and most obvious is that the more tasks managers are able to delegate, the more opportunity they have to seek and accept increased responsibilities from higher-level managers.

Several specific techniques have been suggested throughout the years for helping managers delegate effectively.

1. Establish goals and objectives. Managers must have good skills in planning, particularly in setting realistic achievable objectives.
2. Define responsibility and authority. Subordinates should be clearly informed about what they will be held accountable for and

DELEGATION DO'S AND DONT'S

Do's

- Delegate as simply and directly as possible. Give precise instructions.
- Illustrate how each delegation applies to organizational goals.
- Mutually develop standards of performance.
- Clarify expected results.
- Anticipate what questions your employees may have and answer them in order.
- Discuss recurring problems.
- Seek out employee ideas on how to do the job.
- Accentuate the positive rather than the negative. Be supportive. Exhibit trust.
- Recognize superior performance.
- Keep your promises.

Dont's

- Do not threaten your staff. Effective delegation depends more on leadership skills that position power.
- Do not assume a condescending attitude.
- Do not just give answers. Show an employee how to and why.
- Do not overreact to problems.
- Refrain from criticizing an employee in front of others.
- Avoid excessive checks on progress.

From "Delegation: The Art of Managing," by Patrick J. Montana and Deborah F. Nash, copyright Oct. 1981. Reprinted with the permission of *Personnel Journal*, Costa Mesa, Calif.; all rights reserved.

what part of the organization's resources will be placed at their disposal. If a nutritionist is in charge of the Special Supplemental Feeding Program for Women, Infants and Children (WIC), the total responsibilities include administration of program and outcomes of patient care such as reduction in specific health problems such as anemia and underweight.

3. Motivate subordinates. The challenge of extra responsibility alone will not always encourage subordinates to accept and perform delegated tasks. Managers can motivate subordinates by remaining sensitive to their needs and goals.

4. Require complete work. The manager's job is to provide guidelines, help, and information to subordinates. Subordinates must do the actual delegated work.

5. Provide training. Managers need to teach subordinates how to improve their job performance.

6. Establish adequate controls. Managers should not spend all of their time checking on how well subordinates are doing. A reliable control system (such as weekly reports) should keep time spent in supervising to a minimum.

Barriers to effective delegation. Reluctance to delegate is a barrier to effective delegation. There are a number of reasons that managers commonly offer to explain why they do not delegate: "I can do it better myself"; "My subordinates are not capable." These reasons are often excuses that managers use to hide the real reasons they avoid delegation. Insecurity may be a major cause of reluctance to delegate. Managers are accountable for actions of their subordinates, and this may cause reluctance to take chances and delegate tasks. The manager may feel loss of power if a subordinate does too good a job. In addition, a manager may simply be too disorganized or inflexible to plan ahead and decide which tasks should be delegated to whom or to set up a control system so that subordinates' actions can be monitored. Lack of confidence in subordinates is a third reason managers avoid delegation. Managers who lack confidence in their subordinates—perhaps because of an inflated sense of their own worth—will severely limit their subordinates' freedom to act.

Decentralization

The delegation of authority by industrial managers is closely related to an organization's decentralization of authority. The concept of decentralization and centralization refers to the extent to which authority has been passed down to lower levels (decentralization) or has been retained at the top of the organization (centralization). The greater the amount of authority delegated throughout the organization, the more decentralized the organization is. For example, to the extent that lower-level managers can expend significant amounts for equipment or supplies without first checking with higher-level managers, the organization is more decentralized.

The appropriate amount of decentralization for an organization will vary with time and circumstances.

• • •

We have just discussed the basic elements and importance of organizing. To prepare the community dietitian/nutritionist to organize effectively in a realistic environment, managing organizational change, conflict, and creativity must be discussed before an action plan can be put into effect with any hope of achieving results.

ORGANIZING FOR CHANGING ENVIRONMENTS

What the "best" type of organizational structure is for a given situation has long been an important question for managers in all types of organizations. In this section we will deal with how organizations can be designed so that they "fit" with the environment in which they operate.

Early Approaches to Organizational Design

Classical management writers tried to find the one best way of designing an organization. They tended to favor a bureaucratic, hierarchical structure based on legalized, formal authority and characterized by task specialization. However, such a structure is relatively inflexible and neglects the human and environmental factors that can affect the organization.

Neoclassicists tried to improve the classical model. McGregor (1967) suggested that organization structure based on Theory Y values and Theory X would increase both the productivity and the satisfaction of organization members. Theory Y values include organizations based on assumptions that managers would meet human needs of their members and utilize their potential. Theory X implies that most people have little ambition, desire security above all, and will avoid work. Argyris (1964) argued that there was a need for a more informal organizational design that would give members greater independence and power. Likert and Likert (1976) favored what they called a "system 4" organization structure. It espouses the principle of supportive relationships using group decision making when appropriate and setting high performance goals.

Contingency Approaches to Organizational Design

Contingency approaches to organizational design stress the need to fit an organization's structure to its strategy, technology, environment, and people.

In selecting a strategy and the structure to implement it, managers must consider how the external environment will affect the organization. The relationship between strategy, structure, and environment can be viewed from two major perspectives. In the first perspective the organization is *reactive* to its environment. The strategy formulation process must consider the environment in which the organization operates currently and will be operating in the future. In the second perspective the organization is *proactive* because the strategy formulation process involves choosing the area or markets in which the organization will operate in the long run. Most organizations cannot control the external environment and therefore must adjust to it. However, through their strategies, they can and do choose those parts of the external environment with which they will interact the most and which therefore will exert the most influence such as a product market in a particular part of the country. An organization's strategy will be influenced by the opportunities and threats in its external environment; the goals, values and beliefs of its members and its strengths and weaknesses.

MANAGING ORGANIZATIONAL CHANGE

This section will focus on systematic programs to bring about planned change in organizations and their subunits. Managers are confronted with a somewhat paradoxical situation. On the one hand, they must be responsive to demands for change in work environments. They must anticipate changes, and, viewing their accountability broadly, they must exercise leadership in bringing changes to the organizations they manage. Managers must be "change seekers" and "change agents" (Albanese, 1978). On the other hand, managers must respond to the demands of stability in work environments. Thus managers are "stability seekers" and "stability agents." The paradox is a need for balance. Managers must

create and maintain work environments that balance the demands of both stability and change. Nevertheless, organizational change is bound to occur, given the variety of forces for change that exists both within and outside an organization. The major change in funding nutrition and public health programs from categorical to block grants provided a new way to look at programs in total and also imposed a competitive element in seeking funds for nutrition services. There are two constructive ways that managers can deal with change: *react to it* or *plan for it*. The former is appropriate for the day-to-day decisions a manager must make. The latter approach is necessary when a major part or all of the organization needs to change.

The change agent is the individual who is responsible for taking a leadership role in managing the process of change. Change agents can be

Table 4-1. Methods for dealing with resistance to change

Approach	Commonly Used When	Advantages	Disadvantages
Education + communication	There is a lack of information or inaccurate information and analysis.	Once persuaded, people will often help implement the change.	Can be very time-consuming if many people are involved.
Participation + involvement	The initiators do not have all the information they need to design the change, and others have considerable power to resist.	People who participate will be committed to implementing change, and any relevant information they have will be integrated into the change plan.	Can be very time-consuming if participators design an inappropriate change.
Facilitation + support	People are resisting because of adjustment problems.	No other approach works as well with adjustment problems.	Can be time-consuming, expensive, and still fail.
Negotiation + agreement	Some person or group with considerable power to resist will clearly lose out in a change.	Sometimes it is a relatively easy way to avoid major resistance.	Can be too expensive if it alerts others to negotiate for compliance.
Manipulation + co-optation	Other tactics will not work or are too expensive.	It can be a relatively quick and inexpensive solution to resistance problems.	Can lead to future problems if people feel manipulated.
Explicit + implicit coercion	Speed is essential, and the change initiators possess considerable power.	It is speedy and can overcome any kind of resistance.	Can be risky if it leaves people angry with the initiators.

members of the organization, or they can be consultants brought in from the outside.

Overcoming Resistance to Change

Kotter and Schlesinger (1979) offer six, highly situation-dependent, ways of overcoming resistance to change (Table 4-1).

Education and Communication

One of the most obvious ways to overcome resistance to change is to inform people about the planned change and the need for it early in the process. If the need for and logic of the change are explained—whether individually to subordinates, to groups in meetings, or to entire organizations through elaborate audiovisual education campaigns—the road to successful change may be smoother.

Participation and Involvement

If potential resisters are drawn into the actual design and implementation of the change, it may be better prepared and easier to effect.

Facilitation and Support

Easing the change process and providing support for those caught up in it is another way managers can deal with resistance. Implementing retraining programs, allowing time off after a difficult period, and offering emotional support and understanding may help.

Negotiation and Agreement

Another technique is negotiation with avowed or potential resisters. Examples include initiating union agreements, increasing an employee's pension benefits in exchange for his or her early retirement, or obtaining written letters of understanding from the heads of organization subunits that would be affected by the change.

Manipulation and Co-Option

Sometimes managers covertly steer individuals or groups away from resistance to change. They may manipulate workers by releasing information selectively or by consciously structuring the sequence of events. They may co-opt an individual, perhaps a key person within a group, by giving him or her a desirable role in designing or carrying out the change process. Aside from the doubtful ethics of such a technique, this approach may backfire.

Explicit and Implicit Coercion

Managers may force people to go along with a change by explicit or implicit threats involving loss of jobs, lack of promotion, and the like. Managers also dismiss or transfer employees who stand in the way of change. As with manipulation and co-option, such methods, although not uncommon, are risky and make it more difficult to gain support for future change efforts.

• • •

Overcoming resistance to change will involve using more than one of these six approaches. Which techniques to employ and how to translate them into effective actions will depend on the specifics of the situation.

MANAGING ORGANIZATIONAL CONFLICT AND CREATIVITY

Before the action plan can be developed, two additional issues must be considered: conflict and creativity. In this section we will discuss how conflict can be managed effectively in organizations and how innovation and creativity can be encouraged. As we discuss conflict and creativity, you will see that the two are often connected. Too much or too little conflict can inhibit creativity. Poorly managed conflict can do the same. However, when conflict is well managed, problems can be resolved effectively, and the solutions are more likely to be fresh and innovative.

Conflict, Competition, and Cooperation

The subject of *conflict* has been confused by different definitions and conceptions of the term (Schmidt and Kochan, 1972). We will define conflict in a way that allows us to discuss the constructive, functional aspects of organizational conflict.

Table 4-2. Old and current views of conflict

Old View	Current View
Conflict is avoidable.	Conflict is inevitable.
Conflict is caused by management errors in designing and managing organizations or by troublemakers.	Conflict arises from many causes, including organizational structure, unavoidable differences in goals, differences in perceptions and values of specialized personnel, and so on.
Conflict disrupts the organization and prevents optimal performance.	Conflict contributes to and detracts from organizational performance in varying degrees.
The task of management is to eliminate conflict.	The task of management is to manage the level of conflict and its resolution for optimal organizational performance.
Optimal organizational performance requires the removal of conflict.	Optimal organizational performance requires a moderate level of conflict.

From James A.F. Stoner, Management, ed. 2, © 1982, pp. 408, 593. Reprinted by permission of Prentice-Hall, Inc., Englewood Cliffs, N.J.

Organizational conflict is a disagreement between two or more organization members or groups arising from the fact that they must share scarce resources or work activities and/or from the fact that they have different status, goals, values, or perceptions. Organization members or subunits in disagreement attempt to have their own cause or point of view prevail over that of others.

One of the many semantic difficulties relating to organizational conflict is the distinction between conflict and competition. We distinguish between these concepts on the basis of whether one party is able to keep the other from attaining its goals. *Competition* exists when the goals of the parties involved are incompatible but the parties cannot interfere with each other. For example, two groups may compete with each other to be the first to meet a quota. (Obviously, both teams cannot come in first). If there is no opportunity to interfere with the other party's goal attainment, a competitive situation exists; however, if the opportunity for interference exists, and if that opportunity is acted on, then the situation is one of conflict.

Cooperation occurs when two or more parties work together to achieve mutual goals. Nutrition councils in many states foster the concept of cooperation to meet nutritional needs of their populations. It is possible for conflict and cooperation to coexist. The opposite of cooperation is not conflict, but lack of cooperation. For example, two parties may agree on goals but disagree strongly on how to attain these goals. When we speak of managing conflict, we mean that managers should try to find ways to balance conflict and cooperation.

Changing Views of Conflict

Views of conflict have changed in the last three decades. In the traditional view all conflict is seen as a harmful result of the failure to apply management principles. The current view is that conflict is not only inevitable but sometimes even necessary for the organization to survive. Conflict can often lead to a search for solutions; thus it is often an instrument of organizational innovation and change (Table 4-2). From this perspective, the task of managers is not to suppress or resolve all conflict but to manage it so as to minimize its harmful aspects and maximize its beneficial aspects. A manager also has ample opportunity in an organization to negotiate. When managers or individuals are in tense situations, having the perception that all parties can win if they negotiate allows the parties to manage the delicate conflicting issues (Kasten, 1984).

Types of Conflict

There are five types of conflict possible in organizational life. Conflict between groups in the same organization, conflict between individuals and groups, conflicts within and between individuals, and conflicts between organizations.

Conflict between individuals in the same organization is often attributed to personality differences. More often, such conflicts erupt from role-related pressures (between managers and subordinates) or from the manner in which people personalize conflict between groups ("Your people are always dumping extra work on mine").

Conflict between individuals and groups is commonly related to the way individuals deal with the pressures for conformity imposed on them by their work group. For example, an individual may be punished by his or her work group for exceeding or falling behind the group's productivity norms.

Conflict between organizations has been considered an inherent and desirable form of conflict in the economic systems of the United States and many other countries, at least if the conflict is restricted to economic competition. Such conflict has led to the development of new products, technologies, and services; lower prices; and more efficient use of resources. Government laws and regulatory agencies attempt to promote functional conflict (through antitrust legislation, for example) and manage the dysfunctional aspects of such conflict, such as false advertising.

Sources of Organizational Conflict

The sources of organizational conflict discussed here are related most clearly to intergroup conflict. However, they also apply to some extent to conflict between individuals and between individuals and groups. The major sources of organizational conflict include the need to share scarce resources, differences in goals between organization units, interdependence of work activities in the organization, and differences in values or perceptions among organization units. With the block grant concept of funding, nutrition programs may be competing against environmental services for the same funds; this competition can cause intergroup conflicts.

Some people enjoy conflict, debate, and argument; when controlled, mild discord can stimulate organization members and improve their performance. Some individuals, however, manage to escalate their conflicts, debates, and arguments into full-scale battles. People who are highly authoritarian, for example, or low in self-esteem may frequently anger their colleagues by overreacting to mild disagreements. In general, the potential for intergroup conflict is highest when group members differ markedly in such characteristics as work attitudes, age, and education.

In addition to conflicts created by erratic individuals, intergroup conflict can also result from ambiguously defined work responsibilities and unclear goals. One manager may try to expand the role of his or her subunit; this effort will usually stimulate other managers to "defend their turf." Also, if members of different groups know little about each other's jobs, they may unwittingly make unreasonable demands on each other. These demands may in turn trigger conflict. Ambiguous communications can also cause intergroup conflict, such as when the same phrase has different meanings for different groups.

Managing Professionals

Lebell (1980) labels the managing of professionals as "the quiet conflict." He states that in the interactions between management and employee professionals may reflect undercurrents of disagreement, animosity, and distrust. Unfortunately, such evidence of pervasive, unresolved conflict is seldom recognized or dealt with as such. Differing values and conceptual models may be at the root of the problem. The professional values independence for both self and subordinates (for self-image, creativity, and efficiency), whereas the manager values control and predictability (for self-image and productivity). Management is concerned with coordinating many disciplines for results. The professional seeks an enclave of professionalism to shelter and further a process. The accurate identification of conflict sources will often point the way to appropriate remedies. If these sources of conflict are understood and accepted, it can help eliminate unwanted conflict and/or mitigate its undesirable effects:

- Both manager and employee-professional should recognize the scope of functions and contributions the agency requires.
- Whether an employee is a professional or craftsman, his or her services do not inevitably increase in value each year. Ignoring this economic reality is often the basis of misunderstanding and unnecessary conflict.
- Professionals must perceive and project a realistic picture of what they can accomplish.
- Professionals must further understand that they cannot realistically expect to have all their psychological needs satisfied nor have all their professionally related values and attitudes accepted.

Conflict Resolution Methods

The three conflict resolution methods most commonly used are dominance and suppression, compromise, and integrative problem solving. These methods differ in the extent to which they yield effective and creative solutions to conflict and in the extent to which they leave parties in the conflict able to deal with future conflicts (Stoner, 1982).

Dominance and suppression. Dominance and suppression methods usually have two things in common: (1) they repress conflict, rather than settle it, and force it not to surface in a discussion; and (2) they create a win-lose situation in which the loser, forced to give way to higher authority or greater power, usually winds up disappointed and hostile. Suppression and dominance is manifested in the following ways:

1. *Forcing.* When the person in authority says, in effect, "Cut it out—I'm the boss and you've got to do it my way," argument is effectively snuffed out. Such autocratic suppression may lead to indirect but nonetheless destructive expressions of conflict.
2. *Smoothing.* In smoothing, a more diplomatic way of suppressing conflict, the manager minimizes the extent and importance of the disagreement and tries to talk

one side into giving in. When the manager has more information than the other parties and makes a reasonable suggestion, this method can be effective. However, if the manager is seen as favoring one side or failing to understand the issue, the losing side may feel resentful.

3. *Avoidance.* If quarreling groups come to a manager for a decision but the manager avoids taking a position, no one will be satisfied. Pretending to be unaware that conflict exists is a frequent form of avoidance. Another form is refusal to deal with conflict by stalling and repeatedly postponing action "until more information is available."
4. *Majority rule.* Trying to resolve group conflict by a majority vote can be effective if members regard the procedure as fair. However, if one voting bloc consistently outvotes the other, the losing side will feel powerless and frustrated.

Compromise. Through compromise, managers try to resolve conflict by finding a middle ground between two or more positions. The essence of a workable compromise is that each party achieves some of its objectives and sacrifices others. Decisions reached by compromise are not likely to leave conflicting parties feeling frustrated or hostile. From an organizational point of view, however, compromise is a weak conflict resolution method because it does not usually lead to a solution that can best help the organization achieve its goals. Instead, the solution reached will simply be one that both parties in the conflict can live with (Shea, 1980).

Integrative problem solving. With integrative problem solving, intergroup conflict is converted into a joint problem-solving situation. Together, parties to the conflict try to resolve the problem that has arisen between them. Instead of suppressing conflict or trying to find a compromise, the parties openly try to find a solution they all can accept. Managers who give subordinates the feeling that all members and groups are working together for a common goal, who encourage the free exchange of ideas, and who stress the benefits of finding the optimum solution to a conflict are more likely to achieve integrative solutions.

Organizational Creativity

Just as conflict must be managed to work toward the action plan, so must creativity be considered.

Creativity has become an important part of organizational life. When functional conflict is well managed, the organization is able to find new and better ways—and more creative ways—of accomplishing work. In this age of tough competition, resource scarcity, and high labor and equipment costs, anything that leads to more efficient and effective operations increases an organization's chances of survival and success. Creativity also enables the organization to anticipate change, which has become very important as new technologies, services, and methods of operation make old ones obsolete. By bringing in imaginative visual aids and introducing group problem-solving techniques, the community dietitian/nutritionist may demonstrate great creativity in stressing to groups the importance of nutrition.

Stimulating Individual and Group Creativity

The methods of stimulating creativity discussed here—brainstorming, nominal group process, and creative decision making—are designed to be used in groups. However, the principles that underlie these methods can also help individuals improve their creativity.

Brainstorming. Brainstorming encourages the free flow of ideas without inhibition by prejudgment or criticism. Group members are assembled, presented with the problem, and urged to produce as many ideas or solutions as they can. No evaluation is permitted. Quantity is preferred to quality, and rapid-fire contributions are sought. Even impractical suggestions are well received and recorded, since they may stimulate more useful recommendations.

A comparison was done of the effectiveness of groups and individuals who used the brainstorming technique (Stoner, 1982). (In individual brainstorming the individual produces ideas without criticizing or evaluating them.) It was found that individuals working alone usually developed more and better ideas than the same number of people working together in a group. Despite the free atmosphere of brainstorming sessions, group members still inhibit one another's creativity and thus limit the range of ideas that are produced.

However, brainstorming group sessions, as opposed to individual sessions, are still used in organizations, possibly because managers are unaware of studies citing the negative aspects of this method. It may also be easier for managers to arrange group sessions, which generally are stimulating for the participants, than to induce individuals to brainstorm on their own.

Nominal group process. An extension and modification of the brainstorming approach, the nominal group process removes the vocal interaction that may inhibit some individuals. Group members work alone but in the same room, developing ideas. They then share their lists of ideas, one item at a time, round robin. This approach appears to yield more ideas than brainstorming yet keeps some of the advantages of that technique (Delbecq and Vandeven, 1971).

Creative group decision making. Creative group decision making is appropriate when there is no apparent or agreed-on method of solving a problem. According to Delbecq and Vandeven, creative decision-making groups should be composed of competent personnel from a variety of backgrounds and should be directed by a leader who can stimulate creative behavior. The group problem-solving process is somewhat akin to brainstorming in that discussion is spontaneous, all group members participate, and the evaluation of ideas is suspended at the beginning of the session so as not to discourage suggestions. Whereas brainstorming avoids decision making, reaching a decision is the aim of the creative decision-making group. The creativity of group members is fostered by a permissive atmosphere in which originality, unusual ideas, and even eccentricity are encouraged (Steiner, 1965) (Table 4-3).

Table 4-3. Characteristics of the creative individual and organization

The Creative Individual	The Creative Organization
Conceptual fluency . . . is able to produce a large number of ideas quickly	Has idea people Opens channels of communication Ad hoc devices: suggestion systems, brainstorming: idea units absolved of other responsibilities Encourages contact with outside sources
Originality . . . generates unusual ideas	Heterogeneous personnel policy Includes marginal, unusual types Assigns nonspecialists to problems Allows eccentricity
Separates source from content in evaluating information . . . is motivated by interest in problem . . . follows wherever it leads	Has an objective, fact-founded approach Ideas evaluated on their merits, not status of originator Ad hoc approaches: anonymous communications; blind votes Selects and promotes on merit only
Suspends judgment . . . avoids early commitment . . . spends more time in analysis, exploration	Lack of financial, material commitment to products, policies Invests in basic research; flexible, long-range planning Experiments with new ideas rather than prejudging on "rational" grounds; everything gets a chance
Less authoritarian . . . has relativistic view of life	More decentralized; diversified Administrative slack; time and resources to absorb errors Risk-taking ethos . . . tolerates and expects taking changes
Accepts own impulses . . . playful, undisciplined exploration	Not run as "tight ship" Employees have fun Allows freedom to choose and pursue problems Freedom to discuss ideas
Independent judgment, less conformity	Organizationally autonomous
Deviant, sees self as different	Original and different objectives, not trying to be another "X"
Rich, "bizarre" fantasy life and superior reality orientation	Security of routine . . . *allows* innovation . . ."Philistines" provide stable, secure environment that allows "creators" to roam Has separate units or occasions for generating vs. evaluating ideas . . . separates creative from productive functions

Adapted from *The Creative Organization*, edited by Gary A. Steiner, by permission of The University of Chicago Press © 1965 by The University of Chicago. All rights reserved. In James A.F. Stoner, Management, ed. 2, © 1982, pp. 408, 593. Reprinted by permission of Prentice-Hall, Inc., Englewood Cliffs, N.J.

ORGANIZING FOR ACTION IN NUTRITION SERVICES

To operationalize the conceptual, theoretical, and environmental approaches to organizing, we will now discuss the use of a marketing approach to segment clients and target markets. A marketing approach will be used to develop the action plan, to implement activities, and to achieve the stated objective. An action plan is a step-by-step process delineated to reach the stated outcome.

Marketing

Marketing is a subject of growing interest to not-for-profit organizations, both public and private. Hospitals, colleges, religious organizations, social service organizations, health departments, and other not-for-profit organizations have been experiencing increasing problems in the marketplace: declining numbers of customers and dwindling contributions. Marketing appears to be the management function that offers these organizations hope. Hoover (1983) recently stated that the profession of dietetics needs marketing sophistication. She stated that nutritionists' view that marketing is only advertising or consumer manipulation has probably limited their effectiveness in presenting their product, nutrition. Entrepreneurs have demonstrated that the public wants dietetic services and that such services can be marketed successfully. In a hospital the dietetic service is one of the few services that a patient and family feel qualified to evaluate. The relative importance of a patient's favorable perception of a dietetic service gains new significance if competition with other hospitals is used as one of the mechanisms for cost containment. In these turbulent times not-for-profit organizations strongly depend on the marketplace. Consider the following example. The nation's 7000 hospitals are currently filling only 60% of their beds, down from the rate of 80% in the early 1970s. Fewer patients are being admitted, and their length of hospital stay is falling. Departments such as maternity and pediatrics are especially hard hit because of the falling birthrate. Meanwhile, hospital costs are soaring as a result of rising minimum wages and energy costs. Some

experts have predicted that 100 to 150 hospitals will close in the next 10 years (Kotler, 1982).

Thus, as shown from the data just mentioned, hospitals are experiencing marketing problems. These organizations are confronting changing client attitudes and societal needs, increasing public-private competition, and diminishing financial resources. Board members, public authorities, and citizen groups are questioning administrators of not-for-profit organizations about their organization's mission, opportunities, and strategies. One result is that these administrators are forced to take a hard look at marketing to see what this discipline might offer to keep their organization viable and reliant.

Parks (1984) recently described the application of the marketing process to an extended-degree dietetic program that serves a national audience. The marketing approach was used because dietetic education programs seeking to maintain their enrollment levels find it necessary to adopt more sophisticated marketing strategies. As part of the process, Parks also presented a strategy for initiating a marketing study and marketing orientation by analyzing internal program data. Because using marketing strategies for an educational program is a relatively new concept in dietetics, the model developed by Parks has more extensive implications for dietitians in business health care facilities than for those in private practice.

In this chapter marketing will be discussed in the context of not-for-profit organizations, since most health care providers, specifically community dietitians/nutritionists, are employed in not-for-profit (both public and private) organizations. Although the basic tenets are the same, strategies are different for profit and not-for-profit organizations. (See Kotler [1982] for an excellent treatment of this subject.)

What Is Marketing?

Marketing is the analysis, planning, implementation, and control of carefully formulated programs designed to achieve organizational objectives. It is process similar to program planning, which is used in health services (Chapter 3).

Several things should be noted about this definition of marketing:

1. Marketing is defined as managerial process involving analysis, planning, implementation, and control.
2. Marketing manifests itself in carefully formulated programs, not just random actions to achieve desired results. Marketing takes place before any selling occurs.
3. Marketing seeks to bring about voluntary exchange of values. The marketer seeks to formulate enough benefits for the target market of sufficient attractiveness to produce a voluntary exchange.
4. Marketing is the selection of target markets rather than a quixotic attempt to serve every market and be all things to all people. Marketers routinely distinguish between possible market segments and decide which ones to secure.
5. The purpose of marketing is to help organizations ensure survival and continued health through serving their markets more effectively. In the business sector the major objective is profit making, whereas in the nonbusiness sector other objectives prevail; for example, the county health department wants to improve the level and distribution of health services. Effective marketing entails very specific objectives.
6. Marketing relies on designing the organization's product in terms of the target market's needs and desires rather than in terms of the seller's personal tastes. Local governments that design playgrounds or toll roads without studying public attitudes often find the subsequent level of public usage disappointing. Effective marketing is user oriented, not seller oriented.
7. Marketing utilizes and blends a set of tools called the *marketing mix*—product design, pricing, communication, and distribution.

Not-for-Profit Organization Marketing

Marketing in the not-for-profit sector involves the same marketing principles as for profit marketing; however, the not-for-profit sector offers new and challenging settings for the application of these principles. Four major characteristics of the not-for-profit organization call for special attention in the application of marketing principles:

1. *Multiple publics.* Not-for-profit organizations normally have at least two major publics to work with: their clients and their funders. The former group poses the problem of resource allocation and the latter, the problem of resource attraction. In addition, many other publics surround not-for-profit organizations and call for marketing programs. Business organizations also deal with a multitude of publics, but their tendency is to concentrate their marketing efforts on their customers.
2. *Multiple objectives.* Not-for-profit organizations tend to pursue several important objectives simultaneously rather than only one, such as profits. As a result, strategies are more difficult to formulate. A choice must be made among alternative strategies.
3. *Services versus physical goods.* Not-for-profit organizations produce services rather than goods. Services have the characteristics of being intangible, inseparable, variable, and perceivable.
4. *Public scrutiny.* Not-for-profit organizations are usually subject to close public scrutiny because they provide needed public services, are subsidized, are tax exempt, and in many cases are mandated into existence. They experience political pressures from various publics and are expected to operate in the public interest.

What Are the Characteristics of an Effective Marketing Organization?

With a marketing orientation, the main task of the organization is to determine the needs and wants of target markets and to satisfy them through the design, communication, pricing, and delivery of appropriate and competitive viable services. The organization's effectiveness is re-

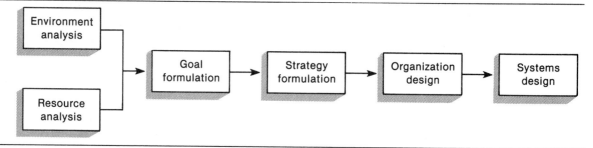

Figure 4-3. Strategic market planning process.
Redrawn from Philip Kotler, Marketing for Nonprofit Organizations, © 1982, pp. 84, 174.
Reprinted by permission of Prentice-Hall, Inc., Englewood Cliffs, N.J.

flected in the degree to which it exhibits five major attributes of a marketing orientation:

1. *Customer philosophy.* Does management acknowledge the primacy of the marketplace and of customer needs and wants in shaping the organization's plans and operation?
2. *Integrated marketing organizations.* Is the organization staffed to carry out marketing analysis, planning, implementation, and control?
3. *Adequate marketing information.* Does management receive the kind and quality of information needed to conduct effective marketing?
4. *Strategic orientation.* Does management generate innovate strategies and plans for achieving its long-run objectives?
5. *Operational efficiency.* Are marketing activities selected and handled in a cost-effective manner?

Organizations that move toward a marketing orientation take on these characteristics vital to their survival and effectiveness. They become more responsive, adaptive, and entrepreneurial.

Strategic Market Planning Process

As discussed in Chapter 2, organizations that want to be adaptive are increasingly turning to strategic planning as the major systematic theory for adapting to change. Marketers define strategic and market planning as the managerial process of developing and maintaining a strategic fit between the organization's goals and resources and its changing marketing opportunities (Kotler, 1982). Figure 4-3 describes the strategic market planning process. We will briefly examine each of the marketing steps.

Environment analysis. The first step is to analyze the environment in which the organization operates, trying to identify the leading trends and their implications for the organization. If the organization is going to adapt, it must determine what to adapt to. Major components of the organization's environment include the following:

1. Internal environment consists of internal publics, board of directors, management staff, and volunteers. The task is to examine the needs, wants, and interests.
2. Market environment consists of other groups and other organizations that the focal organization must monitor trends and changes in the needs, perceptions, preferences, and satisfactions of these key groups.
3. Public environment consists of groups and organizations that take an interest in the work of the focal organization. This environment consists of local publics, media publics, and regulatory agencies whose actions can affect the welfare of the focal organization.

4. Competitive environment consists of groups that compete for attention and publicity from the audiences of the focal organization.
5. Macroenvironment consists of large-scale fundamental forces that shape opportunities and pose threats to the focal organization. The main macroenvironments are demographic, economic, technical, political, and social forces.

The environment analysis is similar to the needs assessment or identifying the problem in the program planning model described in Chapter 3.

Resource analysis. Following the environmental analysis, management should undertake an analysis of its resources and capabilities. The purpose is to identify the major resources that the organization has (its strengths) and lacks (its weaknesses). The organization should pay attention to its distinctive competencies—those resources and abilities which the organization is especially strong in.

Goal formulation. The environment and resource analyses are designed to provide the necessary background and stimulus for management to think about the basic goals of the organization. For every type of institution there is always a potential set of relevant objectives, and the institution makes a choice among them (Chapter 3).

Strategy formulation. Strategy formulation calls for the organization to develop a strategy for seeking its goal. In seeking feasible strategies, the organization should proceed in two stages. First, it should develop a service portfolio strategy, that is, decide what to do with each of its current major services. Second, it should develop a service/market expansion strategy, that is, decide what new services and markets to add. For example, a new service for a hospital and the department of dietetics may be an outpatient clinic with nutrition and exercise as the main focus of a life-style program. New markets would be the persons in the community who are intent on losing weight and exercising.

Organization design. The purpose of strategy formulation is to develop actions that will help the organization achieve its goals in the new environment. The existing organization must be capable of carrying out these strategies. It must have structure, people, and values to implement the strategy successfully.

Systems design. The final step is to install the systems that the organization needs to develop and carry out the strategies that will achieve its goals in the new environment. The three principal systems follow:

1. *Marketing Information System.* The job of effectively running an organization calls for continuous information about customers, marketing intermediaries, suppliers, competitors, publics, and macroenvironment forces. This information can be obtained through sales analysis, marketing intelligence, and marketing research. To be of use, the information must be accurate, timely, and comprehensive.
2. *Marketing Planning System.* Information to be effectively used should be incorporated in a modern planning system. A planning discipline is important if the organization hopes to achieve optimum results in the marketplace. The marketplace planning and control system is described in Figure 4-4.
3. *Marketing Control System.* Plans must be implemented and monitored. The purpose of the marketing control system is to measure the ongoing results of a plan against the plan's goals and to take corrective action before it is too late (Figure 4-4).

Marketing Strategy

Strategic market planning indicates the particular product markets that represent the organization's best opportunities. The organization must develop a marketing strategy for succeeding in each product market. Marketing strategy is the selection of a target market(s), the choice of a competitive position, and the development of effective marketing mix to reach and serve the chosen customers. Marketing mix consists of a particular blend of product, services, price,

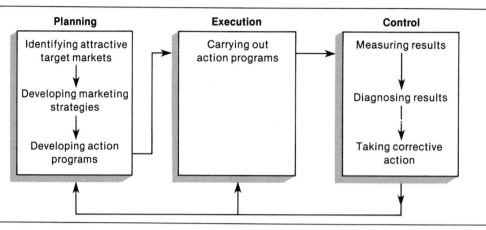

Figure 4-4. The marketing planning and control system.
Redrawn from Philip Kotler, Marketing for Nonprofit Organizations, © 1982, pp. 84, 174.
Reprinted by permission of Prentice-Hall, Inc., Englewood Cliffs, N.J.

place, and promotion that the organization uses to achieve its objectives in the target market.

Social Marketing

The term *social marketing* was first introduced in 1971 to describe the use of marketing principles and techniques to advance a social cause, idea, or behavior (such as a smoking cessation program) (Fox and Kotler, 1980). Social marketing is the design, implementation, and control of programs that seek to increase the acceptability of a social idea or cause in a target program. It relies on concepts of market segmentation, conscience research, concept development, communication, facilitation, incentives, and exchange theory to maximize target group response. Social marketing is also called social cause marketing or public issue marketing.

The effectiveness of social marketing varies with the type of social change sought. Cognitive change is the most responsive to social marketing. Social marketing may also be effective in producing action change, that is, a particular act. Behavioral change, such as the modification of food, smoking, or drinking habits, is harder to achieve. Value change, that is, efforts to modify the value orientation of a target market, is also difficult to effect.

Bloom and Novelli (1983) identify a set of general problems that confront practitioners who attempt to transfer marketing approaches used to sell toothpaste and soap to promote concepts such as smoking cessation, safe driving, and weight control. The problems discussed are identified in the following decision-making areas: market analysis, market segmentation, product strategy, product strategy development, pricing strategy development, channel strategy development, communication strategy development, organizational design, planning, and evaluation. An awareness of these decision-making areas should allow social agency managers to formulate more workable and effective marketing programs.

The process. The social marketing process consists of the following steps: (1) problem definition, (2) goal setting, (3) target market segmentation, (4) concise analysis, (5) influence channel analysis, (6) marketing strategies and tactics, and (7) implementation and evaluation.

A social marketing approach does not guarantee that the social objectives will be achieved or that the costs will be acceptable, but it does represent a more precise way of looking at social objectives. However, social marketing appears to represent a bridging mechanism that links the

A SOCIAL MARKETING PLAN FOR EVERYWHERESVILLE: A START!

Step 1 *Problem Definition*

A. *Environment Analysis*

(The needs assessment completed in Chapter 3 presents most of the information required for the environment analysis.) Everywheresville has a serious problem with cardiovascular disease risk.

B. *Resource Analysis*

The health department in Everywheresville has no funds to complete a cardiovascular disease risk program. Therefore funds must be sought from other sources.

Step 2 *Goal Setting*

The goal might be to develop a pilot cardiovascular disease risk factor program in the southern part of Everywheresville (middle to upper income) by seeking funds from four community organizations in that area—the Heart Association, the American Association of University Women, the grocery chain organization, and the local newspaper—within 6 months.

Step 3 *Target Market Segmentation*

The southern part of Everywheresville has a population of middle- and upper-income groups who have been identified by the work site program at the engineering plant to be at high risk for cardiovascular disease.

Step 4 *Concise Analysis*

Of the 500 employees at the engineering plant, 200 will be targeted to participate in a pilot program. They will be selected on the basis of their degree of risk. The employee mix will include executives, as well as middle management and salaried employees.

Step 5 *Influence Channel Analysis*

The top executives of the engineering corporation are concerned for their employees in terms of healthy lifestyles and in terms of years of productivity in the company. These executives have offered to assist the health department to obtain funds from the four sources listed and to provide additional funding for the project.

Step 6 *Marketing Strategies and Tactics*

To develop a services portfolio, a consultant has been enlisted from the director of public relations for a major organization in the community whose wife is a dietitian and is interested in programs for healthy lifestyles. The consultant has suggested that a task force, composed of members of the agencies and the corporation who donated funds, be developed to assist in completing the marketing plan, including strategies and tactics for this project.

Step 7 *Implementation and Evaluation*

To complete the implementation plan, a great deal of time and effort will be spent on developing a strong evaluation component to determine the outcome of this program. (See action plan for implementation, below, and evaluation, Chapter 7.) This cardiovascular disease risk factor pilot project has stimulated strong community support and involvement.

---

behavior around scientists' knowledge of human behavior with the socially useful implementation of what the knowledge allows. It may offer a useful framework for effective social planning at a time when social issues have become more relevant and critical (Kotler, 1982). We have developed a social marketing plan for Everywheresville in order to apply the concept (box above).

Completing the Action Plan

We have reviewed the various elements of organizing and have segmented the markets. Now we will discuss the development of the action plan.

Steps in the Action Plan

The action plan is a method of organizing that is familiar and useful to the community dietitian/nutritionist. It is a process that determines how each activity will be achieved. For the sake of clarity, an activity is defined as a specific procedure or process, completed at a certain point in time, that is carried out by organization personnel as part of a strategy for reaching the desired objective (Craig, 1978). (A *task* is a specific procedure or process that includes what will be done, when, and by whom.) In the design of the action plan, activities can be divided into five steps.

Step 1: Determine what major activities are needed and in what order they should occur. At this point you are starting with a strategy, a certain way of approaching the problem. What activities need to be done to carry out the strategy? Start by making a rough list of possible activities. Review your force field analysis of helping or hindering forces on p. 62.

SAMPLE STRATEGY. Form a task force composed of community leaders, corporation executives, and health department personnel to develop a plan for a pilot cardiovascular disease risk factor program at the engineering plant in Everywheresville.

A sample list of activities follows:
- Get members to serve on task force.
- Arrange meeting.
- Get task force agreement on general content of plan.
- Task force members get input from groups they represent.
- Get letters of support from advocate groups.
- Distribute rough draft of plan to task force members.

Next you need to order these activities in sequence. One way to do this is to start at the end and think backward, asking a series of questions: "If this is where I want to be, what do I have to do just before I get to this point?" and so on, back to the beginning.

Step 2: Determine a schedule for completing activities. Once activities have been identified, the next step is to set some general deadlines for completing each activity. At this step, you are beginning to assess how much time each stage will take in order to complete the entire process in the desired time. This process means two things:

1. Starting the activity in the form of the process to be completed by a certain point.
2. Placing the activities into a calendar form. This process will show you clearly when one or more activities have to be completed before the next activity can begin.

There are many techniques for scheduling activities. Two of the more common ones include the Gantt Scheduling and the Pert chart (Craig, 1978).

In Gantt Scheduling (Figure 4-5) a bar chart is used to reflect completion dates and activities. Horizontal dotted lines are drawn so their lengths are proportional to the planned duration of each activity. Progress on each activity is monitored by drawing solid lines parallel to and below the dotted lines to show actual duration for completed activities.

Activities are listed in the first column on the left. To use the Gantt technique, one works from left to right, plotting activities as they must occur and establishing a completion date for the job.

The Pert (Program Evaluation and Review Technique) chart is a more sophisticated technique, developed by the U.S. government for keeping track of submarines. This technique is used when it is necessary for many tasks to be accomplished in sequence and in the shortest possible time. It is a technique well suited to group planning, where cooperation is essential to completing many tasks by a deadline. For example, in a community health clinic many areas such as initial client information forms and health and nutrition assessments must be developed before the first client can be seen.

The Pert chart identifies activities, which culminate in events. Working backward from the final deadline, the time needed for each activity is calculated, and deadlines are scheduled for each event. By showing activities that can occur simultaneously and those which must occur in sequence, the chart reveals a critical path, which is the overall time needed to complete the project. An advantage of Pert charting is that it helps group members focus their energies on critical tasks and continually reevaluate the process to see if they are on schedule. A simple Pert chart is shown in Figure 4-6, with the critical path shown as a heavy line.

Step 3: Calculate the resources. Now that the major activities have been laid out in calendar form, it is possible to determine what resources will be needed to carry out the strategy. The primary things to consider are (1) how much

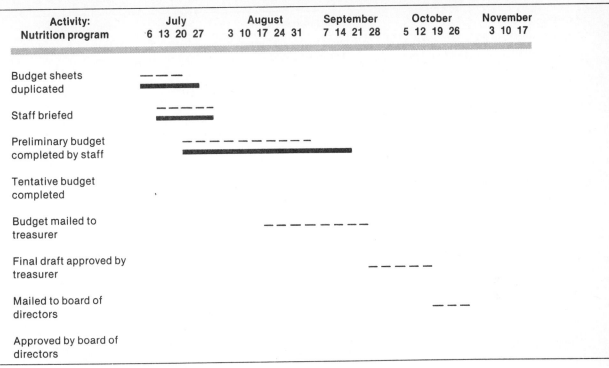

Figure 4-5. Gantt scheduling.
Redrawn from Craig, D.P.: HIP pocket guide to planning and evaluation, Learning Concepts, Inc.
Distributed by University Associates, San Diego, Calif.

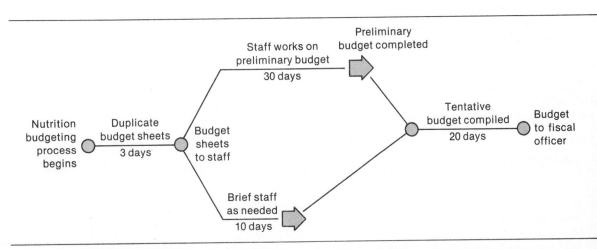

Figure 4-6. Pert chart.
Redrawn from Craig, D.P.: HIP pocket guide to planning and evaluation, Learning Concepts, Inc.
Distributed by University Associates, San Diego, Calif.

Activity	Who Is Responsible	Completion Date
1. Contact potential task force representative and obtain commitment to serve	Chief nutritionist assisted by senior PH nutritionist	February 1
2. Arrange meeting of task force	Senior nutritionist assisted by clerical staff	February 15
3. Identify interest and concern of employees, management, and advocate groups	Task force member: nutritionist (senior) responsible for management interests and concerns	May 1

staff will be needed and (2) what costs are involved. A general or detailed budget should be drawn up at this point.

STRATEGY. Form a task force composed of community leaders, corporation executives, and health department personnel to develop a plan for a pilot cardiovascular disease risk factor program at the engineering plant.

Sample Resources	Six-Month Budget (January to June)
Public health nutritionist (senior) at $20,000/yr plus 20% fringes 1/4 time for 6 mo	$3900
Shift nutritionist's routine tasks to public health nutritionist (1) at $18,000/yr plus 20% fringes 1/4 time for 6 mo	$3150
Clerical time at $4.50/hr average 10 hr/wk for 6 mo	$1170
Miscellaneous (supplies, printing, telephone, travel)	200
	$8420

Step 4: Assign responsibility to someone for each activity. After determining the costs involved and deciding to proceed with the strategy, the next step is to assign responsibility for each of the major activities. The person who is responsible will then proceed with even more detailed planning of how to do that activity.

In the sample strategy, responsibility might be divided as shown above.

Step 5: Plan what specific tasks will be done, who needs to be involved, when the tasks will occur, and what specific resources will be needed. Once major activities have been assigned, the responsible staff person proceeds to detail precisely what has to be done, by whom, how, and when. One way to do this is, again, to work backward from the desired end point. The worksheet below shows the detailed plan.

• • •

TASK PLANNING SHEET

Your strategy: Form task force to develop plan to get the children into health care delivery systems.
Your activity: Get agreement of members to serve on task force.

Tasks	Why	When	Who	Resources
1. List key groups and potential task force members	To make sure all possibilities are considered	January 5	Self	3 hours
2. Go over list with chief nutritionist and agree on whom to approach	Get director's perspective and approval	January 8	Self Chief nutritionist	2 hours
3. Send letters inviting task force members to participate	Official recognition	February 15	Self Clerical	4 hours

CHECKLIST FOR ACTION PLAN

- Flows naturally from problems and objectives
- Clearly describes program activities
- States reasons for selection of activities
- Describes sequence of activities
- Describes staffing of program
- Describes clients and client selection
- Presents a reasonable scope of activities that can be accomplished within the time allotted for the program and within the resources of the applicant

Because a large volume of material has been presented in this section, the checklist above should provide guidelines for pursuing an action plan that is results oriented.

SUMMARY

Organizing includes detailing all the work that must be completed to meet organizational goals, including delegation. In delegating assignments to employees, managers must have a clear understanding of what needs to be completed. It is the managers job to define the scope and responsibility of the work to be done.

Marketing is the planning, implementing, and control of programs designed to achieve organizational objectives. Action planning is the process that determines how each activity will be achieved. A program is organized by using the action plan to state specific activities that must be completed to achieve outcomes.

REFERENCES

Albanese, R.: Managing toward accountability for performance, Homewood, Ill., 1978, Richard D. Irwin, Inc.

Argyris, C.: Integrating the individual and the organization, New York, 1964, Wiley Publishing.

Bloom, P.N., and Novelli, W.D.: Problems and challenges in social marketing In Wendel, R., editor: Marketing 83/84, Guilford, Conn., 1983, Dushkin Publishing Group, Inc.

Craig, D.P.: HIP pocket guide to planning and evaluation, Austin, Tex., 1978, Learning Concepts.

Delbecq, A.L., and Vandeven, A.H.: A group model for problem identification and program planning, J. Applied Behavioral Science 7:4, July/Aug. 1971.

Fox, K.F.A., and Kotter, J.P.: The markets of social causes: the first ten years, J. Marketing, Fall 1980.

Hackman, J.R., and Lawler, E.E.: Employee reactions to job characteristics, J. Applied Psychol. Management 55:269, 1971.

Haimann, T., Scott, W.G., and Connor, P.E.: Management, ed. 4, Boston, 1982, Houghton Mifflin Co.

Hoover, L.W.: Enhancing managerial effectiveness in dietetics, J. Am. Diet. Assoc. 82(1):58, 1983.

Kasten, B.R.: Negotiating in conflict situations, J. Am. Diet. Assoc. 84:1002, 1984.

Kotler, P.: Marketing for non-profit organizations, ed. 2, Englewood Cliffs, N.J., 1982, Prentice-Hall, Inc.

Kotter, J.P., and Schlesinger, L.A.: Choosing strategies for change, Harvard Bus. Rev. 57:2, March/April 1979.

Lagges, J.G.: The role of delegation in improving productivity, Personnel J., p. 776, Nov. 1979.

Lebell, D.: Managing professionals: the quiet conflict, Personnel J. 59:566, 1980.

Likert, R., and Likert, J.G.: New ways of managing conflict, New York, 1976, McGraw-Hill, Inc.

Litterer, J.A.: Organizations: structure and behavior, ed. 3, New York, 1980, John Wiley & Sons, Inc.

McGregor, D.: The professional manager, New York, 1967, McGraw-Hill, Inc.

Miles, R.H.: Macro organizational behavior, Santa Monica, Calif., 1980, Goodyear.

Montana, P.J., and Nash, D.F.: Delegation: the art of managing, Personnel J. 60:784, 1981.

Ouchi, W.G., and Dowling, J.B.: Defining the span of control, Administrative Sciences Q. 19:3, Sept. 1974.

Parks, S.C., Moody, D.L., and Barbrow, E.P.: The marketing concept applied to an educational program, J. Am. Diet. Assoc. 84:1031, 1984.

Scanlon, B.K., and Atherton, R.M.: Participation and the effective use of authority, Personnel J. 60:697, 1981.

Schmidt, S.M., and Kochan, T.A.: Conflict: toward conceptual clarity, Administrative Sciences Q. 17:3, Sept. 1972.

Shea, G.P.: The study of bargaining and conflict behavior: broadening the conceptual area, J. Conflict Resolution 24:4, Dec. 1980.

Steiner, G.A., editor: The creative organization, Chicago, 1965, The University of Chicago Press.

Stoner, J.A.F.: Management, ed. 2, Englewood Cliffs, N.J., 1982, Prentice-Hall, Inc.

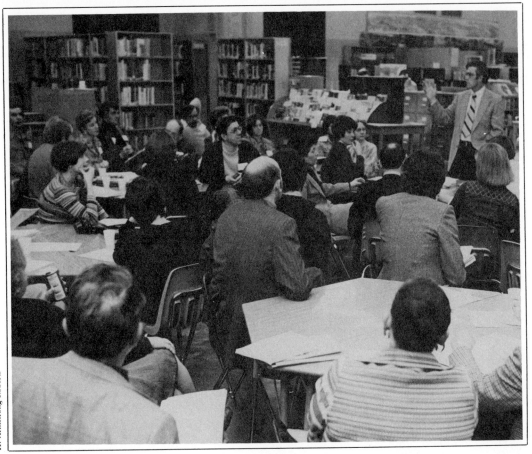

H. Armstrong Roberts

Leading to Achieve Individual and Organizational Goals

GENERAL CONCEPT

Leaders play a critical role in helping groups, organizations, or societies achieve their goals. Leadership abilities and skills in directing an organization are important factors in managers' effectiveness. To a large extent, a manager's leadership ability—that is, a manager's ability to motivate, influence, direct, and communicate with subordinates—will determine his or her effectiveness.

When you finish this chapter, you should be able to
- Identify and describe the theoretical approaches to motivation
- Define and explain the leadership process
- Describe major approaches to the study of leadership
- Distinguish between major leadership styles and determine the style most suitable to productivity
- Define communication and explain why it is important to managers
- Summarize the barriers to interpersonal and organizational communication and explain how they can be overcome

The old adage "Nothing succeeds like success" is not only serendipitous, but also it may have a scientific basis. Researchers studying motivation found that the prime factor in being successful is simply the self-perception among motivated subjects that they are doing well (Peters and Waterman, 1982). Managers in business or in a health care organization may be adept at planning for and organizing the human and physical resources at their command, but unless they can get people in the organization to do what must be done, they will not succeed. In the nutrition field, nutritionists' scientific knowledge may be up to date; however, if they cannot use this information to modify clients' behavior, when appropriate, then they are not successful. To a large extent, a manager's leadership ability—that is, a manager's ability to motivate, influence, direct, and communicate with subordinates—will determine the manager's effectiveness and ultimate success (Figure 5-1).

THE IMPORTANCE OF MOTIVATION

Motivation—that which causes, channels, and sustains people's behavior—has always been an important and perplexing subject for managers. Behavior is basically goal oriented. In other words, behavior is generally motivated by a desire to attain some goal. In nutrition the goal is to provide quality nutrition services to the populations served. The specific goal is not always consciously known by an individual. The drive that motivates distinctive individual behavioral patterns (personality) is to a considerable degree subconscious and therefore not easily susceptible to examination and evaluation (Hersey and Blanchard, 1982).

Many theories exist about what motivates people and why. The theories differ in what they implicitly suggest that managers do to obtain effective performance. In our discussion we will cover both old and new theoretical perspectives on motivation, focusing on current knowledge about motivation and its relationship to work behavior and satisfaction.

Motivation is not the only influence on a person's performance level. Two other factors involved are the individual's *abilities* and his or her understanding of what behavior is necessary to achieve high performance; this factor is called *role perception* (Stoner, 1982). Motivation, abilities, and role perception are interrelated.

MOTIVATION THEORIES

It is useful to review some of the major classifications of motivation theories, since each theoretical perspective will shed light on how motivation influences work performance. Distinctions are made on the basis of control theories, which focus on "the what" of motivation, and process theories, which focus on "the how" of motivation. Reinforcement theories, a third approach, emphasize the way in which behavior is learned.

Control Theories

The control approach is associated with such names as Maslow and McClelland. These men may be familiar, since they have strongly influenced the management field and have affected the thoughts and actions of practicing managers.

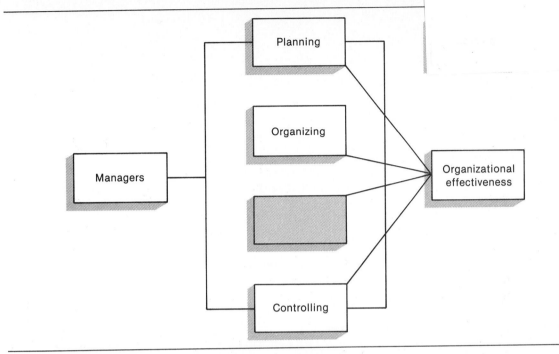

Figure 5-1. Management process.

Maslow's Hierarchy of Human Needs

Maslow (1964), a psychologist, formulated one of the most widely known theories of motivation. The first premise is that humans are wanting animals whose needs depend on what they already have. Only needs not yet satisfied can influence behavior; an adequately fulfilled need is not a motivator. The second premise is that human needs are arranged in a hierarchy of importance. Once a particular need is fulfilled, another "higher" need emerges and demands fulfillment. Maslow's five hierarchies include the following (Figure 5-2):

1. *Physiological needs.* This category consists of the basic survival needs for food, water, and so on.
2. *Safety and security needs.* Once the survival needs are met, attention can be turned to ensuring continued survival by protecting oneself against physical harm and deprivation.
3. *Affection and social activity needs.* This third level is related to the social and gregarious nature of humans. It is somewhat of a breaking point in the hierarchy because it deviates from the physical or quasi-physical needs of the first two levels. This level addresses people's need for association or companionship with others, for belonging to groups, and for giving and receiving friendship and affection.
4. *Esteem and status needs.* These are the needs for self-respect or self-esteem that come from an awareness of one's importance to others.
5. *Self-realization needs.* This highest level of human needs includes the need to achieve one's fullest potential. It exhibits itself in

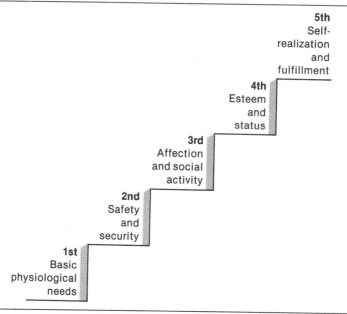

Figure 5-2. Hierarchy of human needs.
From Maslow, A.: Psychol. Rev. 50:4, July 1943. Redrawn from Rakich, J.S., Beaufort, B.L., and
O'Donovan, T.R.: Managing health care organizations, Philadelphia, 1977, W.B. Saunders Co.

the need to be creative and to have the opportunity for self-expression (Rakich, Longest, and Donovan, 1977).

McClelland

McClelland (1961) found that people with a high need for achievement have several characteristics of interest to managers:

1. They like to take responsibility for solving problems.
2. They tend to set moderately difficult goals for themselves and to take calculated risks.
3. They place great importance on concrete feedback on how well they are doing.

Process Theories (Integrating Models)

Rather than emphasizing the control of needs and the driving nature of these needs, the process approach emphasizes *how* and *by what goals* individuals are motivated. In this view needs are

just one element in the process by which individuals decide how to behave.

Basic to process theories of motivation is the notion of *expecting*, that is, what a person anticipates is likely to happen as a result of his or her behavior. For example, if a community dietitian/nutritionist expects that meeting deadlines, such as completing the nutrition budget on time, will earn praise from superiors and that not meeting deadlines will earn disapproval, then the person who prefers praise will be motivated to meet deadlines. Conversely, if a person expects that meeting deadlines will not earn praise, he or she may not be as motivated.

An additional factor in motivation is the *valence* or strength of an individual's preference for the expected outcome. For example, if an individual expects that exceeding case load (reaching more clients with nutrition services) will lead to promotion to supervisor, and if the individual strongly desires to be promoted, then he or she will be strongly motivated to exceed the expected case load.

Expectancy Model: Implications for Managers and Organizations

The expectancy model presents managers with a number of guidelines for motivating subordinates. The following should be considered: (1) determine reward values of each subordinate; (2) determine the performance you desire; (3) make the performance level attainable; (4) link rewards to performance; (5) analyze what factors might counteract the effectiveness of the reward; and (6) make sure the reward is adequate. For example, providing funds to attend a major continuing education workshop to those who have reached their stated objectives is a strong motivator for community dietitians/nutritionists.

In terms of organization the expectancy model has several implications: (1) organizations usually get what they reward, not what they want; (2) the job itself can be made intrinsically rewarding; and (3) the immediate supervisor has an important role in the motivation process.

Methods for Behavior Modification

Four techniques that managers can use to modify the behavior of subordinates are positive reinforcement, avoidance learning, extinction, and punishment.

Positive Reinforcement

A consequence that encourages repetition of a given behavior is positively reinforcing. Primary reinforcers such as water and food satisfy biological needs. Secondary reinforcers, such as praise, promotion, and money, are rewarding because of positive past associations for the individual.

Peters and Waterman (1982) have made the general observation that most managers know very little about the value of positive reinforcement. Many either appear not to value it at all or consider it beneath them or undignified. The evidence from excellent companies strongly suggests that managers who feel this way are doing themselves a disservice. The excellent companies seem not only to know the value of positive reinforcement, but also how to manage it.

The way that reinforcement is carried out is more important than the amount (Skinner, 1971). First, reinforcement should be *specific*, incorporating as much information content as possible. Peters and Waterman (1982) noted that activity-based management by objectives (MBOs) systems are more common in the excellent companies than are financially based MBOs. Second, reinforcement should have *immediacy*; the manager should make comments as soon as possible after the event occurs. Third, the system of feedback should take account of *achievability*. Was the task possible to accomplish? The fourth characteristic is that some of the feedback should come in the form of *intangible* but meaningful attention from top management. Skinner asserts that regular reinforcement loses impact because it comes to be expected. Thus unpredictable intermittent reinforcement works better; moreover, small rewards are often more effective than large ones. Community dietitians/nutritionists must be skilled in working with persons at all levels; for example, in a health department they deal with indigent patients and clients as well as the director of the institution. Therefore positive reinforcement skills must be well developed.

Avoidance Learning

Avoidance learning occurs when individuals learn to avoid or escape from unpleasant consequences. In the workplace a statement such as "When are you going to start carrying your share of the load?" may cause an individual to avoid future criticism by improving his or her performance.

Extinction and Punishment

Extinction and punishment are designed to reduce undesired behavior rather than reinforce desired behavior. Extinction is the absence of reinforcement following undesired behavior. If extinction is repeated, the behavior will eventually disappear or become extinct. Through punishment, managers try to correct improper behavior of subordinates by providing negative consequences. Giving harsh criticisms, denying privileges, and demoting are common forms of punishment in the workplace (Sims, 1980). For example, if a community dietitian/nutritionist has difficulty in relating to a particular community group and is considered insensitive to its needs, he or she should be removed from this area if the objectives are to be accomplished.

LEADERSHIP

The successful organization has one major attribute that sets it apart from unsuccessful organizations: dynamic and effective leadership. Peters and Waterman (1982) state that an effective leader must be the master of two ends of the spectrum: ideas at the highest level of abstraction and actions at the most mundane level of detail. The value-shaping leader is concerned on the one hand with soaring lofty visions that will generate excitement and enthusiasm for tens or hundreds of thousands of people. This idea could be described as a "path-finding" role. On the other hand, the only way to instill enthusiasm seems to be through scores of daily events, with the value-shaping manager becoming an implementer par excellence. In this role the leader is detail oriented and directly instills values through deeds rather than words; no opportunity is too small. Attention to ideas—path finding and soaring visions— would seem to suggest rare, imposing people writing on stone tablets. According to Peters and Waterman, who looked at how leaders shape values, this is not the case. Success in instilling values appears to have little to do with charisma. Rather, it derives from obvious sincere, sustained, personal commitment to the values the leaders sought to implant, coupled with extraordinary *persistence* in reinforcing those values. None of the people they studied relied on personal magnetism; all made themselves into effective leaders.

Management writers agree that leadership is the process of influencing the activities of an individual or a group in efforts toward goal achievement in a given situation. From this definition of leadership, it follows that the leadership process is a function of the leader, the follower, and other situational variables (Hersey and Blanchard, 1982).

It is important to note that this definition makes no mention of any particular type of organization. In any situation in which someone is trying to influence the behavior of another individual or group, leadership occurs. Thus everyone attempts leadership at one time or another, whether his or her activities are centered on a business, educational institution, hospital, political organization, or family.

It should also be remembered that when this definition mentions leader and follower, one should not infer only a hierarchical relationship such as suggested by superior (boss)/subordinate. Any time an individual is attempting to influence the behavior of someone else, that individual is the potential leader and the person he or she is attempting to influence is the potential follower, no matter whether that person is boss, colleague (associate), subordinate, friend, or relative. This is an important concept in the field of nutrition, since nutritionists work with a variety of personnel, both professional and lay.

Leadership Process

We have defined leadership as the process of influencing the activities of an individual or a group in efforts toward goal achievement in a given situation. In essence, leadership involves accomplishing goals with and through people. Therefore a leader must be concerned about tasks and human relationships. Although using different terminology, Barnard (1938) identified these same leadership concerns in his classic work *The Functions of the Executive*. These leadership concerns seem to be a reflection of two of the earliest schools of thought in organizational theory: scientific management and human relations.

Scientific Management Movement

In the early 1900s one of the most widely read theorists on administration was Frederick Winslow Taylor (1911). The basis for his scientific management was technological in nature. He believed that the best way to increase output was to improve the techniques or methods used by

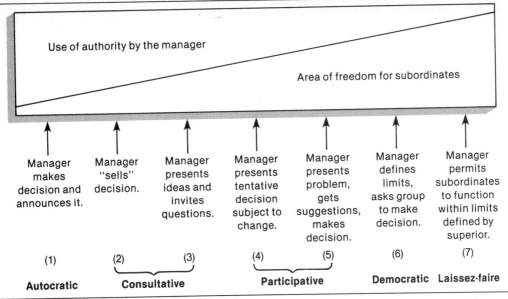

Figure 5-3. Continuum of leader decision-making authority.
Modified from Tannebaum, R., and Schmidt, W.H.: Harvard Bus. Rev. 36:96, March-April 1958.
Redrawn from Rakich, J.S., Beaufort, B.L., and O'Donovan, T.R.: Managing health care organizations, Philadelphia, 1977, W.B. Saunders Co.

workers. Consequently, he has been interpreted as considering people as instruments or machines to be manipulated by their leaders. An example of his preoccupation with instruments was the use of time and motion studies. The result of his technological approach was that workers had to adjust to the management and not the management to workers.

Human Relations Movement

In the 1920s and early 1930s the trend started by Taylor was replaced by the human relations movement, initiated by Elton Mayo (1945) and his associates. These theorists argued that in addition to finding the best technological methods to improve output, it was beneficial to management to look into human affairs. They claimed that the real power centers within an organization were the interpersonal relations that developed within the working unit. The study of these human relations was the most important consideration for management and the analysis

of organization. The organization was to be developed around the workers and had to take into consideration human feelings and attitudes.

In human relations theory the function of the leader was to facilitate cooperative goal attainment among followers while providing opportunities for their personal growth and development. The main focus, contrary to scientific management theory, was on individual needs and not on the needs of the organization.

The recognition of these concerns has characterized the writings on leadership ever since the conflict between the scientific management and the human relations schools of thought became apparent.

Influences on Choice of Leadership Style

Tannenbaum and Schmidt (1973) formulated a continuum basically describing the decision-making authority dimension of leader behavior. The continuum (Figure 5-3) has two polar ends with changing degrees of manager-subordinate decision-making authority. The authors have provided descriptions indicating the degree of decision-making authority held by the manager. At the bottom of the continuum are commonly used labels ranging from *autocratic* to *laissez-faire*.

Autocratic

In the continuum of leader authority in Figure 5-3 the autocratic end represents the manager who makes decisions and announces them to the group. The use of the autocratic style means that the manager has made a decision pertaining to what the purpose of the group activity is, how the group activity is to be structured, and who is to be assigned to what specific tasks.

In health care settings one seldom sees this pure form of the autocratic leader style exercised by administrative personnel. It is often the physician, as the person responsible for the activities required for patient care, who adopts this style. Out of necessity, the physician must make decisions that no one else can. In fact, the physician in health care occupies the unique position of having responsibility via medical staff bylaws and an enormous amount of authority in patient care coordination without having any formal authority delegated by hospital management. The authority responsibility of a physician is far different from that of salaried health care managers (Rakich, Longest, and Donovan, 1977).

Consultative

In the consultative style (Figure 5-3) the manager "sells" the decision or presents ideas and invites questions from subordinates, or both. Specifically, the manager makes decisions concerning the work activity to be carried out—its purpose and how, when, and by whom it is to be done—and attempts to sell the subordinates on the decision.

Participative

In the participative style of leader decision authority the manager identifies the purpose, the problems, and the means by which the activities should be carried out; presents a tentative decision already made or seeks subordinates' opinions; and then makes the final decision. In Figure 5-3 the "Area of freedom for subordinates" is much greater and the "Use of authority by manager" is much smaller than with the autocratic and consultative styles. Participative management is a very powerful motivation because it enables employees to have some measure of influence and control over work-related activities. The work group can influence the decision made concerning work activities and their purposes.

There is a great deal of evidence supporting the contention that a participative leader decision authority style can have a favorable effect on organizational productivity and efficiency. It has become fashionable in recent years for leading management experts to trumpet the potential for learning from the Japanese. Particular attention has been called to the advantages of the Japanese management style and techniques that it practices (Cole, 1981).

Democratic

In the democratic style of leader decision authority the manager defines the limits of the situation and the problem to be solved and asks the group to make decisions. The subordinates have a relatively large "area of decision freedom." The boundaries of activity are set by the manager, who permits the group to make decisions within those restrictions.

Laissez-faire

The term *laissez-faire* was originally coined for the doctrine that government should not interfere in commerce. It is sometimes called "free reign." In the description in Figure 5-3 subordinates are permitted to function within the limits set by the manager's superior. There is no interference within the group by the manager, who although participates in the decision making, attempts to do so with no more influence than any other member of the group. The manager is merely a figurehead. This style of leader decision authority is rarely found in health care organizations.

Quality Circles

The quality circle concept is not a secret weapon; it is a very simple idea that started in Japan in 1962. A quality circle is a small group of employees who meet regularly to identify, analyze, and solve a company's problems (Gryna, 1981). A summary of the characteristics of quality circles is given below. Quality circles are one of the many forms of participative management, a form familiar to some American companies. The quality circle approach developed in Japan incorporates several unique features including problem solution by workers and training for workers in developing problem-solving tools and skills. Quality circles are most likely to succeed in organizations that already have some form of participative management.

Benefits

The benefits of circles fall into the following broad categories: improvement of the attitudes and behaviors of people at all levels of the organization and measurable savings from circle projects. Improved communications has often been mentioned as a major benefit. The circle's effects on an individual's characteristics are noteworthy: (1) it enables the individual to improve personal capabilities, (2) it increases the individual's self-respect, (3) it helps managers change certain personality characteristics, and (4) it helps workers develop the potential to become the supervisors of the future.

As activity of a circle progresses and workers learn problem-solving tools and group participation, it becomes apparent at all levels of management that workers' knowledge of a job is an untapped resource. Supervisors have repeatedly mentioned how surprised they were by work knowledge and creativity. Gryna (1981) describes the procedure for setting up a quality circle group.

TYPICAL CHARACTERISTICS OF QUALITY CIRCLES

Objective

To improve communication, particularly between line employees and managers.
To identify and solve problems.

Organization

The circle consists of a leader and 8 to 10 employees from one area of work.
The circle also has a coordinator and one or more facilitators who work closely with it.

Selection of Circle Members

Participation of members is voluntary.
Participation of leaders may or may not be voluntary.

Scope of Problems Analyzed by Circles

The circle selects its own problems.
Initially the circle is encouraged to select problems from its immediate work area.

Problems are not restricted to quality, but also include productivity, cost, safety, morale, housekeeping, environment, and other spheres.

Training

Formal training in problem-solving techniques is usually a part of circle meetings.

Meetings

Usually 1 hour per week.

Awards for Circle Activities

Usually no monetary awards are given.
The most effective reward is the satisfaction of the circle members from solving problems and observing the implementation of their own solutions.

From Gryna, F.: Quality circles: a team approach to problem solving, ed. 1, New York, 1981, AMACOM.

Problems

In some companies circles have failed. Other companies have had only marginal success. Some early warning signals of failing quality circles are a lack of a reasonable amount of implementation of circle recommendations, slow response to requests made by circles, absenteeism at meetings, postponing circle meetings, and scheduling other meetings at the same time as circle meetings. Part of the support circles need for success is for management to give problems to the circles over which the workers have some control. A problem that management controls is *not* appropriate for circles (Aubrey and Finch, 1982). It is evident from the research, however, that quality circles can make a major contribution to individual workers as well as the entire organization (Takeuchi, 1981).

Guidelines for Using Participative Approaches in Management

To make full use of a participative approach, the following guidelines are suggested by Cole (1980):

1. The importance of the results should be such that there is adequate time to seek opinions from employees.
2. Personnel should have expertise and skill in the matters under consideration. For example, it would be beneficial to ask dietitic technicians for their opinion about an efficient work flow at the clinic they service.
3. The cost of possible error should be considered. When others are asked to participate, there is a risk that mistakes will be made. Obviously, an area such as direct patient care would not lend itself to this method.
4. A quick shift in style is cautioned against. Employees should be prepared for the change in order to reduce skepticism and to build their confidence.
5. Employees must be willing to participate.
6. Finally, the participative style should be used with sincerity and legitimacy.

The goal for health care organizations cannot be long-term maximization of patient care without a reasonable level of participative decision making from the health care team. A large part of the health care field is made up of professionals, and they do not tolerate being left out of the decision process (Rakich, Longest, and Donovan, 1977).

Managerial Grid

The Ohio State University leadership study instituted in 1945 concentrated on two theoretical concepts of leadership, one emphasizing task accomplishment and the other stressing the development of personal relationships (Stogdill and Duoms, 1957). Blake and Mouton (1985) developed these concepts in their Managerial Grid® and have used them extensively in organization and management development programs.

In the Managerial Grid five different types of leadership based on concern for production (task) and concern for people (relationship) are located in four quadrants (Figure 5-4).

Concern for production is illustrated on the horizontal axis. Production becomes more important to the leader as his or her rating advances on the horizontal scale. A leader with a rating of nine on the horizontal axis has a maximum concern for production.

Concern for people is illustrated on the vertical axis. People become more important to the leader as his or her rating progresses up the vertical axis. A leader with a rating of nine on the vertical axis has maximum concern for people. The five leadership styles are described as follows (Blake and Mouton, 1985):

Impoverished. Exertion of minimum effort to get required work done is appropriate to sustain organization requirements.

Country club. Thoughtful attention to needs of people for satisfying relationships leads to a comfortable, friendly organization atmosphere and work tempo. This stage provides more comfort than outcome.

Task. Efficiency in operations results from arranging conditions of work in such a way that human elements interfere to a minimum degree; there is more emphasis on tasks than on people.

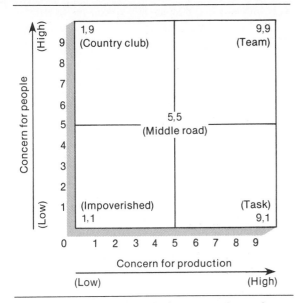

Figure 5-4. The Managerial Grid leadership styles.
Redrawn from Blake, Robert R., and Mouton, Jane S.: The Managerial Grid, III. Houston: Gulf Publishing Co., 1985, p. 12.

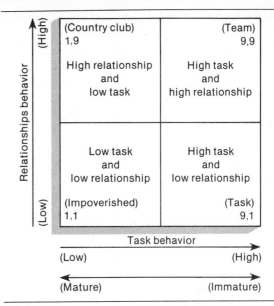

Figure 5-5. Basic leader behavior styles.
Redrawn from Paul Hersey and Ken Blanchard, Management of Organizational Behavior: Utilizing Human Resources, 4th ed., © 1982, p. 89. Reprinted by permission of Prentice-Hall, Inc., Englewood Cliffs, N.J.

Middle-of-the-road. Adequate organization performance is possible through balancing the necessity to get out work while maintaining morale at a satisfactory level.

Team. Work is accomplished by committed people; interdependence through a "common stake" in organization purpose leads to relationships of trust and respect.

The Tri-Dimensional Leader Effectiveness Model

In the leadership models developed by Hersey and Blanchard (1982) the terms *task behavior* and *relationship behavior* are used to describe concepts of consideration and initiating structure. The four basic leader behavior quadrants are labeled high task and low relationship; high task and high relationship; high relationship and low task; and low relationship and low task (Figure 5-5).

These four basic styles depict essentially different leadership styles. The leadership style of an individual is the behavior pattern that person exhibits when attempting to influence the activities of others, as perceived by those others. This leadership style may be very different from how the leader perceives his or her behavior, which we will define as self-perception rather than style. A person's leadership style involves some combination of either task behavior or relationship behavior. The two types of behavior, task and relationship, which are central to the concept of leadership style, are defined as follows:

1. Task behavior. The extent to which leaders are likely to organize and define the roles of the members of their group (followers); to explain what activities each is to do and when, where, and how tasks are to be accomplished.

Table 5-1. How the basic leader behavior styles may be seen by others when they are effective or ineffective

Basic Styles	Effective	Ineffective
High task and low relationship behavior	Seen as having well-defined methods for accomplishing goals that are helpful to the followers.	Seen as imposing methods on others; sometimes seen as unpleasant and interested only in short-run output.
High task and high relationship behavior	Seen as satisfying the needs of the group for setting goals and organizing work, but also providing high levels of socioemotional support.	Seen as initiating more structure than is needed by the group and often appears not to be genuine in interpersonal relationships.
High relationship and low task behavior	Seen as having implicit trust in people and as being primarily concerned with facilitating their goal accomplishment.	Seen as primarily interested in harmony; sometimes seen as unwilling to accomplish a task if it risks disrupting a relationship or losing "good person" image.
Low relationship and low task behavior	Seen as appropriately delegating to subordinates decisions about how the work should be done and providing little socioemotional support where little is needed by the group.	Seen as providing little structure or socioemotional support when needed by members of the group.

From Paul Hersey and Ken Blanchard, Management of Organizational Behavior: Utilizing Human Resources, 4th ed., © 1982, p. 89. Reprinted by permission of Prentice-Hall, Inc., Englewood Cliffs, N.J.

2. Relationship behavior. The extent to which leaders are likely to maintain personal relationships with members of their group (followers) by opening up channels of communication.

Table 5-1 describes briefly one of the many different ways each style might be perceived as effective or ineffective by others.

The Hersey-Blanchard model has generated interest because it recommends a leadership type that is dynamic and flexible, rather than static. According to Hersey and Blanchard (1982), if the style is appropriate, it will not only motivate subordinates but also will help them to move toward maturity. Thus the manager who develops his or her subordinates, increases their confidence, and helps them learn their work will constantly be shifting leadership styles. These leadership models can be applied to the field of dietetics and nutrition, particularly in the area of productivity. By developing subordinates' confidence, the leader may instill a feeling of security. Their data offer a wealth of information for continuing education of community dietitians/nutritionists to become effective leaders.

COMMUNICATIONS

The correspondence on p. 105 is by no means atypical; it is an example of poor communication. Alice Caldwell obviously had not clarified in her own mind what she wanted her memo to accomplish. On the other hand, she clearly wanted Mary's report to be in on time. However, she was aware that Mary was tied up with the new clinic, and she felt the need to offer her an extension. Her unresolved conflict resulted in a stiff, confusing memo that must have frustrated Mary. Mary's memo, in turn, expressed her angry reaction and suggested that she would accomplish both tasks in time by sacrificing quality. The result was that neither the individuals involved nor the organization got what they needed.

The Importance of Communication

The management process of decision making, planning, organization, executing, and controlling depends on effective communication. Without it, plans and objectives would go no farther than the person who originated them; the organization would exist only as a conglomeration of isolated people and departments; the execution

---

MEMO

To: Mary Peterson, R.D.
From: Alice Caldwell, R.D.
Re: Quarterly Report on Nutrition Surveillance
         System Data

As you are aware, your quarterly surveillance report is due in one week. I cannot emphasize how important it is that you get the report in on time. USDA cannot proceed with its review of our WIC program (Supplemental Feeding Program for Pregnant Women, Infants and Children) unless reports from all regional nutritionists are available. However, you seem to be busy with the new WIC clinic and its large case load. If you are unable to complete the report by the due date, you may take an extension. I will have to postpone USDA auditors' visit and will have to explain why our department's reports are incomplete.

MEMO

To: Alice Caldwell, R.D.
From: Mary Peterson, R.D.
Re: Your Recent Memo

Your memo about my quarterly surveillance report came as something of a surprise to me. Frankly, you don't seem to appreciate the amount of work this new clinic requires. I have been working late every day and on weekends and have given up my aerobics class so that we can open the clinic on the date set by the community. I had planned to ask for an extension for the quarterly report, but if the report is that important, I'll make sure you get it on time. I just hope you don't expect the report and the details completed for the clinic to be as good as they should be.

---

of activity could not take place because no one would know what, when, how, and why to do anything; and the controlling process would not exist because there would be no feedback mechanism for measuring performance and expectations.

Communication is defined as the creation or exchange of understanding between a sender and a receiver (Rakich, Longest, and Donovan, 1977). Clearly this definition does not restrict the concept to words alone; communication includes all methods through which meaning is conveyed to others. Even silence can convey meaning and must be considered part of communicating. Communicating is an exchange—a giving and receiving of information. However, the physical exchange is only one part of the process; understanding is the other. Unless people make themselves understood and understand what others are saying, the process cannot work. Figure 5-6 shows the process of communication. A sender transmits information through a communication channel to a receiver. Both sender and receiver have two responsibilities: the sender has to translate information and then choose a medium (pictures, actions, or words) for transmission, and the receiver has to accept that information (seeing, hearing, or reading) and then interpret it.

Oral Communication

In an organization most communication is oral. It is a lot faster to call someone and get an answer than it is to write a memo, send it, and wait for a response. However, saving time is only one aspect of oral communication. Face-to-face conversations are the heart of an effective communication system. Here is where the exchange between sender and receiver works best. No other form of communication—not the telephone, not the intercom—can equal face-to-face contact. Why? The answer is simple: immediate feedback. Whatever the response—a shrug, a smile, any expression—the sender knows immediately how a message has been received. Oral communication is equally effective for the receiver, who can instantly clarify what something means.

Written Communication

The human voice adds meaning and shading that even long pages of written words simply cannot convey. But no matter how effective oral communications are, every organization needs writ-

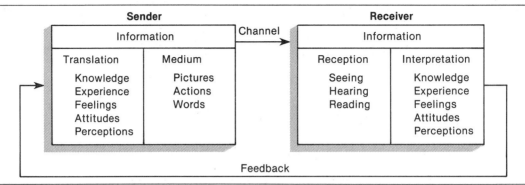

Figure 5-6. The communication process.
Modified from Organizational Communication Behavioral Perspectives, ed. 2, by Jerry W. Koehler, Karl W.E. Anatol, and Ronald L. Applebaum. Copyright © 1981 by Holt, Rinehart & Winston. Reprinted by permission of CBS College Publishing.

ten communications. Letter reports and manuals are a permanent record of what is going on. Finally, there is a question of formality. Written communications carry greater "official" weight than oral ones.

The style that one uses in writing is also important to communications. What is said in a letter or memorandum is partly how it is said. The message, the sender's real intentions, can get lost in the words. Writing a letter is far more than stating the basic message one wishes to give to someone. It is also conveying how the sender wishes to relate to the recipient and what he or she wants the recipient to feel in response. That is important because it may determine what the reader does about the message (Fielder, 1982). These additional means are conveyed through the style one chooses to write with. There is no single style for all occasions. Sometimes it is tactful to be personal, and sometimes it is appropriate to be fairly impersonal. At times it feels right to be simple and direct and at other times roundabout and colorful. One thing is certain: strategy is part of style. The message a person wants to send is partly conveyed in the tone. Any message varies according to the way it is phrased.

Barriers to Effective Interpersonal Communication

A number of common barriers to interpersonal communication have been identified.

Hearing what you expect to hear. Experience may lead you to expect to hear the same message. Workers habitually criticized for their work may hear a statement such as "You did a fine job on that" as a sarcastic put-down, even when it is a genuine compliment. Hearing what you expect to hear can create negative situations and stress in individuals or groups.

Ignoring information that conflicts with what you "know." When you hear a message that disagrees with your preconceptions, you may ignore the message rather than change your ideas or seek some alternative explanation.

Evaluating the source. The meaning you apply to any message is influenced by your evaluation of the message's source. Imagine the different ways you would decode the message "Relax—don't work so hard" if the source were your mother, your boss, your doctor, or someone competing for your job. In this example, evaluating the source may help the receiver to extract the meaning intended by the sender. In many cases, however, consideration of the source of the message will distort the message the receiver actually "hears." Labor-management relations are often fraught with such communication distortions. When neither side trusts the other, even the most positive communications are met with skepticism and are scrutinized for hidden meanings or traps.

Differing perceptions. Words, actions, and events are perceived in light of the receiver's values and environmental pressures. If you congratulate a subordinate for completing a task on schedule, you may generate a feeling of pride and accomplishment. However, if that individual's work group considers meeting schedules a sign of "buttering up the boss," that individual may deliberately begin to delay task completion, to reestablish group identity.

Words that mean different things to different people. Words are symbols. As symbols, they may have different meanings for different people in different situations. The *telephone* to a person who installs telephones may signify job or task; to someone in the hospital, *telephone* may mean the possibility of companionship; to a junior executive moving into a private office for the first time, *telephone* may represent success.

Inconsistent nonverbal signals. Tone of voice, facial expressions, and bodily postures can help or hinder communication.

Effects of emotions. The emotion that dominates your mood—anger, fear, happiness, anticipation—will affect your interpretation of a relevant message. If, for example, you are in an atmosphere where you feel threatened with loss of power or prestige, you may lose the ability to gauge the meanings of messages you receive and will respond defensively or aggressively.

Noise. To function effectively, individuals must "screen out" many of the messages they receive. No person can respond to every sound or gesture, even if he or she is aware of them all. Sometimes, in the process of "screening out" the irrelevant, the relevant is also lost.

Effective Listening

Senders can overcome communication barriers by spending more time listening. Listening re-duces misunderstandings. It allows speakers to adjust their messages to their receivers' response. Listening means putting aside feelings and biases to really hear what is being said. Remember, you do not have to agree with the message, but you must try to understand it. Look for the meaning of the ideas, not the individual's words. Latent (hidden) context is every bit as important as manifest (obvious) context. Do not be afraid to ask, "Is this what you mean?" Questions show that you are interested and you are paying attention (Haimann, 1982). Following are 10 rules for effective listening:

1. *Stop talking.* You cannot listen if you are talking. As Polonius said in *Hamlet*, "Give every man thy ear, but few thy voice."
2. *Put the talker at ease.* Help him or her feel free to talk. This is what a permissive environment is all about.
3. *Show the talker that you want to listen.* Look and act interested. Do not read your mail while someone talks. Listen to understand, not to criticize.
4. *Remove distractions.* Do not doodle, tap, or shuffle papers.
5. *Empathize.* Try to help yourself see the other person's point of view.
6. *Be patient.* Allow plenty of time. Do not interrupt. Do not walk away.
7. *Hold your temper.* An angry person misunderstands words.
8. *Restrict on argument and criticism.* This puts people on the defensive, and they may become silent or get angry. Do not argue. Even if you win, you lose.
9. *Ask questions.* This encourages the talker and shows that you are listening. It also helps to clarify what is being said.
10. *Stop talking.* This is the first and last rule because all the others depend on it. You cannot do an effective listening job while you are talking (Davis, 1981).

Listening requires two ears, one for meaning and one for dealing. Decision makers who do not listen have less information for making sound decisions.

The Use of Humor by Today's Managers

Considering the barriers to communication, one might assume that humorous interchange up and down traditional authoritarian organizational structures would be very limited. However, it appears that the organizational environment of today and tomorrow just might tolerate, and even thrive on, the tension release associated with a laugh.

Malone (1980) has stated that many writers have acknowledged the favorable, even therapeutic, effects of humor. However, few have attempted to relate humor to the functions of management and leadership. Research on this topic could possibly convert an undeveloped resource into a tool that could enhance managing to get things done.

Humor is described as "a process initiated by a stimulus, such as a joke or cartoon, and terminating with some response indicative of experienced pleasure, such as laughter" (Malone, 1980).

With traditional organizational barriers being challenged, aren't there increasing opportunities for the productive use of wholesome humor? Although humor is presently an untested tool, could it possibly be an underdeveloped resource that can contribute to enhancing the satisfaction and productivity of human beings at work?

Moving from Defensive to Supportive Communication

One important approach to overcoming communication barriers is described by Gibb (1961). He suggests that the types of behavior or attitudes people manifest affect the way they communicate. Certain types of behavior will cause individuals to react defensively and will inhibit communication, whereas other types will cause people to feel they are supported, thereby facilitating communication. The two categories of behavior identified by Gibb are listed in Table 5-2. Behavior characterized by any of the qualities in the left column causes defensiveness in the receiver; those in the right column are seen as supportive and hence act to reduce defensiveness. We will briefly discuss each of the six pairs of behaviors.

Table 5-2. Categories of defensive and supportive communication behaviors

Defensive Behaviors	Supportive Behaviors
1. Evaluation	1. Description
2. Control	2. Problem orientation
3. Strategy	3. Spontaneity
4. Neutrality	4. Empathy
5. Superiority	5. Equality
6. Certainty	6. Provisionalism

From Jack R. Gibb, "Defensive Communication, *Journal of Communication*, 11, no. 13 (September 1961), 143. Used by permission of the International Communication Association and the author. In James A.F. Stoner, *Management*, ed. 2, © 1982, pp. 408, 593. Reprinted by permission of Prentice-Hall, Inc., Englewood Cliffs, N.J.

Evaluation-description. If the speaker's manner, expression, tone, or choice of phrase is interpreted as a judgment about or an evaluation of the listener, then the listener may become defensive. This reaction is not unrealistic, since much communication is, in fact, evaluative. Managers will often find it difficult not to pass judgment on subordinates automatically. Conscious effort is sometimes needed to avoid this defense-provoking behavior. Senders should pay careful attention to objectivity in communications ("description").

One should avoid the common tendency to formulate a reply mentally while the other person is speaking, instead of concentrating on trying to listen to what the speaker is actually saying.

Control-problem orientation. Statements, orders, or seemingly simple observations attempting to control other persons imply that the speaker has better judgment and therefore that the listeners are inferior. Methods of communicating an attempt to control may range from a threat-backed command to a simple disapproving frown. Since these methods imply that the receiver is not capable of making a wise decision without direction, they create defensiveness even if the control is accepted. When the sender makes it clear, however, that he or she is trying to join with the receiver in defining and solving a problem, a supportive climate results and an improvement in communication is almost inevitable.

Strategy-spontaneity. If a person thinks someone is "playing games," rather than acting spontaneously, the usual reaction is resistance. Deceit and manipulation can "turn off" that individual to anyone from a potential date to a candidate for governor. Managers who have been superficially involved in sensitivity or human relations training frequently attempt to "act" spontaneously; the listener often senses an underlying insincerity. Genuine and honest communication, however, usually creates a genuine and honest response.

Neutrality-empathy. Communication that demonstrates empathy for the listener will produce highly favorable reactions. Conversely, a cold, clinical attitude will be interpreted as indifference and will lead to stiff, formal, less satisfying interchanges.

Superiority-equality. Individuals who act superior do not usually get cooperative and friendly responses. Those who lecture and admonish will be received coldly. Those who talk as equals, on the other hand, and who indicate they trust and respect their listeners will usually receive honest and forthright replies. Managers who want two-way communication with their subordinates must work hard to keep their rank from getting in the way.

Certainty-provisionalism. When persons try to impress others that they know all the answers and that nothing will shake them from their convictions, listeners are likely to become defensively argumentative or sullenly acquiescent. If, on the other hand, they indicate that they want to hear other perspectives and consider new information, a supportive and cooperative attitude is engendered, and open communication is encouraged.

Communications in Organizations

The effectiveness of organizational communication is influenced by the organization's formal channels of communication and authority structure, by job specialization, and by "information ownership." The formal channels may be rigid and highly centralized, with individuals able to communicate with only a few persons, or they may be loose and decentralized, with individuals able to communicate with each other at any level. Experiments have found that for simple tasks centralized networks are faster and more accurate than decentralized networks, whereas for complex tasks decentralized channels are quicker and more accurate. Group member satisfaction is higher in decentralized networks.

Vertical communication is communication that moves up and down the organization's chain of command. Status and power differences between manager and subordinates, a subordinate's desire for upward mobility, and a lack of trust between manager and subordinates interfere with accurate and complete vertical communication.

Lateral communication improves coordination and problem solving and fosters employee satisfaction. Informal communication occurs outside the organization's formal channels. A particularly quick and pervasive type of informal communication is the "grapevine" (Stoner, 1982).

Overcoming Organizational Barriers to Communication

To deal with barriers to organizational communication, one must first recognize that communication is an inherently complex process. Verbal and visual symbols used to describe reality are far from precise. A simple word such as *job* can be applied to anything from a child's newspaper route to the presidency of the United States. Words such as *achievement*, *effectiveness*, or *responsibility* are even more vague. This imprecision of language (and gestures) is one reason perfect communication is difficult, if not impossible, to achieve.

Another reason communication is inherently difficult is that human beings perceive and interpret reality based on their individual backgrounds, needs, emotions, values, and experiences. Some writers, in fact, believe that most organizational barriers to communication are based on differences in the way people understand the communications they receive.

Comprehending the innate barriers to communication and taking steps to minimize them are therefore the first steps toward improving a manager's ability to communicate effectively.

The American Management Association

TEN COMMANDMENTS OF GOOD COMMUNICATION

1. *Seek to clarify your ideas before communicating.* The more systematically we analyze the problem or idea to be communicated, the clearer it becomes . . . Good [communication] planning must [also] consider the goals and attitudes of those who will receive the communication and those who will be affected by it.

2. *Examine the true purpose of each communication.* Before you communicate, ask yourself what you *really* want to accomplish with your message—obtain information, initiate action, change another person's attitude? Identify your most important goal and then adapt your language, tone, and total approach to serve that specific objective.

3. *Consider the total physical and human setting whenever you communicate.* Meaning and intent are conveyed by more than words alone. . . . Consider, for example, your *sense of timing*—i.e., the circumstances under which you make an announcement or render a decision; the *physical setting*—whether you communicate in private, for example, or otherwise; the *social climate* that pervades work relationships within the company or a department and sets the tone of its communications; *custom and past practice*—the degree to which your communication conforms to, or departs from, the expectations of your audience.

4. *Consult with others, where appropriate, in planning communications.* . . . Such consultation often helps to lend additional insight and objectivity to your message. Moreover, those who have helped you plan your communication will give it their active support.

5. *Be mindful, while you communicate, of the overtones as well as the basic content of your message.* Your tone of voice, your expression, your apparent receptiveness to the responses of others—all have tremendous impact on those you wish to reach. Frequently overlooked, these subtleties of communication often affect a listener's reaction to a message even more than its basic content.

6. *Take the opportunity, when it arises, to convey something of help or value to the receiver.* Consideration of the other person's interests and needs—the habit of trying to look at things from his point of view—will frequently point up opportunities to convey something of immediate benefit or long-range value to him.

7. *Follow up your communication.* This you can do by asking questions, by encouraging the receiver to express his reactions, by follow-up contacts, by subsequent review of performance. Make certain that every important communication has a "feedback" so that complete understanding and appropriate action result.

8. *Communicate for tomorrow as well as today.* While communications may be aimed primarily at meeting the demands of an immediate situation, they must be planned with the past in mind if they are to maintain consistency in the receiver's view; but, most important of all, they must be consistent with long-range interest and goals. For example, it is not easy to communicate frankly on such matters as poor performance or the shortcomings of a loyal subordinate—but postponing disagreeable communications makes them more difficult in the long run and is actually unfair to your subordinates and your company.

9. *Be sure your actions support your communications.* In the final analysis, the most persuasive kind of communication is not what you say but what you do. . . . For every manager this means that good supervisory practices—such as clear assignment of responsibility and authority, fair rewards for effort, and sound policy enforcement—serve to communicate more than all the gifts of oratory.

10. *Seek not only to be understood but to understand—be a good listener.* When we start talking we often cease to listen—in that larger sense of being attuned to the other person's unspoken reactions and attitudes. . . . [Listening] demands that we concentrate not only on the explicit meanings another person is expressing, but on the implicit meanings, unspoken words, and undertones that may be far more significant.

(AMA) has codified a number of communication principles into what it calls the "Ten Commandments of Good Communication." These "commandments," designed to improve the effectiveness of organizational communications, are listed and summarized on p. 110.

The AMA principles provide useful guidelines for how the communication of individual managers can be improved. Management by objectives (MBO) and organizational development, discussed in Chapter 4, can help improve communication in organizations as a whole. MBO emphasizes joint goal setting, performance feedback, and joint problem solving. Thus MBO programs are particularly useful for improving downward communication in organizations and for creating an atmosphere of trust between managers and subordinates. Organizational development approaches attempt to change an organization's climate or culture. Bringing about this change affects the organization's communication system. Successfully applied, organizational development will establish open, objective, and authentic communication between individuals and managers at all levels of the organization.

THE VITAMINS OF HUMAN RELATIONS

No chapter on leadership would be complete for community dietitians/nutritionists without Romero's vitamins for human relations:

Vitamin A. Like blood, the supervisor has to circulate to stay in touch with the organization. One of the ways that leadership is felt is by the supervisor's physical presence. Wearing out the seat of one's pants in a swivel chair is not enough.

Vitamin B. Management and employees are partners, and like all partnerships, theirs must be based on trust to work. Everything is possible if employees feel they are treated with fairness. Anything else divides the working group into pockets of resistance that will collapse the bridge of productive feeling between employees and management.

Vitamin C. Good human relations begin with the understanding that every person is unique.

Vitamin D. This one should be taken in combination with C. No one responds productively to a leader who uses a club. Leaders like that get only the bare minimum of effort and never rouse employees to cooperative activity. The supervisor who is too conscious of authority puts a distance between himself or herself and the employees, and that works against the development of loyalty and cooperation.

Vitamin E. To build respect for one's position, one must keep the promises made to employees. It is a good general rule to make as few promises as possible, but the promises that are made must be kept.

Vitamin G. Successful supervisors are careful to discuss the prospect of change with their employees. This not only gives management the benefit of employee insights and support but also it squashes the rumors that inevitably travel around a shop.

Vitamin P. All people defend themselves against threats to their self-respect, something that must be kept in mind when correcting a performance problem. The objective should be to educate employees without making them afraid to try new tasks. That will win cooperation—something more than respectful yielding. Try starting with a pat on the back to soften the blow of criticism.

Vitamin B_1. If there is any secret to successful supervision, it is the ability to see issues from the other person's point of view. The effort to understand another's position pays off in terms of a willingness to please the supervisor. The value of that is incalculable.

Vitamin B_2. Some supervisors who would not hesitate to give an employee a warning notice never realize the value of praise. All people need the stimulation of praise.

Vitamin B_3. This is the encouragement of ambition and initiative in one's employees. It is a by-product of a regimen of B_1 and B_2.

Vitamin B_4. Accentuate the positive. Enthusiasm is infectious, and a good supervisor gives it to the whole department.

Vitamin B_{11}. Cooperation is a two-way street. Keep that in mind because without it all the fine planning in the world will never be translated into action.

Vitamin B_{12}. This last vitamin is essential, especially for supervisors who have taken all their other vitamins and realized success. Success can be its own worst enemy, accompanied as it often is by self-satisfaction, intolerance, close-mindedness, and egotism.*

*Reprinted, by permission of the publisher, from *Supervisory Management*, Feb. 1982 © 1982 AMACOM, a division of American Management Associations, New York. All rights reserved.

SUMMARY

To achieve individual and organizational goals, managers must have the ability to motivate people to accomplish these objectives. Leadership is the process of influencing activities in efforts toward goal achievement. Various leadership styles are discussed in this chapter, ranging from autocratic to laissez-faire.

Communications is a process of exchange—a giving and receiving of information. Without effective communication, the management process could not be accomplished. Barriers to effective communications are discussed along with several suggestions made for overcoming organizational barriers.

REFERENCES

Aubrey, C., and Finch, W.: Management, professional and clerical quality circles, Paper presented at American Society for Quality Control, Quality Congress Transactions, Milwaukee, 1982.

Barnard, C.I.: The functions of the executive, Cambridge, Mass., 1938, Harward University Press.

Blake, R.R., and Mouton, J.S.: The managerial grid III, Houston, 1985, Gulf Publishing Co.

Cole, R.E.: The Japanese lesson in quality, Technology Rev. 83(7):29, 1981.

Davis, K.: Human behavior at work, ed. 6, New York, 1981, McGraw-Hill, Inc.

Fielder, J.S.: What do you mean you don't like my style? Harvard Bus. Rev. 60:128, May/June 1982.

Gibb, J.R.: Defensive communication, J. Communication 11(13):141, 1961.

Gryna, F.: Quality circles: a team approach to problem solving, ed. 1, New York, 1981, AMACOM.

Haimann, T., Scott, W.G., and Connors, P.E.: Management, ed. 4, Boston, 1982, Houghton Mifflin Co.

Hersey, P., and Blanchard, K.H.: Management of organizational behavior: utilizing human resources, ed. 4, Englewood Cliffs, N.J., 1982, Prentice-Hall, Inc.

Malone, P.B., III: Humor: a double-edged tool for today's managers? Acad. Management Rev. 5(3):357, 1980.

Maslow, A.H.: Motivation and personality, New York, 1964, Harper & Row Publishers, Inc.

Mayo, E.: The social problems of an industrial civilization, Harvard Bus. Rev., May/June 1945.

McClelland, D.C.: The achieving society, Princeton, N.J., 1961, Van Nostrand.

Peters, T.J., and Waterman, R.H., Jr.: In search of excellence, New York, 1982, Harper & Row Publishers, Inc.

Rakich, J.S., Longest, B.B., and Donovan, T.R.: Managing health care organizations, Philadelphia, 1977, W.B. Saunders Co.

Romero, R.G.: The vitamins of human relations, Supervisory Management 27:14, Feb. 1982.

Sims, H.P., Jr.: Further thoughts on punishment in organizations, Acad. Management Rev. 5:1, Jan. 1980.

Skinner, B.F.: Beyond freedom and dignity, New York, 1971, Alfred A. Knopf.

Stogdill, R.M., and Duoms, A.E., editors: Leader behavior: its description and measurement, Research Monograph N88, Bureau of Business Research, Columbus, Ohio, 1957, The Ohio State University.

Stoner, J.A.F.: Management, ed. 2, Englewood Cliffs, N.J., 1982, Prentice-Hall, Inc.

Takeuchi, H.: Productivity learning from the Japanese, California Management Rev. 23:5, Summer 1981.

Tannenbaum, R., and Schmidt, W.H.: How to choose a leadership pattern (revised), Harvard Bus. Rev. 3:162, May/June 1973.

Taylor, F.W.: The principles of scientific management, New York, 1911, Harper & Brothers.

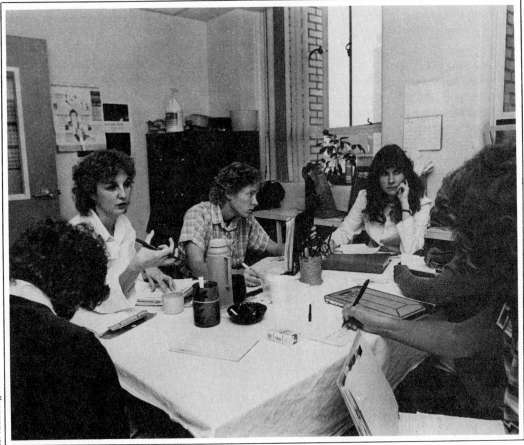

H. Armstrong Roberts

Controlling Nutrition Services for Productivity

GENERAL CONCEPT

Good management requires effective control. Well-planned objectives, showing organization, capable direction, and motivation have little possibility for success unless an adequate system of control exists. One system in health care is program evaluation, the ability to determine the worth or value of efforts expended to achieve a given objective.

When you finish this chapter, you should be able to
- Define the steps in an effective control process
- Explain the importance of evaluation for health care providers and the reasons for completing evaluations
- Describe the various designs that can be employed to effectively evaluate a program
- Design an evaluation for one project by using the case study developed throughout the chapter
- Describe in your case study what to evaluate, what is being measured, and what threats there are to internal validity

THE CONTROL PROCESS

Control (evaluation) is the vitally important process through which managers assure that actual activities conform to planned activities (Figure 6-1) (Stoner, 1982). It involves four basic steps: (1) establishing methods for measuring performance, (2) measuring performance, (3) comparing performance against standards, and (4) taking corrective action (Figure 6-2).

Establishing Standards and Methods for Measuring Performance

For this step to be effective, standards must be specified in meaningful terms and accepted by members of the organization. The method of measurement should also be accepted as accurate. An organization may set an objective to become "a leader in its field"; to do this, the standard must be defined, and a system of measurement must be established. In the field of dietetics, standards of practice have been developed for practitioners in the field. These standards are necessary to deliver quality nutrition services.

Measuring Performance

Like all aspects of control, this is an ongoing repetitive process, with the actual frequency de-

pendent on the type of activity being measured. Accuracy of anthropometric measurements in a preschool clinic may be continuously monitored in a health care setting, whereas progress on long-term expansion objectives of several clinics may be received by top management only once or twice per year. A fault to be avoided, however, is allowing too long a period to pass between performance measurements (Bohrnstedt, 1982).

Comparing Performance Against Standards

This is the easiest step in the control process because the complexities presumably have been solved in the first two steps. Now it is a matter of comparing measured results with the target or standard previously set. If performance matches standard, "everything is under control," and as Figure 6-2 shows, managers do not have to interfere actively in the organization's operations.

Taking Corrective Action

Corrective action should be taken if performance falls short of standards and the analysis indicates that action is required. This corrective action may involve a change in one or more activities of the organization's operations, or it may involve a change in the standards originally established. Unless managers see the control process through to its conclusion, they are merely monitoring performance rather than exercising control.

In designing a control system, managers must decide on the types and number of measurements to be used, who will set the standards, how flexible the standards will be, the frequency of measurement, and the direction that feedback will take (Anthony and Dearden, 1980). In the field of nutrition, standards must be developed for nutritional assessment and nutrition intervention in order to demonstrate outcomes of services.

EVALUATION: HOW TO MEASURE OUTCOMES

One of the major methods used to measure outcomes in health and nutrition programs is program evaluation. Ideally there should be some useful relationship between the process of man-

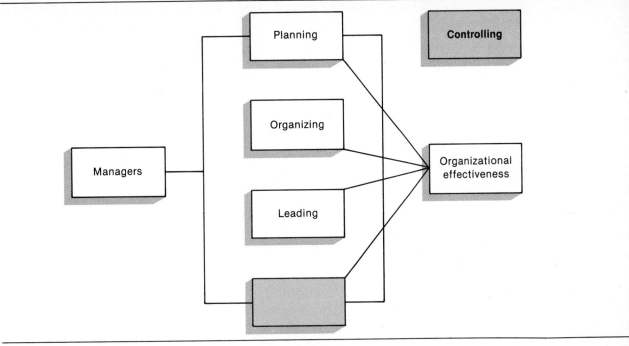

Figure 6-1. Management process.

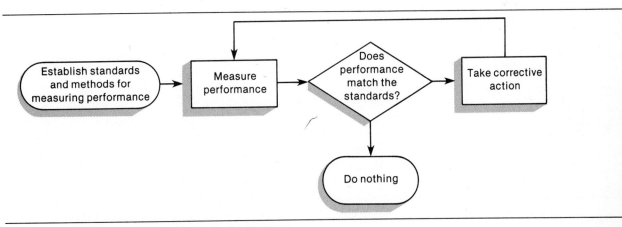

Figure 6-2. Basic steps in the control process.
Redrawn from James A.F. Stoner, Management, ed. 2, © 1982, pp. 408, 593. Reprinted by permission of Prentice-Hall, Inc., Englewood Cliffs, N.J.

aging a program and the process of evaluating it. A program is a collection of activities intended to achieve a common purpose. The process of program evaluation, then, is an effort to judge the extent and efficiency of accomplishment and to find ways of improving outcome (Havens, 1981). A "good" program evaluation, like a "good" program, is one that accomplishes its purposes with reasonable efficiency (Rossi and Freeman, 1982).

What Is Evaluation?

Program evaluation is concerned specifically with determining the worth or values of efforts expended to achieve a given purpose or objective. It is important to realize that everyone constantly makes evaluations or judgments in terms of right or wrong, good or bad, honest or dishonest, practical or impractical. These evaluations occur so frequently and quickly on a day-to-day basis that people are often not consciously aware of this measure. Individuals draw on the full range of their experiences in making these judgments or evaluations, whether these evaluations are objective or intuitive (Cronbach et al., 1980).

Meredith (1976) describes program evaluation as the determination of the degree of progress in achieving program objectives. He states that evaluation can and should be used for both planning and control and thus serves as an all-important feedback link between these crucial functions.

Why Evaluation?

Increasing concern for improving the quality of health care, prospective payment systems, reimbursement mechanisms, and cost containment efforts has focused on the need for developing evaluation strategies for health and nutrition care (Alkin and Solomon, 1982). If consumers and professionals are to feel satisfied that the very best care is being given with the services available, evaluation of quality must occur.

There is a growing demand for the development of methodology to evaluate nutrition and dietetic programs. This demand is related to the desire of all skillful managers to work systematically toward strengthening their programs.

In terms of allocation decisions within both the private and public sectors that ultimately affect the nutrition and dietetic profession, the burden of proof in terms of the effectiveness of services rendered by the profession rests with the profession itself (Tolpin, 1979).

It has been noted that many nutrition programs are not systematically evaluated. Neumann, Neumann, and Ifekwunique (1973) commented that "most people associated with nutrition programs usually feel what they are doing is worthwhile, that the value is clear to all observers and that the best has been accomplished with the resources at hand." Gordon and Scrimshaw (1972) also commented on the comparatively small effort at scientific evaluation of dietetics and nutrition intervention programs: "A curious paradox is evident in the care that laboratory and clinical investigators take to establish the validity of newly apparent facts about nutrition and the common absence of evaluation of public health service programs when those findings are turned to practical use."

Dietetic practitioners must realize that despite the amount of money, materials, manpower, and other often limited resources, evaluations, whether simple or complex, can be accomplished.

To address the issues of evaluation, the first step is to establish the linkage between nutrition factors and health status in a systematic way. To accomplish this, evaluation must be built into the planning process at the initial stages of development and must be an essential component throughout the process. The community dietitian/nutritionist who uses planning and evaluation to assist in solving problems has the best chance of:

- Changing tradition
- Influencing public opinion
- Persuading political leaders or administrators to increase resources to meet nutrition needs
- Improving the rate of success in obtaining the objective and quality of services

- Obtaining personal satisfaction as a professional and feeling a greater sense of accomplishment for efforts

EVALUATION DESIGN

In program evaluation a plan must be developed to select the people to be studied, set the timing of the investigation, and establish procedures for the collection of data. In developing a design, the evaluator can aim at the traditional controlled experiment or at one of the less formalized quasi-experimental designs. The investigation can be of just one project or of a number of projects with the same basic goals. It can deal with the traditional social science variables or with an economic analysis of program cost and benefits (Levine, Solomon, and Hellstern, 1981).

Experimental Model

The classic design for evaluation has been the experimental model, which uses both experimental and control groups. The target population units (individuals, work teams, precincts, students, cities) are randomly chosen to be either the group that gets a program or the control group that does not. Differences are computed, and the program is deemed a success if the experimental group has improved more than the control group. Figure 6-3 illustrates the model graphically.

Usually the control group will receive some program. For example, they may receive the same diet portion of the experiment but not the exercise portion. In cases where no real treatment can be offered to controls, a "placebo" program can be devised that gives the aura but not the substance of service. For example, instead of receiving vitamin C as the experimental group is doing, the control group receives a placebo. This removes the possibility of a Hawthorne or placebo effect—a positive response that is merely a result of the attention that participants receive.

Organizing randomized designs is a highly effective way to rule out the possibility that something other than the program is causing the improvements or setbacks that are observed.

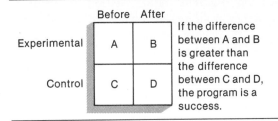

Figure 6-3. Illustration of an experimental model.
Redrawn from Carol H. Weiss EVALUATION RESEARCH: Methods for Assessing Program Effectiveness, © 1972, p. 61. Reprinted by permission of Prentice-Hall, Inc., Englewood Cliffs, New Jersey.

Randomizations protect against possible confusion in analyzing results.

Problems in Action Programs

The controlled experiment is often impossible in action settings. There may be no extra people to serve as controls; the program serves everybody eligible and interested. Even if there are unserved people, program practitioners may refuse to assign any of them to a control condition because they believe in their professional obligation not to deny service. Occasionally, the only possible controls are widely scattered or are unlikely to cooperate with a program that offers nothing in return. The randomized assignment procedure of the experiment also creates problems. Practitioners generally want to assign all people to treatments because their job is to give services.

Use of Experimental Design

The basic need in research is to fit the design to the purpose of the study. Experimental design is a good way to find out how well a particular program achieves its goal. The experiment should be able to offer the optimum design. The essential requirement for a true experiment is the randomized assignment of people to programs. Experimentalists suggest that randomized assignment is much more possible in the real world than many people suspect.

When resources are scarce and some people

must do without, randomization is possible. When new programs are introduced over a period of time, the delayed receivers can become the controls for those who get the programs early. Often, special pilot projects can be designed on an experimental basis.

Quasi-Experimental Design

Quasi-experimental designs are those which do not meet all the strict requirements of the experiment but nevertheless can be satisfactory. Campbell and Stanley (1973) indicate that one of the basic criteria for such designs is the extent to which they protect against the effect of extraneous variables on the outcome measures. The best designs are those which control relevant outside effects and lead to valid inferences about the effects of the program.

Unlike the experimental design, which protects against almost all possible outside effects, quasi-experiments have the advantage of being practical when conditions prevent true experimentation. However, these are not sloppy experiments, since evaluators know in advance what they do and do not control for. Any misrepresentation is understood and allowed for by the evaluator, who draws conclusions carefully.

Two quasi-experimental designs are worth mentioning here: the time series and the multiple time series.

Time Series

The time series design, one of the most attractive quasi-experiments, involves a series of measurements at periodic intervals before the program begins and after the program ends. It is possible to see whether the measures immediately before and after the program are a continuation of previous patterns or whether they indicate a noteworthy change. For example, in the area of nutrition, patients with any disease entity, such as anemia, are followed up via measurements of hemoglobin and hemotocrit. Over a period of time changes in hemoglobin and hemotocrit levels of the patient are observed.

Multiple Time Series

The second kind of quasi-experimental design is the multiple time series, which also has great validity. The evaluator tries to find a group or institution similar to the group in the program and takes the same periodic measurements during the same time span. Thus there is a control group to take care of any effects resulting naturally from the elapse of time. This design appears to be particularly appropriate for evaluations of school programs, such as nutrition education classes taught to students, since repeated testing goes on normally and long series of prescores and postscores are often available (Weiss, 1972).

Nonequivalent Control Groups

Another type of design, and probably the most common design in practice, is the use of a nonequivalent control group. Here there is no random assignment to program and control, as there would be in a true experiment, but available individuals, such as patients in the clinic with similar characteristics, are used in controls. For example, pregnant women attending a WIC clinic could be considered for a nonequivalent control group design. Such nonrandomized controls are generally referred to as comparison groups, since their before and after measures are compared with the program's groups.

Obviously, the evaluator must be aware of possible misrepresentation arising from the control groups, especially if the groups selected for the study had extreme scores such as a group of patients with elevated serum cholesterol levels (Morris and Fitz-Gibbon, 1978). A major problem is how to make the comparison groups as similar to the experimental group as possible.

Matching

Matching procedures are sometimes resorted to, in which members of the experimental and control groups are paired according to available measures. Sometimes the whole experimental group is matched with a similar group at the start of the program. Then the benefits of the program to the experimental group should be clear. However, experience shows that matching is much less satisfactory than randomized assignments because all variables cannot be controlled unless there is randomization.

Self-Selection

Another problem in selecting a comparison group is self-selection. People who choose to enter a program are likely to be different from those who do not. The problem of self-selection sometimes can be overcome if both experimentals and controls are selected from volunteers, and if the volunteers are randomly assigned to either group. This could be a condition for a true experiment. However, even when randomized assignment is not feasible, it is usually better to have some nonequivalent comparison group than no control at all.

Nonexperimental Designs

Sometimes it is impossible to use even a quasi-experimental design. The evaluator then has to resort to one of three common nonexperimental designs: (1) a "before and after" study of a single person, (2) an "after only" study of a program participant, or (3) an "after only" study of participants and nonrandom controls. The inherent weakness is that all of these designs fail to control many of the factors that might explain how observed changes were caused by something other than the program. At their best they can be detailed, provocative, and rich in insight. If the data are collected systematically and with care, they certainly offer more information than would have been possible without any study at all. In all cases, nonexperimental designs leave considerable room for differing interpretations of how much change has occurred and how much of the observed change was caused by the operation of the program. However, with all caveats, there are times when these designs may be worth considering if there are no other alternatives.

One reason for using a nonexperimental design is that it sometimes provides a preliminary look at the effectiveness of a program. If, for example, a before and after study, with all the contamination effects of outside events, maturation, testing, and so on, finds little change in participants, the program is probably having little effect. It may not be worthwhile to invest in more rigorous evaluation.

Often, desirable options may not be available to evaluators. They may not be called in until the program is in midstream, or they may not have access to comparative groups, since a great deal of evaluation is still being done under restrictive, unscientific conditions. It is always useful to consider ways to overcome any basic flaws in an evaluation procedure. This is why the nonexperimental design in public health and in nutrition can be an extremely useful tool (Weiss, 1972).

EVALUATION IN ACTION SETTINGS (SERVICE PROGRAMS)

It must be remembered that evaluation usually takes place while another, more primary, activity is going on—namely, that of the service program. Since evaluation most often occurs in an action setting, it must be adapted to the program environment and cause as little disruption as possible. Some interference is unavoidable, especially in the collection of data, when questions must be asked and answered. If the focus of the evaluation is clear, unnecessary intrusion can be avoided. Weiss (1972) points to three features of an evaluation in an action setting that researchers should be aware of: the tendency of the program to change while it is being evaluated; the relationship between the evaluator and program personnel; the setting of the program, usually within some institution or organization that in some way affects the outcome.

The Changing Program

Conscientious practitioners within a program will change their methods as they discover areas and means for improvements. For example, if there are new techniques developed for nutrition counseling, to effect behavioral change, the practitioner should employ them as soon as possible. Also, there may be changes in clientele and in community conditions. More money may become available; the staff or the political climate may change. All of these factors can affect viewpoints, principles, and the actual activity of the program, whether it is a model or experiment, and especially if it is a complex, long-range program.

The evaluator periodically must step back to observe these changes and also examine records, talk to personnel, and attend meetings having to do with the program. The evaluator, often in some manner an administrator of the program, should be particularly alert to changes in program management. The staff may make changes that they believe will produce more effective results, but the evaluator should be able to see how these fit in with the ultimate objectives.

Even if the evaluator is not in control, he or she still can influence program maintenance. The evaluator has the responsibility of preventing the program from straying from its original concept and operation.

In the model or developmental phase the program must be held stable for experimental evaluation, whereas in other stages less rigidity is acceptable and variable input is not only tolerated but expected (Wortman, 1981). If the reasons for program drifts are classified and analyzed, it seems possible to counteract them to some extent. Weiss (1972) offers these seven suggestions:

1. Take frequent periodic measures of the program's progress. For example, monthly assessing of training, therapy, and other aspects is better than limiting collection of outcome data to one point in time.
2. Encourage clear transitions if a program changes from one approach to another.
3. Clarify and classify the assumptions and procedures of each phase.
4. Keep careful records on persons who participated in each phase, rather than lumping all the participants together. Analyze outcomes in terms of the phases of the program.
5. Try to recycle or recapitulate earlier program phases. Sometimes this happens naturally. Re-

working a phase is a good way to check on earlier conclusions.
6. Seek to set aside funds to get approval for smaller-scale evaluations of at least one program phase or component that will remain stable for a given period.
7. If nothing works and the program continues to meander, consider giving up the evaluation in favor of meticulous analysis of the what, how, and why of events.

WHAT ARE THE ESSENTIAL STEPS IN PROGRAM EVALUATION?

There are several essential steps in the evaluation process of procedure outcomes. Weiss (1972) states that "evaluation is a demanding and necessary business, calling for time, imagination, tenacity and skill."

To set the tone for our discussion and to put planning and evaluation into proper perspective, we present Berg and Muscat's definition of planning (1972): "Planning is generally discussed in terms of a sequence of steps, but in practice it is rather an interactive process that resembles the tango, four steps forward, three steps back with an occasional turn-around."

To get in the mood to tango, Suchman's model for evaluation (1967) will be discussed (Figure 6-4). This model assists in determining what is measured in evaluation; what the elements of planning and evaluation are: how to get to the evaluation process; and how to plan effectively to be able to determine results.

The following case study will be used throughout the model to make the planning and evaluation process dynamic.

CASE STUDY OF OBESITY IN A PRESCHOOL POPULATION

The health-conscious administrator of the new ABC preschool program was concerned about the number of children in the program who appeared "pudgy" and who preferred to sit and play games rather than participate in some of the sports activities planned for them. His concern was heightened when he met several

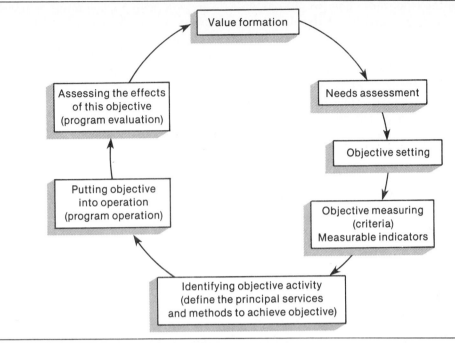

Figure 6-4. Suchman's circular scheme on evaluation.
Redrawn from "Suchman's Circular Scheme on Evaluation," adapted from Evaluative Research:
Principles and Practice in Public Service and Social Action Programs, by Edward A. Suchman.
Copyright © 1968 by Russell Sage Foundation. Reprinted by permission of Basic Books, Inc.

of the parents at a recent school function, many of whom were obese.

There are 35 children in the preschool program, 15 4 year olds and 20 5 year olds. There are 16 boys and 19 girls. The administrator estimates that at least 9 or 10 children are "very overweight." He arrived at this figure through observation (eyeball test) and through review of the height and weight measurements recently taken by the preschool teacher. She brings her bathroom scale to school to take the children's weight, and she used the measuring tape (cloth) from her sewing kit to provide measurements of height.

Lunch is served at the school for all children, and it is prepared by Mrs. Bolscvech, a delightful, large Polish woman who enjoys preparing her native dishes, such as sausage, potato pancakes, sauerkraut, and black bread, for the children.

The school serves a community of approximately 10,000 people, mostly blue-collar workers who are employed by the pickle plant. The employees receive health services from a health maintenance organization (HMO) that was established by the company. The costs of the health services are shared between employer and employees. Approximately 60% of the community are of Polish and Russian ancestry, and approximately 40% are blacks who were born and raised in this midwestern community.

After a discussion with the parents, the administrator has requested the services of the HMO health team (nutritionist, nurse, and physician), who suggested that the children be assessed and that those overweight be enrolled in a five-session counseling program.

The administration of the HMO is willing to provide the necessary personnel, equipment and materials to assist these children up to the maximum of $600 for program development and implementation.

Based on the case study, how would one develop a plan for an evaluation of this program?

Value Formation

In Suchman's scheme for evaluation (Figure 6-4), the first step considered is value formation. Value is defined as attributed or relative worth, merit, or usefulness. Chapter 3 describes values in detail. Thus the recognition of values helps health practitioners establish priorities and hierarchies of importance among needs and goals. Such value orientation occurs in all public services. Value determination on the part of professionals and the public creates the objectives and often the destiny of public service programs.

In the case study the administrator of the preschool program valued the importance of good health practices, such as proper nutrition, maintaining normal body weight, and exercise.

Needs Assessment

The initial step in the planning and evaluation process is the needs assessment. If this step is overlooked, or done carelessly, the rest of the process may end up being completely off base. Therefore a clear description of what the need is and what problem it is going to solve is very important (Chapter 3).

Describing the Need

Describing the need is often called community diagnosis. For a hospitalized patient it is described as the clinical and nutrition assessment to reach a diagnosis to facilitate a plan for care.

Community diagnosis is an attempt to identify as fully as possible what the health problems with nutrition implications are and what resources are currently available (Christakis, 1973). A community, in this instance, could also be a hospital where one is attempting to define the health problems of the total number of patients and the levels of nutrition care required by the patients. This diagnosis then enables the dietetic practitioner to implement solutions. Gathering existing data on these and other fac-

tors will help to determine whether the community's or individual patient's nutrition resources are adequate, what groups or persons are potentially at high risk, and how well community and nutrition-related health needs are being met by existing curative and preventive health programs (Chapter 3).

To complete an adequate diagnosis of a community or patient, one must realize that nutrition problems originate from complex interrelationships between environmental and social factors and the individuals in the community. Christakis (1973) lists 16 areas that pertain to community assessment (pp. 46 and 47).

After compiling data on all or most of the 16 areas, the evaluator is ready to describe the need for a particular effort.

The final achievement of all program planning and evaluation is meeting a need, satisfying a want, or alleviating an existing condition.

A look at the case study reveals that some data are available in 8 of the 16 areas cited in Chapter 3:

1. Demographic information—community of approximately 10,000 people in the Midwest
2. Socioeconomic stratification—mostly blue-collar workers employed by the pickle plant
3. Health statistics resources—morbidity and mortality: limited information is provided here; however, employees of the pickle plant receive health services from the company with a cost sharing plan between employer and employees
4. Local health resources—HMO, preschool facility
5. Dental health—no information
6. Cultural factors—approximately 60% of the community are of Polish and Russian ancestry, and approximately 40% are blacks who were born and raised in this midwestern community
7. Community political organizations—limited information
8. Housing—no information

9. Food supply—only information on lunch at preschool
10. School nutrition program—information on the preschool lunch is provided; the meal described appears to be high in calories
11. Social welfare—no information
12. Transportation—no information
13. Education—limited information
14. Occupational data—major industry is pickle plant
15. Geography and environment—Midwest
16. Surveillance data—none

Obtaining this information is vital before initiating services for these children.

Setting Objectives

One of the most important elements in the planning and evaluation process is developing sound objectives. These objectives should be based on the information collected in the needs assessment. If the objectives are not clear, concise, and measurable, the evaluation will be ineffective, since the evaluator cannot identify where he or she started. Inadequate objectives make results difficult to identify. A major discussion of goals, objectives, outcome, and process appears on pp. 54-57.

Examples of an outcome and process objective for the case study follow:

Outcome. To reduce the amount of obesity in the 4- and 5-year-old children by 80% (8 of 10 children) to their ideal weight, which is 22 kg (40 lb) (50th percentile), in a 6-month period using the existing HMO health and nutrition team

Process. To develop a system that includes nutrition assessment, nutrition counseling for children and their families, and follow-up services on a regularly scheduled basis to alleviate the problem, using the existing HMO health and nutrition team, within a 6-month period

Use of the terms *outcome* and *process* may be called a *hierarchy* of objectives, all working toward the major health outcome.

Objective Measuring Criteria (Measurable Indicators)

The kind of evaluation that is performed depends largely on the type of measures available for determining the accomplishment of the objectives. For example, if the objective states that obesity should be reduced in the preschool children seen at the preschool center, then the community dietitian/nutritionist needs some measures for determining how many children are obese and by what criteria. A criterion (measurable indicator) that could be written for the obese child (4 to 5 years of age) follows:

> Child achieves weight/height equal to or less than 95th percentile when plotted on NCHS growth chart.

Objective measuring has definite implications for quality assurance in dietetics (Chapter 7). The criteria in quality assurance are the yardsticks, the predetermined elements against which service or the dietetic objectives can be compared.

Identifying and Implementing Objectives

The activities used to implement the plan must be systematic and realistic. *Systematic* implies that the steps which are taken to meet objectives should fit together as a cohesive whole. Clearly stating objectives will be a great help in making methods systematic.

Nutrition intervention strategies are considered in this area (Chapter 8). The plan is set for action and actual operation. To operationalize any nutrition plan, the elements of quality nutrition services must be included:

- Nutrition screening and assessment, including anthropometric, biochemical, clinical, medical, dietary, and socioeconomic factors
- Nutrition intervention, including nutrition education/counseling and a plan for the care of each client or patient
- Referral to other service providers
- Evaluation to determine results of services

An example of the steps in an action plan using the preschool case study is included in Figure 6-5.

Objective: To reduce the amount of obesity in 4- and 5-year-old children by 80% (8 of the 10 children) to their ideal weight, which is 18 kg (40 lb) (50th percentile), in a 6-month period using the existing HMO health and nutrition team.

Action steps (method)	Time frame	Personnel responsible
A. Nutrition assessment:		
1. Complete measurements of height and weight for all children in the center using standardized equipment. The scale must be calibrated regularly, and a fixed measuring rod other than that on the scale should be used. Measurements will be taken by two people (nurse and nutritionist), and weight must agree within 100 gm and heights must agree within 0.5 cm.	Within 1 month of program initiation	Nurse and nutritionist
2. Complete skinfold measurement including: a. Thoracic b. Triceps c. Subscapular Measurements will be taken by two people (nurse and nutritionist); skinfold measurements must agree within 0.5 mm.	Within 1 month of program initiation	Nurse and nutritionist
3. Complete a clinical assessment of children.	Within 1 month of program initiation	Physician
4. Complete dietary history including socioeconomic information by using a combination of 24-hour recall and food frequency. Make appointments to discuss the recall with each child's parents or caretaker.	Within 2 months of program initiation	Nutritionist
B. Nutrition intervention:		
1. Develop a patient care plan based on results of nutrition assessment.	Within 1 week after nutrition assessment is completed	Nutritionist
2. Monitor patients on a weekly basis to determine compliance with diet and exercise regimen.	Weekly	Nutritionist
3. Record data at each patient visit.		
C. Evaluation:		
1. Prepare computerized data collection forms to include data from nutrition assessment and intervention information.	Before working with patients on nutrition intervention	Nutritionist and HMO team member
2. Review data collected on a weekly basis and make necessary changes in intervention strategies.	Weekly	Nutritionist
3. Summarize data on a 3-month and 6-month basis to determine if results have been achieved.	3 and 6 months	Nutritionist presents information to HMO team and parents of children

Figure 6-5. Example of action plan for the case study (p. 120).

Assessing the Effects of the Objective-Program Evaluation

Evaluation is concerned with determining values or worth. On the basis of an assessment of an objective-oriented operation, a judgment is made as to whether the activity was worthwhile. This step actually brings one back to the value formation. At the end of the evaluation process one may get a new value, or one may reaffirm, revise, or redefine an old value. The question of what has been accomplished is the issue here. For example, in the preschool case study, did you, as stated in your objective, reduce the amount of obesity in the 4- and 5-year-old children by 80% to the ideal weight in a 6-month period? If you have met this objective, fine. If not, why? What were the obstacles or constraints?

Basic Processes of Evaluation

There are two basic processes of evaluation: measurement and comparison. Measurement is at the core of all evaluation. It has been defined as the assignment of numbers to objects or events according to rules. *Comparison* is defined as the examination of characteristics or qualities to discover similarities or differences.

We will now look at (1) what to evaluate, (2) measures used to do the evaluation, and (3) threats to internal validity.

WHAT TO EVALUATE

There are five distinct categories of evaluation that we will focus on: appropriateness, adequacy, effectiveness, efficiency, and side effects (Deniston, 1972).

Appropriateness relates to the extent to which programs are directed toward those problems which are believed to have the greatest importance. In other words, is it right to use these resources to do these activities and strategies to stress for this objective? One question related to appropriateness might be: Was the situation defined as a problem by program personnel also considered a problem by society?

In the case study how appropriate was the program to reduce obesity in preschool children?

The situation—obese children—was considered a problem by the administrator, parents, and health workers at the HMO. Therefore this would be an appropriate program to pursue.

Adequacy is concerned with the extent of a problem that a particular program intends to eliminate. Are these resources "enough" to carry out the activities? Are you doing "enough" activity to have the strategy to work? Is the strategy "sufficient to accomplish the objective?" Is the objective "big enough" given the size of the problem?

In the case study the problem involves 10 obese children. It appeared that acceptable weight reduction could be obtained in 8, or 80%, of the children. This estimate appears to be adequate. Working with only 1 child out of 10 would be inadequate for this particular situation.

Effectiveness concerns the extent to which preestablished program objectives are attained as a result of program activity. Have you used the resources you planned to, and do they combine to produce the planned activities? Do your activities result in a completed strategy? Was the planned strategy carried out, and has it resulted in the objective being met? To what extent has the objective been met and the problem reduced? In other words, what are the results of your program? Effectiveness must always be determined before efficiency (cost) can be determined, since you must know your results before you can put a price tag on what you accomplished.

In the preschool case study the preestablished objective was to reduce obesity in eight children in 6 months. Suppose, for example, that only seven children showed weight loss. The effectiveness level would then be 88% (7 divided by 8). If it was stated that 8 children would lose weight and only 2 children actually did, the effectiveness rate would only be 25%.

Efficiency relates to the cost in resources of attaining objectives. Could resources be combined efficiently or different resources be used so that the same activities could be produced at lower costs? Could the activity process be changed so that the same activities could be produced at lower costs? How costly is the strategy compared to the benefits obtained? Would another strategy accomplish the same objective at lower costs? How does the actual cost compare with the planned cost for meeting the objective?

For the purposes of the case study, suppose that each of the five parent-child counseling sessions cost $12, which amounts to $60 for each child. With 10 children, the amount of funds—$600—committed by the HMO would cover the cost of the project. Remember that in planning an actual program the cost of assessment and follow-up also needs to be included. However, in this case the administrator budgeted for counseling services and used his budget to fund assessment and follow-up.

Side effects are effects of program operations other than attainment of objectives. They pertain to all possible effects that could have occurred, both positive and negative, anticipated and unanticipated.

At the preschool the impression was that parents became involved in weight reduction sessions and learned methods to control food intake and to cut calories.

WHAT IS BEING MEASURED: THE CHARACTERISTICS OF MEASURES

Consideration must be given to the characteristics of measures in any evaluation scheme, including validity, reliability, precision, completeness, and coverage (Deniston, 1972).

Validity of measures can be viewed as the extent to which the nature of the phenomenon of interest (i.e., the total of all parts, including scientific description) has actually been assessed. Validity tells you whether you are really measuring what you think you are measuring.

In the case study it was decided to measure height, weight, and skinfolds. Do these measurements allow one to estimate body fat in children? Measurements of body density, total body water, and total body potassium are the best indirect research methods for estimating body fat. How-

ever, noninvasive clinical determinations such as height, weight, and skinfold thickness provide acceptable indicators of body fat. Another method, carcass analysis, is hardly practical, since there would be few volunteers. Using the eyeball test alone, as the administrator did, would provide sufficient information to begin an intervention program but would be difficult to use in measuring results with any great accuracy.

Reliability refers to the ability to obtain the same results with repeated measures. Reliability refers to the repeatability of a measurement: would the same person get the same result twice or would two or more people get the same results measuring the same way? Note from the action plan that both the nurse and the nutritionist perform height, weight, and skinfold measurements. These data will assist with testing of reliability of measures.

Precision defines the extent to which a measurement technique can discriminate between differences in magnitude. The ends of this continuum may be labeled *crude* and *precise*. In the case study crude versus precise would refer to the following: measuring skinfold thickness to the nearest 1 mm would be less precise than if it were measured to the nearest 0.5 mm.

Completeness is the extent to which a phenomenon of interest (total of all parts including scientific description) is assessed in totality rather than in part. In the preschool population, consider the extent to which the indices (height, weight, and skinfolds) captured the total concept of body fat rather than some narrow aspect of it. If an evaluator decided to measure only weight, without height and skinfolds, measurements would be less complete.

Coverage is the extent to which measurements are applied to each client or clients. The session in the preschool could conceivably be attended by all parents and children, therefore providing good coverage. If only 2 children out of 10 and 1 parent showed up, the session would have poor coverage.

WHAT CAN GO WRONG: THREATS TO INTERNAL VALIDITY

When we begin to talk about internal validity, the researchers indicate quite readily that the closer one comes to the experimental design in their program the more valid the results. The experimental design addresses control and comparison groups and may be impractical in a delivery system setting (pp. 117 and 118). However, comparison groups may be readily available in a clinic setting where there are people on a waiting list for services—they could be the ready-made comparison group. This situation may assist the evaluator to demonstrate change in the group he or she is working with versus those who have not had the benefit of counseling.

There are several areas that can go wrong if strategies are not properly planned. The threats to internal validity include the following (Campbell and Stanley, 1973):

1. *History*—events may occur in addition to the experimental treatment and thus provide alternate explanations of effects. For example, parents may have already instituted changes in the preschool children's diets when the administrator expressed concern initially. This action would make a difference in the results. It would be important in planning the program to obtain an initial history for each child to determine these events.

2. *Maturation*—events within the respondents produce changes as a function of the passage of time per se such as growth and secular trends. A frequently heard comment from some people is that children get taller and "grow out of their fat." In the preschool program it is important to take accurate height, weight, and skinfold measurements in the initial and follow-up assessments to control for this problem.

3. *Instrumentation (accuracy)*—changes in the calibration of a measuring instrument or changes in the observer's scores may produce changes in the obtained measure-

ments. In the preschool program scales must be properly calibrated, and calipers must be properly adjusted.

4. *Testing*—the effects of taking a test on the scores of a second testing. The parents in the preschool population may have made subsequent changes in a child's diet on their own as a result of the initial assessment, and the school may have instituted a more vigorous program in physical fitness after the initial assessment of the children.

5. *Regression artifacts (statistical regression)* —pseudoshifts occurring when persons or treatment units have been selected on the basis of their extreme scores. When an evaluator selects people with extreme scores, such as obese children, he or she may have trouble with statistical regression. One way to solve this problem would be to involve all preschool children in the assessment and counseling session.

6. *Experimental mortality*—the differential loss of respondents from comparison groups. If some children came to the initial session to be assessed and then dropped out, experimental mortality has occurred.

7. *Selection*—biases resulting from differential recruitment of comparison groups, producing different mean levels of the measures of effects. If a comparison group were to be used, the sample would have to be selected very carefully.

8. *Instability*—unreliability of measures or fluctuations in sampling persons or components. This problem could occur in the preschool program if untrained measurers were used at first and then trained; they would have high reliability afterwards, but their measurements would be unreliable initially. This factor would yield inaccurate data. Another problem that often occurs is improper recording of measurements.

The following checklist may assist in completing the evaluation:

- Reviews precise objectives that were to be accomplished
- Defines evaluation criteria
- Describes data gathering methods
- Explains any test instruments, questionnaires, or indices to be used
- Describes the process of data analysis
- Shows how evaluation will be used for program improvements

USE OF EVALUATION RESULTS: IMPLICATION FOR PROGRAM ADMINISTRATORS

Once the evaluation report, with all its data and findings, is completed, it should be given to the manager of the program. The next issue is the implementation of change, if it is called for. Often there are constraints to change that evaluators should consider as they produce their reports.

The Role of Evaluators

Many researchers see themselves as part of an academic community to whom they look for recognition, rather than part of a practical public service program. After evaluators have determined the results of their investigation, they often do not draw conclusions or propose recommendations for actual implementation of a change for the better. They then may wonder why their work is neglected by practitioners. However, even if evaluators have not followed through with recommendations, it is up to the practical administrators and decision makers to use the data themselves and thus not waste the large amount of time and money that has undoubtedly gone into the evaluation (Levine and Hughes, 1981).

Resistance by the Institution

Sometimes an evaluation report may clearly point to certain revisions, but they are resisted by the program's organization for various reasons. Change is usually difficult and requires some extra effort; it also generally means that more money is spent and the staff is disrupted. These results could involve a revision of roles and rela-

tionships with personnel, the community, and funders. Also, change might mean a reconsideration of basic ideology, commitments, and methodology—areas in which change is particularly difficult and threatening.

Revisions and the Gap Between Evaluation and Action

Because of such natural resistance, certain specific techniques should be employed to overcome it. It is the administrator's role to make an effort to use the results of the evaluation to improve the program and to reward or encourage staff members who co-operate with him or her. Another technique suggested by Weiss (1972) includes early recognition of the need for particular revisions and of those persons who will put them into practice, selection of issues of special concern, involvement of the staff in planning and conducting the revisions, and also the usefulness of an evaluation in disseminating information. Another consideration in implementing revisions should be the timing of the report, especially if it makes use of comparisons of various methods or procedures.

Evaluation results are also of interest to funding agencies. These policy makers are the ones who decide whether or not to continue a program or to decrease or increase its funding. Information on the evaluation should be given to them and also to boards of education, state departments, hospitals, and other public service agencies for the purposes of gaining visibility and publicity for the program being studied and for demonstrating the need and value of evaluation (Wholey, 1981).

Evaluation does not provide all the answers and often presents no clear path for improvement. However, it can show evidence to those in a decision-making capacity. An evaluation can also indicate with some authority what are likely outcomes or consequences of recommended revisions. This feature is of particular interest if a radical revision is suggested by the evaluation.

Another result of the evaluation of nutrition services is accountability. The evaluation process

Table 6-1. Accountability in public health

Responsible Party	Accountable to Whom	In the Area of	For the Purpose of	Measurable by
Program administrators	Public at large	Communicable disease Prevention	Attaining acceptable standards of quality of life	Mortality, morbidity
	Individual consumer	Services provided	Quality, quantity, adequacy of services provided	Mortality, morbidity
	Providers (participants)	Fees, roles in decision making, planning, working conditions	Acceptable life-style, prestige, self-esteem	Provider feedback, staff turnover
	Governmental bodies	Effectiveness, efficiency, adequacy of program	Satisfaction of constituency; funding, legislation	Fiscal, mortality, morbidity assessment; favorable public image
	Parent organization	Program priorities, efficiency, effectiveness	Organizational and financial support to meet consumer needs	Mortality, morbidity, administrative guidelines, standards
	Sister organizations	Communication, cooperation, program assistance	Coordination of efforts to meet community needs; stimulate community interest; better public image	Formation, frequency of meeting of joint councils; degree of cooperation in joint projects
	Professional organizations	Service priorities, patient eligibility, service components, support of professional organizations	Professional recognition; professional and political support	Professional organizations' endorsements and cooperation
	News media	Communication; cooperation	Maintaining public image; political and financial support	Media's support of agency's efforts
	Special interest	Cooperation with efforts in their special interests	Public image, financial and political support	Degree of cooperation sought by special groups

Modified from Your accountability for health—how much is lots? Presented at Forty-first Annual Meeting, Southern Branch American Public Health Association, Louisville, Ky., May 9-11, 1973.

is not complete unless the results are appropriately communicated. *Accountable* may be defined as "being answerable." But questions may arise: Answerable to whom? In what area? For what purpose? Answers to these questions appear in Table 6-1, which demonstrates the wide variety of persons, areas, and purposes that are implicated in the process of accountability.

Negative Evaluation Results

As indicated earlier, and as Elinson (1967) points out, there is a significant tendency for a thorough and objective investigative analysis to show negative results; that is, it shows that the program has little or negligible effect. This tendency has the unfortunate consequence of making program administrators less open to evaluation and more suspicious of its value. Furthermore, large established programs are the ones that are rarely evaluated; rather, it is the smaller, innovative program that is trying to do something new that usually must undergo an evaluation. Often these small programs are just the ones that should be encouraged.

An evaluation with negative results may indicate that the more straightforward aspects of medical, educational, and general social reform have been accomplished but that the more complex problems of efficient use of time and talent need more attention. There are many competing and overlapping programs, and there is a need for interrelated and integrated programs instead of huge, single-issue programs or a number of small, fragmentary programs. Evaluation can be the most useful tool in pointing out the specific needs in the complex area of administration.

Just as any program needs appropriate planning and administration to succeed, so too does useful evaluation. An evaluation is the means by which the success and effects of a program can be measured, and it can point out the direction for beneficial changes in a program. It also helps ensure that the program is responsible to both its clientele and its funders. Although the roles and even the personalities of the evaluator and the program practitioners may seem different, every effort at cooperation and planning together should be made so that the work of both proceeds to produce the most beneficial effects.

Program evaluation is commonly thought of as a dry, fruitless endeavor, extolled in theory but ignored in practice. Under conditions of limited resources, the application of program evaluation is more than an opportunity; it is a necessity. In Chapter 7 we will discuss additional control measures such as budgeting and quality assurance.

SUMMARY

Controlling nutrition services to achieve outcomes is the vital process through which managers ensure that actual activities conform to planned activities. Program evaluation is one of the methods of control used in health services. Although evaluation is a difficult process in action setting because of the changing nature of the program, it is necessary and worthwhile. This chapter addresses the issues of what to evaluate, what is being measured, and what can go wrong in evaluation.

REFERENCES

Alkin, M.C., and Solomon, L.: The costs of evaluation, Beverly Hills, 1982, Sage Publications, Inc.

Anthony, R.N., and Dearden, J.: Management control systems, ed. 4, Homewood, Ill., 1980, Richard D. Irwin, Inc.

Berg, A., and Muscat, R.: An approach to nutrition planning, Am. J. Clin. Nutr. 25:939, 1972.

Bohrnstedt, G.W.: Measurement. In Rossi, P.H., et al., editors: Handbook of survey research, New York, 1982, Academic Press, Inc.

Campbell, D.T., and Stanley, J.C.: Experimental and quasi-experimental designs for research in teaching. In Travers, R.M.W., editor: Second handbook of research on teaching, Skokie, Ill., 1973, Rand McNally & Co.

Christakis, G., editor: Nutritional assessment in health programs, Am. J. Public Health 63(suppl.):1, 1973.

Cronbach, L.J., et al.: Toward reform of program evaluation, San Francisco, 1980, Jossey-Bass, Inc., Publishers.

Deniston, O.L.: Evaluation of disease control programs, USDHHS, Public Health Service, Washington, D.C., March 1972, U.S. Government Printing Office.

Elinson, J.: Effectiveness of social action programs in health and welfare. In Assessing the effectiveness of child health services, Report of the 56th Ross Conference, Columbus, Ohio, 1967, Ross Laboratories.

Gordon, J.E., and Scrimshaw, N.S.: Evaluating nutrition intervention programs, Nutrition Rev. **30**:263, 1972.

Havens, H.S.: Public management forum, Public Administration Rev. **41**:480, 1981.

Levine, L.C., and Hughes, E.F.X.: Research on the utilization of evaluation: a review and synthesis, Evaluation Rev. **5**:525, 1981.

Levine, R.A., Solomon, M.A., and Hellstern, G.N., editors: Evaluation and research and practice: comparative and international perspectives, Beverly Hills, 1981, Sage Publications, Inc.

Meredith, J.: Program evaluation techniques in health services, Am. J. Public Health **66**:1069, 1976.

Morris, L.L., and Fitz-Gibbon, C.T.: Evaluation handbook, Center for the Study of Evaluation, University of California, Los Angeles, Beverly Hills, 1978, Sage Publications, Inc.

Neumann, A.K., Neumann, C.G., and Ifekwunique, A.E.: Evaluation of small scale nutrition programs, Am. J. Clin. Nutr. **26**:446, 1973.

Rossi, P.H., and Freeman, H.E.: Evaluation: a systematic approach, ed. 2, Beverly Hills, 1982, Sage Publications, Inc.

Stoner, J.A.F.: Management, ed. 2, Englewood Cliffs, N.J., 1982, Prentice-Hall, Inc.

Suchman, E.A.: Evaluative research, New York, 1967, Russell Sage Foundation.

Tolpin, H.G.: Costs/benefit analysis: an overview in costs and benefits of nutritional care phase I, Chicago, 1979, The American Dietetic Association.

Weiss, C.H.: Evaluation research, methods of assessing program effectiveness, Englewood Cliffs, N.J., 1972, Prentice-Hall, Inc.

Wholey, J.S.: Using evaluation to improve program performance. In Levine, R.A., editor: Evaluation research and practice: comparative and international perspectives, Beverly Hills, 1981, Sage Publications, Inc.

Wortman, P.M.: Methods for evaluating health services, Beverly Hills, 1981, Sage Publications, Inc.

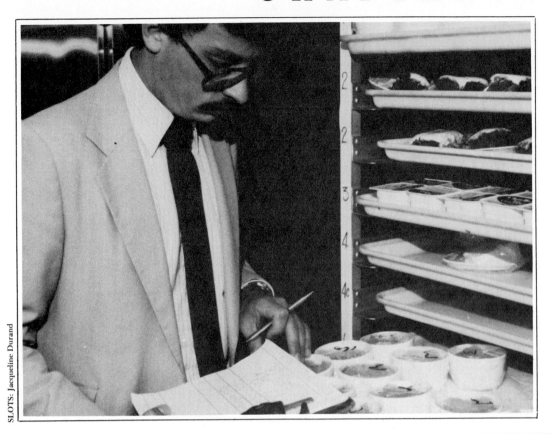

SLOTS: Jacqueline Durand

Quality Assurance, Financial Control, and Cost-Effectiveness/Benefit Measures

GENERAL CONCEPT

Individuals within hospitals or health agencies who complete quality assurance steps can measure and monitor health care to assure that it is effective and efficient to improve consumer outcomes. An understanding of sound financial control is one of the most important responsibilities in health and nutrition administration. Knowledge of cost-effectiveness analysis (CEA) and cost-benefit analysis (CBA) is imperative in today's economic climate. CEA and CBA are analytical techniques that community dietitians/nutritionists should use to allocate resources.

When you finish this chapter, you should be able to

- Define quality assurance and the five principles generic to any quality assurance program
- Identify the differences between quality assurance and evaluation
- Define the steps in developing a quality assurance program
- Describe the elements of a performance budget and indicate the possible advantages and precautions of this type of budget
- Describe the difference between CEA and CBA
- Define the 10 principles of CEA/CBA methodology
- Describe the factors that affect the use of CEA/CBA

Quality assurance, financial control, and cost-effectiveness/benefit analysis are important parts of the controlling process in management (Figure 7-1).

QUALITY ASSURANCE

The major impetus to formalizing and documenting quality assurance activities in health care was the establishment of Professional Standards Review Organizations (PSROs) for the evaluation of the quality of health care services. PSROs were mandated by section 249F of Public Law 92-603 in October 1972 and were required to involve local practicing physicians in the ongoing review and evaluation of health care services provided by Medicare, Medicaid, and Title V (Maternal and Child Health) of the Social Security Act. More recently the Joint Commission on Accreditation of Hospitals (JCAH) has mandated quality assurance as an accreditation requirement. *Guidelines on Dietetic Services*, published by the JCAH (1978), mandates hospitals to document ongoing programs of quality assurance for dietetic services.

The American Dietetic Association (ADA) has provided leadership in the development of quality assurance in dietetic practice since 1973, with the appointment of a Professional Standards Review Committee, which is now called the Quality Assurance Committee. Three documents were completed by ADA committees that are considered the basic references for dietitian/nutritionist practitioners: *Guidelines for Evaluating Dietetic Practice, Professional Standards Review Procedure Manual,* and *Patient Care Audit* (ADA, 1976, 1979).

What Is Quality Assurance?

Quality assurance is defined as a problem-solving approach to measure and monitor health care to assure that it is effective and efficient. The goal of quality assurance is to achieve care that improves consumer outcomes (Kaufman, 1983). A quality assurance program assists practitioners to base decisions for patient care on the most accurate available scientific knowledge and proven practices. The result should be health care that is more predictable and efficient.

Williamson (1979) indicates that a comprehensive quality assurance system is characterized by a deductive problem-oriented approach to achieving outcomes in health care. According to Williamson, the five principles generic to any comprehensive quality assurance system relate to the following:

1. *Motivation.* Quality assurance must be internally motivated; commitment to it is most effectively inspired by the incentive of measured accomplishment.
2. *Administration.* Quality assurance must be integrated into local health care management functions.
3. *Content.* Quality assurance must have a sufficiently comprehensive scope to identify all areas having the greatest need or potential for improvement.
4. *Function.* Quality assurance must be an ongoing improvement activity applying multiple methods most suited to content.
5. *Evaluation.* Quality assurance must ultimately

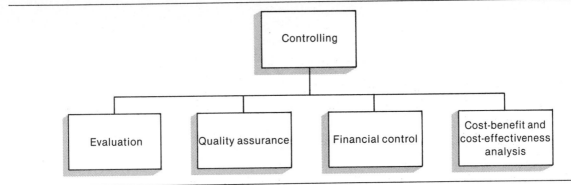

Figure 7-1. Controlling process in managing nutrition services.

be evaluated in terms of health, economic, and social improvements in relation to time, money, and resource expenditures.

Characteristics of Ambulatory Care

Ambulatory care settings, versus acute or inpatient care settings, have unique characteristics that present some challenges in the development of quality assurance efforts (O'Neal, 1978):

1. There is often no distinct episode of illness with clear beginning and end points. The patient's perception of illness may be vague.
2. Access to care is controlled by the client, who can choose to keep or not keep appointments. There may be long periods of time between visits. Surveillance of health problems may be brief and intermittent.
3. Control of the treatment plan and ongoing care are contingent on the understanding, motivation, and active involvement of the client and family.
4. Health or medical records and data systems in ambulatory care settings may not be as well organized as in inpatient care settings. Standards for recording health data may be developed or implemented; there may be less agreement on what to chart, and notations may be brief.

Difference Between Evaluation and Quality Assurance

Quality assurance is one of the control mechanisms available to health providers which at-

tempts to assure that health care is effective and efficient. Evaluation is concerned specifically with determining the worth or value of efforts expended to achieve a given purpose or objective (Chapter 3). Program objectives are a major focus of the evaluation model. *Quality assurance* is defined as the certification of continuous, effective, and efficient care (Owen, 1984). Criteria (predetermined elements against which quality of care or services can be compared) used for quality assurance should be the basis on which the practitioner develops measurable objectives (Figures 6-4 and 7-2).

The nutrition program plan (p. 137), including evaluation, provides the framework for nutrition services and is the initial component required to develop a quality assurance system.

Achieving Quality Assurance in Ambulatory Nutrition Care

The goal of health providers in using quality assurance techniques is to guarantee that nutrition care practices produce favorable patient outcomes. Accomplishing this goal requires:

1. Establishing ambulatory nutrition care standards based on current scientific knowledge and practice
2. Adapting these standards to individual program needs and incorporating these standards into ambulatory nutrition programs

RELATIONSHIP OF QUALITY ASSURANCE TO PROGRAM PLANNING AND EVALUATION

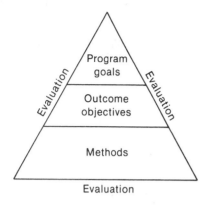

Program planning and evaluation*

Goal:	To improve the nutritional health of infants
Outcome:	90% of underweight infants will be identified for appropriate intervention
Methods:	Height will be measured. Weight will be measured. Growth charts will be plotted.

COMPARE

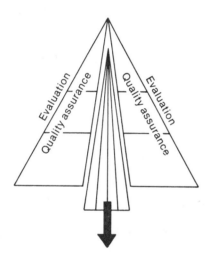

Quality assurance system*

Goal:	Infants at nutrition risk will be accurately identified for intervention.
Outcome:	75% of underweight infants will consume adequate calories to achieve weight for length at or above the 5th percentile within 6 months.
Process:	Sliding foot piece touches bottom of infant's feet at both heels when length measurement is read. Infant is weighed nude.
Structure:	Recumbent length measuring board will agree with 1/16 inch of a standard length statiometer.

*Incomplete examples.

Figure 7-2. Sentinel Site project, Detroit Health Department.
Redrawn from Wong, F.: Description of quality assurance system quality assurance manual for anthropometry. I, Atlanta, 1984, Centers for Disease Control.

ELEMENTS OF QUALITY ASSURANCE INTEGRATED INTO THE NUTRITION PROGRAM

1. *Nutrition program plan* provides the framework for nutrition services. It specifies the structural criteria by including the work plan, budget, and staff.
2. *Professional standards of practice* should be based on appropriate, current research and practice and require continuing review of the nutrition and health care literature.
3. *Policies and procedures* define the specific nutrition services to be provided to defined target populations.
4. *Process and outcome criteria* are standards against which to audit standards of practice. These criteria, written to be concrete, realistic, understandable, measurable, behavioral, and achieveable (RUMBA), are the basis for the program plan objectives.

5. *Documentation/recording of care* is usually in the health/medical record where it can be shared by all health care providers and utilized for audit.
6. *Written audit system* indicates areas to be studied, as well as how, by whom, and how often.
7. *Statistical reporting system* summarizes data on services rendered to patients and includes status of caseload and client outcomes in relation to stated objectives.
8. *Educational plan* for inservice education for staff is designed to help correct any identified problems or deficiencies.

Reprinted from Kaufman, M., editor: Guide to quality assurance in ambulatory nutrition care, Chicago, 1983, The American Dietetic Association.

---

3. Determining program effectiveness and identifying areas of acceptable performance
4. Providing a sense of accomplishment and recognition to those achieving standards of performance
5. Identifying areas of unacceptable performance where improvements can be achieved
6. Initiating action to correct problems associated with inadequate and/or unacceptable performance (Kaufman, 1983)

Quality Assurance in Program Planning and Evaluation

The basic components of a comprehensive nutrition program integrating a quality assurance system are described above.

Criteria used for quality assurance should be the basis for the development of measurable program objectives by the program manager. A program plan should be developed with those involved in its implementation and should specify how the desired results will be achieved. Components of the program plan are described in detail in Chapter 3.

The elements of a nutrition program plan provide the manager with the tools to anticipate results and conduct ongoing evaluation. Measurable objectives based on valid criteria determine the data needed to judge the achievement of the program objectives and focus on program improvement. Process criteria guide the program planner in the selection of methods to achieve desired outcomes and suggest which elements of care require documentation. Program evaluation is conducted to determine whether the methods have been implemented and anticipated results have been achieved. Results of evaluation assist the manager in making decisions on ways to improve the program and provide feedback to the program staff about which methods are effective and which are deficient.

Developing Quality Assurance Measures for Ambulatory Nutrition Services

A complete guide for quality assurance, entitled *Guide to Quality Assurance and Ambulatory Nutrition Care* (Kaufman, 1983), describes in detail the steps to develop a quality assurance program. This is an important document for any community dietitian/nutritionist who is developing a quality assurance program.

Three major aspects of care have been used to measure quality: outcome, process, and structure. Generic criteria, such as program plans and policies and procedures for assessment, are also suggested here for the program in which care is provided to target populations. A definition of outcome, process, and structure follows.*

Outcome

Outcome is the end result or consequence of health and/or nutrition care. Outcomes are considered the ultimate indicators of quality measuring the actual health status of the client. In nutrition care, outcome measures are based on anthropometric, biochemical, clinical, and dietary intake data (Chapter 8). Proximal or intermediate outcome measures are accepted as indicative of short-term changes even though these may not actually measure the correction of nutritional health problems. Intermediate measurements that may be used with varying degrees of validity are changes in client nutrition knowledge, attitudes, and/or eating practices. A complete review of outcome and process objectives is included in Chapter 3.

Process

Although outcomes are the ultimate indicators of success, there are many intervening factors that make it difficult to accurately assess the single impact of nutrition care. Therefore it is necessary and possible to evaluate the process. Process is defined as the sequence of established activities or procedures used by providers in the delivery of health care. In nutrition care, process elements include assessment, establishment of the plan for counseling and education, prescription for food and/or nutrient supplements, referrals, and follow-up. Written policies and procedures or protocols can serve as a basis for identifying key process criteria.

*The material in the following sections (pp. 138-143) is reprinted from Kaufman, M., editor: Guide to quality assurance in ambulatory nutrition care, Chicago, 1983, The American Dietetic Association.

Structure

Structure refers to the personnel, equipment, and facilities required to carry out the processes of health and/or nutrition care. Examples include staff qualifications, staffing ratios, assessment equipment (such as scales or skinfold calipers), educational materials, training aids, space, and laboratory services.

Criteria for Nutrition Services in Health Care Delivery
Program Criteria

A nutrition program plan containing statements of problems, objectives, methods, and evaluation (POME) is written and integrated as a component of the agency's health services plan (process or P). Policies and procedures or protocols on assessment, intervention, and referral are written for the delivery of nutrition services (P).

Patient/Client Care Criteria

An assessment of the client's nutrition status is recorded (P). It includes the following data:
- Anthropometric
- Biochemical
- Clinical/medical/dental
- Dietary
- Socioeconomic

Based on the assessment, the decision for case management (determination of need, provision of anticipatory guidance, provision or referral for counseling, or referral to other providers or services) is documented (P).

A plan of care is developed for each client by the provider with the client who is assessed to require anticipatory guidance or counseling. This plan is written as a component of the client's care record (P).

The client's written plan of care includes the following:
1. Statement of nutrition problem/need
2. Objectives of care
3. Methods of care
4. Provision for follow-up care
5. Evaluation or review of patient's progress (P). (A SOAP [subjective, objective, assessment, and plan] note format can be used.)

Documentation

It is essential to document that the procedures are actually carried out in order to assess the processes of care. Process assessments compare the documented care with what is accepted as optimum practice based on current scientific nutrition knowledge and expert opinion. Similarly recorded laboratory data, anthropometric measures, dietary assessments, knowledge tests, and attitudinal surveys document outcomes.

In ambulatory care, documentation most frequently occurs in the patient's medical record and/or family folder. The problem-oriented medical record (POMR) and SOAP note format for recording information are valuable sources of documentation in quality assurance programs, since this record format organizes the sequence of care provided to the client according to his or her identified needs.

Developing Criteria

An important step in the development of a quality assurance system is to prepare criteria. Criteria are described as predetermined elements or standards against which quality of care or service can be compared. These criteria are developed from professional judgments based on current accepted research. It is necessary that criteria be stated in behavioral terms and that they be measurable and achievable. The sequential steps in developing quality assurance criteria are summarized in Figure 7-3.

Step 1. Selecting the Population

In the development of process and outcome criteria for quality assurance, the target population for whom the criteria will be written must be clearly specified, for example, healthy clients or clients with specific conditions. Ideally an interdisciplinary team of health care providers and consumers concerned with the quality of health and nutrition services should select the target populations. Various group decision-making methods can be used to reach consensus. The Delphi technique and nominal group process facilitate group decision making by allowing all group members to express their ideas equally

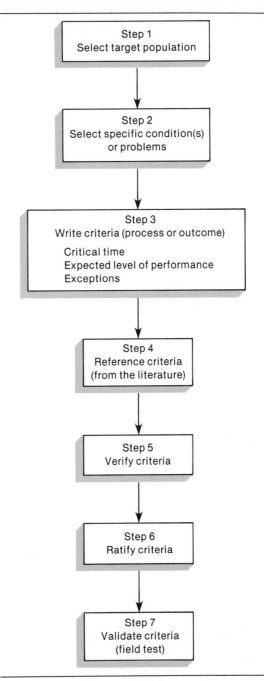

Figure 7-3. Steps in developing quality assurance criteria.

Redrawn from Kaufman, M., editor: Quality assurance in ambulatory nutrition care, Chicago, 1983. The American Dietetic Association.

with no one individual dominating the group or pressuring the group to conform (Delbecq, Vanderven, and Gustafson, 1975). The techniques generally lead to convergence of opinions, satisfaction, and acceptance of the group decision.

Populations that have the greatest potential for achieving benefits and cost-effectiveness in nutrition care exhibit the following characteristics:

1. Target population is at high risk for nutrition and diet-related problems.
2. Problems frequently occur in the population (i.e., statistical evidence documents the problems).
3. The problems are responsive to nutrition intervention, or there is evidence that nutrition intervention will contribute to the solution.
4. Standardization of nutrition management of the problem is generally agreed on by experts and practitioners as being effective.

Step 2. Selecting Specific Conditions

After the population has been selected, parameters that clearly define the population should be specified. For example, healthy children might be defined as "age 1 to puberty, with no current medical complications and a normal height, weight, or weight-for-height between the 5th and 95th percentile on the National Center for Health Statistics growth charts."

Step 3. Specifying Criteria

Again, the nominal group process is a useful decision-making tool to specify the criteria for outcome and/or process. Instructions to the group should emphasize that the criteria should define the essential elements or the key indicators of exemplary nutrition care. Criteria should not be a list of every possible outcome and/or process that is a component of total care. The indicators can be obtained from the nutrition program plan and from policies and procedures used in the practice.

Characteristics of criteria that are most useful in quality assurance are described by the acronym RUMBA:

R = Relevant
U = Understandable
M = Measurable
B = Behavioral
A = Achievable

When a criterion meets the RUMBA characteristics, there is a greater probability that it is a reliable and valid indicator of quality care. Reliability refers to the repeatability of a measurement: "Would the same worker get the same results on repeated trials or would two or more different workers get the same results measuring the same thing?" If the answers are "yes," then the results are reliable. Validity indicates whether the measure is actually measuring what it is intended to measure. A measurement can never be valid if it is unreliable, although reliability does not assure validity (Chapter 6).

Criteria written in behavioral terms should express a single action or the consequence of this action. Behavioral criteria indicate a provider carrying out a procedure (process) or visualize a change in the client's status as the result of care (outcome).

Theoretically, behavioral criteria can be measured and/or verified. However, problems often occur in specifying criteria that can be measured with reliable and valid tools. Reliable and valid measurements require the availability of accurate, unbiased data to verify whether a criterion has been met (Vermeersch, 1979; Vermeersch and Kaufman, 1981).

Measurement depends on explicitly stated criteria that are very precise. Such criteria specify the exact data and methods to be used for verification. An example of an explicit outcome criterion that would be written for a healthy child would be: "Child's 24-hour dietary intake provides nutrients that meet 100% of the Recommended Dietary Allowances (RDA) for protein, calcium, and iron." This criterion clearly states that a 24-hour food intake recall and calculations of nutrients and comparison with the appropriate RDA for the specified nutrients are required for each child to determine whether the criterion has been met.

The challenge is to write criteria that are explicit enough to be reliable yet flexible enough to be achievable.

Critical time. Specifying a time frame for achievement is important for process and outcome criteria. The intent of a criterion could vary depending on the timing in the nutrition care sequence. The critical time specifies the target time by which the process or outcome should be achieved. For example, the critical time for nutrition assessment may be the initial visit. Accomplishment of an outcome such as "Child consumes adequate diet for age" will vary according to the characteristics of the target population. Practitioners must use their best judgments of what critical times are desirable for reaching optimum effects on health status, and comparable, critical times must be stated in actual elapsed time periods such as days, weeks, months, age of child, and trimesters of pregnancy.

Exceptions. There may be anticipated circumstances that prevent the achievement of an outcome or process for certain groups of clients because of conditions beyond the control of the practitioner or the client. Designating exceptions allows for differentiations between process or outcomes not met because of these anticipated circumstances from those not met because of differences in health care. Examples of exceptions would include those clients who are lost to follow-up or those with a complicating health condition requiring different or additional care.

Specifying the expected performance level. The level of expected performance in any health care setting should be specified for each criterion. The ideal and most desirable performance level or standard is 100%. This level of performance means that the criterion is expected to be met for all cases to which it is applied. However, 100% may not be realistic particularly if baseline data indicate that current performance is low. The percentage specified should be based on a level of performance that would reflect desirable practice in the particular care setting. Establishing the percentage level of performance for each criterion indicates the "threshold for action" accepted by staff. If the actual performance level for each criterion falls below that which is expected, there should be a commitment to take corrective action to improve performance. For example, if an essen-

tial procedure (process) should be carried out for each patient and is either not carried out or not recorded at the expected performance level, training can be established to make this a routine procedure.

Step 4. *Referencing the Criteria*

Validity of each written criterion is established by identifying the source in the literature that substantiates its scientific base and/or efficacy and safety. References should be selected that represent the best current research and consensus of scientific thinking.

Step 5. *Verifying the Criteria*

The documentation and methods used to determine if the criteria are met should be identified. Examples of available and appropriate data sources would be patient care records, records of patient interviews, encounter forms, statistical reports, and special surveys or studies. Written instructions must be provided to evaluators to describe how the data will be interpreted and analyzed to judge whether a given case "passes or fails" on each criterion. The verification serves as a guideline to evaluators when the criteria are applied in quality assessment. If more than one evaluator performs the assessment, the verification instructions help assure that auditors are consistent and improve the likelihood that results of the assessment are reliable.

Step 6. *Ratifying the Criteria*

Approval of each criterion by the practitioners is obtained through ratification. Each person involved or affected by the quality assessment should have an opportunity to accept or reject each criterion. Through this ratification process, practitioners contribute to the development of criteria by which their practice will be judged. Ratification encourages willingness to acknowledge a problem and develops commitment to its solution. It can stimulate new thinking, since there is group participation and involvement. It should help clarify any ambiguities that exist in the criteria. Each participant is educated through discussion, exchange of opinions, and

Table 7-1. Model criteria for quality assurance in ambulatory nutrition care for obese infant*

Criteria			
Identify Outcome (O) and Process (P)	Critical Time	Exceptions†	References
1. Infant achieves weight/length equal to or less than 95th percentile when plotted on NCHS growth chart. (O)	Within 6 months after diagnosis of obesity		NCHS growth charts, 1976, Monthly Vital Statistics Rpt. 25(3), 1976.
2. Infant does not lose weight. (O)	After first week and throughout infancy	Acute illness	Fomon, S.J.: Infant nutrition, ed. 2, Philadelphia, 1974, W.B. Saunders Co., Chapter 2. Fomon, S.J.: Nutritional disorders of children, DHEW Publ. No. HSA-77-5104, Rockville, Md., 1977, p. 32.
3. Parent/caretaker identifies sources of excessive calories consumed by infant as compared to agency protocols. (O)	Initial/subsequent visits		Pipes, P.L.: Nutrition in infancy and childhood, ed. 3, St. Louis, 1984, The C.V. Mosby Co., pp. 146-159.
4. Parent/caretaker describes appropriate feeding practices initiated to control weight gain as defined in agency protocols. (O)	At each subsequent visit		Taitz, L.D.: Obesity in pediatric practice: infantile obesity. In Neumann, C.A., and Jelliffe, D., editors: Symposium on Nutrition in Pediatrics, Ped. Clin. North Am. 24:107-115, 1977.

Reprinted from Kaufman, M., editor: Guide to quality assurance in ambulatory nutrition care, Chicago, 1983, The American Dietetic Association.
*Birth to age 12 months; greater than 95th percentile weight for length and sex; no medical complications (physical handicaps, mental retardation, other syndromes).
†Lost to follow-up applies to all criteria.

consideration of the issues. Educational needs of the group are identified.

Ratification can be conducted by simply distributing the prepared criteria to practitioners and asking for their comments. A field test is a more formal means of ratification in which the draft criteria are applied on a trial basis. The field test procedures resemble an actual quality assessment and usually involve an audit of client records. The difference is that the criteria rather than the quality of care are being assessed. The objective is to see if the criteria follow the RUMBA guidelines. Application of the criteria to actual cases helps identify problems with wording, documentation, or verification. Comments from field testers based on their experience with the criteria provide insight on how the criteria

should be revised to achieve more reliable and valid indicators of quality care.

Step 7. Validating the Criteria

The field test is also used to validate the criteria, that is, to determine if the criteria as written are realistic and achievable in the health care setting. A record audit in the field testing shows that percentage of cases meeting each criterion, suggesting whether or not it can be expected to be met by most cases within the health care delivery setting.

Model Criteria for Quality Assurance in Ambulatory Nutrition Care

Vermeersch and Kaufman (1981) conducted a field test on six sets of quality assurance criteria

Table 7-2. Model criteria for quality assurance in ambulatory nutrition care for obese child*

Criteria Identify Outcome (O) and Process (P)	Critical Time	Exceptions†	References
1. Child achieves weight/height equal to or less than 95th percentile when plotted on NCHS growth chart. (O)	Depends on degree of overweight		Fomon, S.J.: Nutritional disorders of children, DHEW Publ. No. HSA-77-5104, Rockville, Md., 1977, p. 64.
2. Child/caretaker identifies sources of excessive calories as defined by agency protocol. (O)	By first month after initiating care		Growth charts with reference percentile for girls and boys age 2 to 18 years, DHEW, Centers for Disease Control, Atlanta, Ga., 1976.
3. Child and/or caretaker identifies kinds, amounts, and frequency of food appropriate to achieve recommended weight/height as defined by agency protocol. (O)	By second month after initiating care		
4. Child consumes types and amounts of foods in frequencies appropriate to achieve recommended weight for height as defined by agency protocol. (O)	By third month after initiating care		Pipes, P.L.: Nutrition in infancy and childhood, ed. 3, St. Louis, 1981, The C.V. Mosby Co., pp. 123-138, 249-254.
5. Child increases and/or maintains appropriate level of physical activity as defined by agency protocol. (O)	By 6 months after initiating care		Mayer, J.: Obesity during childhood. In Winick, M.: Childhood obesity, New York, 1975, John Wiley & Sons, p. 73.
6. Child maintains weight for height equal to or less than the 95th percentile as plotted on NCHS growth chart. (O)	By 1 year after achievement of weight stabilization		Growth charts with reference percentile for girls and boys age 2 to 18 years, DHEW, Centers for Disease Control, Atlanta, Ga., 1976.

Reprinted from Kaufman, M., editor: Guide to quality assurance in ambulatory nutrition care, Chicago, 1983, The American Dietetic Association.
*One year to puberty; weight for height greater than the 95th percentile; no medical complications (physical handicap, mental retardation, other syndromes).
†Lost to follow-up applies to all criteria.

that were developed at the National Conference on Quality Assurance in Ambulatory Nutrition Care in 1979. The purpose of the field test was to determine the reliability and validity of the criteria developed at the conference and to identify problems associated with the use of the criteria when auditing the quality of ambulatory nutrition care. The RUMBA guidelines served as the model for defining the characteristics of reliable and valid criteria. Field test results were obtained from 102 sites in 35 states.

The results of the field test indicated that many of the criteria did not meet the RUMBA guidelines. The characteristics of well-written and poorly written criteria became evident from the number of clinics and auditors from the same clinics who had difficulty interpreting the various criteria and evaluating their consistency.

From this effort, model criteria were developed for the following target population; pregnant woman, normal infant, obese infant, normal child (age 1 to puberty), obese child (age 1 to puberty), normal adolescent, and other adolescent. Tables 7-1 and 7-2 include examples of the obese infant and obese child. Chapters 9 and 10 include model criteria for specific age-groups throughout the life cycle. *Guide to Quality Assurance in Ambulatory Nutrition Care* (Kaufman, 1983) covers the model criteria in detail.

Implementing the Quality Assurance Audit

The patient care audit is the process for retrospectively monitoring the performance of the health care team and is primarily concerned with upgrading patterns of care in a health care setting. Audit techniques provide a mechanism both for documenting appropriate patterns of care and for identifying areas in which improvement is necessary. The steps in a patient care audit are defined by the ADA* (Figure 7-4).

Step 1. Selection of a subject or topic. The patient care audit begins when the members of the interdisciplinary quality assurance team select a topic they consider important for a review. The audit topic can be a population group, a diagnosis, a therapeutic measure, a physical finding, or an abnormal laboratory test result.

Steps 2 and 3. Development of criteria and ratification of criteria. These topics have been discussed on pp. 139-142.

Step 4. Review of charts and identification of problems. This step begins with selecting an appropriate sample of records to review. The careful definition of population in the criteria set to include specific condition, age, sex, and other relevant factors is essential to the performance of this task. The time frame from which records will be selected must be defined and should allow

---

*The material in the following sections (pp. 144-147) is from *Professional Standards Review Procedure Manual.* Chicago: The American Dietetic Association, 1976. Copyright The American Dietetic Association. Reprinted by permission.

for adequate population size to meet statistical requirements for sampling.

An appropriate audit form must be selected or developed to meet documentation requirements, allow for problem analysis, and satisfy the overall purpose for the audit.

The patient care records are reviewed against the established criteria. When a record does not meet the criterion or the critical time, this is indicated on the audit form with the patient's identification number and other information needed for problem analysis.

Step 5. Problem analysis. Several substeps are involved in problem analysis:

1. The audit committee reevaluates each criterion that is not met.
2. The committee lists possible explanations for not meeting the criterion, identifies the data needed to substantiate these explanations, and determines how the data will be collected.
3. The needed data are collected and analyzed to formulate acceptable explanations for not meeting the criteria.
4. The committee revises the list of possible explanations to produce a list of designated performance deficiencies.

Step 6. Development of solution(s) (or remedial strategies). After discussing the explanations that appear to contribute to the performance deficiency, the committee determines alternate strategies to correct the deficiencies, selects one or more of these strategies, and develops an implementation plan. Health professionals will be given training in carrying out the various strategies proposed.

Step 7. Implementation of solution(s). Remedial strategies may suggest corrective actions to be communicated through administrative channels to appropriate staff members, revising protocols, and conducting in-service education for all staff involved in providing the services indicated in the protocol. It is essential to appropriately communicate with all staff responsible for any aspect of the remedial strategy and to involve them in all key steps in planning and carrying out solutions.

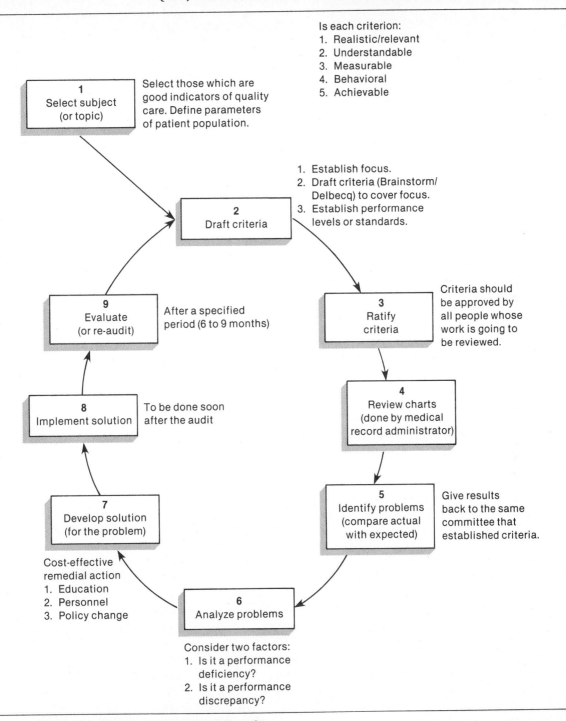

Figure 7-4. Procedure for patient care audit.

From Professional Standards Review Procedure Manual. Chicago: The American Dietetic Association, 1976. Copyright The American Dietetic Association. Reprinted by permission.

SAMPLE GENERAL INFORMATION FORM FOR CLIENT/GROUP AUDIT

Name of agency   Florence Nightingale Clinic

Location   1234 Main Street, Healthville, USA

Audit topic   Antepartum woman

Population   Pregnant women without medical complications who presented for prenatal care
on or after July 1, 1983, who completed pregnancy on or before June 30, 1985.

Number in population   200   % of total clinic population   33%

Sample size   15 cases

Audit conducted from   October 15, 1985   to   October 19, 1985

Audit coordinator   Sally Brown, Nutritionist

Names and titles of auditors

   Auditor 1   Sally Brown, Nutritionist

   Auditor 2   Paula Nevitt, PHN

   Auditor 3   Alex Brown, Health Educator

Criteria	**Means of Verification**
1. The woman's rate of weight gain is: Second trimester—at least 2 lb and no more than 8 lb/mo Third trimester—an average of 0.75 lb and no more than 1 lb/wk	Height and weight recorded each visit: calculate weight gain during pregnancy. Criterion met if gain is between 2 and 8 lb/mo during second trimester and between 0.75 and 1 lb/wk during third trimester
2. The woman achieves or maintains hemoglobin of 11 gm or hematocrit of 33% or more.	Hemoglobin reported in medical record at first visit, end of second trimester, and at term. Field test: criterion met if hemoglobin is above 11 gm at third trimester or at term

Reprinted from Kaufman, M., editor: Guide to quality assurance in ambulatory nutrition care, Chicago, 1983, The American Dietetic Association.

Step 8. Recommendation and communication of audit results. A summary of the specific audit findings, identified performance strengths and deficiencies, explanations of probable factors contributing to the deficiencies, plans for remedial action, and documented actions taken to solve the problem(s) or deficiency(ies) is reported to the appropriate administrative office, program managers, and discipline heads.

Step 9. Re-audit. At a predetermined period after instituting remedial action, a re-audit is conducted. The re-audit determines that the remedial action has been effective and the problem(s) has been corrected. The re-audit involves carrying out step 4, review of charts and identification of problems, as in the initial audit. If problems are still identified, the process would continue using steps 5 to 9.

SAMPLE AUDIT ABSTRACT FORM USING CRITERIA CODES

Name of agency   Florence Nightingale Clinic

Audit topic   Antepartum woman

Auditor number   1

Code: Meets criterion (both criterion and time): +
     Does not meet criterion: − C
     Meets criterion but does not meet critical time: − T
     Exception: E
     Not documented: ND

Case Number	Number Sampled	Criterion 1	2	3	4	5	6	7	8	9
A-765	1	− C	+	+	− T	+	+			
A-926	2	+	+	+	− C	+	−			
B-072	3	− C	+	− C	− C	− C	+			
B-147	4	+	+	+	+	+	+			
B-293	5	E	E	E	E	E	E			
B-476	6	+	− C	− T	− T	+	+			
B-625	7	+	E	− C	− E	− C	+			
B-712	8	− C	+	ND	− T	+	+			
B-901	9	− T	+	− T	ND	+	ND			
B-995	10	ND	− C	− C	− T	− C	+			
C-127	11	+	+	+	+	+	+			
C-349	12	E	E	E	E	E	E			
C-518	13	− C	+	− T	− T	+	− C			
C-701	14	+	+	+	− T	+	+			
A-815	15	+	+	+	+	+	ND			
B-102	16R	− C	ND	− C	ND	ND	ND			
B-24L	17R	+	− C	+	ND	+	+			
B-542	18R		+		+					

Reprinted from Kaufman, M., editor: Guide to quality assurance in ambulatory nutrition care, Chicago, 1983, The American Dietetic Association.

SUMMARY FORM DESCRIBING PERCENTAGE OF CRITERIA MET
AUDIT TOPIC: ANTEPARTUM WOMAN

	Records Not Documented			Exceptions			Meet Criterion		
	Records Audited			Records Audited			Records Audited − Exceptions *(difference should equal the sample size)*		
	Auditor			Auditor			Auditor		
	1	2	3	1	2	3	1	2	3
Criterion	N	%	N	%	N	%	N	%	N	%	N	%	N	%	N	%	N	%
1	1/17	6			2/17	12			8/15	53		
2	1/18	6			3/18	17			11/15	73		
3	1/17	6			2/17	12			7/15	47		
4	3/18	17			3/18	17			3/15	20		
5	1/17	6			2/17	12			11/15	73		
6	3/17	8			2/17	12			11/15	73		
7												
8												
9												
10												

Reprinted from Kaufman, M., editor: Guide to quality assurance in ambulatory nutrition care, Chicago, 1983, The American Dietetic Association.

• • •

Examples of sample procedure forms for a patient care audit are shown on pp. 146-148. The General Information form on p. 146 is completed for each client group being audited. The Audit Abstract form (p. 147) is a tally sheet used by the auditors. The Audit Data summary (above) is used to summarize data from the audit abstract forms from all of the auditors involved. Auditors total the number of records audited and the number of cases coded for each criteria.

Quality Assurance in Inpatient Care Settings or Acute Care Settings

The new *Guidelines on Dietetic Services* published by the Joint Commission on Accreditation of Hospitals (JCAH, 1981) mandates that dietetic services be evaluated. To comply with these guidelines, dietitians/nutritionists are required to document ongoing and completed evaluation studies or audits of dietetic services. Schiller and Behm (1979) have indicated that dietetic audits may be used to assess quality of care or to evaluate the efficiency of a food service. Problems can be clearly identified through an audit, and solutions can be found to improve service and nutritional care. An audit also provides a basis for dietitian/nutritionist accountability.

Dietetic Audits

There are two types of dietetic audits that might prove useful: nutritional care audit (p. 149) and administrative audit (p. 149).

Nutritional care audits may be performed independently or as part of a multidisciplinary effort. The purpose of the audit is to identify a problem and to obtain objective data for analysis. A nutritional care audit might be done in situations when patients often select food items

STANDARDS AND RELATED CRITERIA FOR A NUTRITIONAL CARE AUDIT

Objective: To provide optimum nutritional care for obese patients
Audit topic: Nutritional care of hospitalized obese patients without medical complications

General Standards of Practice

1. Assesses the nutritional needs of clients
2. Records pertinent information in the medical record
3. Evaluates appropriateness of diet orders in relation to other information in the medical record
4. Counsels individuals and families in nutritional principles
5. Adapts dietary plans to the patient's life-style
6. Teaches modified diets to patients as they become well enough to be receptive
7. Develops and implements optimal nutritional plans of care that identify long-range and short-range objectives
8. Evaluates nutritional care with follow-up provided for continuity of care

Audit Criteria

A. Process criteria (what the dietitian does)
   1. Documents in medical record:
      a. Admitting height/weight
      b. Ideal weight
      c. Evaluation of diet history
      d. Notation of relevant laboratory, clinical, or psychosocial data affecting weight
      e. Appropriateness of diet order to achieve realistic weight reduction if specific caloric level is designed by physician
   2. Written physician order for discharge diet and instruction
   3. Documents in medical record:
      a. Diet instruction given
      b. Assessment of patient's willingness to follow diet
      c. Patient's ability to make appropriate food choices in a variety of situations
B. Patient outcome criteria (results of dietetic care)
   1. Weight loss of 2 to 3 pounds in first week and 1 to 2 pounds each week thereafter until ideal weight is achieved
   2. Patient can select balanced diet within caloric restrictions

Reprinted by permission from *Hospitals*, Vol. 53, No. 8, April 16, 1979. Copyright 1979, American Hospital Association.

STANDARDS AND RELATED CRITERIA FOR AN ADMINISTRATIVE AUDIT

Standard: Establishes and maintains standards of food production and service, sanitation, safety, and security
Audit topic: Quality of tray service for hospitalized patients

Criteria

1. Trays are clearly marked with patient name and room number.
2. Patient receives meal according to current diet order.
3. Trays are served accurately according to food items, beverages, and condiments marked on menu.
4. Designated portions of food and beverages are served.
5. Trays are served complete with napkin and appropriate utensils.
6. Trays are free of spillage.
7. Hot food is hot and chilled food is chilled according to established standards both at the point of tray set-up and at the point of delivery to patient.

Reprinted by permission from *Hospitals*, Vol. 53, No. 8, April 16, 1979. Copyright 1979, American Hospital Association.

Table 7-3. Criteria for nutritional care of diabetic patients

Criteria	Data for Audit	
	Dietetic Card File	Medical Record
Assessment		
Interview for diet history; assess intake for calories, total carbohydrate, protein fat, percentage of carbohydrate from simple sugars, caloric and carbohydrate distribution of feedings, ration of saturated to polyunsaturated fat, insulin reactions	Assessment of diet history and appetite status recorded	Assessment of diet history and appetite status recorded
Assess appetite status		
Review medical records to assess appropriateness of diet order	Medical record information recorded; if diet order is inappropriate, record of consultation with physician	
1. Height/weight (determine ideal body weight)		
2. FBS; serum lipids		
3. Urinary glucose, acetone, protein		
4. Medications		
Planning/implementation		
Calculate pattern and plan diet based on patient interview, medical record information, and diet order	Calculation of meal pattern or justification for noncalculation recorded	
Determine nutritional intake for a minimum of 3 days		Nutrient calculations with dietitian's assessment and signature recorded for a minimum of 3 days
Education		
Obtain information related to psychosocial status, ability to purchase and prepare food, educational level. Assess	Assessment of patient's present knowledge of and ability to follow diet record	Assessment of patient's present knowledge of and ability to follow diet recorded
1. Level of previous diet instructions		
2. Patient's comprehension		
3. Patient's attitude and family support of diet		
4. Need for further diet instruction		
Suggest and/or obtain from physician diet order for discharge as soon as feasible		Diet order for discharge written by physician
Provide written and verbal individual and/or group diet counseling	Assessment of diet counseling recorded	Record of instructions given and assessment of patient's willingness and ability to adhere to diet
Arrange appropriate follow-up or continuity of care if needed	Copy of referral attached	Copy of continuity or care form or referral completed by dietitian

Reprinted by permission from *Hospitals*, Vol. 53, No. 9, May 1, 1979. Copyright 1979, American Hospital Association.

Table 7-3. Criteria for nutritional care of diabetic patients—cont'd

| Criteria | Data for Audit | |
	Dietetic Card File	Medical Record
Evaluation		
Continue to monitor effectiveness of diet on regulation of weight, serum glucose, or other given laboratory index (such as serum lipids)		Record of weekly assessment of nutrition intake, body weight, serum glucose, insulin reactions, or other laboratory index
After diet counseling, patient is able to:		Assessment of patient learning outcomes recorded
1. Select 3 days of menus according to individual diet plan		
2. Select a sample restaurant meal according to diet plan		
3. Verbalize a liquid meal plan for sick days		
4. State five foods for the treatment of hypoglycemia		
5. Describe how to contact a dietitian after discharge		
Exceptions		
1. Death		
2. Senility, comatose state		
3. Ineducable or patient does not wish instruction—physician notified		
4. Leaves hospital against medical advice		
5. Hospitalization is less than 3 days		

that are inconsistent with their diet prescription, special dietary products (elemental diets, tube feedings, and dietary supplements) are difficult to obtain, or dietitians need to spend more time in direct patient care.

Another useful dietetic audit is the *administrative audit*. Changes in food service operations can be made and improvements can be observed more rapidly with an administrative audit than they can with a nutritional care audit because the effect of care (patient outcomes) must be observed over an extended period of time (Schiller and Behm, 1979a).

Monodisciplinary Nutritional Care Audit

The monodisciplinary nutritional care audit can be used as a means of monitoring and upgrading the quality of nutritional care (Schiller and Behm, 1979b). Table 7-3 illustrates criteria that have been developed for the nutritional care of diabetic patients (Standards for Dietetic Care, 1979).

Ometer and Oberfell (1982) have developed a model for determining levels of care to identify patients who require increased nutritional support and/or diet education, to determine practices and delineate the degree of care required, and to define role responsibilities of the dietitian and the dietetic technician.

The model encompasses three levels of care. Level I patients are defined as those who have no indicators of possible compromised nutritional status (for example, orthopedic problem: broken ankle in a skiing accident) and for whom the development of nutrition problems during their hospital stay is not anticipated. Level II patients

Table 7-4. General standards of practice and assigned responsibilities by level of care

Activity	Level I R.D.	Level I Technician	Level II R.D.	Level II Technician	Level III R.D.	Level III Technician
Confirm all modified diet orders	—	X	—	X	—	X
Conduct more in-depth assessment	—	—	X	—	X	—
Develop initial care plan	—	X	X	—	X	—
Assess appropriateness of any modified diet orders	X	—	X	—	X	—
Orient patient to diet order	—	X	—	X	—	X
Assist patients with menu selection	—	X	—	X	—	X
Monitor intake through daily meal service rounds	—	X	RD also monitors periodically	X	RD also monitors periodically	X
Provide diet education to include:						
Take booklet to patient	—	X	—	X	—	X
Review rationale and principles	—	X	—	X	X and/or	X
Review foods to use/avoid	—	X	—	X	X and/or	X
Assess patient knowledge of diet and answer questions	—	X	X and/or	X	X	—
Record instruction in medical record with assessment of patient's knowledge	—	X	X and/or	X	X	—
Arrange for follow-up visit if necessary	X	—	X	—	X	—
Chart initial care plan in medical record within 72 hours of admission	—	—	X	—	X	—
Rescreen medical record		X every 7 days	X approximately every 3 days	X	X daily	—
Confer with medical staff about patient's nutritional care	X	—	X	—	X	—
Update plan and document a follow-up note	—	—	X approximately every 7 days	—	X approximately every 3-5 days	—
Document information concerning appetite/tolerance to diet	—	X	—	X	(included above)	
Calculate caloric intakes	—	—	—	X	—	X
Chart caloric intake	—	—	—	X	X and/or	X
Apply anthropometric measures	—	—	—	X	—	X

From Ometer, J.L., and Oberfell, M.S.: Quality assurance. I. A levels of care model. Copyright The American Dietetic Association. Reprinted by permission from *Journal of the American Dietetic Association*, Vol. 81:129, 1982.

are defined as those for whom no laboratory or clinical indicators of possible compromised nutritional status have been documented but for whom there is an increased risk of nutrition problems or deficiencies developing during their hospital stay. Level III patients are defined as having documented indicators of possible compromised nutritional status and/or existing problems, such as diarrhea, which may lead to significant nutrition problems.

Once assigned to an initial level of care, patients are monitored throughout their stay. The dietitian/nutritionist may reassign the patient to another level at any time, the goal being to move the patient from level III to level II to level I. To ensure that goals of each level are achieved, general standards of practice for monitoring and caring for patients by level have been established (Table 7-4).

This level of care model was used for oncology patients. The application of standards of practice for oncology patients allows the clinical dietitian to determine priorities for and delineate the degree of care required and to ensure the delivery of high-quality nutritional care to each oncology patient. Pilot testing has helped delineate role responsibilities and standardize care provided by the dietitian and dietetic technician.

The Administrative Audit

Schiller and Bartlett (1979) distinguish between administrative and nutritional care audits:

1. In administration audits the audit topics may vary to include an entire subsystem: (e.g., procurement, storage, production), whereas in nutritional care audits the topics are classified according to a coding system that is specific and finite.
2. Standards and criteria used in administrative audits differ in breadth and complexity from standards and criteria that are used in nutritional care and planning. Organizing, directing, and controlling are some of the market features that can be used as audit topics.
3. The methods of collecting data are different. Data for nutritional care audits are derived from written documentation in the medical research and dietetic card file. Data for administrative audits may be obtained from observation of activities and from various forms, records, and reports.
4. A fourth difference between the two kinds of audits is that the range of personnel involved is different. Nutritional care audits involve dietitians and dietetic technicians and associates. Administrative audits involve chefs, cooks, bakers, and other kitchen personnel.

Snyder (1981) has developed a model for a food service quality assurance system. He indicates that the industrial concept of quality assurance for the prevention of error by people and equipment is a useful concept and a good base for the development of food service quality assurance systems.

Today's dietitians/nutritionists face many challenges in a rapidly changing environment. None is more demanding than the increasing clamor for improved quality of care while concomitantly reducing costs. To effectively address this need, the community dietitian/nutritionist needs to take an active role in defining nutrition's unique contribution to the community rather than being told what to do and how to do it. Many methods and strategies are available to help community dietitians/nutritionists assume this new role. Planning for quality assurance needs and making appropriate changes will ensure the success of the profession and quality care for consumers.

FINANCIAL CONTROL

Today there is great concern about the health sector and its soaring costs. In 1979 the United States spent $215 billion on the health sector, or 8.9% of the gross national product (GNP). In 1982 the United States spent $322 billion, or 10.5% of the GNP. In just 3 short years health spending increased by 50%—considerably faster than either inflation in the economy or growth in family incomes. Cost containment efforts have been implemented in both the public and private health care sectors. In this chapter two areas of financial control will be discussed: (1) the making of fiscal policy and the principles of budgeting and (2) cost-effectiveness/benefit analyses as a significant part of the controlling process and a tool to enhance decision making (Figure 7-1).

Development of Fiscal Policy

There are important fiscal policy differences between the public and private sectors. In the private sector, decision making can be guided and implemented by considerations that are subject to reasonably accurate escalation. Commodities produced and services rendered in the private sector are sold at prices controlled by cost, demand, and competition in the market. Profit is the basic and controlling motivation (Hanlon and Pickett, 1984). Unfortunately, public affairs do not provide this degree of predetermination and control. Many of the enterprises in the public sector are responses to variable human needs and are not subject to simple or consistent measurement. Taxes are mandatory, and the impact of public services is largely coercive. Under any circumstances, fiscal considerations are involved.

In the public sector, fiscal policy making is the legislature's job, which includes the collection of revenues, the establishment of programs, and the efficient operation of these programs. The actual implementation of these programs involves collection of revenues and disbursement of public money, budgeting, accounting, and purchasing. The health administrator is primarily concerned with the latter three tasks.

Budgeting

A budget is a plan expressed in monetary terms. Budgeting is an important part of the management control process in any organization. Budgets are among the most widely used devices for controlling and coordinating the activities of an organization. It is essential for the health administrator to establish a system of financial bookkeeping that will provide a continuous, accurate, and verifiable account of activities. A departmental budget provides such a system.

Frequently funds are made available, especially to local departments of health, from sources outside the local government. Among these sources are grants or aid from state and federal governments, private foundations, and various voluntary health agencies.

For administrative purposes all monies, regardless of source, should appear in the budget and be placed in the custody of the state or local treasurer. The number of separate funds should be kept at a minimum, since a proliferation of them effectively hampers the development of broad, well-balanced programs (Hanlon and Pickett, 1984).

Purpose of Budgeting

The purpose of a budget in a public health nutrition program is to indicate how and at what rate money is to be expended and thus to regulate expenditures over a period of time. A budget can help prevent waste by showing where the responsibility is for each area of an organization and the coordination and relationship between the aspects. It also can indicate where expansion is possible and if outcomes are not coinciding with projected estimates. Mainly, it can give an early indication of future financial requirements and possibly where such revenue may come from. An informative budget is an essential tool for administrative directors and other persons who are in control of funds.

Budget Preparation

In drafting the budget, the community dietitian/nutritionist should, as early as possible, become thoroughly familiar not only with the budget of the health agency but also with the total budget of the governmental unit of which it is a part and with the methods and forms of budgeting being used. Since the budgets of all governmental agencies have the same general purpose, certain similarities exist in their forms. Following is a summary of the well-accepted basic principles of budgets:

1. Expenditures of a preceding period equal in time to that for which the budget is being prepared (e.g., June-to-June dates). The period should be closed so that actual expenditures as they occurred are stated in this column.
2. Budget of the present period. These figures include only the budget as it was set up, since expenses therein are still being incurred while a budget for the future is being prepared.
3. Changes in the present budget period. These figures should include any significant changes in the present budget that have occurred or that may be anticipated, such as changes in salaries or in departmental organization, which will have the effect of modifying the present budget.
4. Expenditures of the present period, given as actual expenditures to the time the next budget is being made. The actual expenditures and estimates are totaled.
5. Object of expenditure. This column designates each item for which expenditures have been made or are requested. These items should include the salary group classed as permanent, as temporary, or as services secured on a contract basis. Other groups will include materials and supplies, fixed charges, foodstuffs, equipment, and any other divisions of expenditures.
6. Budget requests for the next period. Each item should be arranged in such a manner that comparison with the present budget will be as simple as possible.
7. Comparison between the present and anticipated budgets. Since comparison of present and requested budgets is crucial in the consideration of new budgets, this column should indicate all items for which an increased expenditure is desired, items that are not changed from the present budget, and items that are dropped or in which a decrease in allotment of funds is desired.
8. The adopted budget. At least one column will be necessary for the budget adopted.

As many additional columns should be provided as may be demanded in accordance with the number of official approvals required. This column greatly facilitates the recording of recommendations by different officials empowered to approve one or all phases of the budget previous to its final adoption.

An example of a state budget for the Division of Community Health Services and the Bureau of Nutrition Services, along with the program's goals, appears in Appendix 7-1.

Sometimes it is also necessary to have a budget justification, which is a brief but adequate description of the need and reasons for money for a particular area. This report is especially necessary if a budget analyst must make decisions about giving certain areas priority over others. An example of a state's budget justification for its Bureau of Nutrition Services appears on pp. 166 and 167.

The budget process is continuous and overlapping in that preparation of the budget for the forthcoming fiscal year must begin while the budget for the current year is being executed. The budget cycle has four major phases:

1. The preparation of departmental requests, the evaluation of revenue potential, executive review, the formulation of the budget document, and its transmission to the legislative body.
2. Legislative review and authorization. (This may or may not involve executive veto or approval.)
3. Execution of the budget in accordance with legislative authorization. (This involves translation of the fiscal program into an operational program by the various departments and agencies of government under the general direction and control of the executive.)
4. Postaudit evaluation and review to determine whether expenditures have been made and operations conducted in accordance with legislative intent in conformity with law.

Performance Budgeting

Performance budgeting in effect summarizes the program activities performed in terms of the cost of specified accomplishments. Thus performance budgeting tells what it costs to immunize an individual against a specific disease or to supervise the average food-handling establishment. When such detailed cost analysis or inventory is available for all components or functions in a program, the determination of the cost of the total program becomes possible. One then has a true program performance budget that provides a meaningful indication of the total impact of a program in terms of its cost.

Advantages. The advantages of a program inventory and the resultant performance budget that it makes possible follow:

1. Provides effective tools in planning a well-balanced program
2. Assists in developing short- and long-range program objectives
3. Provides elements for the control of programs and their costs
4. Provides detailed information concerning work volume and unit costs
5. Provides a sound basis for comparing past, present, and future activities, programs, and performance
6. Aids greatly in supporting requests for funds on a demonstrable and realistic basis
7. Discourages "padding" of the budget by program directors
8. Aids in the sound expansion and contraction of program activities
9. Permits personnel to see relationships among activities and programs
10. Provides qualitative and quantitative measures of personnel and department efficiency

Precautions. The program inventory, performance report, performance budget, and program budget are only administrative tools. They must be used properly as aids to administrative evaluation—not in place of it or as ends in themselves. The performance budget specifically must be regarded as a classification of proposed expenditures in terms of accomplishments to be achieved rather than personnel activities, such as nursing visits made, or items purchased. Yardsticks of performance standards have not yet been developed in many important areas. Ideally, there should be standard cost tables and quantitative measurement devices for every important element of the health program.

A basic problem in performance budgeting is that by their very nature preventive medicine and public health deal with negatives, such as cases and epidemics of disease prevented, home or industrial accidents guarded against, and disasters avoided. Attempting to measure the value and efficiency of the efforts applied to such ends is quite different from measuring the cost of gallons of water processed, miles of streets paved, or radios manufactured. To place a monetary value on the prevention of an epidemic is largely conjectural.

When one is thinking about costs in making a performance budget, Hanlon and Pickett (1984) suggest the following guidelines:

1. There should be a record of accumulated costs, reflecting the activity of the program.
2. Fixed costs should be separated from variable costs. In other words, certain expenditures may increase or decrease as the program progresses, whereas others remain fixed.
3. Variable costs should be related to work load and goal achievement so that the efficiency of the program may be determined and appraised.
4. Often a health program's central activity is offering interpersonal services, rather than using many materials, so that the importance and cost of such services far outweighs those of materials.
5. Although specific programs are usually measured, sometimes additional knowledge can be gained if a performance budget is developed for a larger category of programs, such as public health nutrition or laboratory work.

Following is an example of the labor-cost centers that actually or theoretically can be measured (Hanlon and Pickett, 1984):

Maternal Health

$$\frac{\text{(a) Cost of personnel in maternal health clinics per year}}{\text{(b) Number of patient visits per year}} =$$

Cost per maternal patient visit

The numerator (a) is the number of personnel-years of each physician, nurse, community dietitian/nutritionist, and clerk working in or with maternal health clinics (including field follow-up by public health nurses) times the sum of their salaries. The denominator (b) is the number of patient visits to maternal health clinics during the year.

Zero-Based Budgeting

In the normal budgeting process the previous year's level of expenditure is often assumed to have been appropriate. The task of individuals preparing the budget is to decide what activities and funds should be dropped and, more often, what activities and funds should be added (Stoner, 1982). Such a process builds into an organization a bias toward continuing the same activities year after year and well after their reliance and usefulness may have been lost because of environmental changes or changes in the organization's objectives.

Zero-based budgeting (ZBB), in contrast, enables the organization to look at its activities and priorities afresh. The previous year's resource allocations are not automatically considered as the basis for the year's allocation. Instead, each manager has to justify anew his or her entire budget request. ZBB involves allocating an organization's funds on the basis of CBA of each of the organization's major activities. The process involves three major steps:

1. Break down each of the organization's activities into "decision packages." A decision package includes all the information about an activity that managers need to evaluate that activity and compare its costs and benefits to other activities, plus the consequences expected if the activity is not approved and the alternative activities that are available to meet the same purpose.
2. Evaluate the various activities and rank them in order of decreasing benefit to the organization.

3. Allocate resources. The organization's resources are budgeted according to the final ranking that has been established (Linquist and Miller, 1981).

COST-EFFECTIVENESS/BENEFIT

In August, 1983, the *U.S. News and World Report* headline "Soaring Hospital Costs" described a brewing revolt over the cost of health care. This headline depicts the concern about the economic crisis that threatens to undermine medical care for many Americans. The rapid and continuing growth of expenditures in the U.S. medical care system of the U.S. is a central issue in many policy decisions today. Policy makers, health professionals, and consumers are seeking ways to control this growth while simultaneously improving the quality of health care. It is anticipated that by 1993, the bill for health care is expected to top 1 trillion dollars. The nation's 5800 community hospitals are where the largest share of the country's health dollars go. Hospitals receive about 42% of all the money spent on health care, an estimated $150 billion in 1983. All of these conditions are making hospitals a prime target for reform.

One of the most dramatic changes in the hospital industry in recent years has been the growth of investor-owned hospital-management companies. Whereas supporters of investor-owned chains suggest that their growth is attributable to operating efficiencies, critics suggest that it has resulted from pricing and marketing strategies.

Cost-Effectiveness and Cost-Benefit Analysis

Increasingly, the use of cost-effectiveness analysis/cost-benefit analysis (CEA/CBA) is being advocated as a possible means of making the medical care system more efficient. In particular, this technique is suggested for use in health care programs.

Definitions of CBA and CEA refer to formal analytical techniques for comparing the positive and negative consequences of alternate ways to allocate resources. There is a continuum of analyses that examines costs and benefits (USOTA, 1980).

At the end of the continuum are what are referred to as "net cost" studies. In these studies the emphasis is on costs and net cost. At the other end of the continuum are analyses that attempt to relate the use of the technologies under study to specific health-related outcomes and to compare the cost of the technologies to the difference in health benefits. CBA and CEA comprise the entire set of analytical techniques differentiated by the specifics of what costs and benefits are considered and how they are analyzed on this continuum.

Distinctions Between CEA and CBA

The principal distinctions between CEA and CBA lie in the valuation of the desirable consequences of a decision, in the implications of different methods of that valuation, and usually in the scope of the analysis.

In CBA all costs and all benefits are valued in monetary terms. Thus CBA can be used to evaluate the "worth" of a project and would allow comparison of projects of different types (such as dams and hospitals).

In CEA the health-related effects of programs or techniques are not valued in monetary terms, but rather are measured in some other unit (such as years of life gained). A CEA, therefore, does not result in a net monetary value for a project. Instead, it produces a measure of the cost involved in attaining some desirable health-related effect. Conceptually CEA permits direct comparison of only those programs or technologies which share similar objectives.

There are two basic types of health care resource allocation decisions that in theory cover benefits from a CEA/CBA process:

1. *Decisions made within a fixed or prospectively set budget, such as those made by health maintenance organizations (HMOs).* The projects that promise to deliver more benefits for the cost should be more attractive than those projects expected to deliver fewer benefits.
2. *Decisions made in the absence of a direct budget constraint, such as those made for*

Medicare reimbursement in health planning. A function of CEA/CBA in these decisions would be to force consideration of economic factors.

Findings of the Office of Technology Assessment Study

To aid in decisions concerning the possible use of CEA/CBA in federal health programs, the Senate Committee on Labor and Human Resources and on Finance asked the Office of Technology Assessment (OTA) to explore the applications of CEA/CBA to medical technology (OTA, 1980).

Findings of the OTA assessment include the following:

> Performing an analysis of costs and benefits can be very helpful to decision makers because the process of analysis gives structure to the problem, allows an open consideration of all relevant effects of a decision, and forces the explicit treatment of key assumptions. CEA/CBA exhibits too many methodologies and other limitations, however, to justify relying solely on the results of formal CEA/CBA studies in making decisions. *It should not be the sole or prime reason or determinant of a decision.*

These findings support a middle position about CEA/CBA versus the two extreme positions of not being useful at all in decision making and being used as the sole source of information to make decisions. The middle position maintains that the technique could be helpful in structuring information and that this information should be only one of several components of a decision process.

Principles of CEA/CBA Methodology

There is widespread agreement that the following 10 basic *principles* are generally applicable to CEA/CBA:

1. *Define problem.* The problem should be clearly and explicitly defined, and the relationship to health should be stated.
2. *State objectives.* The objective of the technology being assessed should be explicitly stated, and the analysis should address the

degree to which the objectives are expected to be met.

3. *Identify alternatives.* Alternative means (technologies) to accomplish the objective should be identified and subjected to analysis. When slightly different outcomes are involved, the effect this difference will have on the analysis should be examined.

4. *Analyze benefits/effects.* All foreseeable benefits/effects (positive and negative outcomes) should be identified and when possible should be measured. Also when possible and if agreement can be reached, it may be helpful to value all benefits in common terms to make comparisons easier.

5. *Analyze costs.* All expected costs should be identified and when possible should be measured and valued in dollars.

6. *Differentiate perspectives of analysis.* When private or program benefits and costs differ from social benefits and costs (and if a private or program perspective is appropriate for the analysis), the difference should be identified.

7. *Perform discounting.* All future costs and benefits should be discounted to their present value for comparison. Discounting can be thought of as a reverse interest rate.

8. *Analyze uncertainties.* Sensitive analysis should be conducted. Key variables should be analyzed to determine the importance of their uncertainty to the results of the analysis. A range of possible values for each variable should be examined for effects on results.

9. *Address ethical issues.* Ethical issues should be identified, discussed, and placed in appropriate perspective in relation to the rest of the analysis and the objectives of the technology.

10. *Discuss results.* The results of the analysis should be discussed in terms of validity, sensitivity to changes in assumptions, and implications for policy or decision making.

Factors Affecting the Use of CEA/CBA

The stage of development of the technology under study and the type of technology (or function of the technology) are two of the factors that will affect the specific analysis to be used, the uses to which analysis can be put, and the usefulness of resultant information. Other factors are the resultant information; the relative strength or importance of nonanalytical factors, such as politics or equity in the decision to be made; the ability of the sponsors of analysis to implement the results; the existence of adequate data relating to technology; the disease or other problems addressed by the technology or other possible effects of interventions based on analysis; the existence of economic factors that match or run counter to the results of analysis; and the type of discussion to be made (OTA, 1980). Some of the factors that affect the use of CEA/CBA are listed on p. 160.

Potential Users of CEA/CBA

Health care policies and other decisions are made at a variety of levels and in a variety of situations by an extremely broad range of individuals and groups. In theory CEA/CBA results or approaches might be used by any or all of these decision makers.

The box on p. 161 lists many of the decision makers; the list is not exhaustive but should provide an idea of how diverse and numerous the types of decision makers are.

CEA and CBA in Nutritional Care

Responding to the need for CEA/CBA in nutritional care, the ADA commissioned a committee in 1977 to develop a series of research papers that would be used to conduct CBA of nutrition counseling services provided in ambulatory health care settings to attempt to provide the rationale for reimbursement for ambulatory nutritional care services. The Committee to Develop a Research Study on Cost/Benefit of Ambulatory Nutrition Care developed a monograph entitled *Costs and Benefits of Nutritional Care: Phase I* (ADA, 1979).

FACTORS AFFECTING THE USE OF CEA/CBA

Stage of Development of the Technologies Under Study

Tradeoff required between availability/validity of data and ability to affect the future use of the technologies. Both the type of analysis and the usefulness of analysis will be affected.

Nature of Technologies Under Study and Function of Technologies Under Study

In terms of function, diagnostic technologies, for example, often have indirect connections to health outcome and often lend themselves to the net cost type of CEA/CBA. In terms of the physical nature of technologies, surgery, for example, may involve additional uncertainties due to varying skills of surgeons and surgical settings. Both type and use of analysis will be affected, but especially the type or specific methodological elements.

Social, Ethical, or Value Influences in the Decision Environment

Very similar, often overlapping with the above factor. Will affect both the type and uses of the analysis. The example of renal dialysis applies here. Abortion would serve as another example.

Quality of the Analysis

Can be of at least four types:

Analysis subject to inherent methodological limitations (e.g., inability to adequately deal with equity concerns; influence of discount rate chosen on outcome of analysis).

Analysis subject to state-of-the-art limitations (e.g., difficulties in identifying and measuring many costs or effects).

Analysis containing errors of omission or commission. These are errors not due to the state-of-the-art (e.g., failure to discount or perform sensitivity analysis when appropriate).

Analysis subject to data limitations. This factor will affect quality even though the other factors might have been adequately dealt with. Much cost and health outcome data are uncertain, difficult to retrieve, or simply nonexistent.

All four of these factors can affect the quality of analysis, which in turn affects the usefulness of the results.

Ability of Sponsors or Users of Analysis to Implement Results

The usefulness of analysis will naturally depend on the amount of control the user has over the particular technology or situation studied.

Experience/Familiarity of Users with the Type of Analysis Conducted

This factor will affect usefulness in two ways: it will be a direct influence on the acceptability of results, and it will affect the ability of the users to appropriately apply the results.

Existence of Economic Incentives in the Decision Environment

If the economic incentives relating to the use of the technology under study are in accord with the results, their acceptability will be great. If they run counter to the results, the usefulness will be limited, depending on the strength of the economic incentives.

From Office of Technology Assessment: The implications of cost effectiveness analysis of medical technology, Washington, D.C., Aug. 1980, U.S. Government Printing Office.

The committee endeavored to identify the links between nutrition counseling, dietary changes, changes in nutrition, related risk factors, health outcome changes, and the resultant economic benefits. Selected topics reviewed by the committee demonstrate the nutrition/dietary links in pregnancy outcomes, child growth and development, prevention of atherosclerosis, and aging. The role of U.S. food programs is also discussed. Potential economic benefits include reduced use of medical care services, reduced use of institutional and home care services, and improved productivity and time at work.

The committee reported available data that improving nutritional studies and/or changes in diet can modify or defer the development of dis-

PARTIAL LIST OF INDIVIDUALS AND GROUPS MAKING OR INFLUENCING RESOURCE ALLOCATION DECISIONS

Individual physicians and other health care
   professionals
Individual patients
Medical professional societies and boards
Consumer groups
Health industry representatives and organizations
Hospitals, clinics, other health care institutions
Labor organizations
Businesses
Health maintenance organizations
Medicare and Medicaid
Other governmental health care programs
Health systems agencies, state agencies
Professional Standards Review Organizations
Blue Cross and Blue Shield Associations
Other health care insurers, third-party payers
Other quality assurance or utilization review groups
Food and Drug Administration
Rate-setting commissions
Voluntary health organizations
Public health departments
Other state and local health agencies
U.S. Congress, executive agencies, state legislatures
Health care systems, such as the Veterans Administra-
   tion's and the Department of Defense's
Medical schools
Biomedical and health services researchers
Other health-related associations

From Office of Technology Assessment: The implications of cost effectiveness analysis of medical technology, Washington, D.C., Aug. 1980, U.S. Government Printing Office.

ease. The following links have been established: nutrition counseling to diet changes, diet changes to health risk factor changes, and health risk factor changes to health and health status related to economic benefits (ADA, 1979). Each linkage is needed to determine CEA/CBA of nutrition counseling as a component of ambulatory care. Economic returns can accrue when ambulatory nutrition care contributes to reducing the need for costly medical care. For instance, nutrition counseling for patients with juvenile diabetes can prevent the need for emergency hospital care for diabetic coma, or early prenatal nutritional care for high-risk mothers can help prevent the need for delivery in a level III prenatal intensive care center. Economic benefits may occur years later. For example, improved pregnancy outcome that reduces infant mortality will increase productivity in the labor force in 16 to 25 years.

In Figure 7-5 Mason (1979) presents a schematic flow of the links between diet change, risk factors to overcome, health outcomes, and economic benefits. The review shows that improvements in nutritional status during pregnancy may result in more successful pregnancy outcomes.

Examples of Cost-Effectiveness/Benefit Analysis Models

Splett (1982) cited three examples where attempts are being made to determine cost-effective/benefit analysis:

1. The Southwest Kansas Nutrition Program for the Elderly has a goal of providing older Americans with low-cost, nutritionally sound meals at strategically located centers. In meeting this goal the nutritionist identified the need to investigate actual costs to compare cost per meal across 28 service sites.

2. On the West Coast a community health clinic has the multiple objectives of reducing dietitian turnover, increasing revenue, and improving the effectiveness of the outpatient diabetic education program. It was believed that expanded involvement of the dietitian in the diabetic program would be a positive factor in accomplishing these objectives.

3. The United Hospital in St. Paul, Minnesota, developed a therapeutic and educational activity called the "Evening at the Penthouse." This weekly banquet-style dinner aids in preparing the patient for return to home and community. The costs and benefits of the program are presently being analyzed.

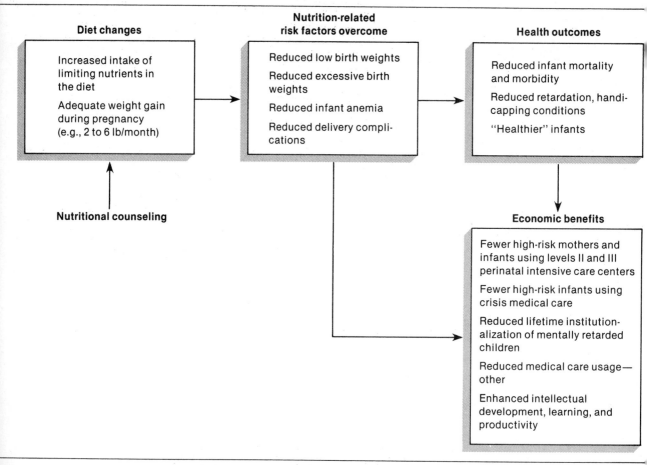

Figure 7-5. Potential economic benefits of nutritional counseling in pregnancy.
Redrawn from Costs and Benefits of Nutritional Care Phase 1. Chicago: The American Dietetic Association, 1979. Copyright The American Dietetic Association. Reprinted by permission.

Dahl (1977), in a study examining the efficiency of comprehensive health care delivery, points out the cost-effective potential of a nutritional component in health care delivery. The study showed that the presence of a nutritional functional area in a comprehensive health care project for children and youth had the net effect of reducing average registrant cost. He stated that an increase in the allocation of funds to the nutritional functional area by 1 percentage point would be likely to reduce total cost per registrant per year about one eleventh of a percentage point. In this comprehensive health care delivery system it was found that the average annual registrant cost of $271.52 was $29.30 lower than it otherwise would have been had there been no nutritional functional area in the comprehensive health program.

Another study by Dahl (1973) indicated that a major source of nutritional care in the absence of a nutritional functional area was the medical functional area. This study showed that an increase of 1 percentage point of nutritional functional area cost (per registrant per year) would decrease medical functional area cost by about one sixth of a percentage point.

Stason and Weinstein (1977) applied cost-effectiveness analysis to the management of hypertension, both to determine how resources can be used most effectively within programs to treat hypertension and to provide a yardstick for comparison with similar resources. Findings revealed that for both sexes, the cost-effectiveness ratio was inversely related to the pretreatment level of diastolic blood pressure. The ratios ranged for men from $3300 at age 20 to $16,300 at age 60, and for women from $850 at age 20 to $5000 at age 60. Ratios could serve to guide the selection of age-specific blood pressure cutoff levels for treatment. In general this study indicated that funds spent to improve adherence to management of hypertension may be a better use of resources than efforts to screen a maximum number of subjects.

REIMBURSEMENT FOR NUTRITION SERVICES

Cost-effectiveness/benefit information on nutrition services is vital if reimbursement for these services is to occur.

Public and private third-party programs include *Medicare* and *Medicaid*. Medicare, which is the largest publicly sponsored health care program, was established to protect those 65 years and over from major and financially debilitating medical bills. Medicaid, the federal and state program that finances the medical care of 29 million poor people like Medicare, was created in 1965 as an amendment to the Social Security Act of 1935 (Chapter 15).

Private programs include Blue Cross/Blue Shield (BC/BS), which was developed in the late 1920s by hospitals and physicians to assure payment of bills. Because of its not-for-profit status, Blue Cross/Blue Shield has traditionally offered complete coverage for lower premiums than other private health insurers. Commercial insurance companies have a variety of health plans that offer their customers whatever benefits they see fit within state and federal laws and statutes.

Since Medicare's inception, the ADA has worked toward the passage of federal legislation that would include, among the benefits offered by home health services agencies, nutrition counseling by dietitians with third-party reimbursement for these services.

Medicare legislation (Title XVIII of the Social Security Act passed in 1964) provided reimbursement for home visits to eligible clients by nurses, home health aides, social workers, and occupational, physical, and speech therapists. Under the Medicare legislation the nutrition services provided to patients in their homes can be funded indirectly as an administrative overhead expense when home health agencies employ a dietitian for staff training or for consulting with other health personnel who provide direct services to clients.

Although the legislation to obtain third-party reimbursement for home health service was introduced in the 93rd, 94th, and 95th Congresses, it was never brought to vote. Members of Congress and administrators in the Social Security Administration have requested data to support the ADA's contention that the benefits of such services would outweigh their costs.

The ADA has used various strategies to pursue third-party reimbursement since the legislative efforts were very productive. The ADA board appointed a committee in 1977 to address the issue of cost-benefits of ambulatory nutrition care. In 1982 the House of Delegates debated the issue of third-party reimbursement in its meeting in San Antonio (Third-Party Reimbursement, 1982). As an outcome of the 1982 meeting, a document was prepared entitled *Nutrition Services Payment System*. This manual was developed as a tool for implementing a fee for service system and for enhancing nationwide payment for nutrition services provided by or under the supervision of registered dietitians (RDs). The purposes of the manual follow:

- To define the services provided by registered dietitians in various practice settings
- To specify uniform codes, terminology, and time estimates for those services
- To provide a framework for implementing the Nutrition Services Payment System, including obtaining fee for service and third-party reimbursement
- To provide guidelines for documenting services in order to assess the cost-effectiveness and cost-benefits of nutrition services

Although it is well-described in ADA literature that the dietitian is the primary practitioner of nutrition care, third-party programs, both public and private, have been slow to recognize the contributions that registered dietitians can offer to beneficiaries. In particular, these programs have been hesitant to reimburse the provider of nutrition services by independent practitioners outside standard institutional settings.

SUMMARY

Assuring quality of nutrition services for clients is one of the major responsibilities of the community dietitian/nutritionist. The elements of quality assurance and the steps to develop a quality assurance program in ambulatory care are described in detail. Developing sound fiscal policy, including the purposes and preparation of budgets, is covered to assist the community dietitian/nutritionist to develop sound fiscal controls. The use of cost effectiveness/cost benefit analysis is described, and their potential use in nutrition care is addressed.

REFERENCES

The American Dietetic Association: Professional standards review procedure manual, Chicago, 1976, ADA.

The American Dietetic Association: Patient care audit, Chicago, 1979, ADA.

The American Dietetic Association: Costs and benefits of nutritional care: phase 1, Chicago, Oct. 1979, ADA.

The American Dietetic Association: Nutrition services payment system manual, Chicago, 1984, ADA.

Dahl, T.: The medical fund: area in comprehensive health care delivery for children and economic analysis, Study Services No. 3.2 (26), Minneapolis, 1973, Minnesota Systems Research, Inc.

Dahl, T.: Economics, management and public health nutrition, J. Am. Diet. Assoc. **70**:144, 1977.

Delbecq, A.L., Vanderven, A.H., and Gustafson, D.: Group techniques for program planning: a guide to nominal group and Delphi processes, Glenview, Ill., 1975, Scott, Foresman & Co.

Deniston, L.O.: Evaluation and cost effectiveness ratios, Ann Arbor, 1978, School of Public Health, University of Michigan.

Kaufman, M., editor: Guide to quality assurance in ambulatory nutrition care, Chicago, 1983, The American Dietetic Association.

Hanlon, J.J., and Pickett, G.E.: Public health administration and practice, ed. 8, St. Louis, 1984, Times Mirror/Mosby College Publishing.

Joint Commission on Accreditation: Guidelines on dietetic services, Chicago, 1978, JCAH.

Joint Commission on Accreditation of Hospitals: New JCAH quality assurance standards and programs, Hospitals **55**:67, 1981.

Linquist, S.C., and Miller, K.B.: Whatever happened to zero based budgeting, Managerial Planning **28**:4, Jan./Feb. 1981.

Mason, M.: Intervention in pregnancy. In The American Dietetic Association: Costs and benefits of nutritional care, phase 1, Chicago, 1979, ADA.

Oberfell, M.S., and Ometer, J.L.: Quality assurance application of oncology standard against a level of care model, J. Am. Diet. Assoc. **81**:132, 1982.

Office of Technology Assessment: The implications of cost effectiveness analysis of medical technology, Washington, D.C., Aug. 1980, U.S. Government Printing Office.

Ometer, J.L., and Oberfell, M.S.: Quality assurance: a level of care model, J. Am. Diet. Assoc. **81**:129, 1982.

O'Neal, E.A.: A framework for ambulatory care evaluation, J. Nurs. Adm., July 1978.

Owen, A.L.: Planning and evaluating nutrition services to ensure quality. In Simko, M., Cowell, C., and Gilbridge, J.A., editors: Nutrition assessment: a comprehensive guide for planning and intervention, Rockville, Md., 1984, Aspen Systems Corp.

Schiller, R., and Behm, V.: Auditing dietetic services: first of a series, Hospitals **53**:122, April 16, 1979a.

Schiller, R., and Behm, V.: Auditing dietetic services: second in a series, Hospitals **53**:105, May 1, 1979b.

Schiller, R., and Bartlett, B.: Auditing dietetic services, Hospitals **53**:118, May 16, 1979.

Snyder, O.P.: A model food service quality assurance system, Food Technol. **71**:67, 1981.

Soaring hospital costs: the brewing revolt, U.S. News and World Report, p. 39, Aug. 22, 1983.

Splett, P.L.: Examining program costs, Community Nutritionist **1**:22, July/Aug. 1982.

Standards for dietetic care of the patient with diabetes mellitus, Columbus, 1979, Department of Dietetics, The Ohio State University Hospital.

Stason, W.B., and Weinstein, M.C.: Public health records at the Harvard School of public health: allocation of resources to manage hypertension, N. Engl. J. Med. **296**:732, 1977.

Stoner, J.A.F.: Management, ed. 2, Englewood Cliffs, N.J., 1982, Prentice-Hall, Inc.

Third-party reimbursement issue paper, House of Delegates, Chicago, Oct. 15, 1982, The American Dietetic Association.

Vermeersch, J.A.: Evaluation of quality assurance standards in ambulatory nutritional care, Proceedings of a National Conference, Durham, N.C., June 1979.

Vermeersch, J.A., and Kaufman, M.: Quality assurance in ambulatory nutrition care, J. Am. Diet. Assoc. **78**:582, 1981.

Williamson, J.: Information management in quality assurance standards development for public health nutrition in quality assurance in ambulatory nutritional care, Proceedings of a national conference, Durham, N.C., June 1979, University of North Carolina Press.

APPENDIX 7-1

STATE PROGRAMS

STATE PROGRAM INFORMATION

Agency: *Department of Health Services*   Program: *Division of Community Health Services (summary)*

Program Description

The Division of Community Health Services is responsible for planning, organizing, coordinating, implementing, and evaluating programs concerned with the delivery of health care to the community. The following services are provided: preventive health care including health education, nutrition, and dental health; detection, diagnosis, and treatment of disease including venereal disease, tuberculosis, immunization, acute disease control, cervical cancer screening, and the State Laboratory.

Program Goal

To provide and promote quality health care to include prevention, detection, diagnosis, and curative services to the hypothetical state in coordination with health care providers.

Program Plans

1. To provide leadership and direction for all programs in Community Health Services with emphasis on evaluation of programs in terms of effectiveness, efficiency, need for expansion, and cost containment or discontinuance. These activities will be monitored on a quarterly basis.

2. To complete a review of the Cancer Hospitalization and Subvention Program in the state and program staff utilizing programmatic review and cost containment measures by January 1986. Recommendations will be made to the Director for further direction of this program.

3. To maintain necessary surveillance systems for monitoring disease occurrence and control activities.

4. To evaluate all licensed laboratory facilities to ensure compliance with licensure statute.

5. To deliver nutrition and supplemental food services to 36,200 individuals and their families, including 1000 older adults, to reduce the prevalence of malnutrition (undernutrition and overnutrition) by 20% in 1 year.

6. To develop educational plans for each Department of Health Services division based on needs, goals, and priorities.

7. To provide dental preventive-education services for 1350 elementary schoolchildren; provide treatment services for 950 indigent elementary schoolchildren; develop and implement multiple topical fluoride mouth rinse programs involving a minimum of 5000 schoolchildren, resulting in a 30% reduction in dental disease.

Continued.

Agency: *Department of Health Services*   Program: *Division of Community Health Services (summary)*

Program Results

1. Implemented a program of staff development in program planning, evaluation, and management by objectives to assist the manager to develop and achieve the objectives established for the division and for their specific program areas.

2. Completed the Medicaid Plan for the Department of Health Services to fulfill federal requirements to obtain these funds.

3. Surveillance activities in Bureau of Disease Control and Laboratory Services resulted in the reporting and processing of 8400 cases and suspected cases of reportable diseases other than venereal disease and tuberculosis.

4. The State Laboratory discontinued selected routine services and diverted resources to more critical areas. Each licensed hospital and independent clinical laboratory in the state was inspected during the year.

5. The Nutrition Program screened 30,230 people in 14 counties and 9 Indian tribes. Screening revealed that 58% of the population had elevated serum cholesterol levels, 13% were anemic, 5.2% were underweight, and 14.6% were overweight. Supplemental food and nutrition instruction was provided to 46,400 WIC recipients: 12,280 infants, 11,800 pregnant and lactating women, and 22,320 children.

6. Health education personnel continued coordination of statewide venereal disease education programs, completing the first statewide venereal disease workshop. Health education personnel identified and began assessment of existing health education programs throughout the state.

7. Eight percent (8%) more children received dental preventive and treatment services; 10% more children received free toothbrushes; 92% more contacts were made at parent and civic group meetings; and 44% more patients received dental services.

STATE PROGRAM INFORMATION

Agency: *Department of Health Services*   Program: *Bureau of Nutrition Services*

Program Description

Plans, develops, and implements nutrition services. Priority for services is placed on the following high-risk groups: women in childbearing years, 0- to 5-year-olds, schoolchildren, adults (parents of children), and the elderly. Services are delivered through five systems—screening, referral, monitoring, aide development, and food delivery—to decrease undernutrition and overnutrition. The bureau administers the special Supplemental Food Program for Women, Infants, and Children (WIC), which reaches 60% of the high-risk population; provides training in nutrition to community health workers, allied health personnel, group care facilities, educational institutions, and the public; formalizes training through community colleges and universities to develop indigenous nutrition manpower.

Program Goal

To develop and provide quality nutrition services as an integral component of health care, thereby improving nutrition and health in the population with a reduction in the number of people requiring sick care services and a decrease in health care costs.

Program Plans

1. To deliver nutrition and supplemental food services to 36,200 individuals and their families, including 1000 older adults, to reduce the prevalence of malnutrition (undernutrition and overnutrition) by 30% in 1 year.

2. To implement the statewide nutrition surveillance system by January 1986 for use by local health-related agencies as a tool for monitoring, program planning, and evaluation.

3. Training in nutrition: (a) 90% of community nutrition workers will be able to develop, implement, and evaluate the client nutrition education plan within 7 months of employment; (b) 60% of nutritionists and dietitians and 3% of other health personnel will participate in at least one training session with evaluation mechanism; (c) 90% of the management personnel in aged, day-care, and other group care facilities referred for nutritional care and/or food service assistance will be followed up to bring at least one previously deficient factor to standard; (d) 75% of those in educational facilities will implement one or more follow-up sessions in which

Agency: *Department of Health Services*

Program: *Bureau of Nutrition Services*

nutrition is related to one or more existing disciplines in the curriculum; (e) 7% of the public will receive nutrition information to improve their diets and/or learn of other sources of help through consultation, group sessions, and mass media.

4. To develop a career ladder for community nutrition workers by June 1986.

Program Results

1. *Screening.* Screened 30,230 people in 14 counties and 9 Indian tribes. Screening revealed that 58% of the population had high serum cholesterol, 13% were anemic, 16.9% were short for their age, 5.2% were underweight, and 14.6% were overweight.

2. *Monitoring.* Follow-up of those at risk resulted in 41.4% of the population decreasing their high serum cholesterol level, 65% of the population overcoming anemia, 44% making improvements in their height measurements, 51% overcoming underweight, and 22% reducing overweight. A survey on outcome of pregnancy in three projects showed that 92% to 100% of WIC mothers delivered full-term mature infants. A computer system to facilitate program evaluation was designed and piloted and will be implemented statewide August 1986.

3. *Referral.* Approximately 4500 referrals were made to and from the nutrition program, utilizing over 100 different agencies.

4. *Supplemental Food and Nutrition Instruction* was provided to 46,400 WIC recipients—12,280 infants, 11,800 pregnant and lactating women, and 22,320 children.

5. *Training.* Trained 132 (100%) community nutrition workers; 7 (100% EPSDT) health assistants; 198 (62%) nutritionists and dietitians; 271 (1.5%) other health personnel; 161 (11.5%) of the personnel in aged and group care facilities; 1061 (0.1%) of those in Educational facilities; 455,733 (20%) of the public through 49 workshops, 84 on-the-job in-service programs, 72,099 individual consultation sessions, 3 seminars, and 31 mass media presentations. A curriculum was designed for the education of community nutrition workers to improve job skills and mobility; 27 (25%) community nutrition workers are enrolled at a community college in a pilot for evaluation.

STATE SUMMARY OF EXPENDITURES AND BUDGET REQUESTS

Agency: *Department of Health Services*

Program: *Community Health Services*

Expenditure Classification	Actual Expenditures 1985-1986	Estimated Expenditures 1985-1986	Increase (Decrease) Requested			Request 1987-1988	Recommended 1987-1988
			A	B	C		
FTE No.	58.00	57.75			8.00	65.75	
Personal services	592.7	717.5	7.2	7.2	111.3	843.2	
Employee related	96.5	115.5	1.1	1.1	11.8	129.5	
Professional services	39.8	31.1	1.4	2.4	5.4	40.3	
Travel—in	41.8	53.3	6.1	3.0	17.1	79.5	
Travel—out	3.0	3.7	0.9	2.4	2.4	9.4	
Food							
Other operating expenditures	359.6	517.2	10.9	25.5	82.0	635.6	
Equipment	19.7	11.0	1.4	1.9	30.7	45.0	
Operations subtotal	1153.1	1449.3	29.0	43.5	260.7	1782.5	
Other	1173.5	1112.3			331.0	1443.3	
Total appropriated	2326.6	2561.6	29.0	43.5	591.7	3225.8	
Add federal funds							
Add other funds	117.3	415.0			(211.5)	203.5	

TOTAL PROGRAM

STATE SUMMARY OF EXPENDITURES AND BUDGET REQUESTS

Agency: *Department of Health Services*   Program: *Bureau of Nutrition Services*

Expenditure Classification	Actual Expenditures 1985-1986	Estimated Expenditures 1985-1986	Increase (Decrease) Requested			Request 1987-1988	Recommended 1987-1988
			A	B	C		
FTE No.	4.75	4.75				4.75	
Personal services	49.5	65.1	0.7	0.6	0.5	66.9	
Employee related	8.0	10.5	0.1	0.1	(0.4)	10.3	
Professional services	1.7	15.1	0.3	0.5		15.9	
Travel—in	5.7	6.0				6.0	
Travel—out	0.3	0.5	0.1	0.2		0.8	
Food							
Other operating expenditures	12.4	24.1	2.1	4.4		91.7	
Equipment		1.3	(0.4)			0.9	
Operations subtotal	77.6	122.6	2.9	5.8	61.2	192.5	
Other	128.8	152.3				263.3	
Total appropriated	206.4	274.9	2.9	5.8	172.2	455.8	
Add federal funds							
Add other funds							
TOTAL PROGRAM							

STATE PROGRAM INFORMATION

Agency: *Department of Health Services*   Program: *Bureau of Nutrition Services*

At A and B level funding: Funds would be insufficient to cover merit increases. Continued lack of opportunity for advancement may result in high staff turnover, especially in the field of nutrition, where nationwide salaries are more competitive.

At C level funding: Five nutrition personnel (4.75 FTEs) will be funded to complete the following duties related to program planning, implementation, and evaluation of nutrition services for 34,795 individuals.

Public Health Nutrition Director

1. Responsible for program planning, direction, and evaluation for delivery of nutrition services to 34,795 clients, which is a 27% increase in the aging and non–WIC-eligible segment of the population over the period between 1986 and 1987.
2. Responsible for directing and implementing the hypothetical state's role in national nutrition surveillance and state-based data collection and analysis for

use by local health-related agencies. Responsible for collection and evaluation of data on nutritional care services for older adults. Overall direction of $10 million federally funded Supplemental Food Program for high-risk pregnant women and children, serving 27,500 clients.

Public Health Nutrition Specialist II (Training Coordinator)

1. Responsible for coordination of statewide training activities through the identification of need, cataloging of resources, planning of programs, and establishment of evaluation tools to provide training in nutrition for the following:
   a. 90% of community nutrition workers will be trained so that they will be able to develop, implement, and evaluate nutrition education plan within 7 months of employment.
   b. 60% of nutritionists and dietitians and 3% of

STATE PROGRAM INFORMATION—cont'd

Agency: *Department of Health Services*   Program: *Bureau of Nutrition Services*

other health personnel should participate in at least one training session with an evaluation mechanism.

c. 90% of the management personnel in aged, day-care, and other group care facilities referred for nutritional care and other group care facilities referred for nutritional care and/or food service assistance will be followed up so that at least one previously deficient factor is brought to standard.

d. 75% of those in educational facilities will implement one or more follow-up sessions in which nutrition is related to one or more existing disciplines in the curriculum.

e. 7% of the public will receive nutrition information through consultation, group sessions, and mass media.

2. Serves as liaison between Bureau of Nutrition services and other Department of Health service bureaus, local health departments, and other health agencies in the areas of training statewide.

3. Responsible for the development and implementation of a career ladder for community nutrition workers in conjunction with the local community college.

Public Health Nutrition Specialist II (75% FTE)

1. Provides technical assistance in public health nutrition for persons 55 years of age and older with services to 1000 aging individuals statewide. Promotes, conducts, and assists in conducting training programs in nutritional care and food services with an evaluation mechanism for 10% of the personnel in aged and group care facilities in 14 counties.

2. Provides information or counseling in nutrition to the public and other agencies statewide.

3. Participates in coordinating field experience throughout the state for master's students, dietetic trainees, and others from 12 university settings in the United States.

Public Health Nutrition Specialist II (Funded by Maternal and Child Health, Assigned to Nutrition)

1. Integrates and coordinates Special Supplemental Food Program (WIC) with existing health department programs of MCH and nutrition in seven counties.

2. Analyzes nutrition surveillance data for seven counties for program planning, evaluation, and monitoring services for cost-effectiveness and contractual compliance.

Secretary III

1. Provides administrative support and prepares a variety of involved statistical and fiscal reports for Public Health Nutrition Director.

2. Maintains correspondence with subvention contractors, other bureaus, and outside agencies and people; maintains filing system for the bureau.

3. Arranges travel schedules, conferences, and presentations for Director.

Clerk Typist II

1. Types reports and correspondence for one nutrition specialist.

2. Other responsibilities include answering telephone, greeting visitors, explaining rules and regulations to public and making appointments.

STATE PROGRAM INFORMATION

Agency: *Department of Health Services*   Program: *Bureau of Nutrition Services*

At B level funding: An additional 2061 cholesterol determinations at $0.78.4 per test* would be completed for $1616. This is the estimated number of tests necessary to screen and follow up the clients to be served at this funding level (34,700 clients). An additional $663 is needed for educational materials.

At C level funding: A total of 34,795 clients would be screened. The additional cholesterol tests would cost $119.* No increase is requested in any category other than institutional supplies.

*Cost per test includes standards and controls.

P·A·R·T II

Delivering Quality Nutrition Services

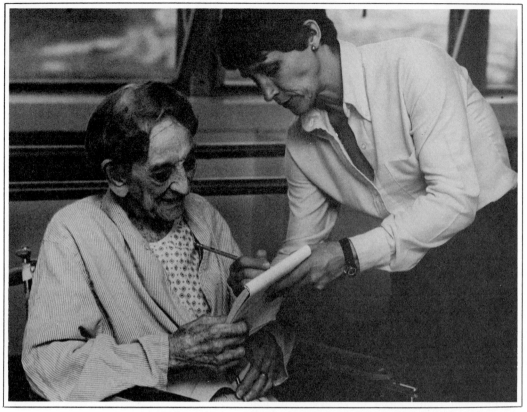

H. Armstrong Roberts

The Elements of Quality Nutrition Services for Prevention of Disease and Promotion of Health

GENERAL CONCEPT

Once nutrition problems are identified through such measures as nutrition surveys and surveillance, then nutrition intervention can be planned. The elements of quality nutrition services include nutrition assessment; dietary, clinical, anthropometric, and biochemical determinations; nutrition intervention, including nutrition counseling and nutrition education; referral for additional services; and evaluation of outcomes.

When you finish this chapter, you should be able to
- Apply the elements of quality nutrition services to an intervention program
- Identify nutrition surveys and nutrition surveillance data that have provided information on the U.S. population
- Discuss the objectives, methodologies, and limitations of dietary studies
- Identify the components of nutrition education
- Describe the food assistance program as part of the referral system

As our nation searches for ways to control health care costs, prevent disease, and improve health care systems and the quality of care for citizens, the science of nutrition becomes an important issue. Adequate food and optimum nutrition are essential to good health. Nutrition is a critical factor in the promotion of health and prevention of disease and in the recovery and rehabilitation from illness or injury. Americans who fail to attain a diet optimum for health can be found at every socioeconomic level.

The nutrition problems of the 1980s can best be described as those of overconsumption of energy and nutrients and undernutrition in high-risk groups. Specific risk factors are identifiable for the major health problems confronting Americans: obesity, cardiovascular disease, pregnancy, infancy and childhood, and dental problems (Chapter 1).

DELIVERING QUALITY NUTRITION SERVICES

The major elements required to deliver quality nutrition services include nutrition assessment; intervention, including preventive treatment and follow-up; referral services; monitoring; and education (Figure 8-1).

In this chapter we will discuss the elements of quality nutrition service in a generic sense, describing the components of each element in detail and reviewing national studies to determine the extent of nutrition problems in the United States. In Chapters 9, 10, and 11 we will describe the elements of quality nutrition services for specific age-groups in the life cycle. Each chapter will contain guidelines for population groups in community nutrition.

Nutrition Surveys in the United States

Although nutrition surveys were being conducted throughout the world, with the first survey commencing in Pakistan in 1956, it was not until the late 1960s that the United States began to address its own nutrition problems. Two surveys were undertaken almost simultaneously to determine the extent of malnutrition in the United States: the Ten-State Nutrition Survey, 1968–1970, and the Preschool Nutrition Survey, 1968–1970. In 1971 a third survey, the first National Health and Nutrition Examination Survey (NHANES), was begun; it was completed in 1974. HANES II started in 1975 and was completed in 1980.

Definitions of Surveys

Nutrition surveys examine the nutritional health of a population group at a particular point in time and thus are considered a cross-sectional examination. The cross-sectional survey provides information on the prevalence or magnitude of a condition or characteristic in a population at a specific time; it does not provide data on the number of persons who may be expected to develop a condition during a period of time.

National Studies on Nutritional Status

In 1968 the CBS television program "Hunger in America" and the publication of *Hunger, U.S.A.* by the Citizens Board of Inquiry into Hunger and Malnutrition shocked the nation by charging that hunger, in the midst of plenty, was a national disgrace. A major effort to determine the ex-

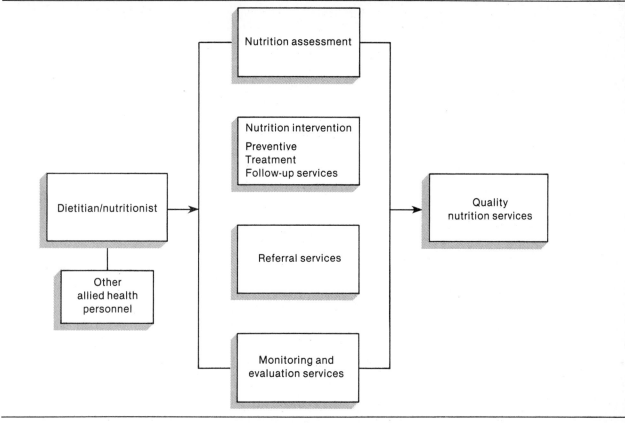

Figure 8-1. Elements of quality nutrition services.

tent of hunger and malnutrition in the United States was the White House Conference on Food, Nutrition and Health held in December 1969 and then a follow-up conference in 1974. The Senate also established a Senate Select Committee on Nutrition Needs, which held hearings on nutrition from 1968 to 1977. One of the major issues evolving from these events was the paucity of data on the nutritional status of the American population. Until 1968 attempts to evaluate the nutritional status of the American population had been confined to small, geographically isolated groups selected to meet the criteria of individual investigators.

Ten-State Nutrition Survey

The first comprehensive attempt to assess the nutritional status of the American people, the Ten-State Nutrition Survey, began in 1968. Approximately 24,000 families were included in the survey. It was conducted through 1970 as a result of an amendment to the Partnership for Health Act in 1967 (USDHHS, 1972).

The results of the Ten-State Nutrition Survey revealed that a significant number of the population surveyed was malnourished or at high risk of developing nutrition problems. The survey showed that malnutrition was found most commonly among blacks, less commonly among Spanish Americans, and least among whites. In general, there was increasing evidence of malnutrition in those persons with the lowest incomes. Although income is a major determinant of nutritional status, other factors such as cultural, social and geographical differences play a significant role in the nutrition level of a population.

Iron deficiency anemia, as evidenced by a high prevalence of low hemoglobin levels, was a widespread problem.

An excess of underweight and undersized children and adolescents was found in all population groups studied, compared with the standards commonly used in the United States. A greater per capita income was associated with greater height, greater body weight, greater thickness of subcutaneous fats, advanced skeletal development, and earlier attainment of maximum stature.

Obesity was found to be prevalent in women, particularly blacks. In some age-groups more than 50% of women were obese.

Poor dental health was also encountered in many segments of the population.

Preschool Nutrition Survey

Another survey of preschool children was conducted from 1968 to 1970 because it was apparent that little was known about the nutritional status of the U.S. population, particularly young children (Owen, Kram, and Garry, 1974).

The primary objective of the Preschool Nutrition Survey (1968-1970) was to provide an overview of descriptive data on nutritional status of a cross-sectional sample of preschool children throughout the United States. About 3400 children between 1 and 6 years of age were studied. This contrasted with the Ten-State Nutrition Survey, which focused on the population presumed to be most at risk because of poverty; the Preschool Nutrition Survey was not designed to determine the prevalence or severity of malnutrition in poor children or in children of any particular racial or ethnic group.

The Preschool Nutrition Survey indicated that evidence of "nutritional risk," that is lower dietary intakes, lower biochemical indices, and

smaller physical size for age, was found among preschool children of lower socioeconomic status. A large segment of the population surveyed was regularly taking vitamin supplements.

It was also evident from the survey that racial, genetic, and socioeconomic factors were important determinants of growth, nutrition, and health (Owen, Kram, and Garry, 1974).

There was a greater prevalence of low-birth-weight infants among Warner Rank I children (lowest socioeconomic rank). Mean hemoglobin values were lower in Warner Rank I and increased progressively in each rank. A mean cholesterol value of 161 mg/dl was found for all children examined and did not change significantly with age. Children in the lower socioeconomic groups, particularly black youngsters, had the highest caries attack rate.

National Health and Nutrition Examination Survey

The National Health and Nutrition Examination Survey (NHANES) programs conducted by the National Center for Health Statistics (NCHS) are unique sources of national data that have been labeled by the Department of Health and Human Services in recent congressional testimony as the "cornerstone" of the proposed National Nutritional Monitoring System (Brandt, 1981).

In 1971 responsibility for monitoring the nutritional status of the population was added to the Health Examination Survey (HES) and then became the NHANES I, conducted from 1971 to 1975. This survey was designed to assess overall health status, with particular emphasis on dental health, skin problems, eye conditions, and the nutritional status of the population 1 to 74 years of age (USDHHS, 1975).

For NHANES II, examinations began in February 1976 and ended in February 1980. Examinations were completed on 21,000 people from 6 months to 74 years of age (Murphy and Muhad, 1982). NHANES II provides the first look at changes in the health and nutritional status of the population over time.

NHANES I findings. Some of the major findings of NHANES I follow:

1. Iron was the nutrient most often found to be below standard in population groups. This deficiency was shown in three age-groups: children 1 to 5 years, for whom the mean measurements were 31% to 40% below the standard; adolescents 12 to 17 years, who were 23% to 33% below the standard; and women 18 to 44 years, who were 41% to 51% below the standard.

2. Black children 6 to 11 years and adults, regardless of race, 45 to 59 years in the lower-income groups also consumed amounts of iron that were below the standard.

3. Most age-groups, regardless of both race and income levels, had calcium, vitamin A, and vitamin C intakes that either approached 90% to 100% of the standard or were above the standard. The exceptions were black women 18 to 44 years, regardless of income levels, who had inadequate mean calcium intakes that were 20% to 23% below the standard, and white women of the same age-group in the lower-income level, who had mean vitamin A intakes 18% below the standard.

4. A higher percentage of white children 1 to 5 years and white women 18 to 44 years in the lower-income group, when compared with black individuals of similar age/sex/income groups, tended to have vitamin A and C intakes that were below the standard. Corresponding percentages in the upper-income group were higher for blacks than for whites.

Findings from NHANES I showed that the average reported consumption of fat was 83 gm on the day the dietary recall was taken (Abraham and Carroll, 1981). Fat represented 37% of the calories consumed daily. Males reported a higher fat intake, a mean of 100 gm per day, than females did (66 gm). The percent of calories from fat was 37% for males and 36% for females.

The major sources of fat in the diet for both males and females age 1 to 74 years in descending order of their percent distribution were meat, milk and milk products, fats and oils, desserts and sweets, and grain products. These food groups provided more than 70% of the fat for each gender and age-group in the population.

Eggs, meat, and milk and milk products were the major source of cholesterol, contributing 77% of the daily intake of cholesterol for males and 74% for females. The desserts and sweets group and the fats and oils group contributed 3% to 6% and 2% to 4%, respectively, of the cholesterol for either gender and all age-groups.

The largest percent of cholesterol intake from meat occurred at ages 18 to 44 years for males and at ages 12 to 17 years for females. The share of cholesterol intake from meat then decreased with age, declining to 21% for males and 23% for females in the oldest age-group (Table 8-1).

Table 8-2 shows the seven food groups that supplied 78% or more of sodium for both genders and all age-groups. Foods such as mustard, catsup, Worcestershire sauce, and other condiments accounted for only 0.2% in the 24-hour recall data because of minimum volume consumption. The data indicate that grain products are the major contributing source of sodium in the 24-hour recall. Milk and milk products were generally the second major source of sodium intake.

NHANES II findings. According to NHANES II, 66% of the U.S. women ages 18 to 30 failed to consume recommended amounts of calcium on any given day. After age 35, the percentage increased to 75%.

Strengths and weaknesses of NHANES I and II data. The methodologies used in NHANES I and II have various strengths and weaknesses and present logistical and conceptual challenges that must be dealt with in collecting, analyzing, and interpreting the data successfully (Murphy and Muhad, 1982).

Some strengths of NHANES programs are significant: (1) the sample is representative of the target population by age, race, sex, income, and region; (2) scientifically acceptable measures are used in the data collection process when possible, and state of the art methods of examination are

Table 8-1. Mean daily dietary cholesterol intake and percent of cholesterol provided by major food groups, by sex and age: United States, 1971-1974

Sex and Age	Mean Cholesterol Intake (mg*)	Source of Cholesterol (%)					
		Eggs	Meat	Milk and Milk Products	Desserts and Sweets	Fats and Oils	Other
Male							
1-74 years	445	35	26	16	4	4	16
1-5 years	301	40	15	25	4	3	14
6-11 years	347	28	19	27	5	3	18
12-17 years	410	23	26	25	5	4	17
18-44 years	521	35	28	13	4	3	16
45-64 years	465	39	27	11	3	4	16
65-74 years	411	45	21	11	4	4	14
Female							
1-74 years	303	34	24	16	5	4	18
1-5 years	274	40	15	26	4	2	13
6-11 years	277	21	20	30	5	3	20
12-17 years	291	25	26	23	6	3	18
18-44 years	311	34	25	13	5	4	19
45-64 years	327	40	25	11	4	4	17
65-74 years	274	40	23	11	5	4	17

From Abraham, S., and Carroll, M.D.: Vital Health Stat. no. 54, Feb. 27, 1981.
*Milligram.

Table 8-2. Mean daily sodium intake and percent of sodium provided by major food groups, by sex and age: United States, 1971-1974*

Sex and Age	Mean Sodium Intake (mg†)	Sources of Sodium (%)							
		Grain Products	Milk and Milk Products	Mixed Protein Dishes	Soups	Meat	Fruits and Vegetables	Fats and Oils	Other
Male									
1-74 years	2701	24	13	12	10	9	7	6	19
1-5 years	1886	20	18	11	12	7	6	6	20
6-11 years	2532	23	6	13	9	7	6	5	22
12-17 years	2965	23	15	14	8	8	6	5	21
18-44 years	3032	23	12	13	9	10	8	6	18
45-64 years	2540	25	11	8	11	10	8	8	19
65-74 years	2229	26	11	6	13	9	8	7	21
Female									
1-74 years	1850	23	14	11	10	8	8	6	19
1-5 years	1721	20	19	12	11	7	6	6	20
6-11 years	2238	23	16	12	10	7	7	5	20
12-17 years	2001	23	16	12	9	8	8	5	19
18-44 years	1863	23	13	13	10	9	8	7	18
45-64 years	1702	24	12	8	11	10	9	7	18
65-74 years	1526	27	13	5	11	7	8	8	21

From Abraham, S., and Carroll, M.D.: Vital Health Stat., no. 54, Feb. 27, 1981.
*NOTE: HANES sodium intake values converted to salt intake values assuming a ratio of 1 gm of salt to 400 mg of sodium.
†Milligram.

used in assessing an illness or condition; (3) regarding the data collection process with respect to content and standardization of procedures, the examinations are conducted in mobile examination centers by a few specially trained staff; (4) a rigorous quality and process control program is used throughout the study, enhancing the ability to evaluate and interpret the results; (5) the data collection procedure and techniques are documented in sufficient detail that subsequent programs may use them to compare data; (6) the results are documented and released in a variety of forms: microdata tapes, vital and health statistics reports, journal articles, and presentation at professional meetings.

Some weaknesses or limitations of methodologies are also important: (1) cross-sectional periodic national probability surveys cannot provide representational local data in sufficient detail to be usable, nor can they address rare conditions (less than 1% or 2%) with acceptable levels of precision; (2) cross-sectional surveys cannot provide casual relationship analyses; (3) surveys have important logical and pragmatic constraints that must be carefully weighed in defining the content of the study; (4) the current level of biomedical knowledge and techniques available for use in population surveys may not provide measures that are sufficiently sensitive or specific; (5) the lengths of data collection and potential effects of seasonality lead to logistical problems and concern in data analysis; (6) the analysis of data must carefully consider the complex survey design and the potential bias caused by nonresponse, which is significant in most population studies using examinations; the examination response rate in NHANES II was 74%.

Nationwide Food Consumption Survey

Since the 1930s, the U.S. Department of Agriculture (USDA) has conducted household food consumption surveys every 10 years. In the last two Nationwide Food Consumption Surveys (NFCS) data have also been collected on the food consumption of households. The 1977-1978 surveys consisted of a 24-hour recall of what was consumed plus a 2-day dietary record of what was eaten.

The 1977-1978 NFCS provided detailed information on the food consumption of households (at home) and the food intake of individuals (at home and away from home) (USDA, 1980).

Nutrient levels and food used by households in 1965 and 1977. Differences in the quantity of food used by households in the spring of 1977 and in the spring of 1965 were reflected in differences in energy and nutrient levels in food used (Cronin, 1980). There was a 10% decline in the level of food energy, probably because of a decreased use of milk and dairy products, breads and cereals, fats and oils, and most foods high in sugar (Table 8-3).

Pao summarized the results of the comparison of the average nutrititive content of the diets of individuals based on the preliminary data from the 1965 and 1977 NFCS and arrived at the following conclusions:

1. Caloric intakes of gender- and age-groups were lower, approximately 10%, in 1977 than in 1965 (Table 8-3).
2. Intakes of infants showed the sharpest drop of all gender- and age-groups from 1965 to 1977 for food energy, protein, fat, and calcium, but a large increase in iron was noted.
3. Intakes of food energy, protein, and fat appear to have decreased the least in older men and women, whereas calcium, vitamin A, and vitamin C intakes were higher in 1977 than in 1965 for this age-group.
4. From 1965 to 1977, intakes of protein declined for all gender- and age-groups except men and women over 65 years of age. Fat intake declined for all gender- and age-groups.
5. Calcium intakes in 1977 were lower than in 1965 for infants, children, and teenagers but were close to or above 1965 levels for six of the eight groups of adults. Average intakes of females 12 years and over were 25% or more below the 1974 Recommended Dietary Allowances (RDA). Several groups of children and males had intakes that averaged about 10% below the RDA.
6. The iron intake of infants in 1977 was more

Table 8-3. Comparison of nutrient level in food used in housekeeping households in the United States, spring 1965 and 1977

Nutrient	Average per Person per Day[*]		Percent Change from 1965[†]
	1965	1977	
Food energy (kcal)	3210	2900	−10
Protein (gm)	106	102	−4
Fat (gm)	154	140	−9
Carbohydrate (gm)	353	307	−13
Calcium (mg)	1110	1070	−4
Iron (mg)	20	20	2
Vitamin A (IU)	7020[‡]	7520	7
Thiamin (mg)	1.6	1.9	18
Riboflavin (mg)	2.4	2.6	7
Preformed niacin (mg)	25	27	8
Ascorbic acid (mg)	100	135	35

From U.S. Department of Agriculture: Family Econ. Rev., Spring 1980.
[*]Average is calculated using a population ratio procedure; 21 meals from household food supplies in a week is equivalent to one person.
[†]Calculated prior to rounding.
[‡]Adjustment made to reflect revised vitamin A value for eggs.

than twice the intake in 1965. However, the average intake of 1 to 2 year olds was much lower—about 45% below the 1974 RDA. Average intakes of females 12 to 50 years were between 35% and 40% below the RDA as in 1965.

7. Vitamin C consumption increased considerably from 1965 to 1977.

8. Average intakes of the following nutrients met 1974 RDA for all gender- and age-groups: protein, vitamin A, riboflavin, and vitamin C. Thiamin and phosphorus intakes met RDA for all groups except one.

9. Vitamin B$_6$ intakes of infants, children, and some groups of teenagers met the 1974 RDA; however, intakes of adult groups were below RDA. Females 15 years and over had average intakes between 35% and 40% below the 1974 RDA. Men and girls 12 to 14 years had average intakes falling 7% to 22% below the standard. These conclusions must be taken with caution because food composition values for vitamin B$_6$ are still in the developmental stage.

10. Average intakes of magnesium were below 1974 RDA for nearly all gender- and age-groups, but food composition values for magnesium are still in the developmental stage.[*]

[*]From Pao, E.M.: Family Econ. Rev., Spring 1980.

NUTRITION SURVEILLANCE

Surveillance, in contrast with survey, implies continuity—"a frequent and continuous watching over." One highly desirable feature of the surveillance system is that a "sample of convenience," that is, data available from any source that accurately describe the sample, can be used effectively.

Uses of Surveillance Data

The usefulness of surveillance information cannot be overemphasized in public health practice. There are six ways in which data from a nutrition surveillance system can be used (Centers for Disease Control, 1975):

1. To define the prevalence of particular nutrition problems in target populations. Flexibility should be built into the system to accommodate additional indices. An example of this flexibility is the Arizona Nutrition Surveillance System, in which serum cholesterol determinations were added to the assessment profile.

2. To facilitate medical care by providing a basis for identifying individuals in need of follow-up treatment.

3. To provide "before" and "after" information so

that the value of intervention and preventive programs, both for individuals and population groups, can be measured. The opportunity to provide data on the result of the program is one of the most important aspects of the surveillance system.

4. To provide data to establish priorities for the allocation of funds and personnel resources.
5. To provide information about the local situation that will enable effective targeting of federal, state, and local feeding programs.
6. To provide a research base for investigating the relationship between various levels of nutritional status and health consequences.

The Nutrition Surveillance System (Centers for Disease Control)

History

In 1973 the CDC began working with five states (Arizona, Kentucky, Louisiana, Texas, and Washington) to develop a system for continuously monitoring the nutritional status of specific, high-risk population groups. These five states recognized the need for timely nutrition-related data on the population served by them for use in program planning and evaluation. The system is based on utilization of readily available data from selected health service delivery programs. Once this nucleus of states demonstrated that the surveillance mechanism was practical and usable, a gradual expansion into other states occurred. Today there are 32 states participating in pediatric nutrition surveillance, encompassing approximately 1 million records of clients per year. Pregnancy nutrition surveillance is active in 18 states, involving approximately 30,000 records of clients per year.

Methods and Procedures

Nutritional status indicators for use in surveillance were selected from those indicators used in nutritional status surveys. The indices used were those which relate to the most widely prevalent nutritional problems and which are inexpensively and routinely obtained by local clinic staff.

Reference standards for the evaluation of surveillance data are derived principally from the national surveys conducted by the NCHS. Although data obtained from surveillance activities may not reflect the same ethnic and geographical composition as the sample drawn for national-level surveys, the data obtained from national samples still serve as a useful reference point in evaluating surveillance findings.

The principal sources of nutrition surveillance data have been programs such as Maternal and Child Health (MCH), Early Periodic Screening, Diagnosis, and Treatment (EPSDT), Supplemental Food Program for Women, Infants and Children (WIC), and Head Start, which have been implemented to improve the health and well-being of high-risk children, particularly minority preschoolers, disadvantaged schoolchildren, and pregnant adolescents. Nearly all health-oriented programs for children require that they be weighed and measured and that hemoglobin or hematocrit levels be determined. These simple and inexpensive determinations are relevant to assessment of the three most common nutrition-related problems documented by the major U.S. nutrition surveys: retardation of linear growth, overweight, and anemia.

Data on other important characteristics, such as age, sex, and ethnic background, are also readily available and can be incorporated into the surveillance mechanism with minimum additional cost and effort. In addition, some health agencies are engaged in measuring serum cholesterol and free erythrocyte protoporphyrin (FEP) levels in the pediatric population; these indicators can be used in surveillance.

Elements

At the local level clinic personnel records are used, providing information on height, weight, hemoglobin or hematocrit, or other pertinent variables for each child screened in a service delivery program. These data are sent to the state health department, where they are edited for obvious measurement errors or inconsistent recording of data and keyed onto computer tapes. These tapes are either processed within the state or sent to the CDC, where the data are analyzed.

The basic analyses are conceptually simple. Each child's height and weight values are compared with the NCHS reference population values and with a set of age- and sex-specific cutoff values for hemoglobin and hematocrit. These comparisons form the basis for the determination of prevalence estimates for anemia, growth retardation, or overweight. The data are then sent back to the states for use at state, district, and local levels.

Monthly printouts, which list all children who were screened and found to have one or more potentially abnormal values, are provided to each clinic.

On a quarterly basis, tables are produced for each reporting clinic. These tables give the numbers and percents of children screened; age, ethnic group, and program distributions; percent and duration of breast-feeding; prevalence of abnormal conditions; and an estimate of the level of probable measurement error. In addition, each state nutrition director receives tables that rank reporting clinics by prevalence of shortness, overweight, thinness, anemia, and probable errors. Similar tabulations are provided annually. As needed, tabulations can be produced showing the proportions of children found to have highly prevalent nutrition abnormalities by the type of program in which they are enrolled (e.g., EPSDT, WIC, MCH clinics).

Guidelines for Interpretation and Reference Data

Comparisons must be made with known values derived from appropriate reference populations to make meaningful interpretations of data. In the CDC system the indices were physical growth of children and anemia.

Height and weight. The reference population used for the height and weight data follow:

Age	Reference Population Data
Birth to 24 months	Fels Research Institute Growth Study
25 to 59 months	Preschool Nutrition Survey
60 to 143 months	National Health Examination Survey I (Cycle II)
144 to 215 months	National Health Examination Survey I (Cycle III)

These data are reasonably representative of the total population of the United States.

The CDC system employs three commonly used methods of comparison for height or weight: height for age, weight for height, and weight for age.

HEIGHT FOR AGE (MEASURE OF SHORTNESS AND TALLNESS). A low height for age is indicated when height for age is less than the 5th percentile of a person at the same sex and age in the reference population. Height for age is the best indication of long-term undernutrition if it has been of sufficient severity and duration to have caused stunting of growth. It is a helpful measure in detecting the short stature that may result from chronic undernutrition in children and their mothers.

WEIGHT FOR HEIGHT (MEASURE OF THINNESS AND FATNESS). Low weight for height is indicated when weight for height is less than the 5th percentile of a person at the same sex and height in the reference population. To determine height-weight for height, the weight for height would be greater than the 95th percentile of a person of the same sex and height in the reference population. Weight for height is an excellent indicator of recent undernutrition or of overnutrition and overweight.

WEIGHT FOR AGE (RATIO OF HEIGHT OBSERVED TO HEIGHT EXPECTED FOR THAT AGE AND SEX). Low weight for age is indicated when weight for age is less than the 5th percentile of a person of the same sex and age in the reference population. Although weight for age determination was used extensively in the past, it is of limited use, since it may be misleading as an index by itself.

Hemoglobin and hematocrit. In the CDC surveillance system the reference values are adapted from the World Health Organization (WHO) study on nutritional anemias and the Ten-State Nutrition Survey. Individuals below these measures are considered to be anemic.

It is useful to array the data as percentage distribution at successive 0.5 gm/dl intervals for hemoglobin and at 1% intervals for hematocrit.

These data are also analyzed according to the percentage of the population at various age intervals that fall below the following specified levels:

Age	Hemoglobin (gm/dl)	Hematocrit (%)
6 to 23 months (both sexes)	10	31
2 to 5 years (both sexes)	11	34
6 to 14 years (both sexes)	12	37
15 years and over (males)	13	40
15 years and over (females), nonpregnant	12	37
15 years and over (females), pregnant	11	34

The cutoff points that are used to define groups with potential nutrition problems have been derived from consultation with many individuals and professional groups (CDC, 1975).

Quality Control

In 1980 over a million records for both screening and follow-up visits were submitted to the CDC Nutrition Surveillance System. Of these, approximately 5% contained errors and were rejected by the system. The most common causes of rejection included invalid clinic or count codes, birth dates later than the date of visit, and invalid ethnic or sex codes. The most common error, invalid clinic codes, was caused primarily by delay in receiving the appropriate codes of new reporting clinics. Improved computer-editing proceedings have been developed and implemented in the surveillance system which identify measurements that may contain errors.

ELEMENTS OF QUALITY NUTRITION SERVICES
Assessment of Nutritional Status

Reliable methods for assessment of nutritional status are needed to (1) determine whether or not impairment of health is the result of inadequate or inappropriate diet, (2) establish the specific nature of any nutritional problem underlying such health impairment, (3) provide knowledge on which to base dietary treatments for improving

health, and (4) permit evaluation of the effectiveness of nutritional treatments or interventions that may be undertaken to improve health (Simopoulos, 1982).

In planning health care delivery for individuals and groups, it is particularly important to identify the nature and extent of common health problems, including nutritional problems. Assessment of nutritional status is assumed to represent only one aspect of total assessment of health. Knowledge of the frequency and severity of nutritional problems in the population who seek care will permit reasonable allocations of resources for solving the more important nutritional problems, thereby contributing to improved health within the community, and will provide a basis for program evaluation (Fomon, 1974).

A successful effort in screening and follow-up of health problems will depend to a large extent on the understanding and motivation of health personnel. Proper application of the methods and interpretation of results require thorough understanding. Motivation for precise recording of results is unlikely to come about unless the importance of the data has been discussed.

Although the primary purpose of screening is the identification of individuals at nutritional risk, assessment of nutritional status of those seeking care will also be of value in providing data regarding nutritional disorders prevalent in the community, in indicating changes with time in prevalence of disorders affecting those receiving care, and especially in identifying individuals with nutritional disorders so that intervention measures may be initiated. The assessment of a community is best determined by correlating results of dietary, clinical, biochemical, and anthropometric studies.

Nutritional Screening and Assessment Process

Figure 8-2 summarizes the screening process (Fomon, 1976). A minimum basic screening effort includes questions about dietary practices, a physical examination including dental examination, measurement of height and weight, laboratory studies including hemoglobin concentration

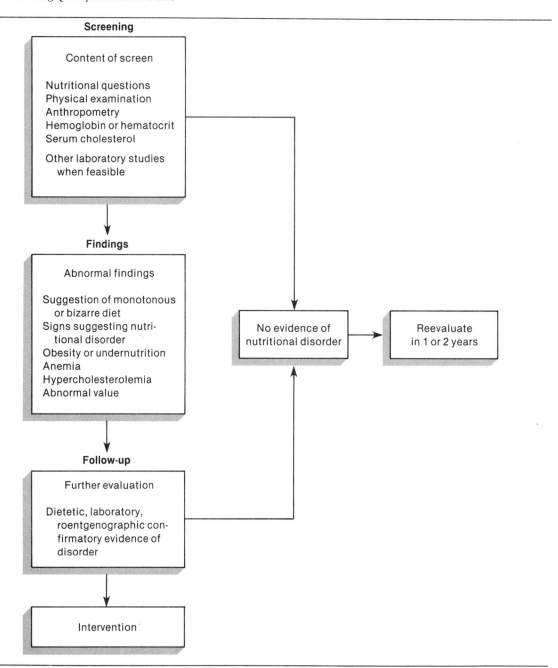

Figure 8-2. Nutritional screening and assessment process.
Modified from Fomon, S.J.: Nutritional disorders of children: screening, followup, prevention, U.S. Department of Health and Human Services, Public Health Service, Health Services Administration, Rockville, Md., 1976, U.S. Government Printing Office.

or hematocrit, and, if feasible, with children over 1 year of age, serum cholesterol (USDHHS, 1978).

If an individual presents no major suspicion of nutritional disorders on the basis of the food and diet questions, physical examination, anthropometric examination, and laboratory studies, there is little likelihood of detecting a nutritional abnormality. The individual will then be given advice regarding the preventive aspects of nutrition and will not be scheduled for further evaluation at that time.

If answers to the dietary screening questions suggest that eating habits are unusual or that the diet itself is unusual or monotonous, the community dietitian/nutritionist should complete a more detailed dietary evaluation. If no evidence of dietary inadequacy is found and if the screening reveals no problem with the physical examination, anthropometric evaluation, and laboratory studies, no further evaluation will be scheduled.

If there is a suggestion of dietary inadequacy, other studies (such as specific laboratory tests to confirm the suspicion and/or dietary counseling) should be indicated. Follow-up in a few months is generally desirable. When suggestive evidence of nutritional deficiency is detected by physical examination, appropriate laboratory studies should be undertaken to determine whether a nutritional deficiency actually exists (USDHHS, 1978).

The assessment of nutritional status may involve several disciplines on the health team. Members of the team should make a clear decision about who will be responsible for specific aspects of the screening/assessment process. However, it is the responsibility of the community dietitian/nutritionist and the physician to review the findings of the screening process to decide whether dietary counseling and follow-up are necessary for management or whether additional studies and procedures are needed.

Data from the following areas should be reviewed in the process of assessing nutritional status of the individual (USDHHS, 1978):

- Information on the family, including socioeconomic data and any community factors that might relate to the problem
- Dietary assessment to determine quality and quantity of individual diets; includes information on dietary intake, food acceptance, meal patterns, methods of food preparation and preservation, and utilization of food assistance programs
- Medical history and current state of health, other data such as medication used, low birth weight, hypertension
- Physical examination and evaluations for signs and symptoms of nutritional status, including dental evaluations when available, height, weight, and other anthropometric measures
- Laboratory studies such as hemoglobin and/or hematocrit, serum ferritin, cholesterol, lipoproteins, urinalysis, stools for ova and parasites
- Special biochemical analysis for serum or plasma albumin, ascorbic acid, alkaline phosphase, urea nitrogen; roentgeographic studies of the wrist

Dietary Methodology

Dietary data constitute an important part of any complete nutrition survey or individual nutrition counseling session in that they provide essential information on nutrient intake levels, sources of nutrients, food habits, preparation practices, and attitudes. They cannot be taken as an absolute indication of adequate nutrition, but they are widely used to obtain presumptive evidence of dietary inadequacies or excesses in individuals, specific population groups, institutions, or other community agencies.

The objectives of the dietary study must be clearly defined, for the objectives determine the appropriate methods to be used in collecting, processing, and interpreting the dietary data (Young, 1981). Questions of sample size and type are fundamental. The size of the sample varies with the objective and the method chosen but also with the classifications to be made in analyzing the data. The method of sampling should be clearly stated, as well as information relative to those unwilling to or unable to cooperate.

Types of dietary studies. In general there are two types of dietary studies, and within each type a variety of methods may be used: those concerned with food usage of families or institutions sharing common food supplies and those concerned with food usage of individuals. Information is obtained whether by food records or by recall of what has been eaten.

HOUSEHOLD OR INSTITUTION. Three household or institution dietary studies are available:

1. Food accounts—a simple running description of food purchased, received as gifts, or produced for household use over a given period of time. These are imprecise and are rarely used today.
2. Food records—a weighted inventory of foods on hand at the beginning and close of the study together with a day-to-day record of food brought into the home or institution over the period of the study with or without an accounting of kitchen and plate waste or food fed to pets. This is the method the USDA used in its early household consumption studies.
3. Food lists—a method by which an interviewer obtains from the person responsible for the food an estimate of the quantities of food used over a given period of time. This is the method used by the USDA in the more recent household food consumption studies (Young, 1981).

INDIVIDUAL. Dietary data on individuals are collected either (1) to obtain average nutrient intake, food intake, or food habits of groups for comparison with other groups; or (2) to obtain nutrient intake of an individual for correlation with clinical or biochemical measurements obtained on that individual.

Studies range from a qualitative type of food habit inquiry to a much more precise quantitative one. Methods used with individuals include the following:

1. An estimation by recall, in which the subject, or in the case of young children, perhaps the parent, recalls the food intake over the previous 24 hours or longer, with dependence on memory

2. Records of food eaten by an individual, kept by weights, household measurements, or estimated quantities over a stated period of time
3. Dietary history, in which by recall or repeated food records or both, the interviewer aims to discover the usual eating patterns over a relatively long period of time; it is a time-consuming process requiring professional personnel
4. Food frequency questionnaires, either self-administered or interviewer administered, as a means of acquiring information on general dietary intake or specific foods or nutrients over a longer period of time at less expense and with less personnel resources; used for epidemiological studies in which people may be grouped according to extremes of intake
5. Weighted intake for precise measurements during which all food eaten is carefully weighed and nutritive values are either calculated from food tables or determined by laboratory analysis of duplicate samples; it is usually used only in research groups with special facilities for collection and analysis

Data collection methods. Whether it is a community dietitian/nutritionist or a nutrition aide who is completing a 24-hour recall, proper training is necessary to obtain maximum information from a client. Actually, for group comparisons, 1-day records on a large number of people will be more revealing of dietary patterns than will studies conducted over long periods on a limited number of people. The 24-hour intake is fairly simple to obtain, either by recall or in a 15- or 20-minute interview conducted by personnel with relatively little technical background.

Certain equipment may be used in conducting the 24-hour recall, such as various sized glasses, spoons, bowls, or food models that will help the client indicate quantities more accurately. A notation of whether an individual has a typical or atypical daily food pattern should be indicated on the form.

The 24-hour intake recall questionnaire and the dietary questionnaire may also be used by trained interviewers under the supervision of a community dietitian/nutritionist experienced in obtaining dietary recalls. The dietary questionnaire is often called a frequency determination, and it can provide both a check on the completeness of the 24-hour recall and additional information on dietary patterns and food practices. Variations appropriate to different cultural groups should be devised. A dietary questionnaire or frequency determination is often useful in individual counseling, as well as in nutrition education and community programs.

INTERPRETING THE DATA. One of the simplest analyses of the 24-hour recall is to compare the client's food consumption with the RDA. If the limitations of the 24-hour recall are kept in mind, gross calculations of nutrient intake are valid. Comparisons with the basic food groups are at best a convenient tool for indicating possible weak areas in the diet, but they have severe limitations if the diet has small variety, unconventional foods, or special cultural components. The use of food composition tables is somewhat more precise but still only a crude quantitative expression of nutrients consumed.

Limitations of dietary history methodology. Failure to meet the RDA standard does not indicate malnutrition, since with the exception of calories, RDA are calculated to be above average physiological requirements for each nutrient. Since RDA are revised periodically, the survey results will be more meaningful for later reference if they are described in terms of absolute quantities of nutrients consumed. The 1980 RDA appear in Table 8-4.

Dietary history methods for epidemiological studies. Interest has recently increased in the role of diet in relation to cancer and other diseases. Because of this heightened interest, emphasis should be placed on the need to conduct effective epidemiological dietary studies focused on the quality of the exposure data. Hankin, Kolonel, and Hinds (1984) designed a dietary history method for use in a case-control study of vitamin A and lung cancer. The method is designed to obtain estimates of the usual frequencies and quantities of 84 major food sources of vitamin A and carotene consumed before symptoms of disease in cases and during the same time period in matched controls. Amounts are estimated from photographs of each item that show three different quantities. A questionnaire that consists of precoded forms for recording the frequencies and usual survey sizes of the 84 items is administered to the client.

The results of the study showed that related to those men with the highest intakes, men who consumed less vitamin A or carotene had a higher risk for lung cancer in a general dose-response fashion. These findings were not apparent in females.

One of the preferred methods for estimating usual dietary intakes of individuals is the diet history questionnaire. In order to provide more information on the reproducibility of the diet history questionnaire in a case-control study, 117 participants in the study were re-interviewed. The reproducibility of a diet history questionnaire was assessed as part of a case-control breast cancer study in Caucasian and Japanese women in Hawaii. The method was designed to estimate the intakes of total and saturated fat, cholesterol, and animal protein. The mean difference in intakes between the two interviews was small and not statistically significant for all four nutrient items among Japanese and Caucasian cases and control cases, whereas the mean difference for all four nutrients was substantial and statistically significant among the Caucasian controls. These findings indicate that the diet history method is reasonably reproducible in three of the four groups of subjects studied (Hankin et al., 1983).

Alternative Approaches to Classic Forms of Consumption Measurement Methods

Two methods recently used include telephone interviewing and market data bases (Schucker, 1982).

Telephone interviewing. Over 50% of consumer data collected by commercial research

Table 8-4. Food and Nutrition Board, National Academy of Sciences–National Research Council Recommended

	Age (years)	Weight		Height		Protein (g)	Fat-Soluble Vitamins		
		(kg)	(lb)	(cm)	(in)		Vitamin A (µg RE)[b]	Vitamin D (µg)[c]	Vitamin E (mg α-TE)[d]
Infants	0.0-0.5	6	13	60	24	kg × 2.2	420	10	3
	0.5-1.0	9	20	71	28	kg × 2.0	400	10	4
Children	1-3	13	29	90	35	23	400	10	5
	4-6	20	44	112	44	30	500	10	6
	7-10	28	62	132	52	34	700	10	7
Males	11-14	45	99	157	62	45	1000	10	8
	15-18	66	145	176	69	56	1000	10	10
	19-22	70	154	177	70	56	1000	7.5	10
	23-50	70	154	178	70	56	1000	5	10
	51+	70	154	178	70	56	1000	5	10
Females	11-14	46	101	157	62	46	800	10	8
	15-18	55	120	163	64	46	800	10	8
	19-22	55	120	163	64	44	800	7.5	8
	23-50	55	120	163	64	44	800	5	8
	51+	55	120	163	64	44	800	5	8
Pregnant						+ 30	+ 200	+ 5	+ 2
Lactating						+ 20	+ 400	+ 5	+ 3

[a] The allowances are intended to provide for individual variations among most normal persons as they live in the United States under usual environmental stresses. Diets should be based on a variety of common foods in order to provide other nutrients for which human requirements have been less well defined.

[b] Retinol equivalents. 1 retinol equivalent = 1µg retinol or 6 µg β carotene.

[c] As cholecalciferol. 10 µg cholecalciferol = 400 IU of vitamin D.

[d] α-tocopherol equivalents. 1 mg d-α tocopherol = 1α-TE.

[e] NE(niacin equivalent) is equal to 1 mg of niacin or 60 mg of dietary tryptophan.

[f] The folacin allowances refer to dietary sources as determined by *Lactobacillus casei* assay after treatment with enzymes (conjugases) to make polyglutamyl forms of the vitamin available to the test organism.

firms today are gathered by telephone and only 10% by personal interviews. The consumer behavior of interest is often relatively simple in nature, such as whether or not a product was purchased or used in a given period. Such interviews can be brief and do not heavily tax the respondent's ability to remember and report accurately.

An example is a Food and Drug Administration (FDA) telephone survey that was conducted for the purpose of estimating the incidence of use of protein supplement products in an adult segment of the population (Schucker, 1982). Consideration of the need for rapid turnaround of information, as well as the presumption that the incidence of protein supplement use by dieters was quite low, led to the conclusion that a telephone probability survey was the most cost-efficient technique for screening a large number of households. Telephone survey costs generally can be expected to average 40% to 50% of the cost of comparable personal interview surveys.

Market data bases. As part of its program of surveillance of the food supply, the FDA periodically obtains access to commercial market data bases that report the nationally projected unit and dollar sales of most packaged foods sold in grocery stores. One application of the data involves analysis of trends in consumer purchases of particular foods and commodity groups (Schucker, 1981). Analyses can be done for individual brands, for combined brands across more

Daily Dietary Allowances,[a] revised 1980

Water-Soluble Vitamins							Minerals					
Vitamin C (mg)	Thia-min (mg)	Ribo-flavin (mg)	Niacin (mg NE)[e]	Vitamin B$_6$ (mg)	Folacin [f] (μg)	Vitamin B$_{12}$ (μg)	Calcium (mg)	Phos-phorus (mg)	Mag-nesium (mg)	Iron (mg)	Zinc (mg)	Iodine (μg)
35	0.3	0.4	6	0.3	30	0.5[g]	360	240	50	10	3	40
35	0.5	0.6	8	0.6	45	1.5	540	360	70	15	5	50
45	0.7	0.8	9	0.9	100	2.0	800	800	150	15	10	70
45	0.9	1.0	11	1.3	200	2.5	800	800	200	10	10	90
45	1.2	1.4	16	1.6	300	3.0	800	800	250	10	10	120
50	1.4	1.6	18	1.8	400	3.0	1200	1200	350	18	15	150
60	1.4	1.7	18	2.0	400	3.0	1200	1200	400	18	15	150
60	1.5	1.7	19	2.2	400	3.0	800	800	350	10	15	150
60	1.4	1.6	18	2.2	400	3.0	800	800	350	10	15	150
60	1.2	1.4	16	2.2	400	3.0	800	800	350	10	15	150
50	1.1	1.3	15	1.8	400	3.0	1200	1200	300	18	15	150
60	1.1	1.3	14	2.0	400	3.0	1200	1200	300	18	15	150
60	1.1	1.3	14	2.0	400	3.0	800	800	300	18	15	150
60	1.0	1.2	13	2.0	400	3.0	800	800	300	18	15	150
60	1.0	1.2	13	2.0	400	3.0	800	800	300	10	15	150
+20	+0.4	+0.3	+2	+0.6	+400	+1.0	+400	+400	+150	[h]	+5	+25
+40	+0.5	+0.5	+5	+0.5	+100	+1.0	+400	+400	+150	[h]	+10	+50

[g] The recommended dietary allowance for vitamin B$_{12}$ in infants is based on average concentration of the vitamin in human milk. The allowances after weaning are based on energy intake (as recommended by the American Academy of Pediatrics) and consideration of other factors, such as intestinal absorption.

[h] The increased requirement during pregnancy cannot be met by the iron content of habitual American diets nor by the existing iron stores of many women; therefore the use of 30-60 mg of supplemental iron is recommended. Iron needs during lactation are not substantially different from those of nonpregnant women, but continued supplementation of the mother for 2-3 months after parturition is advisable in order to replenish stores depleted by pregnancy.

than 400 product classes, or for aggregated across-product classes to 56 food groups.

Clinical Assessment

Nutrition status. Until more sensitive indicators of subclinical malnutrition can be identified, public health practitioners will be unable to identify the more subtle forms of malnutrition. The more overt physical signs and symptoms of malnutrition, however, are clearly defined in dietary malnutrition.

In 1962 the WHO Expert Committee on Medical Assessment of Nutritional Status proposed a classification of physical signs to be used in nutrition surveys. Updated in 1966, this guide has proved valuable (Table 8-5).

Physical signs should be recorded as precisely and practically as possible. In terms of nutritional status, words such as "poor," "fair," or "good" should be avoided unless criteria for these terms are properly identified. An effective teaching tool that can assist the public health practitioner in identifying and standardizing signs of physical deficiencies is a series of color slides, "How to Diagnose Nutritional Deficiencies in Daily Practice" (Sandstead, Carter, and Darby, 1969).

The signs of malnutrition are multiple. One sign will alert the observer to continue with a more careful assessment of the body for other signs (Table 8-5). Environmental factors such as excessive heat, sun, wind, or cold air, lack of per-

Table 8-5. Physical signs of value in clinical assessment of malnutrition

Organ System	Group 1	Group 2
Hair	Lack of luster, thin, sparse, dyspigmentation, easily plucked	
Face	Diffuse depigmentation, nasolabial dyssebacia	
Eyes	Pale conjunctiva, conjunctival xerosis, Bitot's spots, corneal xerosis, keratomalacia	Corneal vascularization, conjunctival injection, conjunctival and scleral pigmentation
Lips	Angular stomatitis, angular scars, cheilosis	
Tongue	Edema, scarlet color, purple color, atrophy of filiform papillae	Hypertrophy of papillae, fissures, geographical tongue
Gums	Spongy, bleeding	Recession
Glands	Thyroid enlargement, parathyroid enlargement	
Skin	Xerosis, follicular hyperkeratosis, petechiae, pellagrous dermatosis, flaky paint dermatosis, edema (subcutaneous)	
Nails	Koilonychia	Transverse ridging
Musculoskeletal	Muscle wasting, craniotabes, frontal or parietal bossing, epiphyseal enlargement, beading of ribs	
Gastroenteric	Hepatomegaly	
Nervous	Psychomotor changes, mental confusion	
Cardiovascular	Cardiac enlargement	

From Owen, G.M.: Physical examination as an assessment tool. In Simko, M., Cowell, C., and Gilbride, J., editors: Nutrition assessment: a comprehensive guide for planning intervention, Rockville, Md., 1984, Aspen Systems Corp. Reprinted with permission of Aspen Systems Corporation.

FEATURES OF MEDICAL HISTORY SUGGESTING MALNUTRITION

1. Recent loss of 10% or more of usual body weight (adults) or failure to gain weight (infant or young child)
2. Restricted intake of food or nutrients
3. Chronic disease
4. Protracted losses of nutrients
   a. Vomiting, diarrhea
   b. Short gut, malabsorption
   c. Renal dialysis
   d. Burns, draining wounds
5. Increased metabolic needs
   a. Burns, trauma
   b. Fever
6. Use of antinutrient or catabolic drugs
   a. Anticancer drugs
   b. Corticosteroids
   c. Antibiotics, anticonvulsants

Modified from Owen, G.M.: Physical examination as an assessment tool. In Simko, M., Cowell, C., and Gilbride, J., editors: Nutrition assessment: a comprehensive guide for planning intervention, Rockville, Md., 1984, Aspen Systems Corp. Reprinted with permission of Aspen Systems Corporation.

sonal hygiene, and various cultural factors can cause or contribute to the physical signs that are associated with malnutrition.

Age of the person being examined also plays a role in the way the signs present themselves and are interpreted. Any physical finding in any age-group that suggests a nutritional abnormality should be considered a clue rather than a diagnosis and should be further explored.

The detailed clinical examination for signs of malnutrition must also include a search for signs related to metabolic diseases that may have a nutritional component. Several important features of the medical history that are suggestive of malnutrition are outlined on p. 190.

Problems in clinical assessment. Two major problems encountered in the clinical assessment of nutrition status are (1) a low rate of prevalence in developed countries, except among high-risk groups; (2) nonspecificity of clinical signs among most populations in these countries, and (3) the substantial differences in the prevalence of physical signs as recorded by different examiners.

Despite these difficulties, physical examinations must be an integral part of most nutrition surveys for the following reasons:

1. Physical examination may reveal evidence of certain nutritional deficiencies that will not be detected by dietary or laboratory methods.
2. The identification of even a few cases of clear-cut nutritional deficiencies may be particularly revealing and provide a clue to other pockets of malnutrition in the community.
3. The nutritional examination may reveal signs of a host of other diseases that merit diagnosis and treatment.

Anthropometric Assessment

Anthropometry, the measurement of body size, weight, and proportions, is one of the most frequently performed child health and nutrition screening procedures. By making accurate measurements and plotting them on standardized growth charts (e.g., NCHS percentile charts), a visual display of growth emerges. Trends revealed through anthropometric data help track individual growth, detect growth abnormalities, monitor nutritional status, and evaluate the effects of nutritional intervention on the treatment of disease (Moore and Roche, 1982).

The American Public Health Association guide *Nutritional Assessment in Health Programs* (Christakis, 1973) recommends the following for anthropometric measurements:

Neonates and infants
  Weight
  Recumbent length (crown-heel)
  Head circumference
  Chest circumference
  Triceps skinfold
Preschoolers
  The same as the preceding category with standing height replacing recumbent length
  Arm circumference
School age through adolescence
  Delete head and chest circumferences
  Standing height
  Otherwise, the same as the preceding categories
Adulthood and aging
  Standing height
  Weight
  Triceps skinfold
  Subscapular skinfold
  Arm circumference

Weight. Body weight should be measured to the nearest 10 gm (½ oz) for infants or 100 gm (¼ lb) for children.

Height and length. Measurements of height and length remain the most important measurement for the assessment of skeletal linear growth. Measures of height or length generally correlate better with socioeconomic status than do measures of weight.

Length is usually indicated for children up to 36 months of age and height thereafter. For length and height measurements a special board such as that designed by Fomon (1974) is highly desirable as opposed to a table. Figures 8-3 and 8-4 illustrate the technique of measuring height.

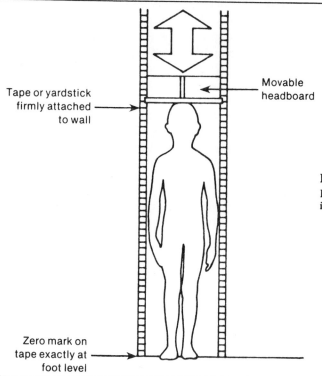

Tape or yardstick firmly attached to wall

Movable headboard

Zero mark on tape exactly at foot level

Figure 8-3. Stature measurement.
Redrawn from A guide to pediatric weighing and measuring, Atlanta, 1977, DHHS Centers for Disease Control.

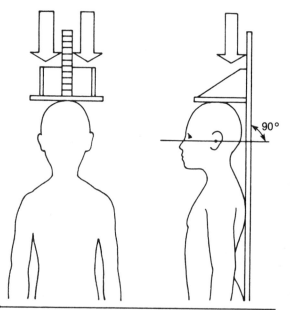

Press headboard firmly against head

90°

Figure 8-4. Stature measurement.
Redrawn from A guide to pediatric weighing and measuring, Atlanta, 1977, DHHS Center for Disease Control.

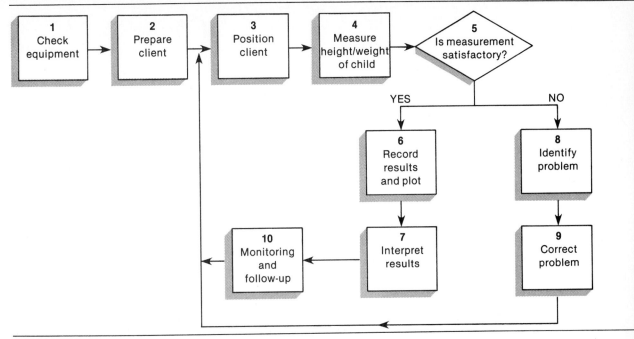

Figure 8-5. Weighing and measuring, training for clinic personnel, flowchart.
Modified from Owen, A.L.: Training manual for weighing and measuring, Sentinel Site Clinic, Detroit, 1980, Detroit Department of Health.

In measuring height, readings are recorded to the nearest 1 cm (¼ in). Recording to the nearest 1.2 to 2.5 cm (½ to 1 in) is too crude, especially for children at borderline levels of low stature. This is done for precision.

Height and weight of individuals over 60 years of age may not be accurate indices of body composition and nutritional status because of osteoporotic changes. Height always should be measured without shoes.

Training for clinic personnel to accurately take, record, and interpret results is essential if other data collected are to be accurate. Figure 8-5 contains a flowchart with 18 points describing the steps to be taken if accurate measurements are completed. This flowchart provides a broad map for persons responsible for measurement of height/stature/weight.

Head circumference. The purpose of the head circumference measurement in infants and toddlers is to screen for microcephaly and macrocephaly. It is considered to be a good index of brain growth, but caution is required when interpreting head circumference data because of familial and general body size factors.

Skinfold. Lean body mass can be determined by calculating triceps skinfold thickness and arm circumference (Figures 8-6 and 8-7). The prevalence of childhood obesity in the United States is at least 10%. The limitations of fatfold measurements have been documented by Tanner (1959); nevertheless, this measurement is currently the most convenient method to assess body fat bulk objectively. More accurate, but expensive, methods exist, but they are not practical outside the research laboratory at the present.

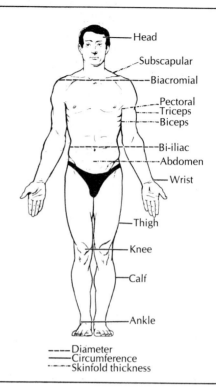

Figure 8-6. Anthropometric measurements used in various formulas for evaluating nutritional status.
From Guthrie, H.A.: Introductory nutrition, ed. 6, St. Louis, 1986, Times Mirror/Mosby College Publishing.

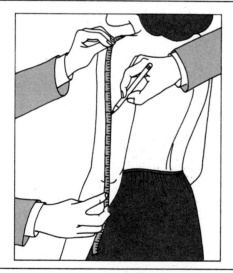
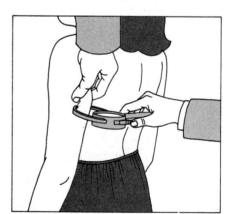

Figure 8-7. Measuring triceps skinfold with calipers.
From Guthrie, H.A.: Introductory nutrition, ed. 6, St. Louis, 1986, Times Mirror/Mosby College Publishing.

Measurements of weight for age and weight for height are used in assessing obesity, but they fail to distinguish muscle and soft tissue bulk from fat. On the other hand, serial weight measurements give a reasonable indication of excessive weight gain and likely obesity (Fomon, 1974).

In general, one limb (left triceps) and one truncal (left subscapular) measure are advised to account for differing distribution of fat. When a single measure is used, triceps has been favored for adolescents. Either the Lange caliper, which is the only one produced commercially in the United States, or the Harpenden, manufactured in England, can be used to record triceps or subscapular skinfold thickness.

Quality control. Erroneous information regarding specific indices such as height and weight measurements can lead to inappropriate conclusions and poor decisions in patient care management. With the CDC surveillance system, certain observations led to questioning of the accuracy of anthropometric data that were collected. Because of accuracy problems, a study was designed by the CDC Bureau of Training and was conducted in Washington. Its purpose was to provide information on the frequency and causes of inaccurate measurements (CDC, 1975). Significant findings included the following:

1. Reference team (two or more persons taking same measurements) results differed considerably from the heights, weights, and lengths obtained by clinic personnel.
2. Clinic measurements of children under 2 years of age tended to show length to be shorter than actual.
3. Although accurate weights are generally obtained, clinics tended to report an artificially high percent of children as being stocky and overweight.
4. Clinic measurements of standing children tended to show height to be taller than actual.
5. Equipment problems were considered to be the principal cause of inaccurate measurements.

6. Technique errors were less significant contributors to measurement inaccuracies.
7. The most common technique error noted was that young children were not properly stretched on the board for measuring.
8. Recording errors contributed significantly to inaccuracy.
9. The number of errors is heavily influenced by motivation of the staff.

This study demonstrated the need to do more careful appraisals of anthropometric measurements on a regularly scheduled basis. Staffs must be trained and kept motivated to perform these measurements accurately. Table 8-6 depicts the common errors of measurement.

Table 8-7 shows some anthropometric measurements applied in nutritional assessment. It also indicates some of the advantages and disadvantages of the particular measurements.

Use of growth charts in child health screening procedures. Although the Stuart-Meredith growth charts have survived for 30 years, their usefulness in contemporary society is limited. Responding to the identified needs of many researchers throughout the country, the NCHS in 1975 compiled data and prepared a series of percentile curves reflecting the growth of contemporary infants, children, and youth in the United States. These recent percentile curves are based on large, nationally representative samples of children. They represent a broad consensus of experts in physical growth, pediatrics, and clinical nutrition.

Anthropometry in the clinical setting. Anthropometry is the most frequently performed child health screening procedure. There have been a number of anthropometric studies with large population groups that have indicated associations between socioeconomic status, dietary adequacy, and growth among young children. Growth charts are effective in facilitating uniformity in clinical appraisal of growth and nutritional status and should help to simplify comparative interpretation of growth data. Growth charts for boys and for girls, prepubescent and 2 to 18 years, are shown in Figures 10-3 and 10-4.

Table 8-6. Common errors of measurement

Measurement	Error
All measurements	Inadequate instrument
	Restless child (procedure should be postponed)
	Reading part of instrument not fixed when value taken
	Reading
	Recording errors
Length	Incorrect age for instrument
	Footwear or headwear not removed
	Head not in correct plane
	Head not firmly against fixed end of board
	Child not straight along board
	Body arched
	Knees bent
	Feet not vertical to movable board
	Board not firmly against heels
Height	Incorrect age for instrument
	Footwear or headwear not removed
	Feet not straight nor flat on vertical platform or wall
	Knees bent
	Body arched or buttocks forward (body not straight)
	Shoulders not straight on board
	Head not in correct plane
	Headboard not firmly on crown of child's head
Weight	Room cold, no privacy
	Scale not calibrated to zero
	Child wearing unreasonable amount of clothing
	Child moving or anxious due to prior misregard
Head circumference	Occipital protuberance/supraorbital landmarks poorly defined
	Hair crushed inadequately, ears under tape
	Tape tension and position poorly maintained by time of reading
	Headwear not removed
Triceps fatfold	Wrong arm (should be left arm)
	Mid-arm point or posterior plane incorrectly measured or marked
	Arm not loose by side during measurement
	Examiner not comfortable nor level with child
	Finger-thumb pinch or caliper placement too deep (muscle) or too superficial (skin)
	Caliper jaws not at marked site
	Reading done too early or too late (should be 2 to 3 seconds)
	At time of reading, pinch not maintained, caliper handle not fully released
Arm circumference	Tape too thick, stretched, or creased
	Wrong arm (should be left arm)
	Mid-arm point incorrectly measured or marked
	Arm not loosely hanging by side during measurement
	Examiner not comfortable nor level with child
	Tape around arm, not at midpoint; too tight (causing skin contour indentation), too loose (inadequately opposed)

Modified from Zerfas, A.J., Shorr, I.J., and Neumann, C.G.: Pediatr. Clin. North Am. 4:253, 1977.

Table 8-7. Some anthropometric measurements applied in nutritional assessment

Measurements	Age Groups	Nutritional Indication	Reproducibility	Advantages	Disadvantages	Observer Error	Interpretation
1. Weight	All groups	Present nutritional status; under and over	Good	Common in use	Difficult in field; can't tell body composition; need accurate age; need proper scales	<100 g in children <250 g in adults	60% severe 60-80% moderate 80-90% mild 90-110% normal 110-120% over 120% & over obese
2. Height	All groups; 7 yr child	Chronic nutritional status (under) Chronic undernutrition in early childhood	Good	Common in use Simple to do in field	Differs by daytime Other factors play a role	<0.5 cm child <3.0 cm in adults	<80% dwarf 80-93% short 93-105% normal >105% giant
3. Head circumference	0-4 yr	Intrauterine and childhood nutrition (chronic undernutrition mental abilities)	Good	Simple	Other factors play a role	<0.5 cm	
4. Mid-arm circumference	All groups	Present under- and overnutrition	Fair	Simple, age independent; child need not be denuded; suitable for rapid survey	No limits for overnutrition; no standard for adult	<0.5 cm	<75% severe 75-80% moderate 80-85% mild >85% normal
5. Skinfold thickness subscapula	All groups	Present under- and overnutrition	Fair	Measure body composition, detect obesity—adults	Needs expensive callipers; difficult with child and in the field	1.0-1.5 mm	Similar to item (1)
6. Weight/ height for age ratio	All ages	Present under- and overnutrition	Good	Index of body build; age independent, 1-4 yr and adults	Need proper scales; need trained personnel		<75% severe 75-85% moderate 85-90% mild 90-110% normal 110-120% over >120% obese
7. Mid-arm/ head ratio	3 mo- 48 mo	Present undernutrition	Good	Simple; age independent; sex independent; any person can do it for field	No standard for adults		<0.25 severe 0.25-0.28 moderate 0.28-0.31 mild 0.31-0.35 normal >0.35% obese
8. Chest/head circumference ratio	1-2 yr	Present undernutrition	Fair or poor	Simple; age independent	For limited age; no classification method		<1 malnourished >1 normal

From Bengoa, J.M.: In Berg, A., Scrimshaw, N.S., and Call, D.L., editors: Nutrition, national development and planning, Cambridge, 1972, The M.I.T. Press. Reprinted by permission of the M.I.T. Press, Cambridge, Mass.

Table 8-8. Growth chart guidelines—weight for height (measurement of thinness and fatness)

Weight-for-Height Chart (Percentiles)	Interpretation	Recommended Intervention and/or Follow-Up
10th to 90th	Normal	Continue to examine at regular intervals, as given in the clinic protocol.
5th to 10th and 90th to 95th	Moderate risk depending on nearness to 5th or 95th percentile	Close attention by a public health worker until a normal consistent pattern of growth is established.
Above 95th	Obesity—depending on body build (musculoskeletal development); when in doubt, measurement of triceps skinfold thickness can be used to distinguish between obesity and extreme muscular development	Remeasure and verify age. Referral to the nutritionist with continual diet and activity counseling.
	Extreme muscular development	No action necessary.
Below 5th	This child may be undernourished; have a disease resulting in a significant weight loss and/or failure to gain weight; be exhibiting a pattern of growth (leaness) that is normal for this particular individual	Remeasure and verify age. Immediate referral to the nutritionist is desirable to determine if the child is malnourished. Close follow-up by the nutritionist and nurse is needed for the child determined to be malnourished and/or extremely underweight, with close periodic examinations until a normal/consistent pattern of growth is established. If a consistent pattern is not established by 3 months, refer child to physician.

From Fleshood, L.: Growth chart guidelines, Nashville, 1980, Tennessee Department of Health, Division of Nutrition and WIC Services.

Table 8-9. Growth chart guidelines—height for age (measurement of shortness and tallness)

Height-for-Age Chart (Percentiles)	Interpretation	Recommended Intervention and/or Follow-Up
5th to 95th	Normal	Continue to examine at regular intervals, as given in the clinic protocol.
95th and above	Probably normal; however, excessively rapid growth may indicate hormonal imbalance	Remeasure and verify age. If excessively rapid growth is maintained after three subsequent measurements at monthly intervals, referral to a physician is advised. Excessively rapid growth mentioned here refers to a rate of growth that is greater than 4 inches (10 cm) in a 3-month period for young infants or greater than 1 inch (2 cm) in a 3-month period for children 1 to 13 years of age.
Below 5th	This child may be chronically malnourished causing significant growth stunting; exhibiting a sign of a variety of diseases that can result in significant growth stunting; exhibiting a pattern of growth that is normal for this particular individual	Remeasure and verify age. Three months of measurements and intervention to determine a pattern of growth. If an improved or a normal/consistent pattern is not established within 3 to 6 months, referral to a physician is recommended.

From Fleshood, L.: Growth chart guidelines, Nashville, 1980, Tennessee Department of Health, Division of Nutrition and WIC Services.

Table 8-10. Growth chart guidelines—weight for age (comparison of actual weight to weight expected for age and sex)

Weight-for-Age Chart (Percentiles)	Interpretation	Recommended Intervention and/or Follow-Up
10th to 90th	Normal	Continue to examine at regular intervals, as given in the clinic protocol.
5th to 10th and 90th to 95th	Moderate risk, depending on height and nearness to 5th or 95th percentile	Remeasure and verify age. Close attention by a public health worker until a normal/consistent pattern of growth is established.
Above 95th	Obesity—depending on height and body build (muscular development). When in doubt, measurement of triceps skinfold thickness can be used to distinguish between obesity and extreme muscular development.	Remeasure and verify age. Plot height for age and weight for height charts to assure that the child is not unusually tall for his or her age. If the child is truly obese, this may be clinically evident; however, the weight for height chart provides documentation. Referral to the nutritionist for continual diet and activity counseling is recommended for the obese child.
	Extreme muscular development	No action necessary.
Below 5th	This child may be undernourished; have a disease that has resulted in significant weight loss and/or failure to gain weight; be exhibiting a pattern of growth that is abnormal for the entire population or reference group but normal for this particular individual	Remeasure and verify age. Plot height for age, weight for height charts to assure that the child is not unusually short for his or her age. Significant underweight for age for height will be clinically evident; however, the weight for height chart provides written documentation. Close follow-up by the nutritionist and nurse is needed for children determined to be malnourished and/or extremely underweight, with close periodic examinations being given until a normal/consistent pattern of growth is established. If normal pattern is not established within 3 months, refer child to physician.

From Fleshood, L.: Growth chart guidelines, Nashville, 1980, Tennessee Department of Health, Division of Nutrition and WIC Services.

Because size at birth may influence size throughout the first several years of life, it is important to obtain the best information possible concerning weight and gestational age at birth. Similarly, among families whose income is considered adequate, the stature of parents must be taken into account when growth of children is evaluated. To facilitate maximum use of the growth chart as one of the assessment tools available to health professionals, the Tennessee Department of Public Health developed guidelines for use by health professionals (Fleshood, 1980). The guidelines aid health department personnel in evaluating the measurement obtained and provide guidance to the community dietitian/nutritionist who is monitoring clients with potential problems affecting growth. Table 8-8 covers measurement of thinness and fatness; Table 8-9 describes measurement of shortness and tallness; and Table 8-10 compares actual weight to the weight expected for age and sex.

Biochemical Assessment

Laboratory methods of nutritional assessment are considered to provide a more objective and precise approach to nutritional status, that is, when compared with community assessment, dietary methodology, or clinical assessment methods.

Often the interpretation of laboratory data is difficult and does not necessarily correlate with either clinical or dietary findings. In contrast, there is a significant degree of correlation between some nutrient intakes and selected biochemical measures (Table 8-11).

Objectives of laboratory assessment. Laboratory tests have two primary purposes, one of which is to detect marginal nutritional deficiencies. Their use is especially important in early detection, before overt clinical signs of disease disappear, thus permitting indications of appropriate remedial steps. Their other purpose is to supplement or enhance other studies such as dietary or community assessment among specific population groups to identify nutritional problems. Table 8-12 indicates biochemical tests applicable to nutrition surveys (Jelliffe, 1966).

In general, laboratory methods indicate deficiencies in the following areas: (1) serum protein, the albumin level; (2) the blood-forming nutrients such as iron, folacin, vitamin B_6, and vitamin B_{12}; (3) water-soluble vitamins such as thiamin, riboflavin, niacin, and vitamin C; (4) the fat-soluble vitamins A, D, E, and K; (5) minerals such as iron, iodine, and other trace elements; and (6) levels of blood lipids, glucose, and various enzymes that are duplicated in heart disease, diabetes, and other chronic diseases.

Generally, two types of tests are employed in laboratory surveys: measurement of circulating levels of nutrients in blood or urine and/or functional tests. After the presence of nutrition problems are recognized, the functional tests measure the effectiveness of the body's use of its nutrient intake. For example, if deficiencies are detected in the urine, measurement of the enzymes, such as the transketolase level in the red blood cells, will provide a more accurate indicator of the degree of severity.

Interpretation of laboratory data. The significance and accuracy of results of biochemical tests are related to standards of collection; methods of transport, and storage, which would include possible exposure to ultraviolet light, heat, and shaking; and the actual technique used, which would include consideration of laboratory controls, using control sera.

The accurate interpretation of results depends on knowledge of the unique metabolism of each particular nutrient, including its storage in the body and the possibility of synthesis in the mode of excretion. The tests employed usually assess one of two aspects of nutritional inadequacy, although their specificity may be less than is at present appreciated. Table 8-13 provides a useful summary of biochemical methods for the practitioner (Fomon, 1976).

The interpretation of laboratory data will always provide areas for some disagreement, since the prime objective is to detect risk of deficiency before clinical evidence of disease develops. Standards may also vary somewhat in specificity and reproducibility according to the methods used. All methods used should be standardized and an appropriate design should be developed so that the results do not vary beyond acceptable limits during the course of the program. Standardization is best accomplished by repeating evaluation of standards that have been previously checked by a recognized standard laboratory. The best single source for advice on standards and controls is the Nutritional Biochemistry Section of the Centers for Disease Control, although there are other laboratories that can be consulted also.

The criteria used in the Ten-State Nutrition Survey are included in Appendix 8-1 for current information and reference purposes. These standards may be modified in the future as better methods and more data about the physiological significance of different intake of various nutrients and their functions are obtained.

Precaution in laboratory evaluation. Certain considerations must be recognized when evaluating the results of laboratory nutritional assessments. Nutrient levels vary from time to time and

Table 8-11. Correlation between dietary intakes and some biochemical variables

Dependent Variable (Biochemical)	Independent Variable (Dietary)	Correlation Coefficient	Analysis of Variance	
			df	F ratio
Urea nitrogen	Protein	.13	1/1270	23*
Ascorbic acid	Vitamin C	.46	1/1351	371*
Riboflavin	Riboflavin	.26	1/1282	97*
Thiamin	Thiamin	.23	1/1305	95*
Vitamin A	Vitamin A	.05	1/1516	4

From Owen, G.M., and Lippman, G.: Nutritional status of infants and young children: U.S.A., Pediatr. Clin. North Am. 24:211, 1977.
*Significant ($p < .001$).

Table 8-12. Biochemical tests applicable to nutrition surveys

Nutritional Deficiency	First Category*	Second Category
1. Protein	Amino acid imbalance test Hydroxyproline excretion test (F) Serum albumin Urinary urea (F)† Urinary creatinine per unit of time (T)	Serum protein fractions by electrophoresis
2. Vitamin A	Serum vitamin A Serum carotene	
3. Vitamin D	Serum alkaline phosphatase (in young children)	Serum inorganic phosphorus
4. Ascorbic acid	Serum ascorbic acid	White blood cell ascorbic acid Urinary ascorbic acid Load test
5. Thiamin	Urine thiamin (F)†	Load test Blood pyruvate Blood lactate Red blood cell hemolysate transketolase
6. Riboflavin	Urinary riboflavin (F)†	Red blood cell riboflavin Load test
7. Niacin	Urinary N-methylnicotinamide (F)†	Load test Urinary pyridone (N-methyl-2-pyridone-5-carbonamide)
8. Iron	Hemoglobin Hematocrit Thin blood film	Serum iron Percentage saturation of transferrin
9. Folic acid Vitamin B_{12}	Hemoglobin Thin blood film	Serum folate (L. casei) Serum B_{12} (E. gracilis)
10. Iodine		Urinary iodine (F) Tests for thyroid function

From Jeliffe, D.B.: The assessment of the nutritional status of the community, Geneva, 1966, World Health Organization; adapted from WHO Expert Committee on Medical Assessment of Nutritional Status, 1963.
(F), In a single urine specimen, preferably fasting; (T), in timed urine specimens.
*Urinary creatinine used as reference for expressing other urine measurements in first category.
†Expressed per gram of creatinine.

Table 8-13. Biochemical methods and remarks regarding interpretation

Substance	Method	Quantity Required	Comment
Hemoglobin (blood)	Cyanmethemoglobin (O'Brien et al., 1968)	20 µl	Concentration of hemoglobin less than 11.0 gm/dl for children below 10 years of age and less than 12.0 gm/dl for older children (less than 13.0 gm/dl for males over 14 years of age) indicates anemia.
Hematocrit (blood)	Capillary tube (O'Brien et al., 1968)	40 µl	Hematocrit less than 34 children below 10 years of age and less than 37 for older children (less than 41 for males over 14 years of age) indicates anemia.
Iron and iron-binding capacity (serum)	Manually by method of Fischer and Price (1964) or automated (Garry and Owen, 1968)	200 µl 10 µl	Concentration of iron, iron-binding capacity and percent saturation of transferrin may require different interpretation in infants than in older individuals.
Free erythrocyte porphyrins (blood)	Method of Piomelli et al. (1976) with filter paper disc	100 µl	Free erythrocyte porphyrin/hemoglobin ratio greater than 5.5 µg/gm indicates iron deficiency.
Total protein (serum)	Microbiuret manually (O'Brien et al., 1968) or automated (Failing et al., 1970)	50 µl	With manual method, a serum blank is desirable.
Albumin (serum)	Electrophoresis on cellulose acetate (Fomon et al., 1970)	10 µl	Concentration of albumin less than 2.9 gm/dl suggests poor protein nutritional status.
Ascorbic acid (plasma)	2.6 Dichloroindophenol reaction manually (O'Brien et al., 1968) or automated (Garry et al., 1974)	20 µl 50 µl	Concentration less than 0.3 mg/dl suggests that recent dietary intake has been low.
Vitamin A (plasma or serum)	Fluorometry (Garry et al., 1970; or Thompson et al., 1971)	200 µl	Concentration less than 10 µg/dl suggests deficiency and concentration less than 20 µg/dl indicates low stores.
Alkaline phosphatase (serum)	Liberation of p-nitrophenol manually (O'Brien et al., 1968) or automated (Morgenstern et al., 1965)	100 µl	Activity greater than 25 Bodansky units/dl is suggestive of rickets.
Inorganic phosphorus (serum or plasma)	Modification of method of Fiske and Subba Row (1925) manually (O'Brien et al., 1968) or automated	50 µl	Concentration less than 4.0 mg/dl is abnormal and suggestive of rickets. However, normal concentration does not rule out the presence of rickets.
Urea nitrogen (serum)	Urease manually (O'Brien et al., 1968) or diacetyl monoxime manually or automated (Marsh et al., 1965)	100 µl 50 µl	Concentration less than 8 mg/dl suggests low recent dietary intake of protein. However, concentrations as low as 3.5 mg/dl are sometimes found in breastfed infants.
Cholesterol (serum)	Manually by method of Carr and Drekter (1956) or automated (Levine and Zak, 1964)	100 µl	Concentration of cholesterol more than 230 mg/dl indicates hypercholesterolemia.

From Fomon, S.J.: Nutritional disorder of children: prevention, screening and follow-up, Washington, D.C., 1976, Pub. no. HSA 76-5612, U.S. Government Printing Office.

Table 8-13. Biochemical methods and remarks regarding interpretation—cont'd

Substance	Method	Quantity Required	Comment
Lipoproteins (serum)	Agarose electrophoresis (Laboratory Methods Committee, 1974)	100 μl	For interpretation, see Fredrickson and Levy (1972).
Creatinine (urine)	Alkaline picrate manually (O'Brien et al., 1968) or automated	100 μl	Serves as reference for other urine determinations.
Riboflavin (urine)	Fluorometry (Horwitz, 1970)	2 ml	Excretion less than 250 $\mu g/gm$ of creatinine suggests low recent dietary intake.
Thiamin (urine)	Thiochrome fluorometry (Horwitz, 1970)	10 ml	Excretion of less than 125 $\mu g/gm$ of creatinine suggests that dietary intake has been low for weeks or months.
Iodine (urine)	Automated ceric ionarsenious acid system (Garry et al., 1973)	5 ml	Excretion of less than 50 $\mu g/gm$ of creatinine suggests low recent dietary intake.

may reflect immediate rather than usual intake. Biological fluid levels and functional operation vary from person to person, even when they have similar diets or are apparently suffering equally from nutritional depletion. Furthermore, intercurrent disease may affect nutrient levels.

It also must be kept in mind that the "cutoff points" selected as representing some degrees of risk of deficiency are and perhaps always will be a somewhat arbitrary decision.

Public health significance and the role of the community dietitian/nutritionist. Community dietitians/nutritionists can help in developing the screening package and should encourage the use of simple accurate tests, keeping in mind the reliability, reproducibility, sensitivity, and specificity of the screening tests. Screening by income criteria alone is not an efficient way of discovering nutritional risk.

Nutrition Intervention

Nutrition counseling, nutrition education, and follow-up services are elements of care provided to patients/clients.

Nutrition Counseling

Nutrition counseling is the process by which patients/clients are most effectively helped to acquire more healthful behaviors (Mason, Wenberg, and Welsch, 1982). In attempting to counsel, consideration should be given to understanding the client's problems and concerns, although others who interact with the client are also important, such as family, peers, colleagues, and the health team.

The screening and assessment results are the first data to be used in determining a client's care plan for nutrition counseling.

Interviewing may be carried out to obtain more information about the client and his or her family as a basis for counseling, to provide new information, to teach new information, to review and strengthen acquired knowledge and desirable habits, or to help the individual set his or her own goals and make decisions. The term *nutrition counseling* is often used in conjunction with clinical practice, whereas *nutrition education* refers to the preventive aspects of nutrition. Chapter 13 describes the elements of counseling and behavioral change in detail.

Nutrition Education

Nutrition education is the process by which beliefs, attitudes, environmental influences, and understanding about food lead to practices that are scientifically sound, practical, and consistent with individual needs and available food resources. Since nutrition is a critical factor in the

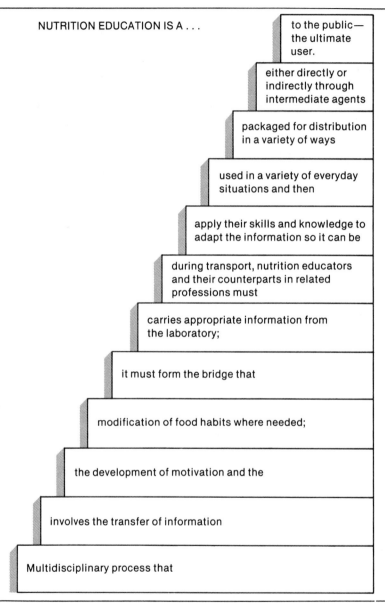

NUTRITION EDUCATION IS A . . .

to the public—
the ultimate
user.

either directly or
indirectly through
intermediate agents

packaged for distribution
in a variety of ways

used in a variety of everyday
situations and then

apply their skills and knowledge to
adapt the information so it can be

during transport, nutrition educators
and their counterparts in related
professions must

carries appropriate information from
the laboratory;

it must form the bridge that

modification of food habits where needed;

the development of motivation and the

involves the transfer of information

Multidisciplinary process that

Figure 8-8. Nutrition education.
Redrawn from Leverton, R.M.: What is nutrition education? Copyright
The American Dietetic Association. Reprinted by permission from *Journal
of the American Dietetic Association*, Vol. 64:17, 1974.

promotion of health and prevention of disease, health providers have a major role in planning and providing nutrition education programs. Nutrition education should be addressed to an individual (or group) at his or her own level, including appropriate cultural adaptations. Because of its preventive aspects, nutrition education should be included at all levels of the health delivery system.

Leverton (1974) has described nutrition education as a multidisciplinary process that involves the transfer of information, the development of motivation, and the modification of food habits when needed. Several steps are required before nutrition education can be effective. Figure 8-8 describes the entire process.

Follow-Up Services

If there is a suggestion of dietary inadequacy, another study (e.g., specific laboratory tests to confirm the suspicion and/or dietary counseling) should be indicated. When suggestive evidence of nutrition problems is detected by physical examination, appropriate laboratory studies should be undertaken to determine whether a nutrition problem actually exists. In some instances an interview with a nutritionist will be desirable in addition to or in lieu of laboratory studies. When laboratory findings confirm clinical signs of nutrition problems, an interview with a nutritionist is essential. Once the problem has been identified at screening (e.g., anemia, obesity, cardiovascular

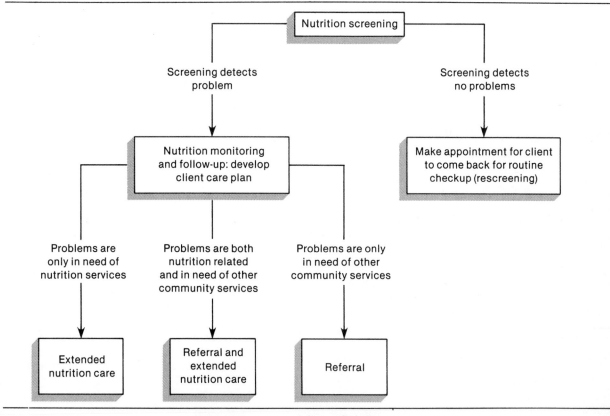

Figure 8-9. Service delivery flowchart.

disease risk), a client care plan must be developed to enable the dietitian/nutritionist to provide the follow-up care. The type of client problem will determine the design of the client care plan, which may be of three different types: a referral to another service, extended nutrition care, or a combination of referral and extended nutrition care. A service delivery flowchart (Figure 8-9) illustrates the generation of each type of client care plan.

All of the client care plans have three common goals: (1) to increase the client's knowledge and skills of his or her needs, (2) to obtain desired behavioral change, and (3) to improve health status and maintain that improvement.

Two tools are valuable aids in developing, implementing, and evaluating the client's individualized care plan:

1. Protocols, developed by the nutrition staff, designate what screening levels constitute risk, at what point and when to make referrals, when to evaluate for health status change, and what subject matter should be covered in client education.

2. The nutrition education plan consists of segments devoted to each nutrition problem that requires intervention. Each segment of the plan should contain (a) behavioral objectives that state what the client needs to know and/or be able to do to help solve his or her health problem(s); (b) learning activities that teach the client to meet the objectives stated in each problem's protocol; and (c) an assessment or a test that enables the nutritionist, nutrition aide, or community worker to determine if the client knows or can perform what is stated in the objective. The plan can then be used with the protocols to (a) select appropriate behavioral objectives that the client needs to meet, (b) select learning activities to teach the client, (c) select an assessment or test to determine if knowledge or skills have been gained, and (d) evaluate to discover whether the client's behavior and health status has changed.

Coordination and Referral System

Referral procedures are essential for continuity of care and to maximize the services available from other sources. Physicians are an integral part of the referral system in the community.

Table 8-14 provides a list of agencies that should be involved in such a system. It is a referral guide for nutrition-related problems that provides information on available community resources such as health service providers, educational institutions, and community groups. A knowledge of these community resources will enhance the patient's care (USDHHS, 1978).

A nutrition referral document should include the following minimum information:

- Client identification, age, address, and telephone
- Name of referring professional or agency with address and telephone
- Diagnosis or reason for referral
- Type of service needed
- Specific diet prescription (if applicable)
- Where nutrition services report is to be sent
- Identification of other consulting professionals presently or recently dealing with the client

A schematic diagram (Figure 8-10) illustrates the nutrition services referral system from community to family and/or from family to community.

Nutrition Information Assistance

Other health care providers may obtain nutrition information from the following state, local, and national sources (USDHHS, 1980):

State and Local Levels
- Public health nutritionist in state and local health departments
- Dietitians/nutritionists in voluntary agencies such as local Diabetes Association, local Heart Association, Visiting Nurse Association
- Dietitians/nutritionists in clinics, health centers, and hospitals
- Dietitians/nutritionists in Head Start programs at the regional, state, and local levels
- Professional organizations such as the American Dietetic Association, Society for Nutrition Educa-

Table 8-14. Referral guide for nutrition-related problems

Problem	Agency	Problem	Agency
Educational	Child day-care facilities School systems Vocational training programs Department of Mental Retardation Veterans Administration Bureau of Indian Affairs Migrant opportunity programs Community action programs	Social—cont'd	Local service and religious organizations Volunteer organizations Mental health services Migrant opportunity programs Community action programs Welfare
Economic	Employment services Vocational training program Rehabilitation programs Welfare, including food assistance programs Religious and other voluntary organizations Bureau of Indian Affairs Social Security	Transportation	Local service and religious organizations Volunteer organizations Migrant opportunity program Community action programs
		Environment	State and county health departments Public service and utility companies Local government officials Agricultural extension programs
Medical	Hospitals Health departments—state, county, and city School nurses Local physicians Crippled Children's services Veterans Administration Hospital Indian Health Service Other local health services	Food	County and City Welfare departments, including food assistance programs Local services and religious organizations Volunteer organizations Migrant opportunities program
Social	Child care facilities School systems Legal aid	Volunteer organizations	Migrant opportunities program Community action programs School Lunch Program Agricultural extension programs

tion, and the American Public Health Association have state or local affiliate chapters
- State Departments of Education (particularly the Nutrition Education Training [NET] Program)
- Local affiliations of the National Dairy Council
- State and local welfare agencies

National Level
- U.S. Department of Health and Human Services, 5600 Fishers Lane, Rockville, MD 20857
  Health Services Administration/Bureau of Community Health Services
  Food and Drug Administration

- U.S. Department of Agriculture, Washington, DC 20250
  Agricultural Research Service
  Consumer and Food Economics Research Division
  Food and Nutrition Service
  Federal, State, and Local Extension Service
- National Research Council, National Academy of Sciences
  2101 Constitution Ave., Washington, DC 20418
- Superintendent of Documents, U.S. Government Printing Office, Washington, D.C., 20401
- American Academy of Pediatrics, 1801 Himna Ave., Evanston, IL 60204

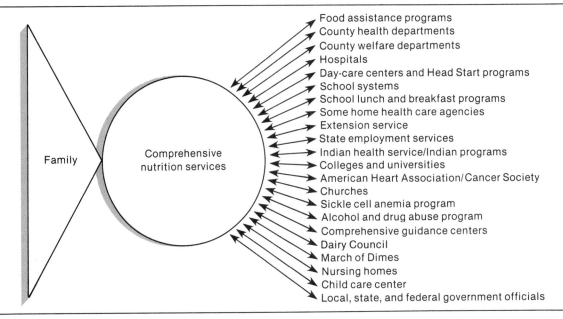

Figure 8-10. Nutrition services referral system.

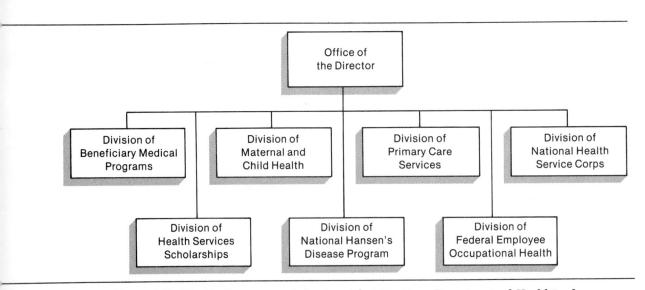

Figure 8-11. Health Resources and Services Administration, Department of Health and Human Services, Bureau of Health Care Delivery and Assistance.
Redrawn from Health Resources and Services Administration, Department of Health and Human Services, Washington, D.C., 1984, U.S. Government Printing Office.

- The American Home Economics Association, 2010 Massachusetts Ave., N.W., Washington, DC 20036
- American Institute of Nutrition, 9639 Rockville Pike, Bethesda, MD 20014
- The American Dietetic Association, 430 North Michigan Ave., Chicago, IL 60601
- The American Medical Association, 535 N. Dearborn St., Chicago, IL 60610
- American Public Health Association, Food and Nutrition Section, 1015 Eighteenth St., N.W., Washington, DC 20036
- Society for Nutrition Education, 21040 Shattuck Ave., Suite 1110, Berkeley, CA 94704

Federal Programs That Support State and Local Nutrition Services

U.S. Department of Health and Human Services. The Bureau of Health Care Delivery and Assistance (BHCDA), housed in the Department of Health and Human Services Health Resources and Services Administration, helps assure that medical care services are provided to persons living in medically underserved areas (MUA) and to persons with special health care needs (Figure 8-11). The bureau also serves as a national focus for providing preventive and specialized health services and for redistributing health care professionals to health manpower shortage areas (HMSAs) to promote a regular source of health services.

Maternal and Child Health Services: Title V of the Social Security Act. Title V of the Social Security Act provides nutrition programs and consultation through the Department of Health and Human Services. The initial legislation authorizing formula grants to states for Maternal and Child Health (MCH) and Crippled Children's Services was the original Social Security Act of August 14, 1935 (PL 74-271). Subsequent amendments earmarked funds for mentally retarded children, initiated Special Projects of Regional and National Significance (SPRANS), established training and research authority, and authorized the Programs of Projects (Maternity and Infant Care, Children and Youth, Dental Care, Intensive Infant Care, and Family Planning). In 1975

the Programs of Projects were merged into the formula grant to states, and in 1981 PL 97-35 created the MCH Services Block Grant.

The MCH Block Grant program is a principal source of support to states, assisting them in their efforts to maintain and strengthen their leadership in planning, promoting, and coordinating health care, including nutrition services, for mothers and children who otherwise do not have access to adequate health care. The MCH Block Grant consolidated the following seven categorical programs into one block that allows each state to develop its own programs and set its own priorities:

- Maternal and Child Health Services/Crippled Children's Services
- Supplemental Security Income (SSI), Disabled Children's Services
- Hemophilia
- Sudden Infant Death Syndrome
- Lead-Based Paint Poisoning Prevention
- Genetic Diseases
- Adolescent Health Services

MCH programs at all levels—federal, state, and local—are continuing their long tradition of working with the private sector, voluntary agencies, educational institutions, state and local agencies, and many other groups. The aim is to encourage initiation of health promotion programs in state and local public health agencies, other ambulatory care organizations, schools, hospitals, and private physicians' offices.

U.S. Department of Health and Human Services, Public Health Service, Office of Disease Prevention and Health Promotion. The offices of the Assistant Secretary for Health and Surgeon General has provided continuing impetus to the health promotion—disease prevention strategy for the nation. The Public Health Service has made significant progress in formulating an agenda for the nation in health promotion, health protection, and disease prevention. *Healthy People*, published in 1979, introduced a set of major goals for improving the health of the American people through the 1980s.

In 1980 the Public Health Service issued a report entitled *Promoting Health, Preventing*

Disease: Objectives for the Nation. Over 227 measurable objectives grouped under 15 priority areas were identified. In 1983 a Public Health Service implementation plan for attaining the objectives for the nation was developed (Chapter 1).

U.S. Department of Health and Human Services, Public Health Service, National Institutes of Health. The Health Education Branch of the Office of Prevention, Education, and Control, National Heart, Lung, and Blood Institute, has provided focus and material development in the area of cardiovascular risk factors for the workplace.

U.S. Department of Agriculture, Extension Service, Expanded Food and Nutrition Education Program (EFNEP). The USDA Extension Service's Expanded Food and Nutrition Education Program (EFNEP) began in 1968. EFNEP helps low-income families, especially those with young children, acquire the knowledge, skills, attitudes, and changed behavior necessary to improve their diets.

In 1970 the program was extended to low-income youth, primarily in urban areas. Youths are taught nutrition-related skills, enabling them to improve the adequacy of their diets.

EFNEP is operating in all states and territories in 961 sites, including cities, counties, and Indian reservations. States select areas for program operation.

State Cooperative Extension Services coordinate and manage EFNEP in states and territories. Program coordinators and food nutrition specialists, based at land-grant universities, provide training and develop resources that serve the needs of county professionals, paraprofessionals, volunteers, and participants. County Extension home economists conduct EFNEP as part of the county home economics program. 4-H youth professionals work with EFNEP.

FUNDING. The program was federally initiated in 1968 by USDA Extension Service with Section 32 funds, then under the Smith-Lever Act in 1970. In 1977 EFNEP received funding under the Food and Agriculture Act and in 1981, under the Agricultural and Food Act.

DELIVERY SYSTEM. County Extension home economists provide on-the-job training and supervise paraprofessionals and volunteers, who teach the EFNEP low-income homemakers and youth. Paraprofessionals often live in the communities where they work. They enroll homemakers in individual or group teaching sessions.

All nutrition education is tailored to the needs, interests, financial resources, ethnic backgrounds, and learning capabilities of EFNEP participants.

EFNEP education programs for youth are tailored to individual age-groups. Youth are taught in groups by paraprofessionals and volunteers.

IMPACT. An EFNEP study conducted in 1979 by Synectics (EFNEP, 1979) showed that:

- EFNEP identifies, enrolls, and teaches families with extremely limited financial resources.
- EFNEP continues to enroll and teach individuals who have poor diets. EFNEP concentrates its teaching on young families.
- The educational level of enrolled homemakers is much lower than the general American population.
- The percent of EFNEP families also receiving food assistance has increased since 1968. EFNEP referrals often come from food stamp offices.

This 1979 study also indicated that EFNEP has a positive impact on the diets and money management habits of program families. Homemakers improve their food and nutrition knowledge, food shopping and budget management skills, and dietary practices. Homemakers add more fruits and vegetables and more breads and cereals to their diets. They grow more food at home and save on food budget expenditures.

Food Assistance Programs

Health care providers should be aware of existing food assistance programs in their localities, since these are an important part of nutrition services available to high-risk groups. Food assistance programs are necessary either to maintain nutritional adequacy or to achieve socially desirable goals for such groups as the poor or for those whose nutritional status is vulnerable because of a rapidly changing and highly complex society—the isolated elderly and schoolchildren.

Most of the major food assistance programs are administered by the USDA through local programs such as National School Lunch Program, School Breakfast Program, Supplemental Food Service, Child Care Food Program, Special Milk Program, Food Stamp Program, Commodity Distribution and the Supplemental Food Program for Women, Infants and Children (WIC). The Department of Health and Human Services administers Nutrition Services Title III, which is a national nutrition program for the elderly. Table 8-15 describes the federally financed food assistance programs, including their purpose and objectives. In this chapter a description will be given of the food assistance programs that address the needs of the family, such as the Food Stamp Program and the Distribution Program. The WIC program, child nutrition programs, and Title III Nutrition Services will be discussed in subsequent chapters.

Food Stamp Program. The Food Stamp Program is a cooperative activity of local, state, and federal governments working together for a healthier America. Under the program, food coupons—commonly referred to as food stamps—are used to supplement the food buying power of eligible low-income households. The program is administered nationally by the USDA Food and Nutrition Service and locally by state welfare agencies. The Food Stamp Program was created to improve the levels of nutrition among low-income households.

PARTICIPANT REQUIREMENTS. The program provides monthly benefits to low-income households to help them purchase a nutritionally adequate diet. To qualify for the program, households must meet eligibility criteria and provide proof of their statements about household finances. U.S. citizens, aliens admitted permanently and legally, and certain other legal aliens may qualify.

The criteria for participation include the following:

- Able-bodied applicants between 18 and 60 years of age must meet certain work requirements.
- All households may have up to $1500 worth of countable resources (checking or savings account, cash, stocks/bonds); households of two or more people may have up to $3000 if at least one member is age 60.
- *All* household members *must* provide a Social Security number; and only households with net monthly incomes at or below 100% of the poverty line may qualify for food stamps; households without elderly or disabled members must also have gross incomes at or below 130% of the poverty line.

The income limits vary by household size and are based on federal poverty levels as provided in the Community Services Block Grant Act and are adjusted each July to reflect changes in the cost of living.

The maximum gross income eligibility standards (July 1, 1984, to June 30, 1985) follow:

Household Size	Continental United States	Alaska	Hawaii
1	540	676	621
2	728	912	838
3	917	1147	1055
4	1105	1382	1271
5	1294	1617	1488
6	1482	1852	1705
7	1671	2087	1921
8	1859	2322	2138
Each additional member	+ 189	+ 236	+ 217

These limits apply to households without elderly or disabled persons.

DETERMINATION OF BENEFIT LEVEL. Net monthly income is used to determine a household's benefit level.

Food stamp net income is figured by adding all of a household's gross income, except that excluded by law, and then subtracting certain deductions.

Table 8-15. Federally financed food assistance programs

Agency/Program	Estimated FY1984 Expenditures (Millions)	Authorizing Act	Purpose of Program	Objectives of Program	Administering Agencies
Department of Agriculture					
Food Stamp Program	11,059.4	Food Stamp Act of 1964 (7 U.S.C. 2011-2027, 2029)	Assist families in providing nutritious meals	Permit eligible households to buy food stamps at less than face value purchase of food at authorized retail stores	USDA Food and Nutrition Service (FNS) and state welfare agencies
Special Supplemental Food Program for Women, Infants and Children (WIC) and Commodity Supplemental Food Program (CSFP)	929.7	Section 17, Child Nutrition Act of 1966 as amended (42 U.S.C. 1786) CSFP Section 4(a) Agriculture and Consumer Protection Act 1973 (7 U.S.C. 612c)	Safeguard the health of high-risk populations by providing specific nutritious foods.	Provide vouchers to purchase foods or provide foods to qualifying pregnant, lactating and postpartum women, infants and children up to 5 years old who are at nutritional risk and are at low income	FNS and state health and tribal agencies
Food Donation/Commodity Distribution Programs	126.1	Section 4(a) Agriculture and Consumer Protection Act 1973 (7 U.S.C. 612c) Section 311 of Older Americans Act of 1965 (42 U.S.C. 303a)	Encourage and maintain the domestic consumption of commodities; prevent the waste of commodities	Use foods donated by USDA to needy persons, institutions, and elderly feeding programs	
National School Lunch Program	2,076.9	Sections 4 and 11, National School Lunch Act of 1946 as amended (42 U.S.C. 1753, 1751-61, and 1766) Section 3 of Child Nutrition Act of 1966 (42 U.S.C. 1733-1785,	Safeguard the health and well being of the nation's children and educate children about proper food habits	Provide meals free or at reduced prices or full pay to children attending a participating school (high school, grade school, or under)	FNS and state educational agencies

Program					
		breakfasts to needy children or those who travel distances	reduced prices to children attending a participating school (high school, grade school, or under)	trition Act of 1966 (42 U.S.C. 1773)	tional agencies
Child Care Food Program	270.5	Initiate, maintain, or expand foodservice programs to children in child care centers and family day care homes	Provide free meals or supplemental snacks to children participating institutions, child care centers, and family day care homes	Section 16, National School Lunch and Child Nutrition Act of 1966 Amendment of 1978 (42 U.S.C. 1766)	FNS, state educational agencies, and public or private nonprofit day care centers
Summer Food Program	88.8	Initiate, maintain, or expand foodservice programs to children in summer camps	Provide meals or snacks to children at participating institutions in poor areas	Section 13, National School Lunch and Child Nutrition Act of 1966 Amendment of 1975 (42 U.S.C. 1761)	FNS, state educational agencies, and public or private nonprofit summer camps
Special Milk Program	19.5	Encourage the consumption of fluid whole milk by children	Provide subsidy for milk served to children in participating schools, child care centers, and summer camps and institutions not participating in other federal subsidized meal programs, free milk to needy	Section 3, Child Nutrition Act of 1966 (42 U.S.C. 1772)	FNS, state educational agencies, and public or private nonprofit day care centers and summer camps

Department of Health and Human Services

Program					
Title III Nutrition Services	584.9	Provide low-cost nutritious meals to the elderly who cannot afford to eat adequately, lack meal preparation skills, have limited mobility, or are lonely	Provide at least one hot meal per day for 5 days a week and social contact for the elderly	Title III of the 1965 Older Americans Act (42 U.S.C. 3045), as amended	DHHS: Human Development Services, Office of Administration on Aging, and state agencies on aging

$15,475.2   Total Federal Expenditures FY84 (est)

From Owen, A.L., Owen, G.M., and Lanna, G.: Health and nutritional benefits of federal food assistance programs. In Costs and Benefits of Nutritional Care Phase 1. Chicago: The American Dietetic Association, 1979. Copyright The American Dietetic Association. Reprinted by permission; updated from Budget of the U.S. Government (appendix), Executive Office of the President, Office of Management and Budget, Washington, D.C., 1984, U.S. Government Printing Office.

The deductions for nonelderly households allowed by law follow:

- An 18% deduction from earned income
- A standard deduction (currently $95) for all households, which was adjusted in October 1984
- A combined deduction (currently $134) for actual dependent care costs and/or excess shelter costs, which was adjusted in October 1984

Households containing an elderly or disabled member are allowed an unlimited excess shelter cost deduction, and the monthly medical expenses of elderly or disabled members above $35 may be deducted from the household's gross income.

U.S. Department of Agriculture Food Distribution Program. Through the Food Distribution Program, the USDA provides foods to help meet many of the nutritional needs of children and needy adults.

The program has a twofold purpose. First, it improves the nutritional quality of the diets of the many people participating in USDA food programs. Second, it helps strengthen the agricultural market for products produced by American farmers.

For example, USDA buys some products grown by the farmers that are in plentiful supply. USDA then distributes these products, through its various Food and Nutrition Service (FNS) programs, to children in schools and child care centers, elderly people, certain needy families, and other special populations (USDHHS, 1980).

FOODS AVAILABLE. The specific foods that USDA donates may vary from time to time depending on what farm products are available. Because of the nutritional needs of participants in programs that receive donated foods, such as the National School Lunch Program, the Commodity Supplemental Food Program, the National Nutrition Services for the Elderly, and the Needy Family Program, USDA purchases and makes available certain types of foods.

Foods generally available include frozen and canned meat and poultry; canned and frozen fruits, vegetables, and juices; dairy products; cereals and grains; vegetable oil and shortening; and peanut products. USDA also provides donated foods, such as infant formula and cereal for children, to meet the special needs of some program participants. When supplying specific cultural groups (such as Indians and participants in the Trust Territory) with commodities, administrators take into consideration the ethnic food preferences of these groups.

USDA has been increasing the kinds of food available for donation. Today more than 50 kinds of foods are donated for distribution to the various programs.

USDA has also increased the amount of time allowed for shipping fruits and vegetables to states. This makes storage easier and allows state programs to offer fresh produce more often.

Monitoring and Evaluation

Health care providers realize that despite the limited amount of money, materials, manpower, and other resources, evaluation, whether simple or complex, can be accomplished. The first step is to establish that linkage between nutrition factors and health status in a systematic way. To accomplish this step, evaluation must be built in to the planning process at the critical stages of development and must be an essential component through the process. Chapters 6 and 7 extensively cover the evaluation process and quality assurance.

The elements of a nutrition program plan provide health care workers with the tools to anticipate results and conduct ongoing evaluation. Results of the evaluation assist program staff in making decisions on ways to improve the program by providing feedback about which methods are effective and which are deficient (USDHHS, 1983).

SUMMARY

In community settings surveys of the nutritional status of the population provide identification of problems to be alleviated. Nutrition surveillance also provides data on specific populations in a community and provides a continuous monitoring of the populations with nutrition problems.

To alleviate nutrition problems once they are identified, a system of nutrition care is implemented. This system includes the following elements: assessment of nutritional status (individual), nutrition intervention, coordination and referral, and monitoring and evaluation to assess outcomes.

REFERENCES

Abraham, S., and Carroll, M.D.: Fat, cholesterol and sodium intake in the diet of persons 1-74 years: advance data, Vital Health Stat. no. 54, Feb. 27, 1981.

Brandt, E.N.: Testimony before the Subcommittee on Department Operations Research and Foreign Agriculture, House Committee on Agriculture and Subcommittee on Science, Research and Technology, House Committee on Science and Technology, June 24, 1981.

Centers for Disease Control, U.S. Department of Health and Human Services: Nutrition surveillance, HEW Pub. no. 77-8295, Washington, D.C., Jan. 1975, U.S. Government Printing Office.

Centers for Disease Control: Nutrition surveillance annual summary: 1980, Atlanta, Nov. 1982.

Christakis, G., editor: Nutritional assessment health programs, Am. J. Public Health 63(Suppl.):1, 1973.

Cronin, F.J.: Nutrient levels and food used by households, 1977 and 1965, Family Econ. Rev., Spring 1980.

Fleshood, L.: Growth chart guidelines, Nashville, 1980, Tennessee Department of Health, Division of Nutrition and WIC Services.

Fomon, S.J., editor: Nutritional disorders of children: prevention, screening and follow-up, DHHS Pub. no. (HSA77-5104), Rockville, Md., 1976.

Hankin, J.H., Kolonel, L.N., and Hinds, M.W.: Dietary history methods for epidemologic studies: application in a case control study of vitamin A and lung cancer, Epidemiology Program, Cancer Research Center of Hawaii, University of Hawaii, Honolulu, Feb. 1984.

Hankin, J.H., et al.: Reproducibility of a diet history questionnaire in a case-control study of breast cancer, Am. J. Clin. Nutr. 37:981, 1983.

Jelliffe, D.B.: The assessment of the nutritional status of the community, Geneva, 1966, World Health Organization.

Leverton, R.M.: What is nutrition education? J. Am. Diet. Assoc. 64:17, 1974.

Mason, M., Wenberg, G.B., and Welsch, P.K.: The dynamics of clinical dietetics, ed. 2, New York, 1982, John Wiley & Sons, Inc.

Moore, W.M., and Roche, A.F.: Pediatric anthropometrics, Columbus, Ohio, Jan. 1982, Ross Laboratories, Inc.

Murphy, R.S., and Muhad, G.A.: Methodologic considerations of the National Health and Nutrition Examination Survey, Am. J. Clin. Nutr. (Suppl.) 35:5, May 1982.

National Academy of Sciences, Committee on Diet, Nutrition and Cancer: Diet, nutrition and cancer, Washington, D.C., 1982, National Academy Press.

Owen, G.M., Kram, K.M., and Garry, P.J.: A study of nutritional status of preschool children in the U.S. 1968-1970, Pediatrics 53(Suppl.):597, 1974.

Pao, E.M.: Nutrient consumption patterns of individuals, 1977 and 1965, Family Econ. Rev., Spring 1980.

Sandstead, H.H., Carter, J.P., and Darby, W.J.: How to diagnose nutritional deficiencies in daily practice, Nutr. Today 4:20, Summer 1969.

Schucker, R.E.: Alternative approaches to classic food consumption measurement methods: telephone interviewing and market data bases. In Simopoulos, A.P., editor: Assessment of nutritional status, Am. J. Clin. Nutr. 35(Suppl.):1306, 1982.

Simopoulos, A.P., editor: Assessment of nutritional status, Am. J. Clin. Nutr. 35(Suppl.):1104, 1982.

Tanner, J.M.: The measurement of body fat in man, Proc. Nutr. 18:148, 1959.

U.S. Department of Agriculture: Nationwide food consumption survey results, Family Econ. Rev., Spring 1980.

U.S. Department of Health and Human Services: The Ten-state nutrition survey in the U.S., 1968-1979, Pub. no. (HSM) 72-8134, Washington, D.C., 1972, U.S. Government Printing Office.

U.S. Department of Health and Human Services: Health and nutrition examination survey (NHANES), Washington, D.C., 1975, U.S. Government Printing Office.

U.S. Department of Health and Human Services: Guide for developing nutrition services in community health program, Public Health Service Bureau of Community Health Services, Rockville, Md., 1978, U.S. Government Printing Office.

U.S. Department of Health and Human Services, Bureau of Community Health Services: Federal and nonfederal resources for nutritional information and services: a selected list, Rockville, Md., 1980, U.S. Government Printing Office.

U.S. Department of Health and Human Services, Department of Agriculture: Nutrition and your health: dietary guidelines for Americans, Washington, D.C., 1980, U.S. Government Printing Office.

U.S. Department of Health and Human Services, Bureau of Community Health Services: Maternal and child health: guide to quality assurance in ambulatory care, Rockville, Md., 1983, U.S. Government Printing Office.

Young, C.M.: Dietary methodology. In Assessing changing food consumption patterns, National Research Council, U.S. Committee on Food Consumption Patterns, Washington, D.C., 1981, National Academy Press.

APPENDIX 8-1

GUIDELINES FOR CRITERIA OF NUTRITIONAL STATUS FOR LABORATORY EVALUATION*

Nutrients and Units	Age of Subject (Years)	Criteria of Status		
		Deficient	Marginal	Acceptable
Hemoglobin (gm/dl)*	6-23 mo	Up to 9.0	9.0- 9.9	10.0 +
	2-5	Up to 10.0	10.0-10.9	11.0 +
	6-12	Up to 10.0	10.0-11.4	11.5 +
	13-16M	Up to 12.0	12.0-12.9	13.0 +
	13-16F	Up to 10.0	10.0-11.4	11.5 +
	16 + M	Up to 12.0	12.0-13.9	14.0 +
	16 + F	Up to 10.0	10.0-11.9	12.0 +
	Pregnant (after 6 + mo)	Up to 9.5	9.5-10.9	11.0 +
Hematocrit (packed cell volume in percent)	Up to 2	Up to 28	28-30	31 +
	2-5	Up to 30	30-33	34 +
	6-12	Up to 30	30-35	36 +
	13-16M	Up to 37	37-39	40 +
	13-16F	Up to 31	31-35	36 +
	16 + M	Up to 37	37-43	44 +
	16 + F	Up to 31	31-37	33 +
	Pregnant	Up to 30	30-32	33 +
Serum albumin (gm/dl)*	Up to 1	—	Up to 2.5	2.5 +
	1-5	—	Up to 3.0	3.0 +
	6-16	—	Up to 3.5	3.5 +.
	16 +	Up to 2.8	2.8-3.4	3.5 +
	Pregnant	Up to 3.0	3.0-3.4	3.5 +
Serum protein (gm/dl)*	Up to 1	—	Up to 5.0	5.0 +
	1-5	—	Up to 5.5	5.5 +
	6-16	—	Up to 6.0	6.0 +
	16 +	Up to 6.0	6.0-6.4	6.5 +
	Pregnant	Up to 5.5	5.5-5.9	6.0 +
Serum ascorbic acid (mg/dl)*	All ages	Up to 0.1	0.1-0.19	0.2 +
Plasma vitamin A (mcg/dl)*	All ages	Up to 10	10-19	20 +
Plasma carotene (mcg/dl)*	All ages	Up to 20	20-39	40 +
	Pregnant	—	40-79	80 +
Serum iron (mcg/dl)	Up to 2	Up to 30	—	30 +
	2-5	Up to 40	—	40 +
	6-12	Up to 50	—	50 +
	12 + M	Up to 60	—	60 +
	12 + F	Up to 40	—	40 +

From Christakis, G., editor: Am. J. Public Health 63(Suppl):1, 1973.
*Adapted from the Ten-State Nutrition Survey.
†Criteria may vary with different methodology.
‡Erythrocyte glutamic oxalacetic transaminase.
§Erythrocyte glutamic pyruvic transaminase.

Nutrients and Units	Age of Subject (Years)	Criteria of Status		
		Deficient	Marginal	Acceptable
Transferrin saturation (%)*	Up to 2	Up to 15.0	—	15.0 +
	2-12M	Up to 20.0	—	20.0 +
	12-M	Up to 20.0	—	20.0 +
	12-F	Up to 15.0	—	15.0 +
Serum folacin (ng/ml)†	All ages	Up to 2.0	2.1-5.9	6.0 +
Serum vitamin B_{12} (pg/ml)†	All ages	Up to 100	—	100 +
Thiamin in urine (mcg/gm creatinine)*	1-3	Up to 120	120-175	175 +
	4-5	Up to 85	85-120	120 +
	6-9	Up to 70	70-180	180 +
	10-15	Up to 55	55-150	150 +
	16 +	Up to 27	27-65	65 +
	Pregnant	Up to 21	21-49	50 +
Riboflavin in urine	1-3	Up to 150	150-499	500 +
	4-5	Up to 100	100-299	300 +
	6-9	Up to 85	85-269	270 +
	10-16	Up to 70	70-199	200 +
	16 +	Up to 27	27-79	80 +
	Pregnant	Up to 30	30-89	90 +
RBC transketolase-TPP-effect (ratio)	All ages	25 +	15-25	Up to 15
RBC glutathione reductase-FAD-effect (ratio)	All ages	1.2 +	—	Up to 1.2
Tryptophan load (mg xanthurenic acid excreted)†	Adults (Dose: 100 mg/kg body weight)	25 + (6 hr) 75 + (24 hr)	— —	Up to 25 Up to 75
Urinary pyridoxine (mcg/gm creatinine)†	1-3	Up to 90	—	90 +
	4-6	Up to 80	—	80 +
	7-9	Up to 60	—	60 +
	10-12	Up to 40	—	40 +
	13-15	Up to 30	—	30 +
	16 +	Up to 20	—	20 +
Urinary N-methyl nicotinamide* (mg/gm creatinine)	All ages	Up to 0.2	0.2-5.59	0.6 +
	Pregnant	Up to 0.8	0.8-2.49	2.5 +
Urinary pantothenic acid (mcg)†	All ages	Up to 200	—	200 +
Plasma vitamin E (mg/dl)†	All ages	Up to 0.2	0.2-0.6	0.6 +
Transaminase index (ratio)†				
EGOT‡	Adult	2.0 +	—	Up to 2.0
EGPT§	Adult	1.25 +	—	Up to 1.25

APPENDIX 8-2

1985 EDITION OF THE RECOMMENDED DIETARY ALLOWANCES

As we go to press, controversy surrounds the 1985 or 1986 edition of the Recommended Dietary Allowances (RDAs). Originally scheduled to be released in the spring of 1985, the RDAs have been delayed by disagreement about the interpretation of certain data.

In a move with broad implications for American eating habits and food assistance programs, the RDA Committee of the National Academy of Sciences has drafted a report calling for lower recommended levels of some vitamins and minerals needed to maintain health. The committee proposed reducing the allowances for vitamins A, C, and B_6, magnesium, iron, and zinc, while raising the RDA for calcium.

The authors of the report said that these recommendations were based on the best available scientific evidence; however, some nutrition experts, including persons asked by the Academy of Sciences to read the report as part of its internal review process, have expressed concern. They said the report on the RDAs could be used by government officials to justify further cuts in food stamps, school lunch subsidies, and other nutrition programs.

Some nutrition experts asserted that the committee's draft report was out of step with the advice of scientists and public health professionals who in recent years have emphasized the role of proper diet in preventing specific nutritional deficiencies as well as reducing the risk of cancer and heart disease.

At the basis of the controversy is an important proposed change in the definition of the RDAs. The new RDAs would be defined as the levels of essential nutrients needed "to protect practically all healthy persons against nutritional deficiencies." The chairman of the RDA committee said the change was made to emphasize what the committee sees as the difference between two approaches to good nutrition. One is based on recommended levels of intake for individual vitamins, minerals, and other nutrients; the other approach is based on a person's overall dietary pattern.

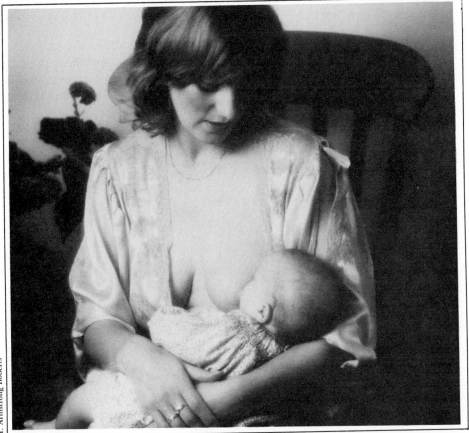

H. Armstrong Roberts

Maternal Nutrition

GENERAL CONCEPT

Pregnancy is one of the most critical and unique periods in the life cycle. The physical and mental health of the mother before and during her pregnancy has profound effects on the status of her infant in utero and at birth.

Throughout much of recorded history, nutrition has been regarded as an important influence on the course and outcome of pregnancy. Many physiological, biochemical, and hormonal changes occur during pregnancy that influence the need for nutrients and the efficiency with which the body uses them. Several of these changes are apparent in the early weeks of pregnancy, which indicates that they are an integral part of the maternal-fetal system. This maternal-fetal system creates the most favorable environment possible for the developing child. The changes are necessary to regulate maternal metabolism, promote fetal growth, and prepare the mother for labor, birth, and lactation (Pitkin, 1983).

NUTRITION-RELATED HEALTH PROBLEMS OF PREGNANT WOMEN

The U.S. Department of Health and Human Services (1980) document *Promoting Health–Preventing Disease* (Chapter 1) identified the following nutrition-related problems affecting pregnant women:
- Poor pregnancy outcomes (and suboptimum mental and physical development of infants and children) associated with inadequate nutrition
- Increased resistance to infection and perhaps certain allergies among breast-fed infants
- The relationship between iron and folic acid deficiencies in pregnant and lactating women and their dietary inadequacies

Specific objectives, to be accomplished by 1990, relating to pregnant women follow (USDHHS, 1980):
- By 1990 the proportion of pregnant women with iron deficiency anemia (as estimated by hemoglobin concentrations early in pregnancy) should be reduced to 3.5%. The USDHHS (1980) reported that in 1978 the proportion was 7.7%.
- By 1990 the proportion of women who breast-feed their infants should be increased to 75% at hospital discharge and 35% at 6 months postpartum. In 1978 the proportions were 45% at hospital discharge and 21% at 6 months postpartum.

IDENTIFYING PROBLEMS IN THE COMMUNITY: PREGNANCY NUTRITION SURVEILLANCE SYSTEM

The Pregnancy Nutrition Surveillance System is part of the CDC Nutrition Surveillance System, which monitors the health of infants, children, and pregnant women seen in public health clinics on a consistent basis. Chapter 8 describes this system in detail.

Birth weight below 2500 gm (5.5 lb) is a standard indication of poor pregnancy outcome. Low birth weight is associated with increased prenatal and infant mortality, poor growth, and increased rates of morbidity up to age 5 years (Food and Nutrition Board, 1982).

Data from the Pregnancy Nutrition Surveillance System have identified black women of all ages and women under the age of 20 years to be at risk for delivering low-birth-weight infants (CDC, 1983; Wong and Trowbridge, 1984).

Pregnant women who smoked were at increased risk; compared with nonsmoking pregnant women, they had nearly double the prevalence of low-birth-weight infants (Table 9-1).

Table 9-1. Prevalence of birth weight below 2500 gm by smoking and ethnic group—1980 Pregnancy Nutrition Surveillance System

Ethnic Origin	Smoking No.	Smoking LBW (%)	Nonsmoking No.	Nonsmoking LBW (%)
White	1,970	8.7	3,075	3.5
Black	852	13.6	2,378	7.5
Hispanic	569	8.6	2,614	4.7
Native American*	84	4.8	2,730	4.4
Asian†	11	—	49	12.2
TOTAL	3,486	9.8	10,846	4.9

From Wong, F.K., and Trowbridge, F.L.: Clin. Nutr. 3(3):94, 1984.
*Native American—American Indian or Alaskan native.
†Includes Southeast Asian refugees.

The combination of smoking and being black placed a pregnant woman in one of the highest risk groups for poor pregnancy outcome.

Data from other sources have found alcohol consumption, low prepregnancy weight, and low pregnancy weight gain to be contributing factors in low-birth-weight outcomes of pregnancy (Food and Nutrition Board, 1982). For both alcohol consumption and smoking during pregnancy, there is evidence of a dose-response effect. A synergistic effect of both smoking and alcohol in increasing the risk of a low-birth-weight infant has also been suggested (Wright et al., 1983). The combination was found to be influential even at the time of conception.

PHYSIOLOGICAL CHANGES IN PREGNANCY

There are several physiological changes that occur during the course of pregnancy, including the following.

Increase in the amount of blood (blood volume). Blood volume increases by almost 50% so that enough oxygen can be available to support the growing fetal and maternal tissues. Thus there is an increase in the need for those nutrients most important for making blood: protein, iron (hemoglobin is a protein with iron in it), folacin, and vitamin B_6. If a woman has sufficient dietary intake and stores of these nutrients before and during pregnancy, she will make this adjustment with little problem; otherwise, anemia may result. To help the body receive more oxygen, other changes occur in addition to blood volume (e.g., breathing becomes faster and deeper, and the heart pumps more blood in a given amount of time).

Changes in gastrointestinal tract. Food moves through the gastrointestinal tract more slowly, allowing the mother to digest food more completely, which in turn helps her to absorb more nutrients from food. Thus absorption of nutrients such as calcium and iron is increased during pregnancy; however, this slower movement of food may lead to constipation.

Changes affecting fluid needs. More fluid is needed by the woman's body because of:

1. Increased blood volume for the mother and development of blood for the fetus
2. Amniotic fluid, which surrounds the fetus in the uterus and protects it from trauma or shock
3. Increased urine output, since the woman is now getting rid of waste products for both herself *and* her baby.

For this reason, a woman needs to drink more fluids during pregnancy—at least eight glasses per day, including water, fruit and vegetable juices, and milk. The pregnant woman should try to avoid caffeine and not drink alcohol-containing beverages and low nutrient beverages such as soft drinks.

Increases in breast tissue and fat stores. The mammary glands in the breast begin to enlarge during pregnancy to allow the milk ducts to prepare for lactation. Fat stores increase in preparation for breast-feeding.

Changes in weight. The woman gains weight as both her tissues and the tissues of the fetus increase and develop. Because of the added tissue, more nutrients in general are required to build new tissue and keep these new tissues healthy. Different nutrients are required in varying degrees; some of the more striking increases are those for protein, folacin, vitamin C, iron, and calcium. Satisfactory progress with regard to

Table 9-2. Recommended daily dietary allowances of some selected nutrients for pregnancy and lactation (National Research Council, 1980 revision)

Nutrients	Nonpregnant Girl 12-14 yr 47 kg (103 lb)	Nonpregnant Girl 14-18 yr 55 kg (120 lb)	Nonpregnant Woman 25 yr 58 kg (128 lb)	Pregnancy Added Need	Pregnancy Girl 12-14 yr	Pregnancy Girl 14-18 yr	Pregnancy Woman 25 yr	Lactation (850 ml daily) Added Need	Lactation 12-14 yr	Lactation 14-18 yr	Lactation Woman 25 yr
Calories	2200	2100	2000	300	2500	2400	2300	500	2700	2600	2500
Protein (gm)	46	46	44	30	76	76	74	20	66	68	64
Calcium (gm)	1.2	1.2	0.8	0.4	1.6	1.6	1.2	0.4	1.6	1.6	1.2
Iron (mg)	18	18	18	*	18 +	18 +	18 +	*	18 +	18 +	18 +
Vitamin A (RE†)	800	800	800	200	1000	1000	1000	400	1200	1200	1200
Thiamin (mg)	1.1	1.1	1.0	0.4	1.5	1.5	1.4	0.5	1.6	1.6	1.5
Riboflavin (mg)	1.3	1.3	1.2	0.3	1.6	1.6	1.5	0.5	1.8	1.8	1.7
Niacin equivalent and tryptophan (mg)	15	14	13	2	17	16	15	5	20	19	18
Ascorbic acid (mg)	50	60	60	20	70	80	80	40	90	100	100
Vitamin D (µg)‡	10	10	5	5	15	15	10	5	15	15	10

From Williams, S.R.: Nutrition and diet therapy, ed. 5, St. Louis, 1985, Times Mirror/Mosby College Publishing.
*Required iron supplement 30 to 60 mg.
†Retinol equivalents.
‡Cholecalciferol; 10 µg equals 400 IU vitamin D.

weight gain is essential to the well-being of the developing fetus. It also serves as a major indicator to the health care provider that the pregnancy is proceeding normally.

NUTRITIONAL NEEDS OF PREGNANT WOMEN

Pregnancy represents a period of high nutrient needs and a purposeful requirement for a positive caloric balance. The diet a pregnant woman consumes should provide the vast majority of her nutrient needs (Brown, 1984). Studies of routine supplementation of healthy pregnant women with vitamins and minerals have failed to show benefits to mothers or infants. Inadequate diets, on the other hand, have been related to clinical problems during the course of pregnancy and to problems during infancy (Rosso and Cramory, 1979). Supplementation with specific vitamins and minerals, when prescribed for a specific problem, may have merit, especially when given in conjunction with dietary counseling.

Although the practice of routine vitamin and mineral supplementation is without rationale, the routine supplementation of iron and folic acid is effective in reducing the incidence of iron deficiency (in both mothers and their infants) and megaloblastic anemia during pregnancy (Food and Nutrition Board, 1970). An additional 30 to 60 mg of iron and 0.4 gm of folic acid are recommended (Food and Nutrition Board, 1980). The nutrients that the mother must consume to supply the fetus and her changing body are reflected in the Recommended Dietary Allowances (RDA) (Table 9-2) for pregnancy. RDA vary with the weight, age, and activity of the woman and should be used only as a guide.

The routine restriction of sodium intake among pregnant women and among women who develop hypertension during pregnancy is contraindicated. The ingestion of alcohol, excessive amounts of caffeine (500 mg or the equivalent of about 4 cups of brewed coffee), and herbal teas that contain natural coumarins is not recommended (Food and Nutrition Board, 1982).

WEIGHT GAIN DURING PREGNANCY

Caloric requirements during pregnancy should be based on rates of weight gain. Because total weight gain is a primary variable influencing in-

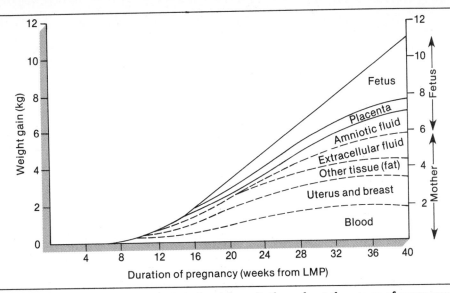

Figure 9-1. Pattern and components of weight gain throughout the course of pregnancy.
Redrawn from Schneider, H.A.: Nutritional support of medical practice, New York, 1983, Harper & Row Publishers, Inc.

fant birth weight and health, a close monitoring of weight gain is recommended. How much women should gain will depend on whether they were underweight, normal weight, or overweight before pregnancy (Brown, 1983, 1984). Current research indicates that weight gains during pregnancy associated with the lowest rates of neonatal mortality are 12 to 16 kg (28 to 36 lb) for underweight women, 11 to 14 kg (26 to 32 lb) for normal weight women, and 9 to 10 kg (20 to 24 lb) for overweight women (Brown et al., 1981). For term babies, the range of birth weights associated with the lowest rates of perinatal and neonatal mortality is 3500 to 4500 gm (7 to 10 lb).

Deviations in Weight and Weight Gain

The patterns and components of weight gain during pregnancy are shown in Figure 9-1. Deviations from usual values for either prepregnant weight or weight gain during pregnancy are relatively common. Figure 9-2 shows a pattern of normal weight gain during pregnancy in women with normal prepregnancy weights. This grid should be used for plotting the pregnant woman's weight throughout pregnancy. Women who are underweight or overweight at time of conception (Table 9-3) should follow a similar pattern of weight gain as normal-weight women during the first trimester. By the twentieth week and thereafter, the underweight woman should have gained 2 or 3 pounds more and the overweight woman 5 or 6 pounds less than the normal-weight woman is expected to gain (Figure 9-2).

Jacobson (1982) summarized the potential hazards for both mother and infant of restricting weight gain to 4 to 6 kg (10 to 15 lb) during pregnancy from a number of surveys and reviews over the past 10 years. It has been shown that the mother's weight gain and prepregnancy weights are the two strongest influences (except gestational age) on birth weight.

The obese woman entering pregnancy faces increased risk of severe complications, notably

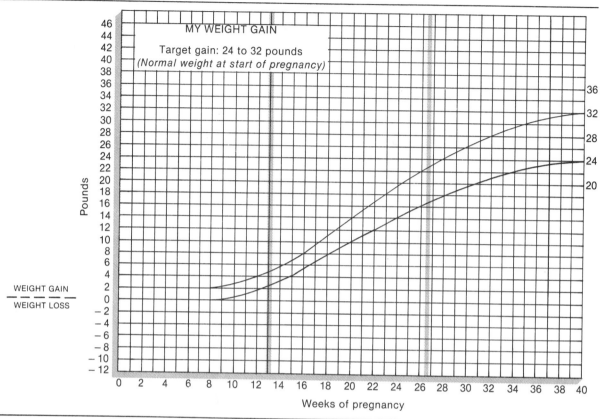

Figure 9-2. Pattern of normal prenatal weight gain.
Redrawn from Brown, J.: Nutrition for your pregnancy: the University of Minnesota guide, Minneapolis, 1983, University of Minnesota Press.

Table 9-3. Recommended weight goals during pregnancy*

Height Without Shoes	Prepregnancy Weight			Height Without Shoes	Prepregnancy Weight		
	Underweight if You Weighed This or Less	Normal Weight Range†	Overweight if You Weighed This or More		Underweight You Weighed This or Less	Normal Weight Range†	Overweight if You Weighed This or More
4'10"	88	89-108	109	5'6"	123	124-150	151
4'11"	91	92-112	113	5'7"	127	128-155	156
5'	94	95-115	116	5'8"	132	133-161	162
5'1"	99	100-121	122	5'9"	137	138-167	168
5'2"	104	105-127	128	5'10"	142	143-173	174
5'3"	108	109-132	133	5'11"	146	147-178	179
5'4"	113	114-138	139	6'	151	152-184	185
5'5"	118	119-144	145				

From Brown, J.: Nutrition for your pregnancy: the University of Michigan guide, Minneapolis, 1983, University of Minnesota Press.
*Your recommended weight gain goal for pregnancy: underweight, 28-36 lb; normal weight, 24-32 lb; overweight, 20-24 lb.
†Normal weight for "thin-boned" women will be closer to the lower end of this range. For "big-boned" women, it will be closer to the higher end.

hypertensive disorders and diabetes mellitus, which have adverse effects on pregnancy outcome. Some have advocated restriction of weight gain in such patients so they conclude pregnancy with a net loss. However, the advisability of such a course seems questionable on several grounds. First, dietary restrictions to limit calories may also result in displacement of other nutrients from the diet. Second, optimum protein utilization in pregnancy apparently requires a minimum of approximately 30 kcal/kg/day. Third, dietary restriction results in catabolism of fat stores, which in turn produces ketonuria.

NUTRITIONAL RISK FACTORS DURING PREGNANCY

To effectively assess the nutritional status of pregnant or lactating women, an understanding of the major risk factors with nutrition implications is needed. Nutritional risk factors include those present at the onset of pregnancy and those which may occur during the course of pregnancy (ACOG and ADA, 1982).

Risk Factors at the Onset of Pregnancy

Adolescence. A pregnant adolescent is considered at high-risk educationally, medically, socially, and nutritionally (Beal, 1981). Girls are at an increased risk if pregnancy occurs within 3 years of menarche. The majority of girls attain physical maturity by 17 years of age, and pregnancy after this age has not been found to present special biological hazards. Thus the course and outcome of pregnancy of girls 17 to 20 years of age resemble those of mature young women (20 to 24 years of age), whereas there is a sharp increase of infant mortality for each year of age under 17.

A pregnant patient under 15 years of age may have had the onset of menses from 1 to 6 years earlier. Her actual chronological age is not nearly as important as her reproductive or biological age (chronological age minus her menarchal age). The adolescent who is less than reproductive or biological year 3 is at particular risk for

reproductive performance. She is still growing, and the pregnancy superimposes additional nutritional demands.

Teenage mothers have a disproportionate number of babies weighing less than 2500 gm (5 lb) at birth. Neonatal, postneonatal, and infant mortality rates are much higher for infants born to young mothers. These rates are greatest among young girls who have repeated pregnancies.

Frequent pregnancies. Three or more pregnancies within 2 years is considered risk. The multiparous woman who has progressed from one pregnancy directly to another is at increased risk. Any patient who has had three or more pregnancies in a 1½ year span is prone to depleted nutrient stores. This situation can potentially compromise maternal and fetal outcome.

Poor reproductive performance. Special attention should be paid to the client's obstetrical history. Poor weight gain in pregnancy, toxemia, a previous stillbirth or low-birth-weight infant, premature delivery, or prenatal infection are all more common in clients who are or have been poorly nourished in the past. As a result, the client with this history may need special nutrition guidance.

Economic deprivation. For the economically deprived, there are several programs to help with the purchase of food or programs that offer supplements, such as the USDA Food Stamp Program and the Supplemental Food Program for Women, Infants and Children (WIC), described in Chapter 8.

Alternate food patterns. A client may enter pregnancy either having been or continuing to be on a fad or otherwise nutritionally inadequate diet. The patient who practices pica may not consume adequate levels of nutrients. Pica is defined as regular and excessive ingestion of nonfood items or of foods with limited nutritional value. The practice often relates to cultural and geographical factors.

Recently the megavitamin diet and various types of vegetarian diets have become popular. With a megavitamin regimen, clients ingest massive amounts of vitamins far above RDA levels. Although there is no documentation that these large amounts of vitamins are beneficial, there is evidence that consumption of large numbers of fat-soluble vitamins, such as vitamins A and D, which are stored in the body, may lead to toxicity. Vitamin dependency can occur in infants whose mothers take megadoses of vitamins C and B_6. Vitamin dependency causes the infant to show deficiency symptoms although the infant consumes levels of nutrients suggested in the RDA. Of particular concern is the strict vegetarian who eliminates all products of animal origin, including meat, poultry, fish, cheese, eggs, and milk, from her diet. The pregnant woman who practices strict vegetarianism may not receive ample quantities of complementary and complete proteins and may not get enough vitamin B_{12}. Intense diet counseling will be required to work out a dietary pattern for a strict vegetarian during the prenatal period.

Smoking, drug addiction, and alcoholism. The patient who is a heavy smoker (more than 20 cigarettes per day), drug addict, or alcoholic (the chronic use of more than 5 ounces of whisky per day or its equivalent from beer or wine) will likely have major physiological problems. As is now known, the effects of smoking during pregnancy include reduction in gestation length, reduced size of the offspring at birth, and an increase in the incidence of prematurity (ACOG and ADA, 1982). Also, individuals who indulge excessively in the use of cigarettes, drugs, or alcohol may not consume sufficient quantities of nutritious food.

There is a high rate of mortality among infants with fetal alcohol syndrome (FAS). FAS occurs in infants born to women who are chronic alcoholics. These infants exhibit specific anomalies of the eyes, nose, heart, and central nervous system that are accompanied by growth retardation, small head circumference, and mental retardation.

Chronic systemic diseases. Medical problems such as anemia, thyroid dysfunction, and chronic medical or surgical gastrointestinal disorders may be associated with interference with the ingestion, absorption, or utilization of nutrients. Drugs used in treating these conditions may also affect the nutrition of the patient by similar interference. Nutrition counseling for patients with such problems should combine nutrition guidelines for prenatal care and diet therapy recommended for that particular medical condition.

Prepregnant weight. If a woman begins pregnancy with a weight that is below 90% of the standard weight for height (less than 152 cm [60 in] in height or 46 kg [100 lb] in weight), she is considered to be at increased risk to enter pregnancy. The patient is also at risk if she is obese, or weighs more than 120% of the standard weight.

Risk Factors During Pregnancy

Anemia of pregnancy. Iron needs during pregnancy are obtained from maternal iron stores, diet, and supplementation. True anemia occurring during pregnancy is most often caused by iron deficiency. Many healthy American women do not have iron stores large enough to meet the demands of pregnancy. Iron supplementation aids greatly in maintaining hemoglobin at normal levels in these patients. During the second and third trimesters of pregnancy, an oral iron supplement of 30 to 60 mg of ferrous salt is recommended. It is also essential, however, that the woman be encouraged to include foods rich in iron and protein in her diet or other deficiencies may appear.

Megaloblastic anemia of pregnancy may be caused by poor food intake, vomiting, or increased demands for folacin. It is characterized by an extremely low red blood cell count and an equally low hemoglobin level and has some of the findings associated with pernicious anemia, with which it may be confused. The administration of folic acid causes a dramatic rise in red blood cells, in hemoglobin, and in appetite. The Committee on Maternal Nutrition suggests a supplement of 400 µg (0.4 mg) of folacin per day (Food and Nutrition Board, 1970).

Toxemia of pregnancy. The cause of toxemia of pregnancy is not known. It is characterized by an elevation in blood pressure, proteinuria, and rapid weight gain caused by edema. There is considerable controversy over the effect of nutrition on the development of toxemia. Toxemia occurs more commonly in pregnant women with poor diets and particularly those with low protein intakes than in those receiving good diets. Tompkins and Wiehl (1951) have shown that supplementation of the diet with protein and thiamin greatly reduces the incidence of toxemia in their patients.

A question has arisen about the relation of salt to toxemia. Robinson (1958), studying over 2000 pregnant women, advised half to increase their salt intake and half to lower it. He found a lower incidence of toxemia in those having the higher salt intake. Mengert (1948) placed 48 patients with proven toxemia either on a high salt diet or a very low one. No difference in the progress of the disease was noted between the two groups of women in this study. The Committee on Maternal Nutrition discourages the routine use of salt restriction and diuretics during pregnancy.

Inadequate weight gain. Normal pregnancy is a time of progressive maternal weight gain. Following are presumptive signs of maternal and fetal malnutrition: (1) failure to gain weight (less than 4 lb [1.8 kg]/mo in last half of pregnancy), (2) actual weight loss, (3) significant nausea and vomiting during early pregnancy, and (4) poor or delayed uterine-fetal growth.

Inadequate maternal weight gain (less than 2 lb [0.9 kg]/mo) in the second and third trimesters has been associated with lowered birth weight and intrauterine growth retardation. It is therefore important to document the progress of weight gain in pregnancy as well as the total amount gained.

Excessive weight gain. Rapid weight gain—3 to 5 lb (1.4 to 2.3 kg)/wk—results only from tissue fluid retention. The patient must be carefully observed for development of preeclampsia.

Excessive weight gain associated with accumulation of fat is less dramatic and is best assessed by evaluating the patient's eating habits and by measuring subcutaneous fat stores by means of skinfold calipers. Sources of calorically rich, but nutritionally poor food should be sought

and eliminated. Weight reduction in pregnancy or lactation by dietary manipulation and/or drug administration is contraindicated because of the potential adverse and possibly toxic effects on fetal nutrition, growth, and development.

The demands of lactation. Increased nutritional demands of lactation can also be a risk factor. If a woman stores between 2 and 3 kg of fat during pregnancy, she will have a reservoir of about 14,000 to 24,000 kcal for lactation needs. Ordinarily fat stores will be gradually used over the first 4 or 6 months of lactation. Without these stores, the nursing mother faces the difficult task of increasing food consumption 50% in order to provide the 1000 kcal required to produce 800 to 900 ml of milk.

Without the demands of nursing, fat stores may remain a permanent addition to the maternal frame and increase the potential for obesity with advancing age and parity. A modest reduction of caloric intake after delivery is appropriate for the woman who does not nurse her infant. This is particularly true if she uses an oral contraceptive agent.

LACTATION

Successful lactation is the end result of numerous interacting factors, including the maturity and anatomy of the newborn, the health and nutrition of the mother, and development of the mammary glands. Physiologically, lactation is controlled by numerous endocrine glands and particularly the pituitary hormones, prolactin and oxytocin, which are influenced by the sucking process and by maternal emotions (Jelliffe and Jelliffe, 1978). The establishment and maintenance of lactation in humans is determined by at least three factors:

1. The anatomical structure of the mammary gland and the development of alveoli, ducts, and nipples
2. The initiation and maintenance of milk secretion
3. The ejection or propulsion of milk from the alveoli to the nipple (Worthington-Roberts, Vermeersch, and Williams, 1985)

Stages of Breast Development

The human breast is a large exocrine gland that uniquely is primarily quiescent during most of a female's life span. It is composed of fat and connective tissues and is lavishly supplied with blood vessels, lymphatics, and nerves. The size of the breast is largely related to the amount of fat present and gives no indication of functional capacity.

Stages of Lactation

Lactation, or more properly the process of breast-feeding, results from the interplay of hormones and the instinctive reflexes and learned behavior by the mother and newborn (Jelliffe and Jelliffe, 1978). Milk initiation (lactogenesis) begins during the latter part of pregnancy when secretion of colostrum occurs as a result of stimulation of the breast alveolar cells by placental lactogen, a prolactin-like substance, and continues after birth as an automatic process.

Although also under complex hormonal control, the continuing secretion of milk is mainly related to sufficient production of the anterior pituitary hormone prolactin and to maternal nutrition. Milk secretion occurs by a process of extrusion from the cells.

Milk ejection involves movements of milk from alveoli, where it is secreted to the mouth of the infant and is an active process within the breast brought about by the let-down or milk ejection reflex.

The last stage of human lactation is the ingestion of milk by the sucking baby. This stage depends on the interaction between mother and newborn and especially on the functioning of the let-down reflex and the existence of neonatal feeding reflexes.

Let-Down Reflex

The most important single function that affects the success of breast-feeding is the let-down reflex (Figure 9-3). It is a complex function that depends on hormones, nerves, and glands, which can be inhibited very early by psychological block. The most efficient stimulus for the milk ejection reflex is sucking of the nipple. Within 1 minute of the onset of suckling the first contraction of the mammary myoepithelium is recorded. Uterine contractions are also stimulated by suckling. The milk ejection reflex is inhibited centrally by cold, pain, and emotional stress. When the infant suckles the breast, he stimulates mechanoreceptors in nipple and areola that send stimuli along nerve pathways to the hypothalamus, which stimulates the posterior pituitary to release oxytocin. It is carried via the bloodstream to the breast and uterus. Oxytocin stimulates myoepithelial cells in the breast to contract and eject milk from the alveolus. Prolactin is responsible for milk production in the alveolus. It is secreted by the anterior pituitary gland in response to suckling. Stress such as pain and anxiety can inhibit the let-down reflex. The sight or cry of the infant can stimulate this reflex.

Management of Successful Lactation and Breast-Feeding

That some mothers choose not to breast-feed indicates some disadvantages of this method. Among these is the problem with the working mother's ability to breast-feed, since day nurseries adjacent to places of work are virtually nonexistent and some employers are punitive in terms of "time off" for maternity leave. From a physiological point of view, the mother may be unable to secrete adequate milk, and she may be constantly fatigued, a common complaint of many mothers. Some other considerations include lack of freedom because of maintaining a feeding schedule, the possibility of breast infection, and a desire to quickly restore the mother's figure to normal.

The health care professional should offer support and assistance to any woman with the least inclination toward breast-feeding. At the same time it seems unwise that strong social pressures should be exerted to coerce women into breast-feeding or that a woman should be made to feel guilty because she elects not to breast-feed.

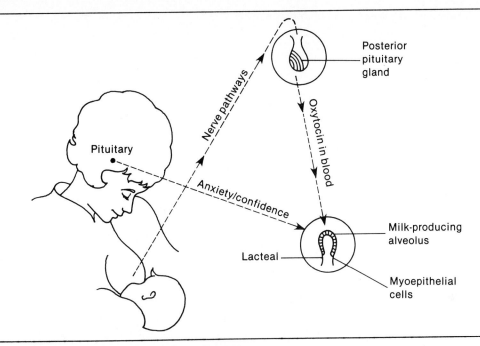

Figure 9-3. The let-down reflex simplified.
Redrawn from Jelliffe, D.B., and Jelliffe, E.F.P.: Psychophysiology of lactation: human milk in the modern world, Oxford, England, 1978, Oxford University Press, Inc.

Common Problems with Nursing

To solve the problems of unsuccessful nursing, one should observe the mother feeding the infant. Most common among these problems include a mother who is uncomfortable or tense, a let-down reflex that will not trigger, or an infant who has a poor suck. Other common problems include sore nipples, plugged duct/breast infection, leaking, and enlargement. Table 9-4 describes some of the problems with possible solutions.

Maternal Nutrition Needs During Lactation

During lactation there is increased need for energy, protein, minerals, and vitamins to cover the cost of secreting milk, to provide the amounts secreted in milk for nourishment of the infant, and to protect the mother's stores. Energy requirement varies with the amount of milk produced, and intake must be regulated for each woman. A woman who is meeting all the needs of a 5 kg (11 lb) infant must secrete about 850 ml of milk providing about 600 kcal daily. Human milk is produced with 80% efficiency, so the requirement for lactation is about 1000 kcal per day. Increased stores of maternal fat during pregnancy provide about one third of the energy costs of lactation during the first 3 or 4 months. Thus the RDA standard is an extra 500 kcal (Table 9-2). If the period of lactation extends beyond 3 months, as it should ideally, then energy intake should be increased to the full amount required. Six months of lactation has an estimated energy cost of about 135,000 kcal, or approximated 100,000 above the amount stored in maternal fat during pregnancy.

Human milk contains about 12 gm of protein

Table 9-4. Common problems encountered during nursing

Problem	Solution
Sore nipples	Vary position of nursing, sitting during one feeding, lying down during the next.
	Dry nipples by exposure to air or sunlight.
	Use lanolin or cooking oil on nipples after feeding.
	To minimize discomfort, rub ice cubes on nipple before nursing.
	Nurse more frequently for shorter periods of time; begin with the less sore nipple.
	Avoid using soap on nipples.
Running out of milk	Nurse more frequently. Avoid giving supplementary bottles until breast-feeding is well established.
	Alternate breasts and empty completely.
	Drink plenty of liquids.
	Eat well and get plenty of rest.
Plugged duct/breast infection	Nurse frequently every 1 to 2 hours; keep affected breast as empty as possible.
	Apply gentle heat on affected area (e.g., hot washcloth).
	Massage gently toward nipple area.
	Wear clothing that is loose and comfortable.
Leaking	Use nursing pads, gauze, handkerchiefs, sanitary napkins, or diapers in bra to absorb leakage from the breast.
	Fold arms and press unobtrusively with the heel of hand to stop leaking.
Engorgement (the breasts become very full and uncomfortable, causing the baby to have difficulty sucking on the breast)	Hot shower and use a warm pack.
	Massage gently.
	Hand expression can be used to get the flow started.
	Hold full breast away from baby's nose to ease sucking.
	Nurse frequently.
Poor let-down reflex	Avoiding unnecessary stresses.
	Avoid fatigue and eat right.
	Nurse frequently.
	Eat properly.
	Consume at least 2 quarts of fluids daily.
	Relax 5 minutes before feeding.
	Get into a routine; nurse in the same place as often as possible.
	If possible, remove distractions (e.g., take the phone off the hook).

Modified from Arizona Department of Health Services, Bureau of Nutrition Services: Lactation protocol, Phoenix, 1983, Arizona Department of Health Services.

per liter. In arriving at the RDA of an additional 20 gm of protein per day during lactation, the National Research Council has assumed that dietary protein is of lower quality than milk protein so that conversion is not 100% efficient and milk production may exceed 1 L/day.

If the mother increases her milk intake by the amount she is secreting for her infant, she will meet her own calcium needs as well as the infant's needs for this nutrient and several other nutrients. Some nursing mothers are found to be in negative calcium and phosphorus balance. This imbalance causes a drain on the mother's stores, but it does not affect milk secretion. The vitamin content of human milk, especially the water-soluble vitamins, partially depends on maternal vitamin intakes. Lactation, like pregnancy, is a period when borderline nutritional status may develop into frank deficiency. Recommended allowances for vitamins during lactation are about 50% more than those for women who are not lactating. Relatively little iron is secreted in milk (0.5 to 1.0 mg/day), and although lactating women usually do not menstruate, there is an added allowance for iron in lactation.

Supplementation

During lactation there is a need to supplement the maternal diet with certain nutrients. As in pregnancy, 30 to 60 mg of elemental iron should be taken daily by all women. This supplement should be continued for at least 2 to 3 months postpartum. Iron supplementation during this period is necessary to replenish maternal iron stores depleted by pregnancy and to replace iron secreted in milk.

Since human milk does not contain an adequate amount of vitamin D, it is advisable to give the infant oral supplements of 400 IU daily. The fluoride content of human milk is low irrespective of the fluoride content of the water supply. An oral supplement of 0.25 mg fluoride is recommended for the exclusively breast-fed infant.

GUIDELINES FOR PATIENT MANAGEMENT

The intervention strategies and outcomes for a pregnant woman include the following (NHCHC and ADA, 1983):

1. Total weight gain for:
   a. Underweight women—12 to 16 kg (28 to 36 lb)
   b. Normal weight women—11 to 14 kg (26 to 32 lb)
   c. Overweight women—9 to 10 kg (20 to 24 lb)
2. Rate of weight gain is 0.9 to 1.4 kg (2 to 3 lb) a month during the first trimester; 1.8 to 2.7 kg (4 to 6 lb) a month during second and third trimesters.
3. Maintain a hemoglobin level of 11 gm or a hematocrit of 33% or more.
4. Urine test for ketones is negative.
5. Reported food intake is appropriate for age and stage of pregnancy.
6. Receive information on substance abuse (alcohol, drugs, tobacco, pica) during pregnancy.
7. Receive information on breast-feeding and appropriate infant feeding alternatives.
8. Iron (30 to 60 mg elemental) supplement is prescribed.
9. Folacin (0.8 to 1.0 mg) supplement is prescribed.
10. Infant's birth weight is greater than 2500 gm.
11. Advised of direct postpartum weight for height, age, and breast-feeding status.

Nutrition Assessment

Every pregnant woman should have a formal assessment of nutritional adequacy. Most often simply a sound and thorough initial history and physical examination, plus the routinely obtained laboratory tests (e.g., urinalysis, red blood cell count, and 2-hour postprandial blood sugar), will be sufficient. Following this up with careful observation of weight gain, several urine checks, and periodic repeat blood counts will often suffice. These procedures are already basic aspects of prenatal care. In addition, assessment of the nutritional status is essential. Basically, three components are vital: recognition of factors that put the patient in a special category of nutritional risk, a nutritionally oriented history and physical examination, and a familiarity with specialized laboratory tests of nutritional adequacy. These special tests are necessary if the patient becomes identifiable at nutritional risk because of the presence of risk factors, significant findings in the history, physical examination, and/or routine laboratory tests or periodic checks during the progressing pregnancy.

An individual assessment of nutrition status must be made at the beginning of prenatal care and supported by continuing evaluation throughout the pregnancy. In planning and delivering health care in the field, the following methods of assessment provide the data necessary to determine need:

1. Clinical observation including medical history:
   Physical examination, pregnancy history, present pregnancy, and chronic disease history
2. Anthropometric measurements:
   Height
   Pregravid (prepregnancy) weight
   Present weight
3. Biochemical/clinical determinations:
   Blood pressure
   Hemoglobin and/or hematocrit
   Mean corpuscular volume
   Mean corpuscular hemoglobin concentration
   Serum iron
   Transferrin
   Serum folate
   Red blood cell folate
4. Dietary observations:
   Dietary intake

History

Data from a history are among the most important elements in nutritional assessment. The standard medical history is a good beginning nutritional assessment. It will help greatly to have clearly in mind the nutritional risk categories. Therefore age, race, marital status, and parity assume nutritional significance. The age of men-

arche is also significant in that it may be delayed by poor nutrition in early childhood. Scanty flow and episodes of amenorrhea in adolescence are sometimes a reflection of poor nutrition in that age group (Aubry, Robert, and Cuenca, 1975). The obstetrical history is especially helpful. Poor weight gain, anemia, excess fluid retention, toxemia, stillbirths, low-birth-weight infants, premature delivery, and perinatal infection are all more common with poor maternal nutrition and should indicate the need for special nutrition evaluation.

Many pregnancies with short interconceptual periods are of concern. The presence of chronic maternal systemic illness with its potential relationship to nutritional adequacy should be thoroughly evaluated. Cigarette smoking, drug, and alcohol habits should be documented in view of their likely effects on nutritional intake, as well as their direct effect on fetal growth and development. Finally, socioeconomic conditions are critically related to nutrition and must be part of the initial obstetrical history.

Physical Examination

Confusion sometimes exists in specific interpretation of physical examination signs during pregnancy. Despite this shortcoming, clinical observations can be useful if they are used in conjunction with the biochemical analysis, anthropometric measurements, and dietary assessment.

Anthropometric Measurements

Several anthropometric measurements are considered good indicators of nutritional well-being if appropriate equipment is available (tape measures, weight scales [beam balance]) and correctly used.

Patients are at nutritional risk if they are less than 85% or more than 120% of their standard weight for age and height. Poor weight gain during pregnancy, especially in low prepregnant weight or low weight for height patients, is a serious indication of inadequate nutrition and is accompanied by a striking increase in low-birth-weight infants. An excessive weight gain—1.4 to

2.3 kg (3 to 5 lb) in a week—is likely to be caused by tissue fluid retention rather than excessive caloric intake. By definition, obesity is a nonpregnant weight above 120% of the ideal for age and body build or a midtriceps skinfold thickness of more than 28 mm. Obesity should not be equated with overall nutrition; excessive caloric ingestion may mask other nutrition problems, such as anemia and inadequate protein intake. The nonnursing postpartum patient needs to reduce her daily caloric intake about 300 kcal (12%) from her prenatal food intake; otherwise she cannot be expected to return to an ideal prepregnant weight status.

Biochemical Determinations

Laboratory data provide vital baseline information for nutritional assessment at the beginning of pregnancy, as well as ongoing monitoring of its course throughout gestation (Food and Nutrition Board, 1977). Although laboratory testing of maternal nutritional adequacy is valuable, it is sometimes very complex. It is valuable because most often laboratory tests will reflect poor nutrition well before it becomes clinically apparent. It is complex because the critical blood or urinary levels are often changed in normal pregnancy, which makes it necessary to have a thorough knowledge of the physiological alterations of normal pregnancy.

The absolute levels of substances in plasma and urine must be interpreted with care for two reasons (Aubry, Robert, and Cuenca, 1975). First, each laboratory's results may vary according to differences in methodology and technique. Local experience and standardization will help greatly to circumvent this problem. Second, the limits of normal values and their distinction from a critical value to define a deficiency state will probably always be a matter of dispute. However, such arbitrary critical levels are valuable when applied with good judgment at the clinical level.

Blood-forming nutrients. Measures of the blood-forming nutrients—iron, folacin, vitamin B_6, and vitamin B_{12}—are important guides for use in preventing and treating anemias often associated with pregnancy. Basic routine tests include measures of hemoglobin and hematocrit levels (Worthington-Roberts, Vermeersch, and Williams, 1985):

- Hemoglobin—less than 11 gm/dl
- Hematocrit—less than 33%
- Mean corpuscular volume—80
- Mean corpuscular hemoglobin concentration—30
- Serum iron—50 mg/dl and percent concentration saturation
- Transferrin—15

Other tests include those for folate deficiency:

- Mean corpuscular volume—100
- Hypersegmented polymorphonuclear leukocytes—3%
- Serum folate—3 ng/dl
- Red blood cell folate—150 ng/dl
- Serum protein—gm/dl

Serum albumin level is important during pregnancy because of its function in helping to maintain normal flow of tissue fluids from the circulating blood through the tissue for nourishment of cells and back into circulation by means of capillary fluid shift mechanisms. A protein deficit contributes to a lowered plasma albumin level and in turn to an inbalance in the fluid shift mechanism, resulting in edema. An acceptable level of serum albumin during pregnancy is 3.5 gm/dl or above.

Other minerals and vitamins. Depending on individual situations, tests of other vitamin and mineral levels may be performed, including determinations of the water-soluble vitamins thiamin, riboflavin, niacin, and vitamin C; the fat-soluble vitamins A, D, E, and K; and other trace minerals.

Blood lipids, glucose, and enzymes. Routine testing for urine sugar and ketone bodies will screen for latent diabetes or gestational glycosuria. Other tests may be performed if there are complicating chronic diseases, particularly heart disease or renal disease.

Table 9-5 summarizes the basic components of nutrition, their metabolic role, the appropriate test, and its interpretation in the face of the

Table 9-5. Nutritional assessment in pregnancy

Nutrient	RDA (Adult Female)			Physiologic and/or Biochemical Role	History and Physical Findings in Deficiency States
	Nonpregnant	Pregnant	Lactating		
Total calories (kcal)	2100	+300	+500	Overall nutrition Energy and metabolism	Dieters, lethargy, weakness, faintness, nausea and vomiting, poor weight gain
Protein (gm)	46	+30	+20	Biosynthesis of cell proteins, cellular integrity, growth	Underweight, underheight, lethargy, anemia, edema, fatty liver
Carbohydrate and lipids				Energy metabolism, biosynthesis of polysaccharides, cholesterol, and steroids	Underweight, underheight, lethargy, anemia, edema
Vitamin A (IU)	4000	5000	6000	Formation of rhodopsin, epithelial integrity, and rod vision	Growth failure, night blindness, xerophthalmia, follicular hyperkeratosis
Vitamin D (IU)	400	400	400	Calcium and phosphate metabolism, bone growth and development	Rickets, stunted growth, osteomalacia or osteoporosis
Vitamin C (mg)	45	60	60	Integrity of intercellular substances, amino acid metabolism, adrenal function	Scurvy, anemia, hemorrhagic disorders, poor wound healing
Vitamin K				Integrity of clotting factors	Hemorrhages
Thiamin (mg)	1.1	+0.3	+0.3	Oxidative decarboxylation reactions	Alcoholism, anorexia, beriberi, polyneuropathy, cardiomyopathy
Riboflavin (mg)	1.4	+0.3	+0.5	H electron transport	Oral lesions, ocular lesion glossitis, dermatitis

From Aubry, R.H., Roberts, A., and Cuenca, V.G.: Nutritional assessment in pregnancy, Clin. Perinatol. 2:214, 1975.
*Criteria from the Ten-State Nutritional Survey.

Laboratory Tests	Normal Range		Findings in Deficiency Status
	Nonpregnant	Pregnant	
Urinary acetone	Negative	Faint positive in AM	Positive
Serum protein, total	6.5 to 8.5 gm/100 ml	6 to 8	<6*
Serum albumin	3.5 to 5 gm/100 ml	3 to 4.5	<3.5*
Blood urea nitrogen	10 to 25 mg/100 ml	5 to 15	<5
Urine urea nitrogen/total nitrogen ratio	>60	>60	<60
FBS	70 to 110 mg/100 ml	65 to 100	<65
2-hr postprandial blood sugar	<110 mg/100 ml	<120	—
Cholesterol	120 to 290 mg/100 ml	200 to 325	—
Vitamin A, serum	20 to 60 μg/100 ml*	20 to 60	<20
Carotene, serum	50 to 300 μg/100 ml	80 to 325	<80*
Serum calcium	4.6 to 5.5 mEq/L	4.2 to 5.2	<4.2 or normal
Serum phosphate	2.5 to 4.8 mg/100 ml	2.3 to 4.6	No change
Alkaline phosphatase	35 to 48 IU/L	35 to 150	No change
Ascorbic acid, serum	0.2 to 2.0 mg/100 ml*	0.2 to 1.5	<0.2
Prothrombin time	12 to 15 sec	12 to 15	Prolonged
Thiamin, blood	1.6 to 4.0 μg/100 ml	—	Decreased
Thiamin, urinary	>55 μg/gm creatinine	—	<50
Lactic acid, blood	5 to 20 mg/100 ml	—	Increased
Riboflavin, urine	>80 mg/gm creatinine	—	<90*

Continued.

Table 9-5. Nutritional assessment in pregnancy—cont'd

| Nutrient | RDA (Adult Female) | | | Physiologic and/or Biochemical Role | History and Physical Findings in Deficiency States |
	Nonpregnant	Pregnant	Lactating		
Niacin (mg)	14	+ 2	+ 4	H electron transport	Pellagra, dermatitis, diarrhea, contusion, oral lesions, anorexia
Pyridoxine (B₆) (mg)	2	2.5	2.5	Coenzyme in amino acid metabolism, etc.	Anemia, polyneuropathy, seborrheic eczema
Folic acid (μg)	400	800	600	Biosynthesis of purine bases, histidine, choline, serine	Glossitis, macrocystic, megaloblastic anemia
Vitamin B₁₂ (mg)	3	4	4	As folic acid, labile methyl groups	Glossitis, peripheral neuropathy, macrocytic anemia
Iron (mg)	18	+ 18	18	Oxygen transport, cytochromes	Anemia, glossitis, achlorhydria
Calcium (mg)	800	1200	1200	Skeletal system bone formation	Osteomalacia
Iodine (μg)	100	125	150	Thyroid function	Goiter, hypothyroidism

physiological alterations of pregnancy. These data are helpful in developing a rational approach to biochemical assessment of nutrition.

Dietary Assessment

Since pregnancy is a time in the life cycle when nutrition is of special importance, it is essential to learn who the mother is, where she is, what her needs are, and how they can best be met. Only in this context can realistic guidance be provided.

Worthington-Roberts, Vermeersch, and Williams (1985) have indicated that dietary assessment in pregnancy involves three basic areas: background data, diet history, and diet analysis.

Background data. Food habits and attitudes cannot be viewed in isolation: life situations and values, as well as physical and emotional factors,

must also be considered. Thus, if nutrition counseling is to be valid, it must be based on an individual plan of care.

A woman's living situation will have an influence on her eating behavior. Therefore information about the home setting, housing, life-style, family members, occupation, general socioeconomic status, food assistance needs, and family roles and attitudes concerning foods are all important. Cultural/ethnic food practices should be explored, including types of food, ethnic dishes, methods of cooking, and taboos associated with pregnancy. Special diet practices such as faddist or unusual patterns are important to determine. Strict vegetarian diets or various forms of pica may be nutritionally unsound. Food allergies and milk or lactose intolerance need to be ex-

Laboratory Tests	Normal Range		Findings in Deficiency Status
	Nonpregnant	Pregnant	
N-methyl nicotinamide	1.6 to 4.3 mg/gm creatinine	2.5 to 6	<2.5*
Kynurenic acid excretion	3 mg/24 hr	—	Increased
Xanthurenic acid excretion	3 mg/24 hr	—	Increased
Folic acid, serum	5 to 21 ng/ml	3 to 15	<3
FIGLU excretion—after 15 gm	<3 mg/24 hr	—	Increased
L-histidine	1 to 4 mg/24 hr	—	Increased
Vitamin B₁₂, serum	330 to 1025 pg/ml	Decreased	Decreased
Methylmalonic acid	<10 mg/24 hr	—	Increased
Hgb/Hct	>12/36	>11/33*	<11/33*
Serum Fe/Fe binding capacity	>50/250 to 400 µg/100 ml	>40/300 to 450	<40/>450
Calcium, serum	4.6 to 5.5 mEq/L	4.2 to 5.2	Normal
Serum thyroxine (T₄)	4.6 to 10.7 µg/100 ml	6 to 12.5	Decreased or normal

plored. The use of all medications and supplements needs to be discussed with the patient.

Diet history and analysis. There are several methods to determine food intake. The two most commonly used that give an overview of the patient's dietary pattern include a recall of foods consumed during the past 24 hours and a food frequency determination describing consumption of food over a period of time.

NUTRITION COUNSELING FOR PREGNANT WOMEN

In attempting to counsel, consideration should be given to understanding the client's problems and concerns, recognizing that others such as family, peers, colleagues, and other members of the health team who interact with the pregnant woman may have considerable influence on her eating habits.

The Arizona Department of Health Services Bureau of Nutrition has developed a plan for nutrition education and counseling that includes objectives of the counseling session and content to be included. Table 9-6 describes this process for the pregnant woman with selected objectives.

To assist the community dietitian/nutritionist and other health care workers in offering the most effective care to the pregnant woman, criteria have been established to provide a systematic approach to obtaining patient outcomes (Guide to Quality Assurance in Ambulatory Nutrition, 1983).

Table 9-7 describes the criteria developed for the pregnant woman in terms of process and out-

Text continued on p. 243.

Table 9-6. Nutrition education for pregnant women

Topic	Objective	Content for Discussion
Weight gain	The client will interpret her weight gain pattern after counselor has plotted it on the weight gain grid.	Counselor explains weight gain grid and helps client determine that the pattern is one of the following (Figure 9-2): excessive weight gain, normal weight gain, slow weight gain, no weight gain, weight loss.
Rate of weight gain	The client will explain rate of weight gain desirable for a healthy pregnancy and total weight that should be gained.	1 to 3 months' gestation = 2 to 3 pounds total 4 to 9 months' gestation = 3 to 4 pounds a month during second and third trimesters Total weight gain should be 20 to 30 pounds.
Components of weight gain	The client will explain components of weight gain during pregnancy.	<table><tr><td>**Component**</td><td>**Pound**</td></tr><tr><td>Fetus</td><td>7½</td></tr><tr><td>Increase in blood volume</td><td>4</td></tr><tr><td>Uterus</td><td>2½</td></tr><tr><td>Placenta</td><td>1</td></tr><tr><td>Fluid around baby (amniotic fluid)</td><td>2</td></tr><tr><td>Increased breast size</td><td>3</td></tr><tr><td>Maternal stores</td><td>4-8</td></tr><tr><td>TOTAL</td><td>24-28</td></tr></table>
Increased nutrient needs	The client will identify the nutrients for which there is need during pregnancy.	Calories—weight gain, growth, energy Protein—growth and development Calcium—fetal bone and tooth development Iron—healthy red blood cells, increase in blood volume for fetus, maternal and fetal iron storage Vitamin A—formation of skin tissue, organs, and cells Vitamin C—formation of tissues Folacin—synthesis (formation) of all cells especially important during periods of rapid growth Other B vitamins—assist in energy production Other nutrients—sodium, iodine, zinc
Risk factors related to pregnancy	Client will explain average risk factors related to her pregnancy.	From the list below the counselor will explain to the client her risk factors: Obesity—short interconceptual period Anemia—teenage pregnancy Multiple births—high parity (i.e., more than 5 pregnancies) Smoking—diabetes or other chronic diseases Alcohol intake—use of drugs or medications (i.e., unless specifically approved by physician) Underweight—poor pregnancy history Toxemia Over 35 years Poor dietary intake

From Arizona Department of Health Services, Bureau of Nutrition: Nutrition education for pregnant women, Phoenix, 1983.

Table 9-7. Model criteria for quality assurance in ambulatory nutrition care for pregnant women*

Criteria Identify Outcome (O) and Process (P)	Critical Time	Exceptions†	References
1. Woman's total weight gain is 20 to 30 lb above her pregravid weight (O)	Time of delivery	Premature delivery	The American College of Obstetricians and Gynecologists and The American Dietetic Association: Assessment of maternal nutrition, Washington, D.C., 1982
2. Woman's rate of weight gain is: 2 to 3 lb during first trimester; 3 to 4 lb/ mo during second and third trimesters. (O)	First trimester Second and third trimesters		Pitkin, R.M.: Assessment of nutritional status of mother, fetus, and newborn, Am. J. Clin. Nutr., 34(Suppl).:662, April 1981.
3. Woman maintains a hemoglobin of 11 gm or a hematocrit of 33% or more. (O)	By third trimester	Non-nutrition-related hemoglobin opathies; hemorrhage; high altitudes	The American College of Obstetricians and Gynecologists and The American Dietetic Association: Assessment of maternal nutrition, Washington, D.C. 1982 Christakis, G., editor: Nutritional assessment in health programs, Washington, D.C., 1973, American Public Health Association.
4. Urine test for ketones is negative. (O)	Throughout pregnancy		Felig, P., and Lynch, V.: Starvation in human pregnancy, hypoglycemia, hypoinsulinemia and hypoketonemia, Science **170**:990, 1970.
5. Woman's reported food intake is appropriate as defined by local protocol for age and stage of pregnancy. (O)	End of second trimester	Late entry to service	Committee on Dietary Allowances, Food and Nutrition Board, National Research Council: Recommended dietary allowances, Washington, D.C., 1980, National Academy of Sciences
6. Woman receives information on substance use and abuse (e.g., alcohol, drugs, tobacco, pica) during pregnancy. (P)	Initial visit	None	The American College of Obstetricians and Gynecologists and the American Dietetic Association: Assessment of maternal nutrition, Washington, D.C., 1982, ADA.

From Kaufman, M., editor: Guide to quality assurance in ambulatory nutrition care, Chicago, 1983, The American Dietetic Association.
*Woman with no medical complication during current pregnancy; pregravid weight 95% to 120% of desirable body weight.
†Lost to follow-up applies to all criteria.   *Continued.*

Table 9-7. Model criteria for quality assurance in ambulatory nutrition care for pregnant women—cont'd

Criteria Identify Outcome (O) and Process (P)	Critical Time	Exceptions	References
7. Woman is given information on breast-feeding and appropriate infant feeding alternatives. (P)	Third trimester	Preterm delivery; adoption	American Academy of Pediatrics: Pediatric nutrition handbook, Evanston, Ill., 1979, AAP.
8. Iron (30 to 60 mg elemental) supplement is prescribed. (P)	Initial visit	Hemolytic anemia	Committee on Maternal Nutrition: Maternal nutrition and the course of pregnancy, Washington, D.C., 1970, National Academy of Sciences.
9. Folacin (0.8 to 1 mg) supplement is prescribed. (P)	Initial visit	None	The American College of Obstetricians and Gynecologists and the American Dietetic Association: Assessment of maternal nutrition, Washington, D.C., 1982, ADA.
10. Infant birth weight is greater than 2500 gm. (O)	Term	Premature delivery; multiple births	Fomon, S.J.: Infant nutrition, ed. 2, Philadelphia, 1974, W.B. Saunders Co. Committee on Maternal Nutrition: Maternal nutrition and the course of pregnancy, Washington, D.C., 1970, National Academy of Sciences.
11. Woman is advised of desirable postpartum weight for height, age, and breast-feeding status. (P)	Third trimester	None	Worthington-Roberts, B., Vermeersch, J., and Williams, S.R.: Nutrition in pregnancy and lactation, ed. 3, St. Louis, 1985, Times Mirror/Mosby College Publishing.

Table 9-8. Daily food guide for pregnant women

Food Group	Recommended Amount (at Least)	Serving Size
Dairy foods (rich in calcium, protein, and minerals): cheese, milk, yogurt, cottage cheese, soybean curd	4 servings	1 serving equals: 1 C milk/yogurt ⅓ C dry milk powder 1½ oz cheese 8 oz soybean curd
Protein foods (rich in protein, iron, fat, and B vitamins): beef, pork, lamb, eggs, chicken, peanut butter, dried beans or peas, cottage cheese, lentils, nuts, seeds	Equivalent of 6 oz	1 oz equals: ¼ C nuts, seeds ½ C beans 1 oz soybean curd (tofu) 1 oz meat or cheese 1 egg ¼ C cottage cheese 2 tbsp peanut butter
"A" vegetables (rich in vitamin A and fiber): carrots, spinach, greens, squash, tomatoes, peppers, broccoli, pumpkin	1-2 servings	1 serving equals: ½ C cooked 1 C raw
"C" fruits and vegetables (rich in vitamin C and fiber): oranges, grapefruit, cantaloupe, strawberries, green chilis, cabbage, tomatoes, lemons, green peppers	1-2 servings	1 serving equals: ½ C juice 1 piece fruit
Other fruits and vegetables (provide other vitamins, minerals, and fiber): bananas, apples, grapes, peas, corn, string beans, potatoes	2-3 servings	1 serving equals: ½ C cooked 1 C raw
Bread and cereals (provide B vitamins, iron, and fiber): breads, tortillas, hot cereals, rice, noodles, macaroni, cold cereals	4 servings	1 serving equals: 1 slice ½ C cooked cereals ½ C rice, pasta
Fats (provide vitamin A and essential fatty acids): butter, margarine, oils, lard, salad dressings, olives, bacon, avocados		As needed to increase calories. Fats are a concentrated form of energy and should be used in moderation since they are naturally supplied in many other foods.
Fluids: Drink at least eight glasses of liquids each day, which would include milk, fruit juices, soups and water. Avoid beverages high in sugar (e.g., soft drinks), alcohol, and caffeine (tea, coffee, chocolate drinks), since these are low in nutrients and may be harmful to the fetus.		

Modified from Arizona Department of Health Services, Bureau of Nutrition Services: Pregnancy protocol, Phoenix, 1983, Arizona Department of Health Services.

VEGETARIAN FOOD GUIDE

General Guidelines

1. Follow nutrition guide for regular food plan during pregnancy.
2. Eat a wide variety of foods, including milk and milk products and eggs.
3. If no milk is allowed, use a supplement of 4 μg of vitamin B_{12} daily. If goat and soy milk are used, partial supplementation may be needed.
4. If no milk is taken, also use supplements of 1200 mg of calcium and 10 μg of vitamin D daily. Partial supplementation will be necessary if fewer than four servings of milk and milk products are consumed.
5. Select a variety of plant foods (especially grains, legumes, nuts, and seeds) to obtain "complete" proteins by complementary combinations, as indicated in the list below.
6. Use iodized salt.

Complementary Plant Protein Combinations*

Food	Amino Acids Deficient	Complementary Protein Food Combinations
Grains	Isoleucine Lysine	Rice + legumes Corn + legumes Wheat + legumes Wheat + peanut + milk Wheat + sesame + soybean Rice + Brewer's yeast
Legumes	Tryptophan Methionine	Legumes + rice Beans + wheat Beans + corn Soybeans + rice + wheat Soybeans + corn + milk Soybeans + wheat + sesame Soybeans + peanuts + sesame Soybeans + peanuts + wheat + rice Soybeans + sesame + wheat
Nuts and seeds	Isoleucine Lysine	Peanuts + sesame + soybeans Sesame + beans Sesame + soybeans + wheat Peanuts + sunflower seeds
Vegetables	Isoleucine Methionine	Lima beans Green beans Brussels sprouts } + Sesame seeds or Brazil nuts or mushrooms Cauliflower Broccoli Greens = millet or rice

From Williams, S.R.: Nutritional guidance in prenatal care. In Worthington-Roberts, B.S., Vermeersch, J., and Williams, S.R.: Nutrition in pregnancy and lactation, ed.3, St. Louis, 1985, Times Mirror/Mosby College Publishing.
*Adapted from Lappe, F.M.: Diet for a small planet, ed.2, New York, 1983, Friends of the Earth/Ballantine.

come criteria, critical time, and exceptions. These criteria provide the basis for an effective counseling session.

There are several tools that are useful in providing nutrition information to the pregnant woman: a daily food guide, sample meal patterns and menus, and information on ethnic preferences and vegetarian diet practices.

Daily Food Guide

A diet consisting of a variety of foods can supply needed nutrients. The increased quantities of essential nutrients needed during pregnancy may be met by skillful planning around a daily food guide that meets RDA. Table 9-8 describes a daily food guide for pregnant women developed by the Arizona Department of Health Services Bureau of Nutrition Services.

Cultural and Social Influences on Food Practices

Consideration of a patient's cultural food preferences increases the communication between counselor and patient, thus providing a greater opportunity to obtain compliance in following a prescribed diet.

Foods basic to almost all vegetarian diets are vegetables, fruits, legumes, nuts, and grains. The use of milk and milk products and eggs varies. The box on p. 242 illustrates combinations of plant foods that are complementary and can make complete protein.

A problem of sufficient income to purchase foods can cause an individual to have a nutritionally inadequate diet. Nutrients such as protein and iron are among those more likely to be deficient in diets of low-income groups. To help improve the nutritional quality of the diet, one should encourage the person with limited income to participate in food programs such as the Special Supplemental Food Program for Women, Infants and Children (WIC) and food stamps (Table 9-10). Nutrition education and counseling are important to ensure the benefits of such programs.

NUTRITION GUIDELINES FOR LACTATION

Guidelines for the lactating mother, including foods, their functions, and daily servings, are indicated in Table 9-9.

Support for Maternal Nutrition

Although there has been significant improvement in the entire area of perinatal health over the last 10 to 12 years, there is still a pressing need for greater emphasis on nutrition in the delivery of perinatal care (Hughes, 1982). To prepare for the future, there is an even greater need to define the scope and current dimensions of the problems in maternal nutrition (Better Health for Our Children, 1981).

REFERRAL FOR ADDITIONAL SERVICES

The major food assistance program for low-income pregnant women in the United States is WIC. In addition, the Food Stamp Program and the Commodity Distribution Program are also available. These programs are described in detail in Chapter 8.

Special Supplemental Food Program for Women, Infants and Children (WIC)

In 1972 Congress authorized the WIC program. I (Owen) worked to develop the WIC legislation and instituted one of the first statewide WIC programs in the country. WIC provides participants with specific nutritious supplemental foods and nutrition education, at no cost. WIC participants are eligible low-income persons who are determined by competent professionals (physicians, nutritionists, nurses, and other health officials) to be at "nutritional risk" because of inadequate nutrition, health care, or both. Federal funds are available to participating state health departments or comparable state agencies. Indian tribes, bands, groups, or their authorized representatives who are recognized by the Bureau of Indian Affairs, U.S. Department of the Interior, or the appropriate area office of the Indian Health Service, U.S. Department of

Table 9-9. Nutrition guidelines for lactation

Food Group	Effect	Daily Servings
Protein		
Animal: Meat, fish, poultry, liver, eggs, milk Vegetable: Beans, peas, nuts, soybean curd, peanut butter	Provide basic building and repairing materials for tissues and cells; important for healthy blood and to fight infections	4
Dairy foods		
Whole, low-fat, or nonfat dry milk, yogurt, cheese	Rich in calcium that helps build strong bones and teeth; aid functioning of heart, muscles, and nerves; help blood coagulate	4-5
Grain products		
Bread, cereals, tortillas, bagels, pasta, rice, crackers	Provide B vitamins that help keep muscles and nerves healthy; often a good source of iron	4-5
Fruits and vegetables		
Vitamin C rich: oranges, citrus, cantaloupes, strawberries, chilis, cabbage, bell peppers	Help body use iron and fight infection	1-2
Leafy greens: broccoli, cabbage, spinach	Promote healthy eyes, skin, teeth, and good vision; a source of vitamin A	2
Other: carrots, potatoes, yams, squash, mushrooms, bean sprouts, apricots, peaches, apples, bananas, pears, plums, dates, berries, grapes, raisins, watermelons	Contain vitamin A and a variety of minerals needed for good health	1-2

Modified from Arizona Department of Health Services, Bureau of Nutrition Services: Pregnancy protocol, Phoenix, 1983, Arizona Department of Health Services.

Table 9-10. Federally sponsored food assistance programs for pregnant women

Program Offered	Purpose	Administering Agencies
Special Supplemental Food Programs for Women, Infants and Children (WIC)	Assist pregnant women, lactating mothers, and children aged 1 to 5 years in obtaining specified nutritious foods	USDA Food and Nutrition Service and state health agencies
Food Stamps	Assist families in providing nutritious meals	USDA Food and Nutrition Service and state welfare agencies
Commodity Distribution Program	Encourage and maintain domestic consumption of commodities, prevent the waste of commodities	USDA Food and Nutrition Service

Modified from Owen, A.L., Owen, G.M., and Lanna, G.: Health and nutritional benefits of federal food assistance programs. In Cost and Benefits of Nutritional Care Phase 1. Chicago: The American Dietetic Association, 1979. Copyright The American Dietetic Association. Reprinted by permission; and Budget of the U.S. Government (appendix), Executive Office of the President, Office of Management and Budget, Washington, D.C., 1984, U.S. Government Printing Office.

Table 9-11. Nutrition assessment and intervention guidelines for pregnant women in community nutrition

Nutritional Assessment Components	Method	Risk and Problems Indicated	Intervention Guidelines	Referral Sources
Anthropometric: weight for height	Use weight-for-height tables to determine prepregnant weight status	Prepregnancy underweight, overweight	Adjust recommended weight to higher-than-average gain for underweight women and lower-than-average gain for overweight women	
Prenatal weight gain	Plot prenatal weight gain on appropriate grid	Inadequate or excessive rate of weight gain; rapid gains may indicate fluid accumulation	Adjust food intake and activity level to correspond with desired rate of weight gain; attempt to separate fluid gain from tissue gain if edema develops; salt restriction is not indicated for the treatment of physiologic edema	Maternal and Infant Care Projects; prenatal care; WIC Program; food stamps
Biochemical Hemoglobin Hematocrit Urine analysis	Standard technique; dip stick for ketones, sugar, and protein spillage	Anemia, gestational diabetes, preeclampsia	Adjust dietary and supplemental iron intake; control blood glucose levels	
Clinical: obstetric history	Questionnaire	Short interval between pregnancies (<1 yr) and nutrient stores depletion; inadequate/excessive weight gain history may be repeated; anemia history may indicate probable reoccurrence; prior oral contraceptive use may increase prenatal need for folic acid and vitamins C and B_6	Replete nutrient stores with adequate diet and supplements if required; adjust diet to include rich food sources of iron, folic acid, vitamins C and B_6 as indicated; provide anticipatory guidance on optimal rate of and total weight gain	Title XIX Early Periodic Screening, Diagnosis, and Treatment Program; Maternal and Child Health Services; state and local health departments; private physicians
Dietary Diet quality and quantity, caffeine and alcohol intake levels Existence of pica	Repeated 24-hour or typical day food recalls; 3-day food record assessments; computerized dietary analysis assessment from a record of food intake; food group intake assessment	Low or excessive nutrient intake levels; excessive consumption of alcohol and caffeine-containing beverages; ingestion of non-food items	Adjust diet to include sources of needed nutrients; discuss possible effects of alcohol on the fetus; provide caution about excessive (>500 mg/day) caffeine consumption	

From Brown, J.E.: Clin. Nutr. 3(3):105, 1984.

Health and Human Services, may also act as state agencies. These agencies distribute funds to the participating local agencies. The funds pay for supplemental foods for participants and pay specified administrative costs, including those of nutrition education.

Eligibility for the Program

Pregnant, postpartum, and breast-feeding women and infants and children up to 5 years of age are eligible if they (1) meet the income standards (a state agency may either set a statewide income standard or allow local agencies to set their own); (2) are individually determined to be at nutritional risk and in need of the supplemental foods the program offers; and (3) live in an approved project area (if the state has a residency requirement) or belong to special population groups, such as migrant farmworkers, Native Americans (Indians), or refugees. Length of residency is not an eligibility requirement. *Nutritional risk* is a term used to indicate abnormal weight gain during pregnancy, a history of high-risk pregnancies, low birth weight (under 2.5 kg [5½ lb]), stunted growth, underweight, obesity, anemia, or an inadequate dietary pattern. When a local agency has limited funds to serve additional participants, applicants are classified according to a priority system based on nutritional need and placed in the program if space becomes available.

Foods Included in the WIC Program

Infants up to 3 months of age receive iron-fortified formula. Older infants (4 through 12 months) receive formula, iron-fortified infant cereal, and fruit juices high in vitamin C. An infant may receive non-iron-fortified or special therapeutic formula when it is prescribed by a physician for a specified medical condition. Participating women and children receive fortified milk and/or cheese; eggs; hot or cold cereals high in iron; fruit and vegetable juices high in vitamin C; and either peanut butter, dry beans, or peas.

WIC provides breast-feeding women with a food package to meet their extra nutritional needs. Women and children with special dietary needs may receive a package containing cereal, juice, and special therapeutic formulas. For a participant to receive this package, a physician must determine that the participant has a medical condition that precludes or restricts the use of conventional foods and requires a therapeutic formula.

The state agency administering the program may use one or all of the following food delivery systems: (1) retail purchase, where participants use vouchers or checks to buy foods at local retail stores authorized by the state agency to accept WIC vouchers or checks; (2) home delivery, where the food is delivered to participants' homes; and (3) direct distribution, where participants pick up the food from a warehouse.

Nutrition Education in WIC

Nutrition education is available to all adult WIC participants, to parents or caretakers of infant and child participants, and, whenever possible, to the child who participates. This nutrition education is designed to have a practical relationship to participants' nutritional needs, household situations, and cultural preferences and includes information on how participants can select food for themselves and their families. The goals of WIC nutrition education are to teach the relationship between proper nutrition and good health, to help the individual at nutritional risk to develop better food habits, and to prevent nutrition-related problems by showing participants how to best use their supplemental and other foods. The WIC program also encourages breast-feeding and counsels pregnant women on its nutritional advantages. Table 9-10 describes the food assistance programs that are available for pregnant women.

Intervention strategies and guidelines for working with pregnant women in the community are included in Table 9-11.

EXAMPLES OF STRATEGIES AT THE LOCAL LEVEL
Effect of an Education Program on the Decision to Breast-Feed

Kaplowitz and Olson (1983) designed a breast-feeding education program for low-income women with a grade school or high school education. The program consisted of a series of five pamphlets mailed to the subjects' homes one at a time over 5 consecutive weeks. An evaluation examined the effect of the program on the pregnant women's decisions about infant feeding. They randomly assigned 44 women to either the experimental or control group. The women in the experimental group received all five pamphlets, whereas the women in the control group did not receive the information. Although the program appeared to be effective in increasing knowledge, it did not cause the women to form more positive attitudes toward breast-feeding or increase the incidence of breast-feeding. The findings suggest that future education programs need to affect both knowledge and attitudes to influence infant feeding decisions.

Evaluation of the Effect of WIC on Birth Weight

Kennedy et al. (1982) completed a retrospective review of WIC and non-WIC medical and nutrition records at nine sites in Massachussetts. A significant proportion of WIC and non-WIC women in this study had maternal biological characteristics that predisposed them to a higher probability of obstetrical complications.

Participant characteristics, including pregravid weight, weight gain during pregnancy, or history of low-birth-weight infants, were found to be significantly associated with birth weight. Sociodemographic factors did not influence prenatal outcome when biological variables were held constant. This study indicates that dietary supplementation in this high-risk prenatal group produced positive and significant changes in birth weight. Concerted efforts should be undertaken as part of the program to locate and certify women as participants early in pregnancy. Early identification of high-risk pregnant women and interaction with health and nutrition services may improve the outcome of pregnancy.

SUMMARY

Optimum nutrition is an integral part of sound maternity care, it is basic to the successful outcome of pregnancy. There are increased nutritional demands during pregnancy. These demands focus on nutrient needs basic to human growth and development, increased intake of protein, vitamins, and minerals to sustain the necessary building process, and sufficient energy input from calories.

To ensure that appropriate nutritional care is provided during pregnancy, an initial individual assessment of nutritional status and need must be made at the beginning of prenatal care, and it must be supported by continuing evaluation and monitoring throughout the pregnancy.

REFERENCES

The American College of Obstetricians and Gynecologists and The American Dietetic Association: Assessment of maternal nutrition, Chicago, 1982, ACOG and ADA.

Aubry, R.H., Robert, M.S., and Cuenca, M.S.: The assessment of maternal nutrition, Clin. Perinatol. 2:207, 1975.

Beal, V.A.: Assessment of nutritional status in pregnancy, Am. J. Clin. Nutr. 34:691, 1981.

Better health for our children, a national strategy report of the Select Panel for the Promotion of Child Health, U.S. Congress and the Secretary of Health and Human Services, vol. I to IV, DHHS (PHS) Pub. no. 79-55071, Washington, D.C., 1981, U.S. Government Printing Office.

Brown, J.E., et al.: Influence of pregnancy weight gain on the size of infants born to underweight women, Obstet. Gynecol. 57:13, 1981.

Brown, J.E.: Nutrition for your pregnancy: the University of Minnesota guide, Minneapolis, 1983, University of Minnesota Press.

Brown, J.E.: Nutrition services for pregnant woman, infant, children and adolescents, Clin. Nutr. 3(3):105, 1984.

Centers for Disease Control: Nutrition surveillance annual survey, 1981, Washington, D.C., Dec. 1983, U.S. Department of Health and Human Services.

Food and Nutrition Board, National Research Council: Alternative dietary practices and nutritional abuses during pregnancy, Washington, D.C., 1982, National Academy Press.

Food and Nutrition Board, Committee on Maternal Nutrition: Maternal nutrition and the course of pregnancy, Washington, D.C., 1970, National Academy of Sciences.

Food and Nutrition Board, Committee on Maternal Nutrition: Maternal nutrition and the course of pregnancy, summary report, Washington, D.C., 1970-1975, National Academy of Sciences.

Food and Nutrition Board, National Research Council: Laboratory indices of nutritional status in pregnancy, Washington, D.C., 1977, National Research Council.

Food and Nutrition Board, National Research Council: Recommended dietary allowances, ed. 9, Washington, D.C., 1980, National Academy of Sciences.

Hughes, M.: Healthy mothers, healthy babies, J. Am. Diet. Assoc. 80:215, 1982.

Jacobson, H.N.: Maternal nutrition in the 1980's, J. Am. Diet. Assoc. 80:216, 1982.

Jelliffe, O.B., and Jelliffe, E.F.P.: Human milk in the modern world, Oxford, England, 1978, Oxford University Press.

Kaplowitz, D.O., and Olson, C.M.: The effect of an education program on the decision to breastfeed, J. Nutr. Ed. 15:61, 1983.

Kennedy, E.T., et al.: Evaluation of the effect of WIC supplemental feeding on birth weight, J. Am. Diet. Assoc. 80:3, 1982.

Mengert, W.F.: Fetal and neonatal mortality, causes and prevention, Am. J. Obstet. Gynecol. 55:660, 1948.

National Association of Community Health Centers: Quality assurance in ambulatory nutrition, Chicago, 1983, The American Dietetic Association.

Pitkin, R.M.: Obstetrics and gynecology. In Schneider, H.A., Anderson, C.E., and Coursin, D.B., editors: Nutritional support of medical practice, New York, 1983, Harper & Row Publishers, Inc.

Robinson, M.: Salt in pregnancy, Lancet 1:178, 1958.

Rosso, P., and Cramory, C.: Nutrition and pregnancy. In Nutrition: pre- and postnatal development, New York, 1979, Plenum Publishing Corp.

Tompkins, W.T., and Wiehl, D.G.: Nutritional deficiencies as a causal factor in toxemia and premature labor, Am. J. Obstet. Gynecol. 62:8989, 1951.

U.S. Department of Health and Human Services, Public Health Service: Promoting health, preventing disease: objectives for the nation, Washington, D.C., 1980, U.S. Government Printing Office.

Wong, F.L., and Trowbridge, F.L.: Nutrition surveys and surveillance: their application to clinical practice, Clin. Nutr. 3(3):194, 1984.

Worthington-Roberts, B.S., Vermeersch, J., and Williams, S.R.: Nutrition, pregnancy, and lactation, ed. 3, St. Louis, 1985, Times Mirror/Mosby College Publishing.

Wright, J.T., et al: Alcohol consumption, pregnancy and low birthweight, Lancet 1:663, 1983.

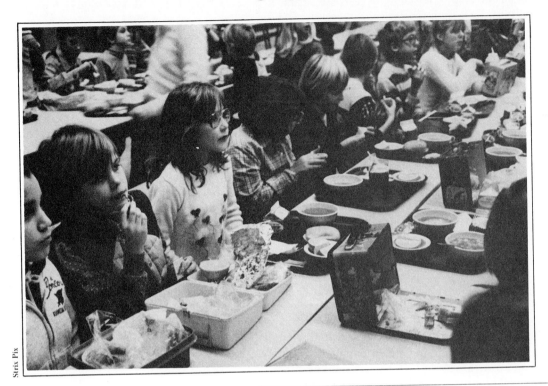

Strix Pix

Guidelines for Nutrition Services for Infants, Children, and Adolescents

GENERAL CONCEPT

Nutrition is an important component of the health care of infants, children, and adolescents. Infants grow rapidly and have requirements for protein, energy, and other essential nutrients that are higher per unit of body weight than at any other time in childhood. Thus the infant's increase in size is among the most dramatic developmental changes occurring during the first year of life. A young child's growth rate slows considerably after the first year of life. Preschoolers' rate of growth is also slow. As a result, toddlers and preschoolers require less food, since their appetites decrease. Adolescence is a time of emotional, physical, social, biological, and educational transitions. The adolescent's health and nutritional needs should be viewed in the context of children seeking to establish their identity in a changing adult world.

Nutrition plays a vital role in the growth and development of infants, children, and adolescents. Since the early 1900s, publicly funded nutrition services have blossomed, wilted, and reblossomed depending on economic conditions and political climate. However, our society continues to strongly value the importance of adequate nutrition during the vulnerable periods of infancy, childhood, and adolescence (Brown, 1984).

NUTRITION-RELATED HEALTH PROBLEMS OF INFANTS, CHILDREN, AND ADOLESCENTS

The U.S. Department of Health and Human Services (1980) has identified several nutrition problems that affect infants and children: iron deficiency anemia in high-risk groups, suboptimum mental and physical development associated with inadequate nutrition, dental caries, and increased resistance to infection in children. Table 10-1 describes additional health-related problems of infants, children, and adolescents.

Specific objectives to be accomplished by 1990 relating to infants, children, and adolescents follow (USDHHS, 1980).

Infants. By 1990, growth retardation of infants caused by inadequate diet should be eliminated in the United States as a public health problem. In 1972-1973 it was estimated that 10% to 15% of infants and children of migratory workers in certain poor rural populations suffered growth retardation as a result of dietary inadequacies. By 1990, the proportion of women who breast-feed their infants should increase to 75% at hospital discharge and 35% at 6 months postpartum. In 1978 the proportions were 45% at hospital discharge and 21% at 6 months postpartum. By 1990, almost all routine health contacts with health professionals should include some element of nutrition education and counseling.

Children and adolescents. By 1990, the mean serum cholesterol level in children ages 1 to 14 should be 150 mg/dl or below. In 1971-1974, for children ages 1 to 17, the mean serum cholesterol level was 176 mg/dl. For a smaller population sample in 1972-1975, the mean blood plasma cholesterol level in children ages 10 to 14 was about 160 mg/dl.

IDENTIFYING PROBLEMS IN THE COMMUNITY: PEDIATRIC NUTRITION SURVEILLANCE SYSTEM
Conditions Related to Deficiencies

The Pediatric Nutrition Surveillance System (CDC, 1982) identified that iron deficiency anemia was prevalent in high-risk groups including young children. Low-income children, ages 2 to 5 years, and blacks had a higher prevalence of low hemoglobin and hematocrit levels. Data from nutrition surveillance for the period 1976 to 1982 generally suggested a modest decline in the prevalence of low hematocrit and hemoglobin levels among white, black, and Hispanic children entering publicly supported health programs (Wong and Trowbridge, 1984).

Growth Stunting

With the exception of Southeast Asian children, blacks under 1 year of age had the highest prevalence of low height for age in the Pediatric Nutrition Surveillance System (CDC, 1982). There is

Table 10-1. Health problems and related nutritional risk factors

Health Problems	Related Nutritional Risk Factors
Infants and children	
Growth retardation, underweight	Dietary inadequacies
Elevated serum cholesterol	Excessive total fat, saturated fat, and cholesterol intake
Dental caries	Excessive, frequent consumption of sweets, lack of fluoride
Iron deficiency anemia	Malnutrition, inadequate dietary iron intake
Infection	Malnutrition
Obesity	Caloric consumption exceeds caloric need
Constipation	Low fiber intake
Adolescents	
Hypertension	Overweight, excessive sodium intake, low potassium intake
Underweight	Undernutrition
Obesity	Caloric consumption exceeds caloric need
Dental caries	Excessive, frequent consumption of sweets
Infection	Malnutrition
Iron deficiency anemia	Early introduction of whole cow's milk, malnutrition, inadequate dietary iron intake
Elevated serum cholesterol	Excessive total fat, saturated fat, and cholesterol intake

From Brown, J.E.: Clin. Nutr. 3(3):104, 1984.

similarity in the height growth of children of other ethnic groups in this age-group. Children with a history of low birth weight had a higher prevalence of growth stunting and of thinness (low weight for height), even at 2 to 4 years of age, in comparison to their counterparts of normal birth weight.

In contrast to results for infants, black children in the CDC Pediatric Surveillance System had the lowest prevalence of short stature by ages 2 to 4 years, reflecting a more rapid rate of growth in early childhood (Figure 10-1). Growth stunting increased in prevalence with age among Hispanic and Native American children. In the period from 1976 to 1982 trends from surveillance suggested a modest decline in the prevalence of growth stunting among children under 2 years of age in all ethnic groups. However, no consistent trends were observed among children 2 to 5 years of age.

Dietary Deficiencies

In the 1977-1978 Nationwide Food Consumption Survey (NFCS) potentially low intakes were documented for nutrients such as iron, calcium, vita-

min B_6, and magnesium (Human Nutrition Information Services, 1982). The highest-risk group included females from adolescence through old age; this group had deficient intakes of all four of these nutrients. People on weight reduction diets, particularly if they were dieting for extended periods of time, comprised another high-risk group for inadequate nutrient intake. Low income was also associated with poor intakes of some nutrients.

Young children had deficient intakes of iron. The iron intake of children ages 1 to 2 years was less than half of that of children under 1 year of age. For infants, there was a threefold increase in iron intake between the 1965 and 1977 surveys. This factor was attributed to the higher consumption of iron-fortified formulas and cereals. A similar finding of low iron intake in young children was observed in the first National Health and Nutrition Examination Survey (NHANES I).

Conditions Related to Excesses or Imbalances

In the CDC Pediatric Nutrition Surveillance System findings (1982), Hispanic and Native

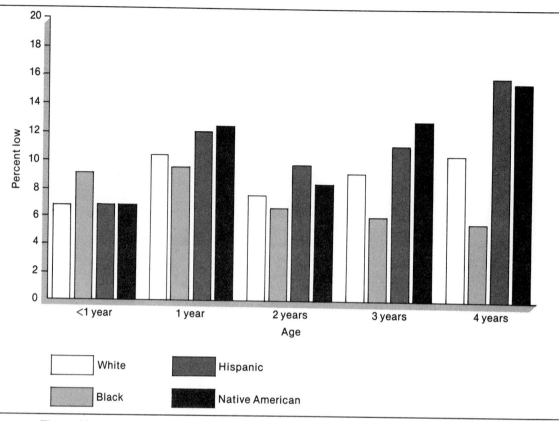

Figure 10-1. Prevalence of low height for age among children screened in selected states, CDC Pediatric Nutrition Surveillance System, 1982.
Redrawn from Wong, F.L., and Trowbridge, F.L.: Clin. Nutr. 3(3):94, 1984.

American children had higher prevalences of obesity than other ethnic groups, except in infancy (Figure 10-2). Trends from 1976 to 1982 showed a modest decline in the prevalence of overweight in children under 2 years of age for all ethnic groups. In contrast, no consistent pattern of change is observed in the 2 to 5 year age-group.

INFANTS
Physical Growth

The infant's increase in size is among the most obvious developmental changes occurring during the first year of life. Following birth, the new-born progresses from a weight of 1 to 4 kg (2 to 8 lb) to a mature weight of approximately 70 kg (154 lb). Average weight gain in the first year is 7 kg (15 lb), about one half of which occurs in the first 4 months of life. Approximately 61,000 kcal are required to achieve the 3.5 kg (7 lb) growth between birth and 4 months of age (Owen and Paige, 1983).

Approximately 33% of calories consumed are used for growth during the first 4 months. This rapid growth in the healthy term infant during the first 4 months of life requires more energy, protein, and other essential nutrients per unit

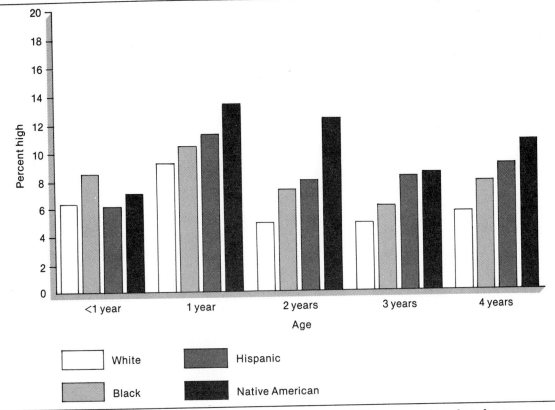

Figure 10-2. Prevalence of high weight for height among children screened in selected states, CDC Pediatric Nutrition Surveillance System, 1982.

Redrawn from Wong, F.L., and Trowbridge, F.L.: Clin. Nutr. 3(3):94, 1984.

of body weight than at any other time in infancy or childhood. These needs can be met completely through the use of human milk and/or formula.

At about 5 months of age the infant enters a transitional period characterized by a decreased rate of growth and an increased level of caloric expenditure for physical activity, developmental readiness, and physiological capacity. Although total nutrient requirements continue to increase as a result of growth, the decreasing requirement for energy and protein pertinent to body weight reflects the progressive decrease in rate of growth.

By age 8 or 9 months, solid foods provide a significant source of energy and other nutrients to supplement the basic intake from human milk or formula.

Physiology of Infant Nutrition

The enormously complex, yet efficient, gastrointestinal mechanism required for the absorption of nutrients and maintenance of health are well developed at birth, but not mature. All the secretions of the digestive tract contain enzymes especially suited to the digestion of human milk.

The ability to handle foods other than milk

Table 10-2. Digestion in infancy

Location	Function	Effect on Feeding
Birth to 3 months*		
Salivary	Lactose not produced in salivary secretions; amylase not available in significant quantities.	Salivary enzymes play no role in digestion of milk.
Gastric	Hydrochloric acid and pepsin precipitate casein into curds separate and acidify whey protein.	Beginning of protein digestion; carbohydrate digestion partly begins; fat indigested in the stomach.
Intestinal	Pancreatic and intestinal enzymes digest proteins into amino acids, reduce carbohydrates to monosaccharides, and split fatty acids from triglycerides in the small intestine.	Protein from human milk is 95% digested, and a similar percentage of protein is digested from commercial formulas, which are heat treated and sufficiently dilute to produce a soft curd.
	Disaccharidases are present in the border of the intestinal mucosa.	Human milk and commercial formulas; carbohydrate digested here.
	Pancreatic amylase is present in small quantities.	Complex carbohydrates poorly utilized.
	Pancreatic lipase is present in sufficient quantity.	Eighty percent of human milk fat is digested at birth, and almost 95% is digested by 1 month.
	Lipase is naturally found in human milk, which is activated by bile salts.	Digestion of fats from commercial formulas equals that of human milk.
		Fat from other sources (butterfat) is poorly digested.
4 to 6 months†		
Salivary	Ptyalin aids digestion to starch.	As solid foods are added to the diet, ptyalin plays a role in the digestion of starches.
Gastric	Functions already mature (occurs soon after birth with hydrochloric acid and pepsin for digestion of milk and nonmilk foods).	Aids in digestion of milk and nonmilk foods.
Intestinal	Enzymes previously lacking are produced in larger quantities and digest nonmilk food substances. More putrefactive bacteria occur in intestinal flora as solid foods increase amount of protein in lower gastrointestinal tract.	Amylase production increases and provides better utilization of starch-containing foods. Increased production of amylase coincides with observed increase in infant's utilization of iron from cereals and nonmilk foods.

From Willis, N.H.: Infant nutrition, birth to 6 months, a syllabus, Philadelphia, 1971, J.B. Lippincott Co.

*The capacities for salivary, gastric, pancreatic, and intestinal digestion increase with age, indicating what may be a natural pattern for the introduction of various sources of solid foods.

†The major changes in digestive capacity that occur at 4 to 6 months involve principally salivary and intestinal functions. Gastric capacities are usually adequate soon after birth and do not change significantly after the third month of life.

Table 10-3. Minimum requirements, advisable intakes, and recommended allowances of selected nutrients for infants: birth to 6 months and 6 to 12 months

Nutrient	Minimum Requirement		Advisable Intake		Recommended Allowance	
	0-6	6-12	0-6	6-12	0-6	6-12
Protein (gm/100 kcal)	1.6	1.4	1.9	1.7	1.9	1.9
Protein (gm/kg)	1.8	1.5	2.2	1.8	2.2	2.0
Vitamins						
A (RE)	75	75	150	150	420	400
D (μg cholecalciferol)	2.5	5	10	10	10	10
E (mg α-TE)	2	2	3	3	4	4
K (μg)	5	5	15	15	12	15
C (mg)	10	10	20	20	35	35
B₁ (mg)	0.1	0.2	0.2	0.2	0.3	0.5
B₂ (mg)	0.1	0.4	0.4	0.4	0.4	0.6
Niacin (mg NE)	2.0	4.5	5	5	6	8
B₆ (mg)	0.1	0.2	0.4	0.4	0.3	0.6
Folacin (μg)	50	50	50	50	30	45
Minerals						
Sodium (mEq)	2.5	2.1	8	6	10	21
Chloride (mEq)	2.3	2.1	7	6	8	13
Potassium (mEq)	2.4	2.0	7	6	16	21
Calcium (mg)	388	289	450	350	360	540
Phosphorus (mg)	132	110	160	130	240	360
Magnesium (mg)	16.5	13.5	25	20	50	70
Iron (mg)	7	7	7	7	10	15

From Owen, G.M., and Paige, D.M.: Infancy. In Paige, D.M., editor: Manual of clinical nutrition, St. Louis, 1983, The C.V. Mosby Co.

depends on the physiological development of the infant. The capacities for salivary, gastric, pancreatic, and intestinal digestion increase with age, indicating what may be a natural pattern for introduction of various sources of solid foods. During the first 3 months salivary fluids seem to play a limited role in the digestion of milk. They become more important when solid foods are added to the diet. Table 10-2 describes the process, functions, and effects of digestion from birth to 6 months of age. The major changes in digestive capacity that occur at 4 to 6 months involve salivary and intestinal functions. Gastric capacities are usually adequate soon after birth and do not change significantly during this period.

Psychosocial Development

The mother's feeding practices from birth determine the infant's exposure to tactile stimulation, which is essential to the infant's physical and emotional growth. Appendix 10-1 describes the neuromuscular and psychosocial development of the infant (up to 12 months) with implications for feeding.

Nutrient Requirements

Requirements for infants less than 6 months of age usually are based on the nutrients consumed by healthy, thriving infants who are breast-fed by healthy, well-nourished mothers (Owen and Paige, 1983). In Table 10-3 minimum requirements, advisable intakes, and recommended di-

Table 10-4. Ranges of daily intakes of nutrients by 3-month-old infants exclusively breast- or formula-fed*

Nutrient	Breast-Fed		Formula-Fed†	
	10th Percentile	90th Percentile	10th Percentile	90th Percentile
Protein (gm/kg)	1.4	2.0	2.0	3.2
Vitamins				
A (RE)	380	600	455	715
D (μg)	0.4	0.6	7	11
E (mg α-TE)	1	1.5	7	11
K (μg)	10	16	22	34
C (mg)	30	45	35	65
B_1 (mg)	0.1	0.2	0.4	0.6
B_2 (mg)	0.3	0.4	0.6	0.9
Niacin (mg NE)	1	1.5	5.5	8.5
B_6 (mg)	.05	.08	0.3	0.4
Folacin (μg)	35	56	56	87
Minerals				
Sodium (mEq)	4.5	7.2	10.5	16.7
Chloride (mEq)	7.5	12	13.1	20.7
Potassium (mEq)	8.5	13.5	15.7	24.6
Calcium (mg)	225	360	415	650
Phosphorus (mg)	95	150	323	509
Magnesium (mg)	27	42	32	50
Iron (mg)	0.4	0.6	9	14

From Owen, G.M., and Paige, D.M.: Infancy. In Paige, D.M., editor: Manual of clinical nutrition, St. Louis, 1983, The C.V. Mosby Co.
*Estimates of levels of intakes of various nutrients are based on average composition (amount of nutrients) of human milk and formulas in relation to the 10th and 90th percentiles of energy intakes of infants involved in a longitudinal growth study.
†Iron-fortified Enfamil or Similac.

etary allowances (RDA) for selected nutrients are summarized. The minimum requirement is the smallest amount of a nutrient needed to protect the individual from undernutrition attributable to deficiency. The term *advisable intake* applies to levels of intake somewhat in excess of the estimated requirement (Fomon, 1974). The RDA for most nutrients represent a value well above the average estimated requirement and encompasses the range of variability observed in individual requirement estimates.

RDA (Food and Nutrition Board, 1980) for infants up to 6 months old are based primarily on the amounts provided by human milk, but in some cases the allowances may exceed those levels to provide for infants receiving formula. RDA for infants 6 months to 1 year of age are based on consumption of formula and increasing amounts of solid foods. In contrast to the allowances for specific nutrients, the allowance for energy is based on average needs of the population groups under consideration, and no adjustment is made for individual variability.

For the infant up to 6 months of age, average energy needs are met at an intake of 115 kcal/kg/day, and for the 6- to 12-month-old infant, 105 kcal/kg/day.

Sources of Nutrients

Ranges of nutrient intakes for healthy infants who are exclusively breast-fed or bottle-fed during the early months of life are shown in Table 10-4 (Owen and Paige, 1983). Breast-fed infants at the lower end of the energy intake distribution consume several nutrients in amounts very close to the estimated requirements. Nutrients in human milk tend to be more bioavailable than the same nutrients in formula, cow's milk, or solid foods.

Human milk. Levels of some nutrients secreted in human milk vary with maternal diet, stages of lactation, duration of lactation, and individual biochemical variability among women (Jelliffe and Jelliffe, 1979). Caloric density and relative proportions of protein, fat, and carbohydrate in colostrum, transitional milk, and mature human milk vary considerably. Recent research has shown that neither maternal diet nor nutritional status has little effect on relative proportions of protein, fat, and carbohydrate in mature human milk. The malnourished woman may be able to produce milk of acceptable quality, although the quantity may be limited. In the healthy, well-nourished mother, the fatty acid composition of milk fat is determined primarily by the diet.

There is a 30% decrease in protein content of human milk between the first and sixth months of lactation (Lonnerdal, Forsum, and Hambraes, 1976). During the same time lactose content does not change; concentrations of calcium, phosphorus, zinc, iron, and sodium and potassium chloride all decrease 10% to 20% (Fomon, 1974). Studies of mineral content of milk from women 1 to 31 months postpartum showed that levels of some trace metals, particularly zinc, declined substantially over time. Levels of iron and copper decreased only moderately after the first 6 months.

Vitamin D and iron appear to be deficient in human milk. In the United States vitamin and mineral supplements are used widely during pregnancy and postpartum, especially during lactation. Thus variations in maternal diet appear to have a limited effect on levels of fat-soluble vitamins (A, D, E, K) in human milk. Variations in maternal intake of water-soluble vitamins (B vitamins and ascorbic acid) are reflected in levels of these vitamins in human milk. Vitamin B_{12} deficiency has been reported in a 6-month-old infant breast-fed by his vegan mother.

IMMUNOLOGICAL BENEFITS OF BREAST-FEEDING. In the past decade there has been considerable research on the nonnutritional aspects of human milk, especially its immunological and other protective constituents. Secretory immunoglobulin A (IgA) in mammary glands and human milk is largely derived from maternal gut associated with lymphoid tissue.

Secretory IgA resists the proleolytic action of the infant's gastroenteric secretions, diminishing antigen contact with the intestinal mucosa until the infant's own antibody responses develop. Lysozymes, lactoperoxidases, and lactoferrin are protein macromolecules in human milk that may be important host resistance factors for the infant. The importance of these immunological, cellular, and enzymatic components of human milk to the infant are indisputable where circumstances preclude preparation, storage, and feeding of a nutritionally adequate and hygienically safe formula.

OTHER NONNUTRIENT COMPONENTS OF HUMAN MILK. Drugs taken by the lactating woman may reach her infant via the milk she produces. The amount of drugs secreted into human milk depends on the lipid solubility of the medication, mechanisms of transport, degree of ionization, and changes in plasma pH. The higher the lipid solubility, the greater the concentration in human milk.

Prepared formulas. The majority of infants who are bottle-fed receive formulas composed of cow's milk protein, vegetable oils, and added carbohydrates. These products meet the infant's nutritional needs during the first 6 months of life (Table 10-5).

COW'S MILK. The major difference between cow's milk and human milk is the greater concentration of proteins and minerals and lower concentration of lactose in cow's milk. The higher ratio of whey proteins (lactalbumin and lactoglobulin) to casein in human milk versus cow's milk has not been shown to be of nutritional significance for the infant (Owen and Paige, 1983).

Butterfat in cow's milk is less well digested and absorbed by the infant than is human milk

Table 10-5. Nutrient composition of human milk and proprietary infant formulas and recommended levels for full-term and low-birth-weight infants (per 100 calories)

Nutrient	Minimum Level Recommended[a]	Human Milk	Enfamil (Mead-Johnson)	Similac (Ross)	SMA (Wyeth)	Enfamil Premature Formula	PM60/40 (Ross)
Protein, gm	1.8[b]	1.3-1.6	2.2	2.2	2.2	3.0	2.22
Fat, gm	3.3	5	5.6	5.4	5.3	5	5.6
Carbohydrate, gm	—	10.3	10.2	10.7	10.7	11	10.2
Ash, gm	—	0.28	0.45	0.61	0.37	0.64	0.3
Vitamin A, IU	250	250	310	296	389	312	296
Vitamin D, IU	40	3	62	59	59	63	59
Vitamin E, IU	0.3(0.7)[c]	0.3	3.1	2.5	1.3	2	2.5
Vitamin K, μg	4	2	8.6	8.1	8.1	9.4	8.1
Vitamin C, mg	8	7.8	8.1	8.1	8.1	8.5	8.1
Thiamin, μg	40	25	78	96	99	80	96
Riboflavin, μg	60	60	150	148	148	90	148
Niacin, μg	250	250	1250	1036	1405	1250	1080
Vitamin B_6, μg	35[d]	15	62	59	59	60	59
Folic acid, μg	4	4	15.6	15	7.4	30	15
Pantothenic acid, μg	300	300	470	444	296	500	444
Vitamin B_{12}, μg	0.15	0.15	0.23	0.22	0.15	0.3	0.22
Biotin, μg	1.5	1.0	2.3	—	2.1	2.3	4.4
Inositol, mg	4	20	4.7	—	—	4.7	24.4
Choline, mg	7	13	15.6	—	14.8	7	12.1
Calcium, mg	50	50	69	75	62	117	59
Phosphorus, mg	25[ef]	25	47	58	46	59	30
Magnesium, mg	6	6	7.8	6.1	7.4	10.4	6.2
Iron, mg	1[g]	0.1	1.9	1.8	1.8	0.16	0.2
Iodine, μg	5	4–9	15.6	14.8	9.6	7.9	6.2
Copper, μg	60	60	94	89	67	90	89
Zinc, mg	0.5	0.5	0.78	0.74	0.5	1	0.74
Manganese, μg	5	1.5	16	5	22	25	5
Sodium, mg	20[f]	24	31	34	21	39	24
Potassium, mg	80	81	102	118	78	110	86
Chloride, mg	55	55	62	74	53	85	59
Renal solute load, mOsm	—	11.3[h]	14.5	15.4	13.2	18.7	13.8

Modified from American Academy of Pediatrics: Pediatric nutrition handbook, Evanston, Ill., 1979, The Academy.

[a] Fed. Reg. 49:14396-14402, 1984.
[b] Protein quality not less than 70% of casein. Lesser quality requires proportionately greater minimum amount of protein.
[c] At least 0.7 IU of vitamin E per gram of linoleic acid.
[d] At least 15 μg of vitamin B_6 per gram of protein.
[e] Calcium/phosphorum ratio not less than 1:1 and not more than 2:0.
[f] Some evidence of higher requirement for low-birth-weight infant.
[g] In iron-fortified formula.
[h] Calculated by method of Ziegler and Fomon.

fat. Cow's milk or evaporated milk meets the infant's needs for most of the B vitamins and for vitamins A and K. Most cow's milk is fortified with vitamin D, but it contains inadequate amounts of vitamins C and E, iron, and copper to serve as the only source of nutrition for the infant. In addition to the nutritional inadequacies of whole cow's milk or evaporated milk, there are problems related to curd formation (relatively high casein content), digestibility of fat, and potential excess renal solute load because of the relatively high levels of protein (urea) and minerals (sodium, potassium, chloride, phosphorous) excreted in the urine.

Solid food. The introduction of solid foods should be delayed until the infant is approximately 5 months old. By this age, the healthy youngster will be able to sit with some support, control his head, and show some hand-eye coordination. During the next 6 or 7 months, as solid foods are introduced, human milk or formula provides a progressively small share of total calories; by age 9 to 12 months approximately one third and one half of calories, respectively, will be supplied by solid foods (Andrews, Clancy, and Katz, 1980). Solid foods supply nearly one half of the total protein and iron intake even though the infant receives an iron-fortified formula. If an isocaloric amount of human milk were substituted for the iron-fortified formula, approximate total intakes of protein, iron, and calcium would be 20 gm, 10.5 mg, and 550 mg, respectively. Solid foods would account for one half the calcium, two thirds the protein, and essentially all the iron in the infant's diet (Owen and Paige, 1983).

Recent Trends in Infant Feeding Practices

The 1970s saw important changes in patterns of infant feeding. Currently, about one half of 1-week-old infants are breast-fed, and one half receive infant formulas. The average duration of breast-feeding has been extended so that nearly one fourth of 6-month-old infants are still breast-fed. Similarly, formula feeding has been extended so that nearly 60% of infants are being fed prepared formulas at 6 months of age while only 25% are fed cow's milk at this age.

It appears that 65% to 75% of infants receive supplemental vitamins and minerals during the first year of life (Andrews, Clancy, and Katz, 1980). In general, the use of vitamin supplements increases with socioeconomic status.

An excellent review of the epidemiological evidence reporting the effects of infant feeding methods on infant health and recent trends in infant feeding methods was described in a report of the Task Force on the Assessment of the Infant Feeding Practices and Infant Health (AAP, 1984).

Health Consequences of Infants at Nutritional Risk
Iron Deficiency

Iron deficiency is one of the most common nutritional deficiencies in North America. Although signs of anemia appear after 12 months of age, they have their genesis in inadequate iron nutrition during the first year of life. Prolonged iron deficiency eventually results in iron deficiency anemia. In infants 6 to 24 months of age anemia is defined as a hemoglobin concentration less than 11 gm/dl.

Obesity

Infantile obesity has been defined by some as weight above the 95th percentile in relation to height, age, sex, and body build. Infantile obesity is commonly secondary to excessive intake of food. Poor infant feeding practices and misuse of solid foods, such as introducing them too early, can readily contribute to overfeeding.

Atherosclerosis

Much more information is needed to document the role of dietary cholesterol in normal growth and development. Until such information is available, a safe guide is to pattern dietary intake in the early months of life on the nutrients found in human milk. For any infant, either healthy or with a familial lipid disorder, there would appear to be no particular advantage in consuming solid food during the first 5 or 6 months of life and no particular advantages in the use of foods high in saturated fats or cholesterol during the second 6 months of life.

Guidelines for Patient Management

The expected outcomes of care for a normal infant include the following:

- Infants maintain acceptable weight/length between the 5th and 95th percentile when plotted on the National Center for Health Statistics (NCHS) growth grid.
- Infants do not deviate more than 25 percentile points from the established pattern of growth (height and weight).
- Infants' hemoglobin levels are equal to or greater than 10 gm or hematocrit levels are equal to or greater than 31% or 11 gm hemoglobin or 34% hematocrit.
- Infants consume human milk or iron-fortified formula.
- Infants consume solid food in accordance with stages of neuromuscular readiness and growth.
- Infants' food intake is nutritionally adequate for age and/or stage of development.

Nutrition Screening and Assessment

Nutritional Disorders of Children: Prevention, Screening and Follow-Up is a useful guide to assist the community dietitian/nutritionist and other health care providers to perform nutritional assessments of infants and children (Fomon, 1976). Nutritional assessment and intervention guidelines for infants and children are presented in Table 10-6.

Anthropometric Assessment

Anthropometric measurements recommended for neonates and infants include weight, recumbent length (crown-heel), head circumference, triceps skinfold, and upper arm circumference.

Appraisal of body size and pattern of growth is a fundamental part of pediatric care. Abnormal size and growth are commonly associated with malnutrition or disease. Evaluation of growth helps in the detection and diagnosis of disorders of infancy and childhood. Discussion of an infant's growth is often the starting point for effective dialogue with that child's parent or caretaker.

In 1975 the NCHS compiled data and prepared a series of percentile curves reflecting the growth of contemporary infants, children, and youth in the United States. These charts should be effective in facilitating uniformity in the clinical appraisal of growth and nutritional status and should help to simplify comparative interpretation of growth data. Figures 10-3 and 10-4 are examples of growth charts for boys and girls, prepubescent and 2 to 18 years.

Tables 10-7 and 10-8 include the NCHS percentiles for length, weight, and head circumference for boys and girls up to 36 months of age.

Weight. Body weight should be measured to the nearest 10 gm (½ oz) for infants or 100 gm (¼ lb) for children. A beam balance scale should be used. The infant's clothes should be removed before he or she is weighed. The infant should be placed in the center of the weighing surface (Figure 10-5). Zero should be checked before every session and when the scale is moved. The scales should be calibrated at least every few months using reference weights.

Length. Recumbent length is measured for children younger than 24 months or for children between 24 and 36 months of age who cannot stand unassisted (Moore and Roche, 1982). The measurement should be made on an examining table using a length measuring device with a headboard and a movable front board that are perpendicular to the table surface. Length is recorded as the distance between the headboard and frontboard when the infant has been positioned properly. Two people are required for measuring an infant's length (Figure 10-6). Length should be recorded to the nearest 0.1 cm (⅛ in).   *Text continued on p. 271.*

Table 10-6. Nutrition assessment and intervention guidelines for population groups in community nutrition

Nutritional Assessment Components	Method	Risks and Problems Indicated	Intervention Guidelines	Referral Sources
Infants and children				
Anthropometric Height for weight Height for age Weight for age Head circumference (to age 2 years) Skinfold thickness	Beam balance scale (nude or lightly dressed), measuring board and nonstretch tape; status using National Center for Health Statistics (NCHS) growth grids; skinfold calipers using standardized technique and validated predictive equation or nomogram	Undernutrition, malnutrition; stunting, failure to thrive (height for age <5th percentile); severe malnutrition (above plus head circumference <5th percentile or a significant drop in range on growth grid); overweight, obesity (weight for height >95th percentile), percent body fat >95th percentile	Refer and report cases of child abuse; refer children and families to food assistance programs; adjust dietary intake to increase weight gain, or stabilize intake until overweight is compensated by increases in height; adjust activity level	Private physicians; WIC Program; Children and Youth Program; Services for the Handicapped; Regional Center for High-Risk Newborns; Title XIX: Head Start; Child abuse and neglect centers; food stamps; Commodity Distribution Program
Biochemical Hemoglobin Hematocrit Serum cholesterol	Standard technique	Malnutrition, anemia, elevated serum cholesterol (≤ 150 mg/dl)	Improve dietary iron intake, supplement with iron, reduce cholesterol intake, apply additional serum cholesterol lowering methods as indicated	
Clinical Birth weight for gestational age	Beam balance scale, digital scale, reference standard	Intrauterine growth retardation, large for gestational age	Adjust feeding to meet nutritional needs based on gestational age and catch-up group potential; rule out hypoglycemia in small and large newborns	
Blood pressure	Monitor in children over 3 years of age	"Higher than normal" blood pressure	Weight management, reduction of dietary salt intake if excessive	
Dietary Dietary quantity and quality Feeding development	Interview or questionnaire on food groups, food recall, or record analysis	Malnutrition, underweight, overweight risk; abnormal development of feeding and motor skills	Adjust dietary intake to meet nutrient needs; progress toward normal feeding developmental milestones	
Adolescents				
Anthropometric Height Weight Skinfold thickness	Beam balance scales, nonstretch tape, calipers; NCHS growth grids for boys and girls 3 to 18 years of age; assess weight status using weight-for-height grid; assess percentage body fat using a reference standard; assess growth velocity using reference standard	Short stature, underweight, overweight	Adjust dietary intake and activity level	Prenatal care; WIC Program; Maternal and Infant Care Program; physical fitness program and recreational facilities
Biochemical Hemoglobin Hematocrit Serum cholesterol	Standard techniques	Malnutrition, anemia, elevated cholesterol	Adjust diet, iron supplementation as indicated	Physician, psychologist, or guidance center
Clinical Blood pressure Dental disease	Standard techniques	"Higher than normal" blood pressure, dental caries	Weight management, salt reduction, reduction in sticky sweets consumption	Drug treatment centers; Alcoholics Anonymous; Neighborhood health center
Dietary: dietary quality and quantity	3-day food record, diet history (computerized nutrient analysis)	Malnutrition	Adjust diet to meet requirements	Adolescent clinics; nontraditional alternative health centers

From Brown, J.E.: Clin. Nutr. **3**(3):105, 1984.

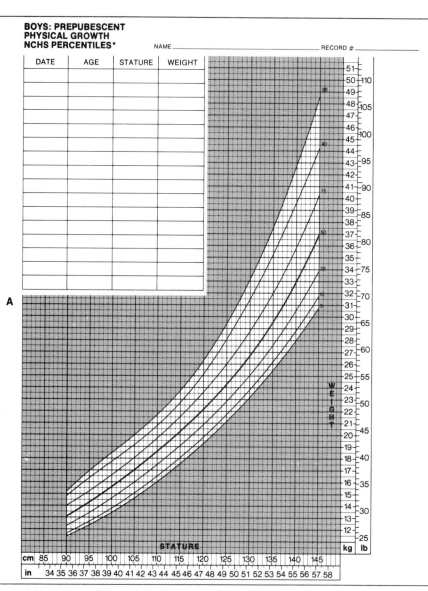

Figure 10-3. A, Physical growth NCHS percentiles in prepubescent boys. **B,** Physical growth NCHS percentiles in boys ages 2 to 18 years.
From Ross Laboratories, Inc., Columbus, Ohio.

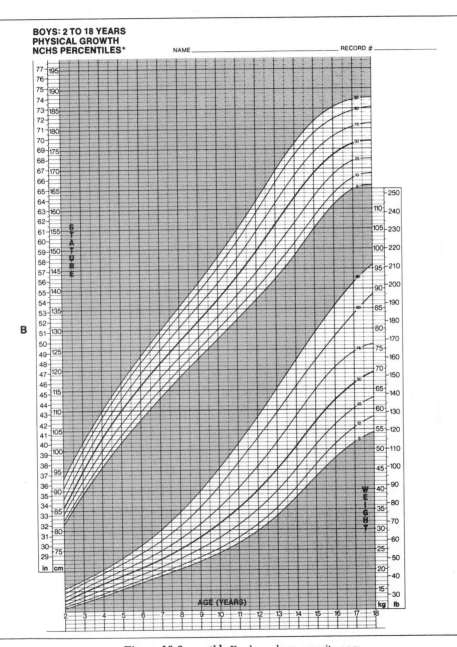

Figure 10-3, cont'd. For legend see opposite page.

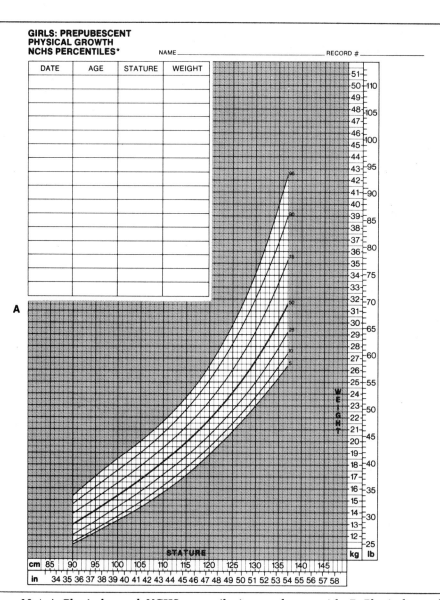

Figure 10-4. A, Physical growth NCHS percentiles in prepubescent girls. **B,** Physical growth NCHS percentiles in girls ages 2 to 18 years.

From Ross Laboratories, Inc., Columbus, Ohio.

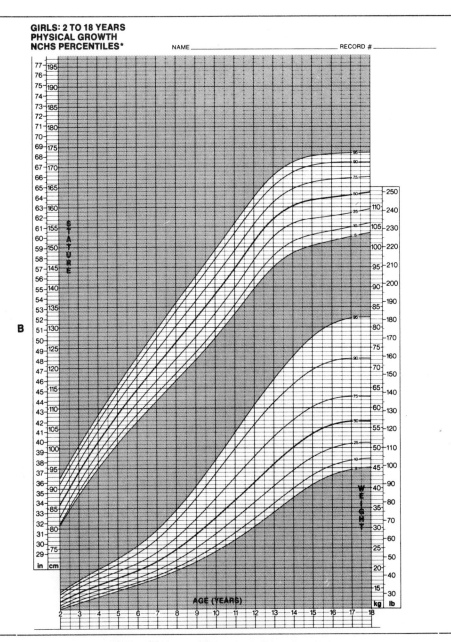

GIRLS: 2 TO 18 YEARS
PHYSICAL GROWTH
NCHS PERCENTILES*

NAME_____   RECORD #_____

Figure 10-4, cont'd. For legend see opposite page.

Table 10-7. NCHS percentiles for length, weight, and head circumference for age: boys, birth to 36 months

| Age (Months) | Percentile | | | | | | | Measurement |
	5th	10th	25th	50th	75th	90th	95th	
Birth	46.4	47.5	49.0	50.5	51.8	53.5	54.4	Length (cm)
	18¼	18¾	19¼	20	20½	21	21½	Length (in)
	2.54	2.78	3.00	3.27	3.64	3.82	4.15	Weight (kg)
	5½	6¼	6½	7¼	8	8½	9¼	Weight (lb)
	32.6	33.0	33.9	34.8	35.6	36.6	37.2	Head C (cm)
	12¾	13	13¼	13¾	14	14½	14¾	Head C (in)
1	50.4	51.3	53.0	54.6	56.2	57.7	58.6	Length (cm)
	19¾	20¼	20¾	21½	22¼	22¾	23	Length (in)
	3.16	3.43	3.82	4.29	4.75	5.14	5.38	Weight (kg)
	7	7½	8½	9½	10½	11¼	11¾	Weight (lb)
	34.9	35.4	36.2	37.2	38.1	39.0	39.6	Head C (cm)
	13¾	14	14¼	14¾	15	15¼	15½	Head C (in)
3	56.7	57.7	59.4	61.1	63.0	64.5	65.4	Length (cm)
	22¼	22¾	23½	24	24¾	25½	25¾	Length (in)
	4.43	4.78	5.32	5.98	6.56	7.14	7.37	Weight (kg)
	9¾	10½	11¾	13¼	14½	15¾	16¼	Weight (lb)
	38.4	38.9	39.7	40.6	41.7	42.5	43.1	Head C (cm)
	15	15¼	15¾	16	16½	16¾	17	Head C (in)
6	63.4	64.4	66.1	67.8	69.7	71.3	72.3	Length (cm)
	25	25¼	26	26¾	27½	28	28½	Length (in)
	6.20	6.61	7.20	7.85	8.49	9.10	9.46	Weight (kg)
	13¾	14½	15¾	17¼	18¾	20	20¾	Weight (lb)
	41.5	42.0	42.8	43.8	44.7	45.6	46.2	Head C (cm)
	16¼	16½	16¾	17¼	17½	18	18¼	Head C (in)
9	68.0	69.1	70.6	72.3	74.0	75.9	77.1	Length (cm)
	26¾	27¼	27¾	28½	29¼	30	30¼	Length (in)
	7.52	7.95	8.56	9.18	9.88	10.49	10.93	Weight (kg)
	16½	17½	18¾	20¼	21¾	23¼	24	Weight (lb)
	43.5	44.0	44.8	45.8	46.6	47.5	48.1	Head C (cm)
	17¼	17¼	17¾	18	18¼	18¾	19	Head C (in)

Table 10-7. NCHS percentiles for length, weight, and head circumference for age: boys, birth to 36 months—cont'd

Age (Months)	Percentile							Measurement
	5th	10th	25th	50th	75th	90th	95th	
12	71.7	72.8	74.3	76.1	77.7	79.8	81.2	**Length (cm)**
	28¼	28¾	29¼	30	30½	31½	32	Length (in)
	8.43	8.84	9.49	10.15	10.91	11.54	11.99	**Weight (kg)**
	18½	19½	21	22½	24	25½	26½	Weight (lb)
	44.8	45.3	46.1	47.0	47.9	48.8	49.3	**Head C (cm)**
	17¾	17¾	18¼	18½	18¾	19¼	19½	Head C (in)
18	77.5	78.7	80.5	82.4	84.3	86.6	88.1	**Length (cm)**
	30½	31	31¾	32½	33¼	34	34¾	Length (in)
	9.59	9.92	10.67	11.47	12.31	13.05	13.44	**Weight (kg)**
	21¼	21¾	23½	25¼	27¼	28¾	29½	Weight (lb)
	46.3	47.7	47.4	48.4	49.3	50.1	50.6	**Head C (cm)**
	18¼	18½	18¾	19	19½	19¾	20	Head C (in)
24	82.3	83.5	85.6	87.6	89.9	92.2	93.8	**Length (cm)**
	32½	32¾	33¾	34½	35½	36¼	37	Length (in)
	10.54	10.85	11.65	12.59	13.44	14.29	14.70	**Weight (kg)**
	23¼	24	25¾	27¾	29¾	31½	32½	Weight (lb)
	47.3	47.7	48.3	49.2	50.2	51.0	51.4	**Head C (cm)**
	18½	18¾	19	19¼	19¾	20	20¼	Head C (in)
30	87.0	88.2	90.1	92.3	94.6	97.0	98.7	**Length (cm)**
	34¼	34¾	35½	36¼	37¼	38¼	38¾	Length (in)
	11.44	11.80	12.63	13.67	14.51	15.47	15.97	**Weight)kg)**
	25¼	26	27¾	30¼	32	34	35¼	Weight (lb)
	48.0	48.4	49.1	49.9	51.0	51.7	52.2	**Head C (cm)**
	19	19	19¼	19¾	20	20¼	20½	Head C (in)
36	91.2	92.4	94.2	96.5	98.9	101.4	103.1	**Length (cm)**
	36	36½	37	38	39	40	40½	Length (in)
	12.26	12.69	13.58	14.69	15.59	16.66	17.28	**Weight (kg)**
	27	28	30	32½	34¼	36¾	38	Weight (lb)
	48.6	49.0	49.7	50.5	51.5	52.3	52.8	**Head C (cm)**
	19¼	19¼	19½	20	20¼	20½	20¾	Head C (in)

Table 10-8. NCHS percentiles for length, weight, and head circumference for age: girls, birth to 36 months

| Age (Months) | Percentile | | | | | | | Measurement |
	5th	10th	25th	50th	75th	90th	95th	
Birth	45.4	46.5	48.2	49.9	51.0	52.0	52.9	**Length** (cm)
	17¾	18¼	19	19¾	20	20½	20¾	Length (in)
	2.36	2.58	2.93	3.23	3.52	3.64	3.81	**Weight** (kg)
	5¼	5¾	6½	7	7¾	8	8½	Weight (lb)
	32.1	32.9	33.5	34.3	34.8	35.5	35.9	**Head C** (cm)
	12¾	13	13¼	13½	13¾	14	14¼	Head C (in)
1	49.2	50.2	51.9	53.5	54.9	56.1	56.9	**Length** (cm)
	19¼	19¾	20½	21	21½	22	22½	Length (in)
	2.97	3.22	3.59	3.98	4.36	4.65	4.92	**Weight** (kg)
	6½	7	8	8¾	9½	10¼	10¾	Weight (lb)
	34.2	34.8	35.6	36.4	37.1	37.8	38.3	**Head C** (cm)
	13½	13¾	14	14¼	14½	15	15	Head C (in)
3	55.4	56.2	57.8	59.5	61.2	62.7	63.4	**Length** (cm)
	21¾	22¼	22¾	23½	24	24¾	25	Length (in)
	4.18	4.47	4.88	5.40	5.90	6.39	6.74	**Weight** (kg)
	9¼	9¾	10¾	12	13	14	14¾	Weight (lb)
	37.3	37.8	38.7	39.5	40.4	41.2	41.7	**Head C** (cm)
	14¾	15	15¼	15½	16	16¼	16½	Head C (in)
6	61.8	62.6	64.2	65.9	67.8	69.4	70.2	**Length** (cm)
	24¼	24¾	25¼	26	26¾	27¼	27¾	Length (in)
	5.79	6.12	6.60	7.21	7.83	8.38	8.73	**Weight** (kg)
	12¾	13½	14½	16	17¼	18½	19¼	Weight (lb)
	40.3	40.9	41.6	42.4	43.3	44.1	44.6	**Head C** (cm)
	15¾	16	16½	16¾	17	17¼	17½	Head C (in)
9	66.1	67.0	68.7	70.4	72.4	74.0	75.0	**Length** (cm)
	26	26½	27	27¾	28½	29¼	29½	Length (in)
	7.00	7.34	7.89	8.56	9.24	9.83	10.17	**Weight** (kg)
	15½	16¼	17½	18¾	20¼	21¾	22½	Weight (lb)
	42.3	42.8	43.5	44.3	45.1	46.0	46.4	**Head C** (cm)
	16¾	16¾	17¼	17½	17¾	18	18¼	Head C (in)

Modified from National Center for Health Statistics, Health Resources Administration, U.S. Department of Health and Human Services, Hyattsville, Md., 1978, U.S. Government Printing Office. Reprinted with permission of Ross Laboratories, Columbus, OH 43216, from Pediatric Anthropometry, © 1982 Ross Laboratories.

Table 10-8. NCHS percentiles for length, weight, and head circumference for age: girls, birth to 36 months—cont'd

Age (Months)	5th	10th	25th	50th	75th	90th	95th	Measurement
12	69.8	70.8	72.4	74.3	76.3	78.0	79.1	**Length (cm)**
	27½	27¾	28½	29¼	30	30¾	31¼	Length (in)
	7.84	8.19	8.81	9.53	10.23	10.87	11.24	**Weight (kg)**
	17¼	18	19½	21	22½	24	24¾	Weight (lb)
	43.5	44.1	44.8	45.6	46.4	47.2	47.6	**Head C (cm)**
	17¼	17¼	17¾	18	18¼	18½	18¾	Head C (in)
18	76.0	77.2	78.8	80.9	83.0	85.0	86.1	**Length (cm)**
	30	30½	31	31¾	32¾	33½	34	Length (in)
	8.92	9.30	10.04	10.82	11.55	12.30	12.76	**Weight (kg)**
	19¾	20½	22¼	23¾	25½	27	28¼	Weight (lb)
	45.0	45.6	46.3	47.1	47.9	48.6	49.1	**Head C (cm)**
	17¾	18	18¼	18½	18¾	19¼	19¼	Head C (in)
24	81.3	82.5	84.2	86.5	88.7	90.8	92.0	**Length (cm)**
	32	32½	33¼	34	35	35¾	36¼	Length (in)
	9.87	10.26	11.10	11.90	12.74	13.57	14.08	**Weight (kg)**
	21¾	22½	24½	26¼	28	30	31	Weight (lb)
	46.1	46.5	47.3	48.1	48.8	49.6	50.1	**Head C (cm)**
	18¼	18¼	18½	19	19¼	19½	19¾	Head C (in)
30	86.0	87.0	88.9	91.3	93.7	95.6	96.9	**Length (cm)**
	33¾	34¼	35	36	37	37¾	38¼	Length (in)
	10.78	11.21	12.11	12.93	13.93	14.81	15.35	**Weight (kg)**
	23¾	24¾	26¾	28½	30¾	32¾	33¾	Weight (lb)
	47.0	47.3	48.0	48.8	49.4	50.3	50.8	**Head C (cm)**
	18½	18½	19	19¼	19½	19¾	20	Head C (in)
36	90.0	91.0	93.1	95.6	98.1	100.0	101.5	**Length (cm)**
	35½	35¾	36¾	37¾	38½	39¼	40	Length (in)
	11.60	12.07	12.99	13.93	15.03	15.97	16.54	**Weight (kg)**
	25½	26½	28¾	30¾	33¼	35¼	36½	Weight (lb)
	47.6	47.9	48.5	49.3	50.0	50.8	51.4	**Head C (cm)**
	18¾	18¾	19	19½	19¾	20	20¼	Head C (in)

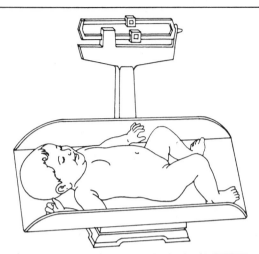

Figure 10-5. Weighing an infant.
Redrawn with permission of Ross Laboratories, Columbus, OH 43216, from Pediatric Anthropometry, © 1982 Ross Laboratories.

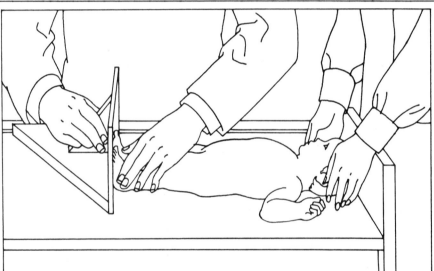

Figure 10-6. Measuring the length of an infant.
Redrawn from U.S. Department of Health and Human Services: A guide to pediatric weighing and measuring, Atlanta, 1977, CDC.

Head circumference. An insertion tape provides adequate positioning and fixation of the tape around the head. Springy hair should be compressed. A hair layer 0.6 cm (¼-in) thick around one half of the head will theoretically increase head circumference by almost 2.5 cm (1 in). Increments in head circumference at various age levels are shown in Tables 10-7 and 10-8.

Skinfold thickness. Skinfold thickness has been proposed as a useful index of relative fatness of the body, since subcutaneous adipose tissue is a major component of body fat (Owen, 1982). The thickness of the skin and subcutaneous fat can be measured with calipers. In 1968 the Committee on Nutrition, American Academy of Pediatrics, suggested that before techniques of measuring skinfold thickness were promulgated as a practical clinical tool for assessing relative fatness of individual children, basic reference data should be collected (Committee on Nutrition, 1968). Between 1963 and 1974, the NCHS pooled skinfold thickness measurements and upper arm girth of about 20,000 children ages 1 to 17 years in the United States and developed smoothed percentiles to serve as reference data. The smoothed percentiles are shown in Table 10-9.

In a report of a small conference convened to discuss the data pooled by the NCHS, it was emphasized that the percentiles described the skinfold thicknesses of American children and adolescents and should not be considered "norms" or "standards" (Owen, 1982). The NCHS skinfold thickness percentiles (Figures 10-7 and 10-8) are based on data from National Health Examination Surveys (NHES) Cycles II and III and NHANES I (Johnson et al., 1981). It is considered inappropriate to conclude that a skinfold thickness above or below some arbitrary percentile is unacceptable because available information is inadequate to define risks of relative fatness. Finally, it was suggested that skinfold thickness should probably not be used as a routine screening measurement in well child care. However, it is operationally reasonable to limit measurements of skinfolds during infancy and childhood to individuals whose weight for stature is greater than the 90th percentile or less than the 10th percentile. Skinfold measurements are useful in the follow-up and monitoring of individual children who are identified as having a potential or real problem of obesity (Owen, 1982).

METHODS OF MEASURING TRICEPS SKINFOLD THICKNESS. Triceps skinfold thickness is a measurement of a double layer of skin and subcutaneous fat on the back of the upper arm. It is a convenient-to-measure, useful index of body fat. Measurement of triceps skinfold thickness requires a flexible, nonstretchable tape measure and a skinfold caliper. A Lange, Harpenden, or Holtain caliper or a reliable plastic caliper (Adipometer, Ross Laboratories, Inc.) is suitable.

Triceps skinfold thickness is measured on the back of the left arm and midway between the shoulder and elbow. This measurement may be difficult to obtain in infants, and much patience is required. The infant should be held in a semiupright position on the lap of the mother or an attendant. The infant's right side should be adjacent to the mother's body, with the infant's head erect. The infant's left hand should be gently restrained, with the elbow flexed 90 degrees and the forearm pressed gently against the infant's abdomen. The tape should be used to locate the midpoint between the left shoulder and elbow placement of the caliper jaws.

At a level about 1 cm above the midpoint, a vertical fold of skin and subcutaneous tissue is grasped between the thumb and index finger. The long axis of the skinfold should be parallel to the long axis of the arm. The skinfold should be pulled gently away from the underlying muscle and held while the jaws of the caliper are placed over it at the previously marked midpoint. Variability of repeated triceps skinfold measurements will be large if they are made at different sites (e.g., above, below, to the right of, or to the left of the marked point). To avoid reading error caused by parallax, the person making the measurement should look down on the caliper, which is held horizontal.

Table 10-9. Increments in skinfold thickness in various age intervals

Age Interval (Months)	Percentiles	S.D.	Triceps (mm) Boys	Triceps (mm) Girls	Subscapular (mm) Boys	Subscapular (mm) Girls
1-3		− 2	− 0.6	− 0.9	− 1.8	− 1.4
	10		0.7	0.1	− 0.5	− 0.7
	25		1.5	1.4	0.2	0.5
	50		2.5	2.5	1.4	1.6
	75		3.6	3.4	2.2	2.6
	90		4.7	4.4	3.1	3.4
		+ 2	5.8	5.9	4.6	4.6
3-6		− 2	− 1.5	− 1.7	− 3.3	− 2.3
	10		− 0.1	− 0.1	− 1.5	− 1.2
	25		0.8	0.7	− 0.7	− 0.6
	50		1.8	2.1	0.2	0.2
	75		2.8	3.3	1.2	1.1
	90		3.6	4.4	2.3	2.0
		+ 2	5.3	5.9	3.9	2.9
6-9		− 2	− 3.0	− 3.5	− 2.9	− 3.3
	10		− 1.7	− 2.2	− 1.5	− 2.0
	25		− 0.7	− 1.1	− 0.8	− 1.1
	50		0.2	− 0.2	0.0	− 0.2
	75		1.4	0.8	0.8	0.5
	90		2.6	1.6	1.9	1.2
		+ 2	3.8	3.3	3.1	2.7
9-12		− 2	− 3.7	− 3.6	− 3.2	− 2.5
	10		− 2.4	− 2.4	− 1.4	− 1.6
	25		− 1.5	− 1.4	− 0.6	− 1.0
	50		0.0	− 0.2	0.0	− 0.3
	75		1.2	1.0	0.7	0.4
	90		2.4	2.1	1.8	1.1
		+ 2	3.5	3.2	3.2	1.9
12-18		− 2	− 3.2	− 3.0	− 3.3	− 3.1
	10		− 2.0	− 2.2	− 2.1	− 2.1
	25		− 1.0	− 0.9	− 1.0	− 1.3
	50		− 0.1	0.2	− 0.4	− 0.6
	75		1.4	1.3	0.4	0.2
	90		2.3	2.1	1.3	1.5
		+ 2	3.6	3.4	2.7	2.1
18-24		− 2	− 3.4	− 3.0	− 3.2	− 2.7
	10		− 2.0	− 2.0	− 1.7	− 1.6
	25		− 1.3	− 0.8	− 1.2	− 1.1
	50		0.0	0.1	− 0.5	− 0.6
	75		1.2	1.2	0.2	0.2
	90		2.4	2.5	0.9	0.9
		+ 2	3.4	3.4	2.4	1.7
24-36		− 2	− 3.5	− 4.2	− 2.9	− 3.5
	10		− 2.3	− 2.7	− 1.9	− 1.8
	25		− 1.2	− 1.2	− 1.2	− 0.9
	50		− 0.2	0.3	− 0.6	− 0.4
	75		1.2	1.3	0.0	0.3
	90		2.3	2.3	0.4	1.2
		+ 2	3.3	4.2	1.5	3.3

Data of Karlberg et al., 1968; from·Fomon, S.J.: Infant nutrition, ed. 2, Philadelphia, 1974, W.B. Saunders Co.

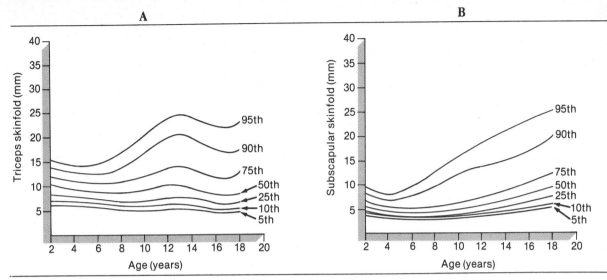

Figure 10-7. A, Triceps skinfold by age percentiles (NCHS) for boys 2 to 18 years. **B,** Subscapular skinfold by age percentiles (NCHS) for boys 2 to 18 years.
Redrawn from Owen, G.M.: Am J. Clin. Nutr. 35:629, 1982, © Am. J. Clin. Nutr., American Society for Clinical Nutrition.

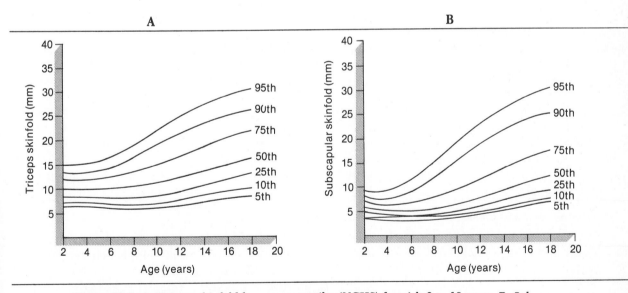

Figure 10-8. A, Triceps skinfold by age percentiles (NCHS) for girls 2 to 18 years. **B,** Subscapular skinfold by age percentiles (NCHS) for girls 2 to 18 years.
Redrawn from Owen, G.M.: Am. J. Clin. Nutr. **35:**629, 1982, © Am. J. Clin. Nutr., American Society for Clinical Nutrition.

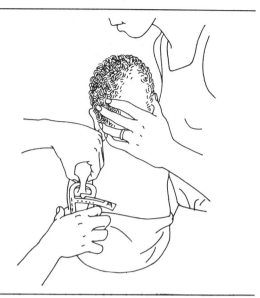

Figure 10-9. Measuring triceps skinfold thickness with an Adipometer.
Redrawn with permission of Ross Laboratories, Columbus, OH 43216, from Pediatric Anthropometry, © 1982 Ross Laboratories.

When an Adipometer skinfold caliper is used, force should be exerted with the thumb and index finger until the lines on the caliper are aligned (Figure 10-9). After 2 to 3 seconds, the measurement should be read and recorded to the nearest millimeter (mm). The caliper may take longer to stabilize on edematous tissue. Other skinfold calipers, such as Lange, Harpenden, and Holtain, require pressure to open the jaws before applying them to the skinfold.

Biochemical Assessment

Laboratory indicators of current dietary intake and of the nutritional status of young children are presented in Table 10-10.

Dietary Assessment

The box on p. 276 provides a questionnaire on infants up to 1 year of age that is designed to identify infants who may be at nutritional risk because of unusual eating habits. The questions are designed to select from among a large group of infants those few (perhaps 5% or 10%) receiving a diet most likely to be deficient or excessive in one or more nutrients and who are in need of further dietary evaluation and counseling. The dietitian/nutritionist will review all completed questionnaires and decide which children are likely to profit from an interview with the community dietitian/nutritionist. It is important to note that the questions are not meant to determine the child's recent intake of calories, protein, iron, or specific vitamins.

Clinical Assessment

The physical examination may reveal signs of a host of other diseases that merit diagnosis and treatment. Table 8-5 indicates the physical signs indicative of suggested malnutrition.

Nutrition Intervention and Counseling
Guidelines for Feeding the Normal Infant

Based on current knowledge there is an optimum feeding schedule to match the special nutritional needs and unique physiological characteristics of the infant during the first year of life. The concensus of current research from most sources covered previously in the chapter indicates the need for providing guidelines regarding feeding practices.

The first 6 months. Human milk should be used as the sole source of food for the first 6 months. The breast-fed infant should receive the following supplements:

Iron (7 mg daily from ferrous sulfate or other preparations of high bioavailability)
Vitamin D (400 IU daily)
Fluoride (0.25 mg daily)

Infants fed commercially prepared iron-fortified formula do not require supplements except fluoride (depending on fluoride content in local drinking water). Infants receiving evaporated milk formulas should receive supplements of vitamin C (20 mg) and iron (7 mg) daily.

Solid foods should not be introduced before 5 to 6 months of age.

Table 10-10. Laboratory indicators of current dietary intake and of nutritional status of the young child

Dietary Component	Current Intake	Nutritional Status	Comments
Protein	Serum or urine urea nitrogen	Serum albumin	Urea nitrogen in serum or urine correlates reasonably well with current net intake of protein if renal function is normal. Creatinine values in serum <6 mg/dl or in urine <8 mg/gm suggest low recent intake of protein. Serum albumin is a rather insensitive and nonspecific indicator of protein status, but values <3.2 gm/dl suggest a poor protein nutritional status.
Iron	Transferrin saturation	Hemoglobin, hematocrit, cell indices	Levels of transferrin saturation (iron/total iron-building capacity × 100) <16% suggest iron deficiency even when the concentration of hemoglobin is <10.5 gm/dl. Hemoglobin concentration >10.5 gm/dl (hematocrit 32%) is suggested as lower limit of normal for 6-year-old child. A mean corpuscular hemoglobin concentration (MCHC) <30 gm/dl of packed erythrocytes suggests iron deficiency.
Vitamin A	Serum carotene	Serum vitamin A	Approximately one half of total vitamin A intake from foods is supplied by fruits, vegetables, and cereal grains in the form of carotene. A level of serum carotene <40 µg/dl suggests low net intake of carotene. A level of serum vitamin A <20 µg/dl suggests low stores in vitamin A or may indicate failure of transport of retinol out of liver into blood.
Ascorbic acid	Serum ascorbate or whole blood ascorbate	Leukocyte ascorbate	At usual levels of intake of ascorbic acid from foods there is good correlation between intake and serum ascorbate; levels in serum <0.3 mg/dl suggest that recent intake has been low. Whole blood ascorbate levels <0.3 mg/dl indicate low intake and reduction in body pool of ascorbic acid. Leukocyte ascorbic acid levels <20 mg/100 gm suggest poor nutritional status.
Riboflavin	Urinary riboflavin	Erythrocyte glutathione reductase	There is a reasonably good correlation between intake and urinary excretion of riboflavin. Excretion of <250 µg/gm creatinine suggests low recent intake of riboflavin. Glutathione reductase-FAD (flavin-adenine dinucleotide) effect expressed as a ratio >1.2 suggests poor nutritional status.
Thiamin	Urinary thiamin	Erythrocyte transketolase	Excretion of <125 µg/gm creatinine suggests low intake of thiamin. Transketolase-TPP (thiamin pyrophosphate) effect expressed as a ratio >15 suggests poor nutritional status.
Folacin	Serum folacin	Erythrocyte folacin, formiminoglutamic acid (FIGLU)	Level of serum folacin <6 µg/dl suggests low intake. Levels of erythrocyte folacin <20 µg/dl or increased excretion of FIGLU in urine following a histidine load suggests poor nutritional status.
Iodine	Urinary iodine	Protein-bound iodine (PBI)	Urinary excretion of <50 µg/gm creatinine suggests low recent intake of iodine. PBI <3 µg/dl suggests poor nutritional status.

From Owen, G.M., and Lippman, G.: Nutritional status of infants and young children: U.S.A., Pediatr. Clin. North Am. 24:211, 1977.

QUESTIONNAIRE 1: INFANTS (FROM BIRTH TO AGE 1 YEAR)

	Yes	No
Is the baby breastfed?	☐	☐
If yes, does he also receive milk or formula?		
If yes, what kind? _____		
Does the baby receive formula?	☐	☐

If yes, Ready-to-feed ☐
     Concentrated liquid ☐
     Other ☐
   How is formula prepared (especially dilution)?

_____

_____

	Yes	No
Is the formula iron-fortified?	☐	☐
Does the baby drink milk?	☐	☐

If yes, Whole milk ☐
     2% milk ☐
     Skim milk ☐
     Other ☐
Specify _____

_____

How many times does he eat each day, including milk or formula? _____

	Yes	No
Does the baby usually take a bottle to bed?	☐	☐

If yes, what is usually in the bottle? _____

If the baby drinks milk or formula, what is the usual amount in a day?
   Less than 16 oz ☐
   16 to 32 oz ☐
   More than 32 oz ☐

Please indicate which, if any, of these foods the baby eats and how often.

	Never or hardly ever (less than once a week)	Sometimes (not daily but at least once a week)	Every day or nearly every day
Eggs	☐	☐	☐
Dried beans or peas	☐	☐	☐
Meat, fish, poultry	☐	☐	☐
Bread, rice, pasta, grits, cereal, tortillas, potatoes	☐	☐	☐
Fruits or fruit juices	☐	☐	☐
Vegetables	☐	☐	☐

From Fomon, S.J.: Nutritional disorders of children: prevention, screening, and follow-up. DHHS Pub. no. (HSA) 77-5104, Bureau of Community Health Services, Washington, D.C., 1977, U.S. Government Printing Office.

Table 10-11. Federally sponsored food assistance programs for infants, children, and adolescents

Program Offered	Purpose of Program	Administering Agencies
Special Supplemental Food Program for Women, Infants and Children (WIC)	Assist pregnant women, lactating mothers, and children aged 1 to 5 years in obtaining specified nutritious foods	Food and Nutrition Services (FNS) and state health agencies
School Lunch Program	Provide lunch free or at reduced prices to children attending participating schools; safeguard the health and well-being of the nation's children and educate children about nutritious food habits	FNS and state educational agencies
School Breakfast Program	Provide a nutritious breakfast free or at reduced prices to needy children attending participating schools	FNS and state educational agencies
Child Care Food Program	Initiate, maintain, or expand the provision of free meals and snacks to children in participating child care centers	FNS and state educational agencies and public or private not-for-profit day-care centers
Food Stamp Program	Assist families in providing nutritious meals	Administered by U.S. Department of Agriculture, FNS, and state welfare agency

Modified from Owen, A.L., Owen, G.M., and Lanna, G.: Health and nutritional benefits of federal food assessment program. In Costs and Benefits of Nutritional Care Phase 1. Chicago: The American Dietetic Association, 1979. Copyright The American Dietetic Association. Reprinted by permission; and Budget of the U.S. Government, 1984 (appendix), Executive Office of the President.

After 6 months. Human milk should be used up to 1 year. If breast-feeding is not possible, an iron-fortified commercial formula should be used throughout the first year.

Between 5 and 6 months of age, the introduction of solids should begin. Iron-fortified dry cereal commercially prepared for infants should be introduced first and fed daily until 18 months of age to assure adequate iron intake. Other foods such as fruit and vegetables commercially prepared or home prepared should then be introduced, but no more than one or two new foods in the same week.

If breast-feeding is continued beyond age 5 to 6 months, some foods that are relatively rich in protein should be included. Milks of reduced fat content are not recommended.

Supplements

IRON. Full-term infants born to well-nourished mothers have a 4- to 6-month iron store in the liver. The American Academy of Pediatrics states that, in the normal infant, the addition of iron-fortified cereal at 6 months of age will supply adequate amounts of iron to prevent iron deficiency anemia. Three tablespoons of iron-fortified infant cereal mixed with formula, breast milk, or water provides 7 mg of iron, the suggested level of supplementation per day. This iron supplement also can be in the form of iron drops prescribed by a physician. Foods can contribute the additional nutrients needed by the infant.

FLUORIDE. The usual source of fluoride is the water supply. Because breast milk contains very small amounts of fluoride and breast-fed infants consume little fluoridated water, there is a need for adding fluoride to the diets of these infants. Breast-fed infants should be referred to the pediatrition for a prescription.

Referral

The food assistance program available to infants includes the Special Supplemental Food Program for Women, Infants and Children (WIC). The WIC program is described in detail in Chapter 9. Table 10-11 describes the food programs available to infants and children (see also pp.

Table 10-12. Model criteria for quality assurance in ambulatory care of normal infant*

Criteria			
Identify Outcome (O) and Process (P)	Critical Time	Exceptions†	References
1. Infant maintains acceptable weight for length between the 5th and 95th percentile on NCHS growth chart (O)	Birth to 12 mo		NCHS growth charts, 1976, Monthly Vital Statistics Rep., vol. 25, no. 3, 1976.
2. Infant does not deviate more than 25 percentile points from his or her established pattern of growth (weight for height) on NCHS growth chart (O)	Birth to 12 mo		Fomon, S.J.: Nutritional disorders of children, DHEW Pub. no. HSA-77-5104, Rockville, Md., 1977, U.S. Government Printing Office.
3. Infant's hemoglobin is equal to or greater than: Hemoglobin / Hematocrit 10 gm / 31% or 11 gm / 34%	4 to 12 mo	Higher altitudes	Centers for Disease Control: Ten-State nutrition survey, 1968-1970, IV. Biochemical, DHEW Pub. no. HSM-72-8132, Atlanta, 1980, CDC. Centers for Disease Control: Nutrition surveillance, annual summary, 1978. Atlanta, 1980, CDC. Fomon, S.J.: Nutritional disorders of children, DHEW Pub. no. HSA-77-5104, Rockville, Md., 1977, U.S. Government Printing Office.

Reprinted from Kaufman, M., editor: Guide to quality assurance in ambulatory nutrition care, Chicago, 1983, The American Dietetic Association.
*Birth to age 12 months; weight/length from 5th up to and including the 95th percentile; no medical complications (physical handicaps, mental retardation, or other syndromes).
†Lost to follow-up applies to all criteria.

210-214). Other areas for referral include the private physician, Early and Periodic Screening, Diagnosis, and Treatment (EPSDT) programs, Head Start, and child abuse and neglect centers.

Assuring Quality of Health and Nutrition Care for Infants

Quality assurance standards have been developed for the normal infant (Table 10-12). These standards provide a basis for evaluating the quality of care.

CHILDREN

A young child's growth rate slows considerably from the first year of age. Toddlers (1 and 2 years old) gain only from 2 to 4 kg (5 to 10 lb) each year. Preschoolers (3 through 4 years old) have even a slower rate of growth, averaging from 1 to 2 kg (3 to 5 lb) each year. As a result of this significant slowing down in growth, the toddler and the preschooler require less food and their appetites decrease. This often is mistaken as poor appetite.

Between ages 1 and 2, children learn to feed themselves independently. They progress from eating with their hands to using utensils. Messiness and spilling are the rule during the first half of the second year, but by age 2, hand-to-mouth coordination has noticeably improved. Children should be allowed to try new skills over and over again.

Hallmark characteristics of a toddler are curiosity and independence. Explanation of the environment is enabled by the child's increasing mobility, manipulation, and trying out of various skills.

During the preschool years (ages 3 to 5) there is a greater increase in height relative to weight; the chubby toddler becomes a leaner preschooler. Each child will grow at his or her own rate as determined by heredity, state of health, and nutritional adequacy of the diet (Endres and Rockwell, 1985).

The mid-childhood years (from age 6 to the onset of puberty) are relatively stable, compared to the preschool and adolescent periods, with regard to growth rate and behavior. Height and weight vary greatly among children because of genetic and environmental influences, but for an individual child, growth is usually slow and steady. In spite of a relatively slow growth rate, nutrition still plays an important role by (1) furnishing the energy needed for the vigorous activities of this age-group, (2) helping to maintain resistance to infection, (3) providing building materials for growth, and (4) providing adequate nutrient stores to assist in adolescent growth.

Nutritional Requirements

Energy. Energy requirements in a child must allow for (1) basal metabolism, (2) specific dynamic action of food, (3) losses in excreta, (4) muscular activity, and (5) growth (Paige and Owen, 1983). The average energy requirement for basal metabolism during the first 12 to 18 months of life is 55 kcal/kg body weight. Thereafter the requirement on a weight-specific basis declines to an adult level of 25 to 30 kcal/kg. Energy allocated to activity on a weight-specific basis rises initially with age, from an average of 20 kcal/kg to 28 kcal/kg, between the first and fourth years. By 9 to 10 years of age, the allocation for activity has dropped back to 20 kcal/kg. The energy requirements for growth decline with increasing age. At age 3 months, the infant requires 28 kcal/kg; at 9 to 12 months, 6 kcal/kg; from 2 to 5 years, 2 kcal/kg; and from 9 to 17 years, 1 kcal/kg.

Protein. On a weight-specific basis, protein requirements decrease from the first month of life through childhood and adolescence. The decrease is most precipitous during the first 6 months of life. Safe levels of protein intake approximate 2.2 gm/kg/day below age 6 months; 2.0 gm/kg/day at 6 to 11 months; and 1.76 gm, 1.50 gm, 1.20 gm/kg/day at ages 1-3-4-6-7-10 years, respectively (Food and Nutrition Board, 1980).

Lipids. During the early months of life, fat provides nearly one half of the calories in the infant diet. This is especially true during the period of exclusive breast-feeding. Generally after the nursing period about one third of calories should be from fat. It is not clear whether in children without a family history of hyperlipidemia, diets low in saturated fats reduce the likelihood of adult atherosclerosis. Despite the absence of direct evidence, it seems prudent to recommend limiting the ingestion of saturated fats.

Minerals. The three major groups of minerals include (1) sodium, potassium, calcium, and magnesium; (2) chlorine, phosphorus, and sulfur, and (3) iron, iodine, and trace elements. Sodium and potassium requirements for growing children are met easily, since most foods contain an abundant supply. Calcium required during growth is estimated to be 50 mg to 70 mg/kg/day. A calcium intake of 1 gm/day provides an ample margin of safety. Exact magnesium requirements are not known. Almost 16% of ingested magnesium is retained. The usual diet is assumed to contain an adequate amount of magnesium.

Iron. The importance of this mineral in the diets of infants and children has long been recognized. Up to 6 months of age, the full-term infant's iron stores, which were deposited in fetal life, are generally adequate for body needs (e.g., the production of hemoglobin). After that age, body stores must be resupplied by the diet to ensure prompt blood formation. The usual hemoglobin level at birth is high, 16 to 18 gm/dl of blood, and falls normally to a level of 10 to 11 gm at 3 to 4 months of age. The hemoglobin level should be 11 gm or more thereafter.

The daily requirement for iron in infancy is at least 6 mg/day beginning at birth, or 8 mg/day if supplements are begun at 3 months of age (Fomon, 1974).

Table 10-13. Characterization of anemia with or without iron deficiency

	Hemoglobin (gm/dl)	Mean Corpuscular Volume (iron)	Percent Saturation Transferrin (iron/TIBC × 100)	Ferritin (ng/ml)
Iron deficiency anemia	<11	<72	<15	< 7
Borderline iron deficiency anemia	<11	±72	<20	<12
Iron deficiency without anemia	>11	<72	<15	< 7
Anemia without iron deficiency	<11	>72	≥20	≥12
NORMAL	>11	>72	≥20	≥12

Nutrition-Related Problems

Of all the manifestations of nutrition problems in this age-group, anemia and obesity are the most common.

Anemia. Primarily the lack of dietary iron is seen most often among children in lower socioeconomic groupings. The lack of dietary iron may be the result of parental ignorance of the importance and sources of iron, poverty that restricts the amount and variety of foods available, or the difficulty of providing recommended levels of iron in the diet under the best of circumstances. A few instances are recorded of anemia resulting from the exclusive use of a milk diet, which is low in iron, after the first 6 months of life.

Characterization of anemia with or without iron deficiency is shown in Table 10-13. Treatment of anemia of childhood usually involves the therapeutic use of iron salts at levels providing from 30 to 100 mg of iron a day, often in conjunction with ascorbic acid, until hemoglobin levels have been restored to normal levels. This regimen is followed by the use of a diet high in iron-rich foods such as meat, green leafy vegetables, and enriched cereals. The child who suffers from anemia is usually lethargic, tires easily, and is highly susceptible to infection.

Obesity. Overnutrition represents the other end of the spectrum. Childhood or juvenile onset obesity is a particular problem because it is extremely difficult to treat and tends to persist into adulthood. The combination of parents, who may unwittingly establish a pattern of overfeeding, and inactivity attributes to the problem of obesity. Working with children on appropriate food habits and exercise is essential. Encouraging a child to adopt a pattern of eating that allows him to grow into his or her weight has met with more success than attempting to bring about an actual weight loss.

Feeding Patterns

In reviewing the food habits of any child, it is important to keep in mind nutritional requirements, culture, socioeconomic status, and family dynamics as they influence the individual. By age 18 months to 2 years, many toddlers are quite adept at feeding themselves. Individual dietary preferences appear, and the child should be allowed to choose food he or she likes. Toddlers often prefer small, frequent feedings of finger foods and often reject or simply pick at a prepared meal. This behavior should not alarm the parent, nor should it be perceived as a challenge to parental authority.

Parents who are distraught over eating patterns of 2- and 3-year-old children often can be reassured that psychogenic anorexia and atypical (by adult standards) eating behavior are normal during this period of experimentation.

Parents should be made aware that the period of maximum growth has been completed by the end of the first year; between ages 1 and 5 years growth slows and is reflected by a proportional decline in nutrient intake on a weight-adjusted basis.

By age 5 years, children can effectively use a knife and fork. There are increased opportunities for socializing through school experiences with exposure to new foods and new practices. Asking children to assist in preparing or serving a new food often will permit them to overcome reluctance to experiment with new foods. Table 10-14 describes food intake according to food groupings and the average size of servings at different age levels.

Guidelines for Patient Management

The expected health outcomes for a normal child include the following (Kaufman, 1983):

1. Child maintains weight for height between 5th and 95th percentile on NCHS growth chart.
2. Child maintains height for age between 5th and 95th percentile on NCHS growth chart.
3. Child does not deviate more than 25 percentile points from his or her established growth pattern (height or weight) on NCHS growth chart.
4. Child's hemoglobin and/or hematocrit determinations are within acceptable levels (p. 260).
5. Child consumes types and amounts of food in frequencies appropriate for age and weight for height.

Nutrition Assessment and Screening
Anthropometric Assessment

The following anthropometric measurements should be completed for a preschool child:

Weight
Stature (standing height)
Head circumference
Chest circumference
Triceps skinfold

For a school-age child through adolescence the following measurements should be taken:

Delete head and chest circumference
Stature (standing height)
Triceps skinfold

Weight. Children who can stand without assistance are weighed standing on the scale and wearing only light-weight undergarments (Figure 10-10). The scale should be in an area that ensures privacy. The child stands over the center of the platform of the scale with heels together.

The reading is made when the child is standing still. Weight of a child should be recorded to the nearest 100 gm (0.1 kg or ¼ lb). Consistency of techniques and choices of weight units are important to avoid unnecessary sources of errors.

Stature. Children between 2 and 3 years of age can be measured in the recumbent or standing position, depending on their ability to cooperate during the procedure. It is essential to note whether length or stature (standing height) was measured because length is greater than stature by up to 2 cm (nearly 1 in). Thus integration of measurements will be difficult if it is not known whether length or stature was measured or, if length was measured on one occasion and stature on another.

Children over 3 years of age should be measured standing (Figure 10-11). Measurements of stature require a measuring stick or a nonstretchable tape attached to a vertical, flat surface, such as a wall. A guide for a right-angle headboard also is needed. Movable measuring rods attached to platform scales are too unsteady to ensure accurate measurement (Moore and Roche, 1982). The child should wear only underclothes, so that the stance can be seen clearly, and stand with bare heels close together, legs straight, arms at the sides, and shoulders relaxed. Two people may be needed to measure the stature of an uncooperative child, but usually only one is required. The child's knees should be straight with heels on the floor and with head, shoulder blades, buttocks, and heels touching the wall.

The child should be asked to stand tall, take a deep breath, and look straight ahead "so the line of vision is perpendicular to the body." Then the headboard is lowered against the guide onto the crown of the head. The measurer's eyes should be level with the headboard to avoid errors. With the headboard in place, the measurement is read and recorded to the nearest 0.1 cm (⅛ in). NCHS growth charts should be used to monitor the child's growth (Figures 10-3 and 10-4).

Head circumference. Head circumference should be measured routinely in infants and children until they are 36 months of age (Figure 10-12).

Table 10-14. Food intake for good nutrition according to food groups and the average size of servings at different age levels

Food Group	Servings per Day	Average Size of Servings at Each Age Level					
		1 Year	2-3 Years	4-5 Years	6-9 Years	10-12 Years	13-15 Years
Milk and cheese (1.5 oz cheese = 1 cup milk)	4	½ cup	½-¾ cup	¾ cup	¾-1 cup	1 cup	1 cup
Meat group (protein foods)	At least 3						
Egg		1 egg	1 egg	1 egg	1 egg	1 egg	1 or more
Lean meat, fish, poultry (liver once a week)		2 tbsp	2 tbsp	4 tbsp	2-3 oz (4-6 tbsp)	3-4 oz	4 oz or more
Peanut butter			1 tbsp	2 tbsp	2-3 tbsp	3 tbsp	3 tbsp
Fruits and vegetables	At least 4, including:						
Vitamin C source (citrus fruit, berries, tomato, cabbage, cantaloupe)	1 or more (twice as much tomato as citrus)	⅓ cup citrus	½ cup	½ cup	1 med. orange	1 med. orange	1 med. orange
Vitamin A source (green or yellow fruits and vegetables)	1 or more	2 tbsp	3 tbsp	4 tbsp (¼ cup)	¼ cup	⅓ cup	¾ cup
Other vegetables (potato, legumes)	2 or more	2 tbsp	3 tbsp	4 tbsp	⅓ cup	½ cup	¾ cup
or							
Other fruits (apple, banana)		¼ cup	⅓ cup	½ cup	1 medium	1 medium	1 medium
Cereals (whole grain or enriched)	At least 4						
Bread		½ slice	1 slice	1½ slices	1-2 slices	2 slices	2 slices
Ready-to-eat cereals		½ oz	¾ oz	1 oz	1 oz	1 oz	1 oz
Cooked cereal (including pastas, rice, etc.)		¼ cup	⅓ cup	½ cup	½ cup	¾ cup	1 cup or more
Fats and carbohydrates	To meet caloric needs						
Butter, margarine, mayonnaise, oils (1 tbsp = 100 calories)		1 tbsp	1 tbsp	1 tbsp	2 tbsp	2 tbsp	2-4 tbsp
Desserts and sweets (100-calorie portions): ⅓ cup pudding or ice cream, two 3-inch cookies, 1 oz cake, 1⅓ oz pie, 2 tbsp jelly, jam, honey, sugar		1 portion	1½ portions	1½ portions	3 portions	3 portions	3-6 portions

From Bennett, M., and Hansen, A.: Nutritional requirements. In Nelson, W., editor: Textbook of pediatrics, Philadelphia, 1969, W. B. Saunders Co.

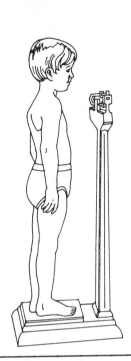

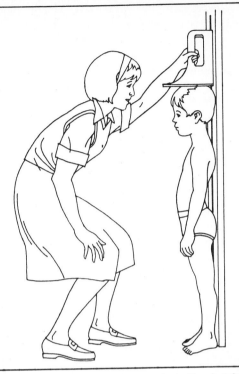

Figure 10-10. Weighing a child.
Redrawn with permission of Ross Laboratories, Columbus, OH 43216, from Pediatric Anthropometry, © 1982 Ross Laboratories.

Figure 10-11. Measuring stature (standing height).
Redrawn with permission of Ross Laboratories, Columbus, OH 43216, from Pediatric Anthropometry, © 1982 Ross Laboratories.

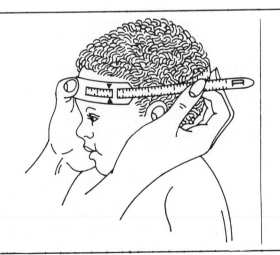

Figure 10-12. Measuring head circumference.
Redrawn with permission of Ross Laboratories, Columbus, OH 43216, from Pediatric Anthropometry, © 1982 Ross Laboratories.

Triceps skinfold thickness. Triceps skinfold thickness is a measurement of a double length of skin and subcutaneous fat on the back of the upper arm. Figure 10-9 describes the method for measurement in children.

Biochemical Assessment

Since anemia is a problem in this age-group, the initial screening should include hemoglobin and hematocrit determinations. Acceptable levels follow:

Age	Hemoglobin	Hematocrit (%)
12-23 months	10	31
2-5 years	11	34
6-12 years	12	37
or		
6 months-10 years	11	34
10-14 years	12	37

Serum cholesterol levels are often completed using 160 mg/dl as a cutoff point for children ages 2 through 17 years.

Guidelines for nutritional assessment and intervention in infants and children are described in Table 10-6.

Dietary Assessment

Techniques of dietary assessment are discussed in detail in Chapter 8.

Clinical Assessment

Screening children for hypertension has become routine in many clinics. For children 3 through 17 years the following cutoff points are used (Arizona Department of Health 1983):

Degree of Risk	Cutoff
Moderate	Diastolic blood pressure ≥75th percentile but <90th percentile
High	Diastolic ≥90th percentile but <100th percentile
Extremely high	Diastolic ≥100 mm Hg or systolic ≥120% of 95th percentile

Nutrition Intervention, Counseling, and Education

Nutrition education is emphasized in school curriculums both in elementary and secondary schools. This effort should be encouraged for all schoolchildren. The National Dairy Council's program developed for elementary school children has been successful in fostering this objective.

The pediatrician's office and the health clinic are available to children and their parents for nutrition and medical services.

Referral

Several food assistance programs are available to children including the WIC, School Breakfast, School Lunch, and Food for Child Care. In addition, food stamps and commodity foods are available to these families. Table 10-12 briefly describes these programs. In addition, Table 8-15 describes the food program in detail.

Assuring Quality of Health and Nutrition Care for Children

Quality assurance standards have been set for the normal child (Table 10-15). These standards provide a basis for evaluating the quality of care (Kaufman, 1983). Guidelines for population groups in community nutrition that serve infants and children are shown in Table 10-15.

ADOLESCENTS

Adolescence, the transition from childhood to adulthood, is accompanied by a series of physical, physiological, biochemical, hormonal, and psychosocial changes. A time of wide variability in norms of growth, it lasts nearly a decade with no specific beginning or end. Progress in the individual is characterized by orderly sequence, but there is marked variation between sexes and between individuals in timing, intensity of change, and deviation of the process.

This progressional period is usually described in two phases: pubescence and adolescence. *Pubescence*, which includes the adolescent growth spurt (average age is 9 to 13 years for fe-

Table 10-15. Model criteria for quality assurance in ambulatory nutrition care of normal child*

Criteria Identify Outcome (O) and Process (P)	Critical Time	Exceptions†	References
1. Child maintains weight for height between 5th and 95th percentile on NCHS growth chart. (O)	1 year-puberty	Less than 2500 gm birth weight until 18 months	Fomon, S.J.: Nutritional disorders of children, DHEW Pub. no. HSA-77-5104, Rockville, Md., 1977, U.S. Government Printing Office.
2. Child maintains height for age between 5th and 95th percentile on NCHS growth chart. (O)			Growth charts with reference percentile for girls and boys age 2 to 18 years, DHEW, Atlanta, 1976, Centers for Disease Control.
3. Child does not deviate more than 25 percentile points from his or her established growth pattern (height or weight) on NCHS growth chart. (O)	1 year-puberty	None	Fomon, S.J.: Nutritional disorders of children, DHEW Pub. no. HSA-77-5104, Rockville, Md., 1977, U.S. Government Printing Office.
4. Child's hemoglobin and/or hematocrit determinations are within acceptable levels as outlined below. (O)			

Hemoglobin	Hematocrit (%)			
10 gm	31	12-23 months	High altitudes	Centers for Disease Control: Nutrition surveillance, annual summary, 1978, Atlanta, 1980, CDC.
11 gm	34	2-5 years		
12 gm	37	6-12 years		Fomon, S.J.: Nutritional disorders of children, DHEW Pub. no. HSA-77-5104, Rockville, Md., 1977, U.S. Government Printing Office.
or				
11 gm	34	6 months-10 years		
12 gm	37	10-14 years		
5. Child consumes types and amounts of foods in frequencies appropriate for age and weight for height as specified in agency protocol. (O)	1 year-puberty	None	Pipes, P.L.: Nutrition in infancy and childhood, ed. 3, St. Louis, 1984, The C.V. Mosby Co.

Reprinted from Kaufman, M., editor: Guide to quality assurance in ambulatory nutrition care, Chicago, 1983, The American Dietetic Association.
*One year up to puberty; weight for height from 5th up to and including the 95th percentile for age and sex; no medical complications (physical handicaps, mental retardation, other syndromes).
†Lost to follow-up applies to all criteria.

males and 12 to 16 years for males), begins with the first increase in hormone secretion and appearance of secondary sex characteristics (increase in breast size in females and external genitalia in males and appearance of pubic hair) and ends when sexual reproduction becomes possible. *Adolescence* (average age is 10 to 17 years for females and 12 to 21 years for males) is the period beginning with the appearance of sexual maturity and terminating with the cessation of growth in stature.

Adolescence is thought of as a nutritionally vulnerable period for two reasons. First, the dramatic increase in physical growth and development during the transition from childhood to adulthood creates great demands. Although

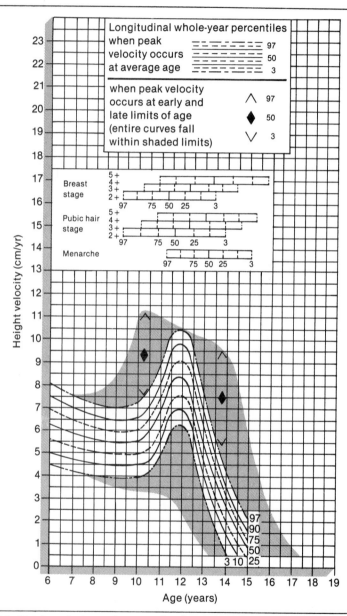

Figure 10-13. Height velocity and stages of puberty in girls.
Redrawn from Paige, D.M., and Owen, G.M.: Childhood and adolescence. In Paige, D.M., editor: Manual of clinical nutrition, St. Louis, 1983, The C.V. Mosby Co.

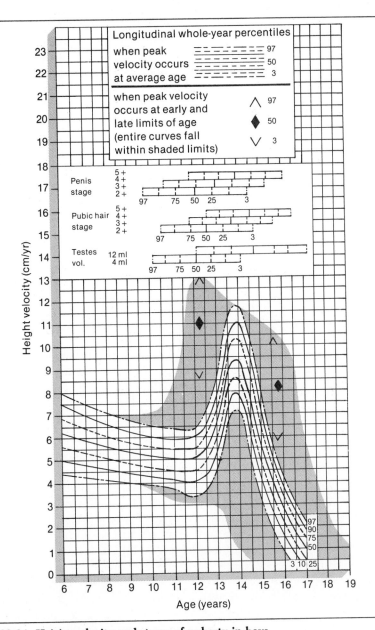

Figure 10-14. Height velocity and stages of puberty in boys.

Redrawn from Paige, D.M., and Owen, G.M.: Childhood and adolescence. In Paige, D.M., editor: Manual of clinical nutrition, St. Louis, 1983, The C.V. Mosby Co.

there is a gradual movement from pubescence to adolescence, there are a few identifiable points of demarcation. During pubescence, which lasts an average of 2 to 3 years, there is a peak velocity of increase in stature and weight preceding menarche in girls and spermatogenesis in boys.

In normal healthy girls, on the average, the growth spurt begins at 9.6 years; peak height velocity at 11.8 years; stage 2 breast development at 11.2 years; and menarche at 12.4 years. Normal variations around the mean are noted, as for any biological phenomenon, but menarche before 9 years and after 16 years of age is considered outside the normal range (Figure 10-13) (Tanner, 1981).

Males begin their pubescent growth spurt approximately 2 years later than females. The onset of male adolescence is accompanied by production of gonadotropin, which stimulates enlargement of the testes in the 9- to 12-year age range. Skeletal growth continues at an accelerated rate, reaching a peak of approximately 10.3 cm (4 in) at age 14.1 years (Figure 10-14). Associated changes in muscle mass, voice, and physical skills are noted. Linear growth almost ceases at approximately age 18 years, although some individuals continue to grow taller well into their twenties (Paige and Owen, 1983).

Hormonal Influences

Although the sex hormones exert a major controlling influence, many other hormones participate in adolescent development. Growth hormone, somatotropin, a polypetide produced by the pituitary, is highly species specific and is necessary for growth, but its role in adolescent growth is still unresolved. Growth hormone stimulates protein anabolism at the cellular level. The thyroid hormones, triiodothyronine (T_3) and thyroxine (T_4), influence overall body growth and skeletal maturation. The metabolic effects of these thyroid hormones include increases in oxygen consumption, heat production, nitrogen retention, protein synthesis, glucose absorption, glycolysis, and gluconeogenesis.

Insulin has an indirect effect on growth,

increasing the uptake and metabolism of glucose, glycogenesis, and the synthesis of fatty acids. It also stimulates the transport of amino acids into the cells and catalyzes the incorporation of amino acids into protein.

Estrogens influence the development and maintenance of secondary sex characteristics and reproductive functions. They result in significant morphological, physiological, and behavior changes by regulating the secretion of follicle-stimulating hormone (FSH) and luteinizing hormone (LH) by the pituitary, thereby increasing uterine weight and inducing vaginal cornifications.

Progesterone, secreted by the corpora lutea of the ovarian cortex, causes changes in the uterine endometrium and is responsible for the cyclic changes in the vagina and also acts in the maturation of breast function.

The physiological sequence of development that occurs during the growth spurt results in a high demand for calories and nutrients to support optimum growth.

Nutrient Requirements

For practicality, the RDA during the adolescent period are divided by chronological rather than maturational or biological age-groups: 7 to 10 years (prepubescent), 11 to 14 years (junior high), 15 to 18 years (high school), and 19 to 22 years (college), with separation by sex after 11 years of age (Food and Nutrition Board, 1980). The RDA for males and females ages 11 to 14 years and 15 to 18 years are shown in Table 10-16.

There are little direct experimental data on which to base nutrient requirements for adolescents. Except for energy, values such as the RDA are extrapolated from infant data and/or adult values. Nutrient needs are greatest during the pubescent growth spurt and gradually decrease as the individual achieves physical maturity. The adolescent growth spurt contributes about 50% to adult body weight and 15% to final adult height. The peak energy value for females is at 7 to 10 years (2400 kcal), but for males it is much later and of greater magnitude, 2900 kcal

Table 10-16. Recommended dietary allowances for adolescents

	Males		Females		Pregnant Females	
	11-14 yr	15-18 yr	11-14 yr	15-18 yr	11-14 yr	15-18 yr
Weight (kg)	45	66	46	55	46	55
Energy (kcal)	2700*	2800	2200	2100	2500	2400
Protein (gm)	45	56	46	46	76	66
Vitamin A (μg RE)	1000	1000	800	800	1000	1000
Vitamin D (μg)	10	10	10	10	15	15
Vitamin E (mg TE)	8	10	8	8	10	10
Vitamin C (mg)	50	60	50	60	70	80
Folacin (μg)	400	400	400	400	800	800
Niacin (mg)	18	18	15	14	17	16
Riboflavin (mg)	1.6	1.7	1.3	1.3	1.6	1.6
Thiamin (mg)	1.4	1.4	1.1	1.1	1.5	1.5
Vitamin B_6 (mg)	1.8	2.0	1.8	2.0	2.6	2.6
Vitamin B_{12} (μg)	3.0	3.0	3.0	3.0	4.0	4.0
Calcium (mg)	1200	1200	1200	1200	1600	1600
Phosphorus (mg)	1200	1200	1200	1200	1600	1600
Iodine (μg)	150	150	150	150	175	175
Iron (mg)	18	18	18	18	30-60	30-60
Magnesium (mg)	350	400	300	300	450	450
Zinc (mg)	15	15	15	15	20	20

From Food and Nutrition Board, National Research Council—National Academy of Sciences: Recommended dietary allowances, ed. 9, Washington, D.C., 1980, U.S. Government Printing Office.
*See RDA, 1980, for range of energy needs.

at 19 to 22 years. The male thus has a higher allowance for energy within which to meet the requirements for other essential nutrients. The female, whose energy needs are less, must select foods of high nutrient density to meet all of her nutrient needs without exceeding the energy allowance.

Energy

The requirements for energy vary widely from one individual to another, not only because of different timing and magnitude of somatic growth, but also because of variations in physical activity.

Age or weight alone is not a useful predictor of energy needs. Combinations of kilocalories-kilograms-age and kilocalories-kilograms-centimeters are more useful tools. Using a single measure, height in adolescence best expresses energy requirements because it usually correlates well with physiological development.

Protein, Carbohydrate, and Lipids

The protein allowances, like those for energy and other nutrients, follow the growth pattern. The highest protein allowance for males begins at 15 years (56 gm) and persists through adulthood; for females the protein allowance peaks at 11 to 18 years (46 gm), with a decrease to 44 gm in adulthood. Most adolescents consume protein in excess of these amounts. Limitation of either protein or energy during the accelerated phase of growth has been demonstrated repeatedly to inhibit growth.

No allowances have been established for carbohydrate or lipids. Carbohydrate is of particular importance to the adolescent who participates in athletic competition.

Vitamins and Minerals

The paucity of information concerning vitamin requirements of adolescents is emphasized by several authors. With the increase in energy demands, rate of tissue synthesis, and skeletal

Table 10-17. Index of Nutritional Quality (INQ)* of menu items offered by a hamburger chain†

Item	Protein	Vitamin A	Vitamin E	Ascorbic Acid	Vitamin B_6	Vitamin B_{12}
Regular hamburger	2.5	0.4	0.1	0.3	0.5	1.5
Regular cheeseburger	2.5	0.5	<0.1	0.2	0.4	1.2
Large hamburger	3.0	0.2	<0.1	0.2	0.7	2.0
Large cheeseburger	2.9	0.6	0.1	0.2	0.5	1.7
Double patty hamburger	2.3	0.3	<0.1	0.2	0.4	1.3
Fish sandwich	1.8	0.2	0.7	0.4	0.2	0.7
Apple pie	0.3	0.1	0.1	0.3	0.3	<0.1
Cherry pie	0.3	0.3	<0.1	0.2	<0.1	<0.1
Cookies	0.5	<0.1	0.2	0.2	<0.1	<0.1
Chocolate shake	1.4	0.4	0.3	0.3	0.4	0.9
Vanilla shake	1.5	0.5	0.3	0.3	0.4	1.1
Strawberry shake	1.4	0.4	0.3	0.3	0.4	0.9
Egg on English muffin	2.5	0.5	0.2	0.2	0.4	0.9
Hot cakes and syrup	0.6	0.2	0.2	0.2	0.1	0.7
Scrambled eggs	3.5	1.4	0.6	0.2	1.1	1.7
Pork sausage	2.3	0.1	0.2	0.1	0.7	0.7
English muffin, buttered	1.0	0.3	<0.1	0.1	0.2	<0.1
French fries	0.5	0.1	<0.1	1.9	0.9	<0.1

From Shannon, B.M., and Parks, S.C.: Fast foods: a perspective on their nutritional impact. Copyright The American Dietetic Association.
*Percent of nutrient requirement supplied by each item, as purchased, divided by percent of energy requirement supplied by each item, as items in which the protein was predominantly high quality (animal origin). This included all items except the pies, cookies, hot cakes, buttered (origin). The energy requirement was set at 2200 kcal daily.
†Nutrient compositions on menu items determined by WARF Institute, Inc., Madison, Wisconsin, 1975.

growth associated with adolescence, it can be expected that vitamin needs are elevated.

To meet the increased energy demands, higher than normal adult levels of thiamin (B_1), riboflavin (B_2), and niacin (B_3) are necessary. Folacin and vitamin B_{12}, both required for tissue growth, have increased requirements. In addition, skeletal growth necessitates adequate vitamin D intake. Vitamins A, C, and E are all essential to keep this new tissue in working order.

Calcium needs are greater during adolescence than in either childhood or adulthood. It is during the growth spurt that about 45% of the adult skeletal mass is formed. Consequently, the RDA standard for calcium increases from 800 mg for children 7 to 10 years to 1200 mg for both males and females 11 to 18 years of age. The need to consume good sources of calcium such as dairy foods is important for bone health during adolescence and beyond.

Perhaps the most controversial allowances during adolescence are for iron. The RDA recommend an intake of 18 mg/day by both males and females from 11 to 18 years. In contrast, the Canadian Dietary Standard is 14 mg/day for females after 13 years; the male allowance reaches 14 mg at 16 to 18 years. The FAO/WHO standard provides a range at all ages that depends on bioavailability of the food iron. These ranges for the male are 9 to 18 mg at 13 to 15 years and 5 to 9 mg after 16 years; the ranges for females are 12 to 24 mg/day at 13 to 15 years and 14 to 28 mg from 16 years into adulthood (FAO/WHO, 1972).

The need for iron increases during the adolescent growth spurt, particularly for males, because of the expansion of blood volume and muscle mass. Females require less iron for growth but must replace iron lost in menstrual flow. Iron needs are related closely to lean body mass, with males requiring 42 mg of iron per kilogram of weight gain; females need 31 mg of iron per kilogram of weight gain. When growth is rapid,

Folacin	Thiamin	Riboflavin	Niacin	Calcium	Iron	Magnesium	Zinc	Copper
0.3	1.5	1.1	2.2	0.5	1.4	0.4	1.0	0.4
0.3	1.2	1.3	2.0	1.1	1.1	0.4	1.0	0.1
0.3	1.0	1.3	2.6	0.4	1.5	0.5	1.5	0.3
0.2	1.0	1.5	3.2	1.1	1.0	0.5	1.4	0.3
0.2	1.0	0.9	1.7	0.7	1.0	0.4	1.1	0.3
0.2	1.0	0.9	1.1	0.6	0.5	0.4	0.2	0.2
0.3	0.1	0.1	0.5	0.1	0.3	0.1	<0.1	0.1
<0.1	0.1	0.1	0.2	0.1	0.2	0.1	<0.1	0.2
<0.1	1.4	1.0	0.3	0.1	0.6	0.2	0.1	0.1
0.4	0.5	3.1	0.2	2.0	0.3	0.8	0.5	0.5
0.4	0.5	2.7	0.2	2.4	0.1	0.6	0.5	0.2
0.4	0.5	2.5	0.2	2.2	0.1	0.6	0.5	0.3
0.4	1.5	2.2	1.3	1.2	1.1	0.4	0.7	0.3
0.1	1.0	1.2	0.9	0.7	0.6	0.3	0.2	0.3
1.1	0.6	4.8	0.3	0.7	1.7	0.4	1.2	0.4
<0.1	1.8	0.9	3.5	0.2	0.6	0.2	0.9	0.3
0.3	1.7	1.0	3.8	1.0	1.0	0.4	0.3	0.4
0.1	1.0	0.2	1.5	0.1	0.3	0.6	<0.1	<0.1

Reprinted by permission from Journal of the American Dietetic Association, Vol. 76:242, 1980.
purchased. The nutrient requirements were set as the U.S. RDA for each nutrient except protein, in which case the requirement was set at 45 gm for English muffin, and French fries. In these cases, the requirement was set at 65 gm, because the protein was predominantly low quality (plant

males require more iron than do menstruating females, but once growth slows down, the female's iron needs surpass those of the male.

Although iron is most easily absorbed from meat, absorption from plant sources, such as beans and green vegetables, can be enhanced threefold when these foods are eaten with foods high in ascorbic acid. To meet the RDA of 18 mg, adolescents consciously must select iron-containing foods of high iron availability.

Zinc is necessary for growth and sexual maturation. Four hundred milligrams of this mineral are retained per day by the male and a little less by the female. It has been shown that many adolescents consume far less than needed, especially girls, who often consume less than half the RDA.

Psychological and Environmental Influences

Many factors infringe on and modify the adolescent's diet. Most teenagers are preoccupied with physical appearance and peer acceptance. A strong desire to be lean and to have a particular body image can result in inappropriate weight reduction, dietary aberrations, and selective widely distributed nutrient deficiencies. In adolescent females such behavior may lead to anorexia nervosa, which is willful self-starvation.

Another problem associated with inappropriate weight loss in females is amenorrhea thought to be caused by the change in the ratio of lean body mass to body fat. At particular risk are female athletes, particularly swimmers and dancers who train intensely, with loss of body fat and concomitant gain in lean body mass.

On the other hand, adolescents who exercise infrequently run a high risk of becoming obese. Lack of exercise, coupled with boredom that results in increased food intake, puts the adolescent in double jeopardy for excessive accumulation of body fat.

Fast-foods, fad diets, skipped meals, snacking, and high carbohydrate foods are facts of life

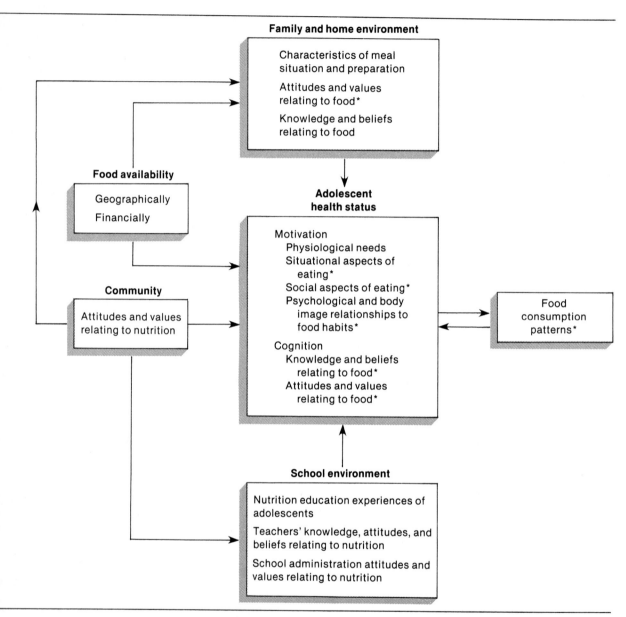

Figure 10-15. Interrelationships of factors influencing adolescent food consumption patterns. ∗ = Factors investigated in the survey described and conducted in Edmonton.
Redrawn from Lund, L.A., and Burk, M.C.: A multidisciplinary analysis of children's food consumption behavior, University of Minnesota's Agriculture Experimental Station Technical Bulletin 265, Minneapolis, 1965, University of Minnesota Press.

Table 10-18. Model criteria for quality assurance in ambulatory care of normal adolescent*

Criteria			
Identify Outcome (O) and Process (P)	Critical Time	Exceptions†	References
1. Adolescent's weight/height does not differ by more than 25 percentile points as plotted on NCHS growth chart. (O)	Throughout puberty and adolescence		Barnes, H.V.: Physical growth and development during puberty (appendix 1), DHEW Pub. no. 79-5234, Adolescent Health Care: A Guide for BCHS Supported Programs and Projects, U.S. Government Printing Office.
2. Adolescent's hematocrit and hemoglobin meet acceptable standards as follows. (O)			

Hemoglobin	Hematocrit			
12 gm	37%	10-14 years	Higher altitudes:	Fomon, S.J.: Nutrition disorders of
13 gm	41%	14 + male	nonnutrition	children, DHEW Pub. no. HSA-77-
12 gm	37%	14 + female		5104, Rockville, Md., 1977, U.S.

			Government Printing Office
3. Adolescent consumes appropriate types and amounts of foods as defined by agency protocol. (O)	Throughout puberty and adolescence		Committee on Dietary Allowances, Food and Nutrition Board: Recommended dietary allowances, Washington, D.C., 1980, National Academy of Sciences.

Reprinted from Kaufman, M., editor: Guide to quality assurance in ambulatory nutrition care, Chicago, 1983, The American Dietetic Association.
*Puberty and adolescence; no medical complications (chronic diseases, physical handicaps, mental retardation, or other syndromes); not underweight or overweight; non-regnant.
†Lost to follow-up applies to all criteria.

in our society. Condemnation of such dietary practices does little to win the adolescent's confidence. Many fast-foods (Table 10-17) are adequate sources of energy and of selected nutrients. However, continued intake of a single class of foods eliminates variety and balance, whereas skipping meals habitually can result in a low intake of selected nutrients or uncontrolled eating binges. Both practices are unhealthy.

When nutritional guidance is needed it should be provided without preconceived or culturally induced bias about the importance or quality of a particular food. A rational approach is to determine the nutritional contribution of the particular food to the adolescent's overall daily needs. Figure 10-15 describes the interrelationships of factors influencing adolescent food consumption patterns.

Guidelines for Patient Management

The outcomes expected in working with adolescents include the following:

1. Weight/height does not differ by more than 25 percentile points from his/her established growth patterns as plotted on NCHS growth chart.
2. Hematocrit and hemoglobin meets acceptable standards as follows:

Age	Hemoglobin	Hematocrit
10-14 years	12 gm	37%
14+ males	13 gm	41%
14+ females	12 gm	37%

3. Adolescents consume appropriate types and amounts of food.

Nutritional Assessment

Assessments for adolescents are comparable to those described for children (p. 281).

Anthropometric assessment. Height, weight, and skinfold thickness measurements should be completed (pp. 281 and 284).

Biochemical assessment. Because iron deficiency is prevalent among adolescents, hemoglobin and hematocrit determinations should be completed (p. 284). In addition, assessments of serum cholesterol levels should be completed.

Clinical assessment. Blood pressure should be completed along with information on drug and alcohol consumption, including tobacco. Table 10-6 describes the guidelines for nutritional and intervention for adolescents.

Referral

Pregnant adolescents may be referred to prenatal care, maternal and infant care programs, and food assistance programs, such as WIC, Food Stamps, and School Lunch, which are described in Table 10-11. In addition, physical fitness programs and bonafide weight reduction programs are also available in the community.

Assuring Quality of Health and Nutrition Care for Adolescents

Quality assurance standards have been set for the normal adolescent (Table 10-18). These standards provide a basis for evaluating the quality of care (Kaufman, 1983).

REFERRAL FOR ADDITIONAL SERVICES
Food Assistance Programs

The major food assistance programs for low-income infants, children, and adolescents include the following:

- Special Supplemental Food Program for Women, Infants and Children (Chapters 8 and 9)
- School Breakfast Program
- School Lunch Program
- Child Care Food Program
- Summer Food Service Program

Children's Nutrition Program

The National School Lunch Program, enacted through the National School Lunch Act of 1946, is the parent of all other child nutrition programs. This federally assisted national lunch program fulfilled two very different needs. On the one hand, farmers wanted to increase consumption of their surplus commodities, and the lunch program was a good market for these foods. On the other hand, with the outbreak of World War II, the United States discovered that many of the draftees had nutrition-related health problems that prevented them from serving in the military. Through the School Lunch Program, Congress sought to avoid similar problems in the future, creating the program as a measure of national security, to safeguard the health and well-being of the nation's children. (In 1962 additional funds were authorized so that children who could not afford the full price of lunch would be able to receive free or reduced-price lunches. In 1970 Congress instituted uniform national income guidelines for free and reduced-price meals so that all children, regardless of family income, would be able to enjoy the benefits of a school lunch program.)

The School Breakfast Program was established as a pilot program by the Child Nutrition Act of 1966. This pilot program grew out of Congressional concern for poor children who came to school hungry and children who had to travel long distances to get to school.

Concern about hunger in the United States led to bipartisan congressional efforts to better meet the nutritional needs of children. In 1975 Congress made the School Breakfast Program a permanent program and stated that it should be made available in all schools where it was needed to provide adequate nutrition. In 1968 the Special Food Service Program for Children was added to the National School Lunch Act, to provide meals to preschool children in day-care centers and family day-care homes and to poor children during the summer months when school meals are not available. In 1975 this program was divided into the Child Care Food Program and the Summer Food Service Program; in 1978 the Child Care Food Program was made a permanent program. Finally, in 1972 the WIC program was added to the Child Nutrition Act as a pilot program to provide supplemental foods to nutritionally vulnerable low-income pregnant women, their infants, and young children. Congress acknowledged that providing supplemental foods during critical times of growth and development would prevent further health problems. In 1974 WIC was made available nationwide.

EXAMPLES OF STRATEGIES AT THE LOCAL LEVEL
North Carolina Public Health Nutrition Program

The North Carolina Public Health Nutrition Program is one of the largest units in the country, employing 245 public health nutritionists throughout the state. Eighteen of these positions are at the state level, and over 200 nutritionists serve the local communities. WIC funds 80% of these positions; the remaining 20% comes from such programs as Title III, Maternal and Child Health, Crippled Children's Services, Family Planning, Chronic Disease, and county funds.

Barbara Ann Hughes, Director of the Nutrition and Dietary Services Branch, credits the growth of services and staff in North Carolina to well-balanced administrative strategies and networking (Hughes, 1983). She and her staff have created a strong local, regional, and state partnership, which is the basis for planning, consolidating, developing policy, and evaluating efforts. When decisions affecting individuals statewide are to be made, a task force is formed with broad representation of the group affected by the decision. Individuals in these task forces are other health professionals. Some examples of their accomplishments using this strategy include development of a nutrition education clearinghouse, development of nutrition food service centers, and development of a training program for entry-level public health nutritionists.

The concept of participative management in its broadest sense has paid great dividends for North Carolina. Through networking the North Carolina program has established a support system for their services. They have creatively united organizations and individuals who ordinarily have no operational base to bring about collectively a greater change for the good of society.

Infancy and Preschool

To address the question of feeding practices in infancy and the prevalence of obesity in preschool children, Wolman (1984) interviewed parents of 262 infants. The age of each infant at the introduction of solid foods and whether he or she was breast-fed were recorded. Four years later, the heights and weights of as many children as possible were collected. More than 80% of the parents introduced solid food during the first 2 months of life. The longer the duration of breast-feeding, the later solids were likely to be introduced. However, the time of the introduction of solids was not related to the prevalence of obesity. Neither breast-feeding itself nor the duration of breast-feeding was related to the prevalence of obesity in the children studied. More research is needed not only on the solid food intake of infants but also on their total intake and activity level. The identification of early predictions of obesity would be extremely helpful to nutrition practices.

A nutrition education curriculum was developed and tested for use by preschool caregivers. Purposes of developing the curriculum were to (1) give preschool caregivers a basic nutrition background through programmed self-instructional units, (2) incorporate nutrition education into existing parts of a typical preschool day, and (3) provide learning activities designed to help preschool children relate food and nutrients to health (Davis et al., 1983). This study demonstrated that early childhood caregivers will use a nutrition curriculum that complements the existing preschool day format, is easy to use, and requires minimum basic instruction for the caregiver.

Nutrition Education for Students Grades 3 to 12

Singleton and Rhoads (1984) studied a proportionately stratified sample of Louisiana students to determine their nutrition hemoglobin as influenced by selected variables. The 3309 students in grades 3 to 12 were interviewed individually with the use of a pretested questionnaire.

Nutrition knowledge was assessed by a test of 15 selected nutrition concepts and the identification of the basic food groups needed daily. A majority of the students judged the study of nutrition in schools to be important. However, only 40.5% of the sample reported currently studying this science, with 15% studying it as an elective subject. A positive relationship existed between scores and grade divisions (3 to 6, 7 to 8, and 9 to 12), correct identification of food groups needed daily, and number of sources and activities used to learn about nutrition. Thus nutrition instruction, which is varied, innovative, and includes student's participation, does improve knowledge of this science.

Adolescent Project

As part of a community weight control program for adolescents, two different 14-week treatment approaches were offered: a behavioral approach without energy restriction and a behavioral approach combined with energy restrictions. Fifty youths were recruited, 14 to 16 years old and up to 55% above ideal weight (Ikeda et al., 1982). Twenty-seven participants completed the program and were available for 1-year follow-up. In comparison to ideal body weight, 3 gained weight, 12 maintained weight, and 12 lost weight during the program. At 1-year follow-up, 11 had lost weight, and the other 4 had maintained or gained weight. We found no difference in the results of the two approaches. Comparison of pretest and posttest results revealed significant improvement in knowledge about weight control among those who completed the program. There was a strong positive correlation between gain in cognitive knowledge and drop in percent overweight. Participants indicated that the program

had been most helpful by increasing individual awareness of eating and exercise habits.

SUMMARY

A healthy child grows at a genetically predetermined rate that may be compromised or accelerated by undernutrition, imbalance of nutrient intake, or overnutrition. Physical growth is one of the major criterion used to assess the nutritional status of infants and children.

Nutrition assessment, counseling, and education provide the framework for quality nutrition care. These components of nutrition services should be considered integral parts of health programs that provide both food and nutrition services to infants, children, and adolescents.

REFERENCES

American Academy of Pediatrics: Report of the task force on the assessment of the scientific evidence relating to infant feeding practices and infant health, Pediatrics (Suppl.), Oct. 1984, p. 74.

Andrews, E.M., Clancy, K.L., and Katz, M.G.: Infant feeding practices of families belonging to prepaid group practice health plan, Pediatrics 65:978, 1980.

Arizona Department of Health Services: Cardiovascular disease protocol, Bureau of Nutrition Services, Phoenix, 1983, Arizona Department of Health.

Brown, J.E.: Nutrition services for pregnant women, infants, children, and adolescents, Clin. Nutr. 3(3):104, 1984.

Centers for Disease Control: Nutrition surveillance annual summary, 1980, U.S. Department of Health and Human Services, Washington, D.C., Nov. 1982, U.S. Government Printing Office.

Centers for Disease Control: Nutrition surveillance annual summary 1981, U.S. Department of Health and Human Services, Washington, D.C., Nov. 1982, U.S. Government Printing Office.

Committee on Nutrition, American Academy of Pediatrics: Measurement of skinfold thickness in childhood, Pediatrics 42:538, 1968.

Davis, S.S., et al.: A nutrition education program for preschool children, J. Nutr. Ed. 15:1, March, 1983.

Endres, B.E., and Rockwell, R.E.: Food, nutrition, and the young child, ed. 2, St. Louis, 1985, Times Mirror/Mosby College Publishing.

FAO/WHO: Requirements of ascorbic acid, vitamin D, vitamin B_{12}, folate and iron: report of a joint FAO/WHO expert committee, WHO Technical Report Series no. 452, Geneva, Nov. 1972, World Health Organization.

Fomon, S.J.: Infant nutrition, ed. 2, Philadelphia, 1974, W.B. Saunders Co.

Fomon, S.J.: Nutritional disorders of children: prevention, screening and follow-up, DHHS Pub. no. (HSA) 76-5612, Rockville, Md., 1976, U.S. Government Printing Office.

Food and Nutrition Board: Recommended dietary allowances, rev. ed. 9, Washington, D.C., 1980, National Academy of Sciences–National Research Council.

Hughes, B.A.: Managing nutrition programs and services: the North Carolina local, regional and state network, Paper presented at a meeting of the American Public Health Association, Dallas, Nov. 14, 1983.

Human Nutrition Information Services: Food and nutrient intakes of individuals in 1 day: low income households, Nov. 1977-March 1978, Washington, D.C., 1982, U.S. Government Printing Office.

Human Nutrition Information Services: Nationwide Food Consumption Survey 1977-1979, preliminary report no. 11, U.S. Department of Agriculture, Washington, D.C., 1982, U.S. Government Printing Office.

Ikeda, J.P., et al.: Two approaches to adolescent weight reduction, J. Nutr. Ed. 14:3, Sept. 1982.

Jelliffe, D.B., and Jelliffe, P.E.F.: Early infant nutrition. In Winich, M., editor: Nutrition: pre- and post-natal development, New York, 1979, Plenum Publishing Corp.

Johnson, C.L., et al.: Basic data on anthropometric measurements, regular measurements of the hip and knee joints for selected age groups (1-74 years of age), U.S., 1972-1975, 1981.

Kaufman, M., editor: Quality assurance in ambulatory nutrition care, Chicago, 1983, The American Dietetic Association.

Lonnerdal, B., Forsum, E., and Hambraes, L.: A longitudinal study of the protein, nitrogen and lactose contents of human milk from Swedish well nourished mothers, Am. J. Clin. Nutr. 29:1127, 1976.

Moore, W.M., and Roche, A.F.: Pediatric anthropometrics, Columbus, Ohio, 1982, Ross Laboratories, Inc.

Owen, G.M.: Measurement, recording and assessment of skinfold thickness in childhood and adolescence: report of a small meeting, Am. J. Clin. Nutr. 35:629, 1982.

Owen, G.M., and Paige, D.M.: Infancy. In Paige, D.M., editor: Manual of clinical nutrition, Pleasantville, N.J., 1983, Nutrition Publications, Inc.

Paige, D.M., and Owen, G.M.: Childhood and adolescence. In Paige, D.M., editor: Manual of clinical nutrition, Pleasantville, N.J., 1983, Nutrition Publications, Inc.

Tanner, J.M.: Growth and maturation in adolescence, Nutr. Rev. 39:43, 1981.

U.S. Department of Health and Human Services, Public Health Services: Health promotion, disease prevention: objectives for the nation, Washington, D.C., 1980, U.S. Government Printing Office.

Wolman, P.G.: Feeding practices in infancy and prevalence of obesity in preschool children, J. Am. Diet. Assoc. 84:436, 1984.

Wong, F.L., and Trowbridge, F.L.: Nutrition surveys and surveillance: their application to clinical practice, Clin. Nutr. 3(3):94, 1984.

APPENDIX 10-1

NEUROMUSCULAR AND PSYCHOSOCIAL DEVELOPMENT IN INFANTS

Neuromuscular	Psychosocial	Implications for Feeding
Birth to 1 Month		
Sucking and swallowing reflex present at birth.	Early emotional and psychological and social attachment of mother and infant may determine future aspects of infant's personality.	Oral reflex is a definite adaptive food-seeking reflex for survival.
Stimulus in mouth leads to rhythmical sucking and swallowing pattern.		On satiety, infant withdraws head from breast or bottle and falls asleep.
Tongue protrusion predominates.	Mother's feeding practices determine exposure of tactile stimulation, which is essential to infant's physical and emotional growth.	If infant's needs are satisfied through food and love, trust develops between child and mother.
		Feeding is the main means for infant to establish human relationship with mother.

From Owen, A.L., Pipes, P., and Lee, S.L.: Infant feeding guide, Bloomfield, N.J., 1979, Health Learning Systems.   *Continued.*

Neuromuscular	Psychosocial	Implications for Feeding
Month 2		
Corners of mouth are well approximated but not very active in sucking. An open gap separates the lateral portions of the lips. Opens mouth widely to grasp nipple once it has touched lips. Hands often open. Tonic grasp disappearing.	Infant recognizes mother's face. Infant learns to equate mother with food. Strong emotional bond develops between mother and infant and can be viewed as beginning of social interaction of infant.	Infant is an individual who shapes his own behavior and feeding schedule. Infant learns to equate mother with food. Infant eats about five times per day and sleeps through the night.
Month 3		
Lip movement begins to refine; lower lip pulls in; may smack lips. Tongue protrusion still present but may swallow with less protrusion. Infant can hold onto an object without focusing on it. By end of third month, control of head and eyes is achieved.	More tactile stimulation exists with breast-fed infant. Basic trust factor (if established) is manifested in infant responses to mother. Infant ceases to cry with hunger when mother approaches. Infant stares into mother's face on feeding; shows response to human voice.	Infant recognizes bottle or breast as source of food. Milk runs out of the sides of the mouth when nipple is withdrawn. Infant still does not readily accept the cup.
Month 4		
Smacking and pouting of lips. True negative pressure suck begins. Grosser back and forth movement of tongue and mandibular action beneath nipple disappears. Maintains grasp when object placed in hand. Rooting reflex gone. Bite reflex disappearing. Lifts head and chest when placed on stomach.	Infant in self-control. Breast-feeding is significant in emotional development of infant. Infant vocalizes through musical cooing; smiles and increases body activity. Can distinguish familiar people and knows mother's voice.	Important to watch infant for readiness of introduction of solid foods, since their introduction may influence life-long dietary behavior. Schedule should be developed for the individual infant on demand to prevent overfeeding. Self-demand feeding satisfies hunger in a natural way. Breast-feeding creates a more intense sense of intimacy and closeness because of skin contact. Feeding considered a psychocommunication and sociocultural exchange between mother and baby.
Month 5		
Beginning of hand-eye coordination is seen. Head is steady now when infant is in a sitting position. Lower lip becomes more active. Lips purse at the corners and nipples are held more firmly.	Infant anticipates feeding. Infant turns head aside to surroundings when satisfied. Seeks out social stimulation and smiles to get attention. Development of hunger rhythm occurs.	Feed only as long as infant desires. Beginning to sit when propped up. Feed infant when he is hungry. Infant will open mouth for spoon and close mouth over it. Food is secured through sucking from the spoon.

Neuromuscular	Psychosocial	Implications for Feeding
Strong sucking has developed. Parts lips in process of shifting foods and in swallowing. Tendency to eject food from mouth because of dominance of tongue projection. Bite reflex disappears. Munching stage evolves. Normal swallowing occurs. Gag reflex strong until chewing of solids. Pats and holds bottle or breast.	Strengthening of trust is through feeding.	Spoon feeding is difficult because of tongue projection as spoon is removed. Considerable spilling milk running from the mouth.

Month 6

Neuromuscular	Psychosocial	Implications for Feeding
Lower lip moves into internal position. Lips purse together at corners. Draws in lower lip when spoon is removed. Pouts lips in process of shifting food in the mouth and during the swallow. Normal bite begins. Sucking is volitional. Tongue is held poised in gutteral position. Mouth poses to receive the spoon. Hand and arm movements refine, and finger-feeding is seen. Takes objects to mouth. Helps with the spoon. Can sit with support.	Hungry infant who is fed learns to trust parents, and the foundation for a healthy personality is facilitated. Interaction with others during feeding influences infant's acceptance and response to food. Infant will show a preference for the individual who gives him the most care. By the end of 6 months, crucial attachment rather than responsiveness occurs.	Holding and cuddling the baby during bottle-feeding encourages warm communication between parent and infant. Developmentally infant is ready for solid foods; any attempt to feed solid foods before this time can be viewed as a form of force-feeding. Stages of addition of solid food to infant's diet should be individualized to infant. Food should never be forced on infant. Use a small spoon that easily fits into infant's mouth.

Month 7

Neuromuscular	Psychosocial	Implications for Feeding
Keeps mouth tightly closed. Chewing begins with action of tongue moving food around in the mouth. Normal gag reflex present. Starts eating solids without choking. Teeth erupt. Good lateral movement of tongue. Reaches with one hand instead of two. Transfers objects from hand to hand. Holds bottle alone.	Infant is more active socially. Expresses wishes for contact but may also refuse it. Attachment to mothering person is shown by infant's recognition of and pleasure in being with her. Develops self-awareness and awareness of surroundings; is developing own personality.	Soft, chewable foods may be introduced. Introduce solids at a time when infant is in a more sociable and experimental mood. Do not force new food if infant cries or fusses at the time it is introduced; wait until infant is in a better mood.

Continued.

Neuromuscular	Psychosocial	Implications for Feeding
Month 8		
Sits freely without support and has good head and body control. Licks spoon with lips. Bites a nipple, spoon, or rim of cup. Chokes easily when drinking from a cup. Inferior scissor grasp developed. Reaches for spoon or cup with hand and head. Expresses satiety by playing, razzing of the lips, or moving his arms actively.	Infant becomes vocal and initiates social contact and mimics adult behavior. Mother's attitude is important in developing self-demand feeding schedule.	Feeding time is one of social interaction for infant. Feeding begins to occur in a regular pattern. Infant should be allowed to use hands in feeding. Infant shows eagerness or cries when food is prepared. Infant may fuss or push food away when he does not like it.
Month 9		
Drinks from bottle independently. When drinking from cup, fluids spill from corners of mouth. Infant can bite off correct amount of food. Table foods are easily chewed. Teeth: eruption of lower and upper lateral incisors. Pincer movement of thumb and forefinger developed. Has developed coordination of hands.	Demonstrates separation anxiety when separated from mother. Necessity of fixing a schedule may cause tension and conflict.	Set a feeding pattern, maintaining a variety of foods so all nutrients will be included in diet.
Month 10		
Tongue is drawn back within mouth and may be depressed in anticipation of feeding. Tongue projection may occur again around 1 year when child explores with tongue to lick food morsels off lower lip. Can handle bottle alone; shown by grasping bottle and bringing it to mouth. Pincer grasp is becoming apparent with infant grasping small objects of food with thumb and index finger. Pokes with index finger at nipple or at food in dish. Finger-feeds small pieces.	Infant mimics adult model in behavior and vocalizes for attention. Expresses needs and feelings. During feeding, infant demands a plaything to keep hands busy. On final satiety, infant turns head to one side and keeps lips pursed.	Infant may be offered fruit juices by the cup. Offer bite-sized pieces of food for infant to pick up in self-feeding.

Neuromuscular	Psychosocial	Implications for Feeding
Month 11		
Infant begins to walk, holds to stand, and cruises.	Infant shows an understanding of adult words and gestures such as "Give it to me" and "Hand it over."	May introduce more table foods.
Feeding behavior matures.		Provide small bite-sized pieces of food for the infant to eat by finger-feeding.
Drinks fairly continuously, four to five swallows at a time.	During feeding, hands rest on side or tray top and by the end of the meal, infant is ready to play.	Encourage self-feeding with help.
Drinks fluids from a cup that is held for him; may begin to hold cup.		
Begins self–spoon feeding with help.		
Finger-feeding; much of meal-time is messy.		
More interested in feel of food than finger-feeding; may put food back into dish.		
Chewing is more refined.		
Month 12		
Pattern of feeding solid foods has changed from sucking to rotary chewing.	Infant becomes quieter on feeding and shows a growing interest in self-feeding.	Finger-feeds most of meal.
Upper lip draws in.		Begins self-feeding with utensils.
Lower lip sweeps over food on upper lip.		
Deliberate spitting occurs.		
Tongue projection may occur again as tongue becomes freer and child explores with it.		
Tongue is drawn back within mouth and may even be depressed in anticipation of feeding.		
Increased neuromotor coordination occurs.		
Rotary chewing is present in solid food eating.		

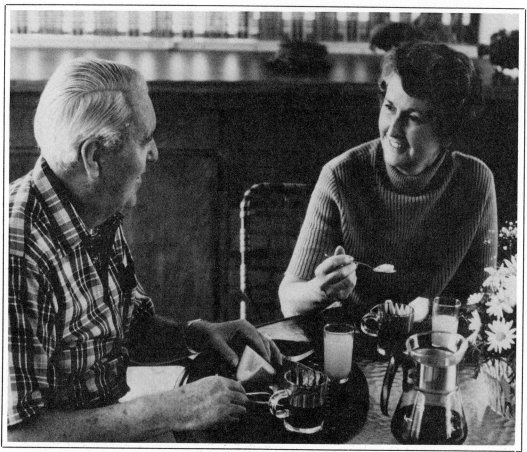

H. Armstrong Roberts

Adults and the Elderly

GENERAL CONCEPT

Maintenance of health and prevention of acute and chronic disease are primary goals for adults and the elderly. The objectives of health promotion need to be understood, accepted, and acted on as early as possible. Most nutrition-related diseases can be successfully avoided or at least maximally delayed if preventive practices and life-style modifications are instituted early in life and followed over the long term.

OBJECTIVES

When you finish this chapter, you should be able to

- Cite examples of the 1990 objectives for the United States as they relate to the adult and elderly population
- Review the energy and nutrient needs of adults and the elderly
- Understand the risk factors for nutrition-related diseases in this population
- Review components of nutrition screening and assessment in adults and the elderly
- Interpret the guidelines for patient management in the adult and elderly population
- Develop an innovative strategy for a nutrition intervention program for the elderly at the local level

A 1984 study by The Administration on Aging sought to identify the health concerns of older Americans by examining attitudes and concerns about physical fitness, nutrition, accidents, smoking, and drugs. The major finding was that older people want information on health practices rather than nutrition knowledge. Nutrition and chronic illness were issues of widespread concern and ranked high in the list of 11 concerns (CNI, Aug. 23, 1984):

Diet/nutrition/overweight
Exercise/staying active
High blood pressure/salt intake
Heart condition/heart attacks/cholesterol
Arthritis/mobility
Eyesight/cataracts/glaucoma/night driving
Loss of hearing
Medication/side effects/lack of information
Dementia/Alzheimer's disease
Circulatory problems/strokes
Diabetes

NUTRITION-RELATED HEALTH PROBLEMS OF ADULTS AND THE ELDERLY

The U.S. Department of Health and Human Services (1980) document *Promoting Health—Preventing Disease* (Chapter 1) identified goals and objectives for combating nutrition-related problems affecting adults and the elderly:

Healthy Adults

Goal: To improve the health of adults, and, by 1990, to reduce deaths among people age 25 to 64 by at least 25%, to fewer than 400 per 100,000.

Healthy Older Adults

Goal: To improve the health and quality of life for older adults and, by 1990, to reduce the average annual number of days of restricted activity due to acute and chronic conditions by 20%, to fewer than 30 days per year for older people ages 65 and older.

Improved health status

- By 1990, at least 60% of the estimated population having definite high blood pressure (160/95) should have attained successful long term blood pressure control (i.e., a blood pressure at or below 140/90 for 2 or more years). [High blood pressure control rates vary among communities and states, with the range generally being from 25% to 60% based on current data.]
- By 1990, the cirrhosis mortality rate should be reduced to 12 per 100,000 per year. [In 1978, the rate was 13.8 per 100,000 per year.]

Reduced risk factors

- By 1990, the prevalence of significant overweight (120% "desired" weight) among the U.S. adult population should be decreased to 10% of men and 17% of women, without nutritional impairment. [In 1971-74, 14% of adult men and 24% of women were more than 120% of "desired weight.] By 1990, 50% of the overweight population should have adopted weight loss regimens, combining an appropriate balance of diet and physical activity.
- By 1990, the average daily sodium ingestion (as measured by excretion) by adults should be reduced at least to the 3 to 6 gm range. [In 1979, estimates ranged between averages of 4 and 10 gm sodium. NOTE: One gm salt provides approximately 0.4 gm sodium.]

- By 1990, the mean serum cholesterol level in the adult population aged 18 to 74 should be at or below 200 mg/dl. [In 1971-74, for male and female adults ages 18 to 74, the mean serum cholesterol level was 223 mg/dl. For a smaller population sample in 1972-75, mean blood plasma cholesterol levels were about 211 mg/dl for males ages 40 to 59 and about 210 mg/dl for females ages 40 to 59.]
- By 1990, the proportion of adults 18 to 65 participating regularly in vigorous physical exercise should be greater than 60%. [In 1978, the proportion who regularly exercise was estimated at over 35%.]
- By 1990, 50% of adults 65 years and older should be engaging in appropriate physical activity (e.g., regular walking, swimming or other aerobic activity). [In 1975, about 36% took regular walks.]
- By 1990, the proportion of adults who smoke should be reduced to below 25%. [In 1979, the proportion of the U.S. population that smoked was 33%.]*

Nutrition is an important aspect of healthful behavior and a major component of general well-being throughout the life cycle. The adult years are often the most fulfilling and active stage of life. During adulthood life-styles are established, values are examined, new responsibilities are assumed, careers take direction, and families are started. Yet nutritional studies of this age-group have been more often a part of epidemiological investigations of chronic disease than self-contained assessments of nutritional status. More recently there has been a growing interest in nutrient and energy requirements of the elderly. This is probably a result of an admitted lack of knowledge in this area, which is succinctly reflected in the Recommended Dietary Allowances, where nutrient allowances are separated in the age categories of "23 to 50" and "51 and over" (FNB, 1980).

*Modified from Healthy people: the Surgeon General's report on health promotion and disease prevention, (PHS) Publication No. 79-5507, U.S. Department of Health and Human Services, Washington, D.C., 1979, U.S. Government Printing Office.

The early years of adulthood often represent a picture of nutritional robustness, exemplified in the special procreational requirements of women, the emerging popularity of vegetarianism, and the exaltation of physical fitness. But the processes of aging and disease are already in progress. Biological age changes form a continuum: rates of loss of lean body mass and organ function are linear from age 20 on. Age changes in physiological functions are shown in Figure 11-1.

Evidence now indicates that major chronic diseases that account for morbidity and mortality in later life have their pathological onsets many decades earlier. Because of improved care, the vast majority of those affected by chronic disease now are able to survive the acute health crises of early and middle years. The life expectancy at birth increased from 40 years in 1900 to 74.6 years in 1982 as a result of decreasing childhood mortality through the control and prevention of infectious disease and the decreasing age-specific death rates for mature adults. Life expectancy is still 69.3 years for blacks, a rate whites achieved about 30 years ago.

There has been a slow, steady increase in the adult and elderly population in both sexes from 1970 to 1982. Although the adult age-group of 18 years and over has increased by 26%, the 65 years and over group has increased by over 34%.

In 1970 there were 20 million persons 65 years and older; this number increased to 27 million by 1982. The most marked increase, over 38%, occurred among women 65 years and older as shown in Table 11-1, which gives a summary of age and sex structure for the United States in 1970, 1980, and 1982 for the adult and elderly groups (U.S. Department of Commerce: Current Population Report, 1983).

This increase in the elderly population has given rise to two special areas of study. *Geriatrics*, the branch of medicine dedicated to the care of the aging, as well as the aged, is concerned with prolonging life through the prevention and treatment of disease. *Gerontology* is the study of the psychological, sociological, economic, physiological, and medical aspects of aging.

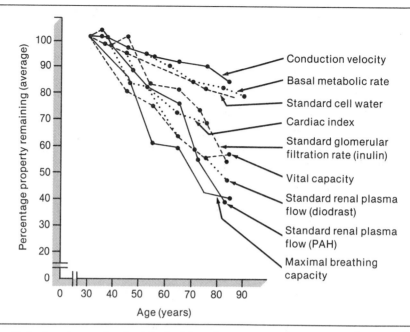

Figure 11-1. Age changes in physiological functions, expressed at percent of mean value, at age 30.
Redrawn from Shock: N.W.: J. Am. Diet. Assoc. **56**:491, 1970.

Mounting evidence suggests that personal health practices contribute to physical health status and longevity. More concerned than ever with health, many adults are adopting regimens that reflect increased physical activity and diets that are lower in fat, salt, and sugar and higher in complex carbohydrates and fiber. This trend also saves on the cost of groceries, particularly meat and poultry, which now account for over 40% of U.S. food expenditures (CNI, Dec. 6, 1984). The average life span—a rough measure of a healthy, productive life—is the highest in the history of the United States. The concept of wellness implies more than the absence of clinical disease; it also means optimum mental and physical performance and disease resistance. Chronic diseases of middle age account for 75% of all deaths in the United States. Among these are the nutrition-related diseases summarized in Table 11-2.

Comparative studies of elderly populations have shown that in industrialized societies there is a wide range of physical capacity and functional ability. A study of several countries, including the United States, Great Britain, Denmark, Israel, Poland, and Yugoslavia, reports that about 75% of the elderly are ambulatory or report only minimal impairment of ability for performance of tasks related to daily living; 12% to 24% are homebound; 2% to 4% are bedridden; and 4% to 8% are living at home (not bedridden) but need help with simple physical tasks (Kane and Kane, 1980).

Institutionalized elderly who are handicapped by chronic disease have less support available from community services (including nutrition services), family members, and friends. They are also more impaired in their access to mental health and social resources (Roe, 1983).

Table 11-1. Population distribution by age*

Age	Population			Percent Distribution			Population Change (1970 to 1982)	
	7-1-82	4-1-80	4-1-70	7-1-82	4-1-80	4-1-70	Number	Percent
Both sexes								
18 years and over	169,292	163,305	134,692	73.0	71.9	65.9	34,600	25.7
65 years and over	26,824	25,549	19,980	11.6	11.3	9.8	6,844	34.3
Male								
18 years and over	80,885	77,944	64,534	71.6	70.5	64.5	16,355	25.3
65 years and over	10,778	10,305	8,370	9.5	9.3	8.4	2,408	28.8
Female								
18 years and over	88,403	85,361	70,158	74.2	73.2	67.2	18,245	26.0
65 years and over	16,046	15,245	11,610	13.5	13.1	11.1	4,436	38.2

From U.S. Bureau of the Census, Current Population Reports, Series P-25, No. 929, 1983.
*Numbers are in thousands and include armed forces overseas.

Table 11-2. Nutritional risk factors associated with leading causes of death in the United States

Cause of Death	Primary Nutritional Risk Factors
Diseases of the heart	Elevated blood cholesterol level; excessive caloric intake; excessive total fat and saturated fat intake
Stroke	Excessive salt intake; excessive caloric intake
Cancer* (breast, cervical, and colon cancers)	Excessive total fat intake; excessive meat intake; low fiber intake
Cirrhosis of liver	Excessive alcohol intake; malnutrition
Diabetes mellitus (adult onset)	Excessive caloric intake
Influenza, pneumonia	Malnutrition

Modified from Brown, J.E., and Dodd, J.: Community Nutritionist, Nov./Dec. 1983. In Lee, S.L.: Clin. Nutr. 3(3):109, 1984.
*Certain types of diets, those rich in vitamins A, C, E, and beta-carotene, have been associated with protection against cancer.

Table 11-3. Nutritional risk factors associated with the development of some health problems

Health Problem	Primary Nutritional Risk Factors
Anemias	Low iron and folacin intake
Infection	Malnutrition
Dental caries	Excessive, frequent consumption of sweets; lack of fluoride
Obesity	Excessive caloric intake
Hypertension	Excessive caloric intake; excessive sodium intake; low potassium intake
Osteoporosis	Low calcium and vitamin D intake
Diverticulitis, constipation	Low fiber intake
Underweight, growth failure	Undernutrition
Iatrogenic malnutrition	Undernutrition in hospitalized patients

Modified from Brown, J.E., and Dodd, J.: Community Nutritionist, Nov./Dec. 1983. In Lee, S.L.: Clin. Nutr. 3(3):109, 1984.

The development of other acute and chronic health problems is also attributed to unhealthy diets, as shown in Table 11-3. Only recently have significant insights been gained into the causes and many risk factors involved in chronic diseases and the tangible, applicable preventive measures.

THE AGING PROCESS: PHYSIOLOGICAL CHANGES

The aging process characterizes all of life. Because one of the effects of aging is the gradual loss of functioning cells from many organs and tissues, it seems reasonable to assume that these effects could be counteracted or at least minimized by following nutrition guidelines. How one ages depends on the interaction between the genetic makeup of the individual and a host of environmental factors, including nutrition.

Once the body has reached physiological maturity, the process of growth and increased functional capabilities of the organs and tissues of earlier years is reversed. This is slow at first, until the rate of degenerative changes outweighs growth. Along with the degenerative change comes impaired functioning of many organs of the body. Although some physiological characteristics such as fasting blood glucose levels, blood pH, and blood osmolarity are maintained even into advanced old age, most physiological functions show gradual decrements in average values over the entire life span, beginning by age 30 (Figure 11-1).

Individual differences are large, and the range of values for most functions increases with age (Shock, 1982). Values for resting cardiac output among subjects carefully screened to exclude all of those showing evidence of heart disease show a much greater range among a group of 70-year-old subjects than is found among a group of 20-year-old persons. With aging differences among subjects of the same age increase so that age alone is a poor predicator of physiological performance in adults. Age decrements vary greatly among different organ systems and physiological performances. Taking the average

values for 30-year-old subjects as 100%, resting cardiac output falls by 40% over the age span of 30 to 90 years in contrast to maximum breathing capacity, which falls by 60% to 70% over the same age span. In contrast, fasting blood glucose level does not change at all, and basal oxygen uptake falls by only 15% on the average (Shock, 1982).

A summary of the physiological changes that may affect the nutritional status in some segments of the adult and elderly population is shown in Table 11-4.

NUTRITIONAL NEEDS OF ADULTS AND THE ELDERLY

As stated earlier, there is much to learn about the nutrition needs of adults, especially the elderly. In the past, studies of this age-group have often been a part of chronic disease epidemiology, although reports are beginning to be published about the needs of well, ambulatory groups of older persons. Research that is underway should soon produce new data.

The National Institute of Health (NIH), the major agency for the support of the biomedical and behavioral aspects of nutrition research and training, has spent $8.2 million on nutrition and aging in fiscal year 1980. In addition to NIH-funded research on nutrition and aging, the U.S. Department of Agriculture (USDA) has established at Tufts University a Human Nutrition Research Center on Aging. The mission of the Center on Aging is to examine the relationship between nutrition and aging:

1. How nutrition influences various body functions as people age
2. The role of nutrition in retarding or advancing the development of chronic disabilities and disorders associated with aging
3. The optimal nutritional needs of older persons to maintain good health and function (Simopoulos, 1982)

Individuals vary with regard to nutrient requirements. Even after adjustment of required estimates for such variables as age, sex, body size, physiological state, and voluntary activity, an

Table 11-4. Physiological changes with age that may affect nutritional status in some segments of the adult and elderly population

Physiological Changes	Potential Effect on Nutritional Intake/Status	Implications for Intervention
Nutrient-drug interactions	May decrease absorption or utilization of nutrients; may increase requirement for certain nutrients	Stress importance of taking medicine as prescribed and following instructions explicitly
Debilitating diseases	Impair appetite, mobility, attitudes, and other factors that affect food consumption	Nutrition education: stress importance of maintaining food and water intake in absence of feeling hungry
Neuromuscular changes—general frailty, poorer balance and reaction time	Decreased mobility affects food buying and preparation; accidents increase	Maintain RDA for protein and encourage moderate exercise
Gastrointestinal and sensory changes, including sense of taste, reduced gastric secretions, constipation, and smell	Impaired food intake, digestion, and absorption of some nutrients	Pay particular attention to iron, vitamin B_{12}, calcium, and fiber intake; encourage food preparation techniques to make meals attractive and appetizing
Skeletal changes; loss of bone mass, osteoporosis, periodontal disease	Difficulty in eating from tooth loss; decrease in food intake; fragility of bones: decreased mobility and increased fractures	Maintain RDA for calcium and vitamin D (some authorities recommend 1.5 gm calcium/day)
Increased blood pressure	Diagnosis of high blood pressure and limits on salt intake, plus drugs that impact on nutrient utilization	Nutrition education: encourage adherence to diet prescribed by dietitian or physician, promote use of other seasonings for flavor and palatability
Decreased kidney functions	May require special diets; may affect production of vitamin D; affects excretion of toxic metabolites and drugs	Nutrition education: stress importance of diet prescription from dietitian or physician
Deteriorating vision	Difficulty reading labels and prices; loss of interest in shopping skills; difficulty in reading recipes; loss of interest in cooking	Nutrition education: group shopping, demonstrations, large print on materials; use familiar dishes and recipes
Decreased basal metabolic rate and decrease in ratio of muscle to fat tissue in body composition	Decrease in energy requirements; increased body weight if caloric intake is not adjusted; less muscle tone	Stress maintenance of ideal body weight and encourage moderate exercise; stress importance of foods with high nutritional value

Data from Winick, M.: Mod. Med., Feb. 15, 1978; Perri, K.: Physiological bases for the nutritional needs of the elderly, term paper, Biology of Aging, University of Michigan, 1976; Posner, B.: Nutrition and the elderly, Lexington, Mass., 1979, Lexington Books. In Lee, S.L.: Clin. Nutr. 3(3):111, 1984.

Table 11-5. Recommended Dietary Allowances for adults 23 to 50 years old and the elderly

Nutrient	Men	Women
Calories*		
Age 23 to 50	2700	2000
Age 51 to 75	2400	1800
Age 76 +	2040	1600
Protein* (gm)	56	44
Vitamin A (RE)	1000	800
Vitamin D (μg)	5	5
Vitamin E (mg)	10	8
Vitamin C (mg)	60	60
Thiamin† (mg)	1.2	1.0
Riboflavin† (mg)	1.4	1.2
Niacin† (mg)	16	13
Vitamin B_6 (mg)	2.2	2.0
Folacin (μg)	400	400
Vitamin B_{12} (μg)	3.0	3.0
Calcium (mg)	800	800
Phosphorus (mg)	800	800
Magnesium (mg)	350	300
Iron† (mg)	10	10
Zinc (mg)	15	15
Iodine (μg)	150	150

Estimated safe and adequate daily dietary intakes of selected minerals

Sodium (mg)	1100-3300	
Potassium (mg)	1875-5625	
Chloride (mg)	1700-5100	

Modified from Food and Nutrition Board, National Academy of Sciences—National Research Council Recommended Dietary Allowances, ed. 9, revised 1980.

*Both caloric and protein guidelines are for standard-sized men and women. Caloric intake may vary according to physical activity and body size, whereas the protein allowance is based on a requirement of 0.8 gm/kilogram of body weight per day. In addition to the nutrients listed in the RDA, fiber and water are important factors to consider.
†The values are slightly higher for some nutrients. For men ages 23 to 50 the requirements are thiamin—1.4 mg, riboflavin—1.6 mg, and niacin—18 mg. The iron requirement for women is 18 mg.

element of individual variability remains. The factors that influence the nutritional requirements and intake of adults and older individuals are those which affect intake, digestion, absorption, storage, and metabolism of nutrients and elimination of waste products. In the absence of detailed metabolic or other studies, it is impossible to describe a person's true requirement for a nutrient. Conversely, it is possible, from past studies, to describe a range of requirements that characterize populations with selected characteristics as shown in the Recommended Dietary Allowances (RDAs) (Table 11-5).

Energy

It is generally assumed from available data that energy requirements decrease with age but that there is little or no change in the need for protein and the micronutrients. The National Academy of Sciences/National Research Council (NAS/NRC) has suggested that adults reduce caloric consumption by 10% between the ages of 51 to 75 years and an additional 10% to 15% after 75 years of age, unless the level of physical activity necessitates a larger or smaller caloric intake.

Protein

The National Research Council recommends that an intake of 0.6 gm of high quality or 0.8 gm of protein of mixed quality per kilogram of body weight be maintained throughout adulthood. Although the RDA for protein (44 gm for women and 54 gm for men) may be provided, with reduced calorie intake protein may be diverted to be used as a source of energy rather than into the synthesis of body proteins.

Because the total amount of protein synthesized daily declines only slightly with age, an intake greatly in excess of the RDA is considered undesirable because of the added burden of excreting urea from the deamination of protein by less efficient kidneys. On the other hand, protein is used primarily for maintenance of cells and for synthesis of enzymes needed for digestion and cellular metabolism. Thus some researchers suggest a higher intake of protein to maintain nitrogen balance and to provide the necessary B vitamins and micronutrients. It is generally recommended that the elderly receive about 12% to 14% of their total calories as protein (Food and Nutrition Board, 1980).

Carbohydrate and Fiber

Carbohydrates are an important source of nutrients and fiber. No recommended allowance has been established for carbohydrates, but a minimum intake of 50 to 100 gm is suggested. The upper limit for carbohydrate intake is based on a person's total caloric needs with a recommendation of about 58% of total calories. Considerable attention is directed to the importance of dietary fiber because it provides bulk in the diet and aids in elimination. Because there is potential risk of lessened absorption of mineral elements as a result of high dietary fiber intake, a moderate amount, but not an excessive amount, of fiber seems appropriate.

Fat

Dietary fat serves as a carrier for fat-soluble vitamins and provides essential fatty acids. Except for these needs, which can be met by a diet containing 15 to 25 gm of appropriate food fats, there is no specific requirement for fat as a nutrient. An expert panel convened by the National Institutes of Health recommended that all Americans, especially those considered to have high cholesterol levels, adopt a diet that derives at most 30% of its calories from fat with no more than 10% each from saturated, monounsaturated, and polyunsaturated fats and a maximum of 300 mg of cholesterol a day (NIH Consensus Development Conference, 1984b).

Water

Although it does not make specific recommendations for adults and the elderly, the NAS/NRC suggests total daily water intake of 1 ml/kcal for adults under normal circumstances. Obligatory urinary nitrogen output per unit of body weight is similar in older and younger persons. However, because the number of nephrons is less in the aged, the solute load per nephron is increased. Adequate water to facilitate excretion of this solute load is vital. Adults and the elderly should be encouraged to consume adequate quantities of fluids, especially water.

Vitamins and Minerals

Requirements for most vitamins and minerals remain essentially the same for older persons as for younger adults (Table 11-5). Evidence suggests that calcium intake be increased from 800 to 1400 mg, especially for postmenopausal women as a result of decreased absorption of calcium and the possible role of calcium deficiency in the development of osteoporosis (NIH Consensus Development Conference, 1984a).

Iron requirements for older persons are lower than for any other age-group. This recommendation is made on the basis that no physical growth occurs in old age and women no longer menstruate. However, the prevalence of anemia has been reported to increase among some elderly persons. Whether this is a result of increased need for iron, vitamin B_{12}, or folacin or a combination of these nutrients is not clear. Regular use of medications such as aspirin or physical conditions that cause blood loss warrant an assessment of levels of iron and other minerals. It is still not known if changes in the gastrointestinal tract associated with the aging process may affect the availability and absorption of iron from food.

Salt

A high salt intake is well established as one of the risk factors associated with hypertension, a chronic condition common among adults and the elderly. Although a high intake is associated with the risk of hypertension, the actual risk of a stroke as a result of hypertension is less for the elderly than for other age-groups. Although there may be a genetic predisposition to salt as a factor in hypertension, it seems appropriate as a public health measure to suggest a decrease in the use of salt during cooking and at the table.

SUPPLEMENTATION AND FADDISM

The changes in vitamin requirements with aging are so poorly documented that it is difficult to quantify their effect on nutrient needs. Yet the use of supplements in the age-group is an enormous cost to those who can afford it least and thus merits discussion.

Older persons and adults are concerned about their health and are highly motivated to take steps they believe will help maintain a sufficient level of health. The issue of supplementation of vitamins and minerals is controversial and often emotional. For the average adult who consumes a variety of foods, supplementation is not necessary except, perhaps, for calcium supplementation.

The primary nutritional findings of a 5-year study of 350 members of a healthy elderly population in Albuquerque indicated wide use of vitamin supplements. Fifty-seven percent of the men and 61% of the women routinely ingested one or more vitamin or mineral supplements (Garry et al., 1982). Ascorbic acid was the vitamin supplemented most, although more than 90% of the population received at least 100% of the RDA from diet alone. Median supplemental intake of ascorbic acid was 830% of the RDA for men and 570% of the RDA for women. Vitamin supplementation varied considerably from one nutrient to another as well as among subjects taking a specific supplement. Median supplemental intake ranged from a high of more than 1800% of the RDA for vitamin E to less than 20% of the RDA for phosphorus. Of the water-soluble vitamins, folic acid was the supplement consumed in lowest absolute amounts relative to the RDA. Of the women in the group that took supplements, 50% still received less than 100% of the RDA for calcium.

Typically, as Garry's study indicated, nutrient supplementation was inappropriate. Those nutrients lacking in the diet (calcium and folic acid) were not provided by the ingested supplements, whereas nutrients that were found in adequate amounts in the diets (ascorbic acid) were the same nutrients contained in the supplements.

Because the amount of money spent on supplements may represent an appreciable proportion of the money available for food, guidance is needed to help those who would profit from supplements to choose the correct ones, although making the proper food choices is preferred. The elderly are particularly vulnerable to misinformation and food faddism. The public in general and the elderly in particular should not have unrealistic expectations of what nutrition can accomplish. Any program in nutrition education at the community level should introduce the subject of quackery and food faddism. Americans of all ages, adults and the elderly in particular, are paying a high price for worthless nostrums, ineffectual and potentially dangerous devices, treatments given by unqualified practitioners, unneeded diet supplements, and other alluring products or services that make misleading promises to cure disease and contribute to longevity.

The fad of popular crash weight control gimmicks is perhaps the most costly of all nutrition quackery. Constantly in search of a panacea that will drop pounds overnight, the obese continue to try liquid protein diets, kelp and vinegar, spirulina, diet pills, and other concoctions that constantly appear. The nutritional adequacy of 11 published weight reduction diets is discussed in the section on obesity.

DIET-DRUG INTERACTIONS

Drug therapy is common among the adult and elderly population, whether it be prescription drugs or over-the-counter drugs purchased for self-medication. In addition to influencing dietary intake, drugs affect the metabolism of nutrients including intestinal absorption, plasma-binding and transport, peripheral utilization, transport across cell membranes, intracellular reactions, storage in tissues, turnover, and elimination and excretion. Drugs are an important cause of malnutrition in addition to their other side effects. A review of drug-diet interactions shows that alterations in the absorption and/or use of folate and vitamins B_6 and B_{12} account for the largest proportion of drug-induced nutritional deficiencies (Roe, 1976). Drugs can induce malabsorption through a number of mechanisms (Table 11-6).

Common prescription drugs that can lead to nutritional depletion include digitalis, the

Table 11-6. Primary intestinal absorptive defects induced by drugs

Drug	Usage	Malabsorption or Fecal Nutrient Loss	Mechanism
Mineral oil	Laxative	Carotene, vitamins A, D, and K	Physical barrier Nutrients dissolve in mineral oil and are lost Micelle formations ↓
Phenolphthalein	Laxative	Vitamin D, Ca	Intestinal hurry K depletion Loss of structural integrity
Neomycin	Antibiotic to "sterilize" gut	Fat, nitrogen, Na, K, Ca, Fe, lactose, sucrose, vitamin B_{12}	Structural defect Pancreatic lipase ↓ Binding of bile acids (salts)
Cholestyramine	Hypocholesterolemic agent Bile acid sequestrant	Fat, vitamins A, B_{12}, and D, Fe, K	Binding of bile acids (salts) and nutrients (e.g., Fe)
Potassium chloride	Potassium repletion	Vitamin B_{12}	Ileal pH ↓
Colchicine	Antiinflammatory agent in gout	Fat, carotene, Na, K, vitamin B_{12}, lactose	Mitotic arrest Structural defect Enzyme damage
Biguanides Metformin Phenformin	Hypoglycemic agents (in diabetes)	Vitamin B_{12}	Competitive inhibition of B_{12} absorption
Para-amino salicylic acid	Antituberculosis agent	Fat, folate, vitamin B_{12}	Mucosal block in B_{12} uptake
Salicylazosulfapyridine (Azulfidine)	Antiinflammatory agent in ulcerative colitis and regional enteritis	Folate	Mucosal block in folate uptake

From Roe, D.A.: Drug-induced nutritional deficiencies, Westport, Conn., 1976, AVI Publishing Co.

diuretics, and indomethacin, which is used to treat arthritis (Roe, 1983). Aspirin in high doses can cause damage to the lining of the gastrointestinal tract, leading to blood loss and the development of iron deficiency anemia. The abuse of cathartics, a health problem in the United States, has resulted in severe malabsorption syndromes. Mineral oil leads to deficiency of fat-soluble vitamins A, D, and K. Laxative abuse, combined with intake of drugs such as phenolphthalein, can cause malabsorption, potassium deficiency, and protein deficiency through excessive loss of protein from the gastrointestinal tract. Antacid abuse can result in phosphate deficiency and can also contribute to osteomalacia (Roe, 1983).

Certain dietary habits of elderly persons may reduce the availability of minerals. For example, iron absorption is reduced in heavy tea drinkers; zinc and iron absorption may be reduced by high-phytate foods such as oatmeal. The aging process itself may reduce the rate of drug metabolism so that drugs that contribute to nutrient depletion may remain in the body longer. Continuing examination of the complex interactions among drugs, food, and nutrients is important. There should be an awareness that there is a synergistic relationship between nutrients and drugs. The impact of drug-induced dietary changes (fatigue, anorexia, etc.) may aggravate the efficacy of drug therapy and further compromise the nutritional status of the elderly. Reducing the number of drugs prescribed and encouraging high-nutrient diets for those who are vulnerable will help decrease the possibility of drug-induced malnutrition. The pharmacist can often provide guidance on ways to minimize undesirable nutrient-drug interaction.

POVERTY AND OTHER SOCIOLOGICAL CONCERNS

Changes in social situations and life-style may affect food intake. For example, death of a family member or close friend, retirement, or physical impairment may result in social withdrawal. In addition, physical and physiological status may impose limitations on food and nutrient consumption. Perhaps the most devastating factor is the economics of aging, which plays a determinant role on the nutritional status of the older person. Adjustment to a lower income after retirement from paid employment commonly limits allowable food expenditures.

The Social Security Act of 1935 and its amendment, which established Medicare and Medicaid programs in 1965, have provided some measure of economic security. The Older Americans Act, first passed by Congress in 1965, was expanded in 1972 by Title VII, which authorized funding of local community projects to provide nutritious meals to persons 60 years and older. Among this target population, special emphasis was to be placed on reaching senior citizens in the greatest economic need and those whom age or infirmity had isolated from ordinary social contact.

In the Comprehensive Older Americans Act Amendments of 1978, nutrition programs were again authorized and funded under an expanded Title III. These funds are channeled from the Administration on Aging in Washington through various state offices on elderly affairs to local agencies on aging. The local agencies, designated by law to be planning and not service delivery agents, normally then contract with nonprofit community groups to provide nutrition and other services to senior citizens.

The primary objective of Title III of the Older Americans Act is the development of comprehensive and coordinated community-based health and social service systems to foster independent living among older Americans. Services provided by Title III to meet this objective include congregate and home-delivered meals, information and referral outreach, transportation, legal guidance, employment information, escorts, counseling, adult day care, education, home health care, and homemaker support.

Community-based long-term care, another community service, is "a coordinated continuum of diagnostic, therapeutic, rehabilitative, supportive, and maintenance services that address the health, social, and personal needs of individuals who have restricted self-care capabilities" (Monteith, 1983).

The number of older Americans living in poverty today is the same (4.9 million) as in 1972, but they comprise a smaller proportion of an older population that is growing rapidly. The U.S. Department of Commerce's 1978 statistics of the black population reported that one of every three elderly blacks lives at or below the poverty level. Aged blacks are about three times as likely to be poor as elderly whites: 32% of all blacks 60 years and older lived in poverty in 1978 in contrast to 11% of elderly whites. As seen in Figure 11-2, the largest group living below the poverty level in 1982 was black women over the age of 72 years who lived alone (CNI, Sept. 13, 1984).

Both the Ten-State Nutrition Survey and the First Health and Nutrition Examination Survey (NHANES) in 1970 confirmed that blacks over the age of 60 are especially nutritionally vulnerable. Food, for example, absorbs more of the budget of the black family than it does for the white family with a comparable income. Food stores in black neighborhoods tend to carry higher priced items than those in white neighborhoods. This is a result of high crime, theft, and security costs in supermarkets located in black neighborhoods.

The common nutrient deficiencies found among blacks include insufficient amounts of vitamins A and C, iron, and calcium, probably as a result of lower intakes of fruits, vegetables, lean meats, and dairy products.

Culture, too, plays a role. Each person brings

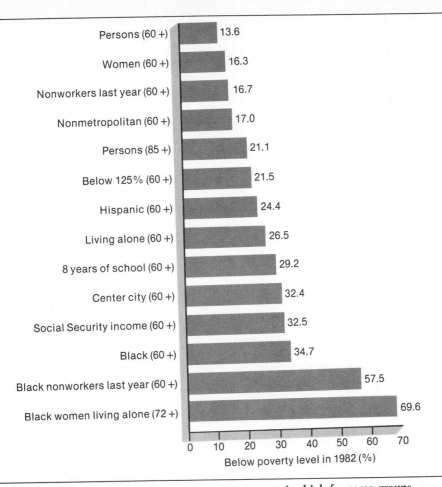

Persons (60 +) — 13.6
Women (60 +) — 16.3
Nonworkers last year (60 +) — 16.7
Nonmetropolitan (60 +) — 17.0
Persons (85 +) — 21.1
Below 125% (60 +) — 21.5
Hispanic (60 +) — 24.4
Living alone (60 +) — 26.5
8 years of school (60 +) — 29.2
Center city (60 +) — 32.4
Social Security income (60 +) — 32.5
Black (60 +) — 34.7
Black nonworkers last year (60 +) — 57.5
Black women living alone (72 +) — 69.6

Below poverty level in 1982 (%)

Figure 11-2. Poverty among the elderly. Poverty remains high for some groups.
Redrawn from Community Nutrition Institute: Poverty among elderly tightens grip on women, Sept. 13, 1984.

to old age all those cultural attitudes and beliefs that have resulted from many years of socialization within an ethnic group. Cultural heritage includes a value system, a world view, and a normative structure. The way in which an individual integrates these elements results in a unique personality. Life-style, attitudes, and behavior affect dietary intake and nutritional status. Although the biological needs for food, water, sleep, air, and elimination are universal, the ways in which they are met are quite different.

Not only do food preferences vary according to ethnicity, but older persons also differ in their eating habits from younger persons within the same ethnic group. For example, the much discussed "soul food" of the southern black may be enjoyed by the 70-year-old because of its pleasant associations from earlier years but may be disliked by the 45-year-old because it reminds that person of an environment he or she is trying to forget.

GUIDELINES FOR PREVENTION OF NUTRITION-RELATED DISEASES

Mounting evidence suggests that personal health practices do contribute to the well-being and longevity of population groups. Although this concept is far from new, recent studies further document the importance of prevention. A study of 7000 adults followed up for 5½ years showed that life expectancy and health are significantly related to the following basic health habits: (1) eating three meals a day at regular times and no snacking; (2) eating breakfast every day; (3) moderate exercise two or three times a week; (4) adequate sleep of 7 or 8 hours a night; (5) no smoking; (6) moderate weight; and (7) no alcohol or only moderate use (Belloc and Breslow, 1972).

Obesity

In the United States, the greatest longevity is associated with below-average weights in the population under consideration, providing the lower weights are not associated with a history of significant medical impairment. If persons are followed up for a sufficient time, obesity at the time of entry into a prospective study is an independent risk factor predictive of premature cardiovascular morbidity and reduced life expectancy (Simopolous and Van Itallie, 1984).

Figure 11-3 shows the percentages of obese persons by age, sex, race, and income (Lowenstein, 1982). In the 65- to 75-year-old age-group the percent of obese women was significantly greater than the percentage of obese men. White men had higher percentages of obesity than black men in both income groups. In contrast, black women showed significantly higher percentages of obesity in the poverty group than did white women.

In the past obesity was associated with coronary heart disease because of its impact on cardiovascular risk factors such as hyperlipidemia and hypertension. However, findings suggest that the duration of obesity has an important bearing on the putative relationship between body weight and longevity. When data from the Framingham Study were analyzed using a 26-year interval between measurements of obesity and subsequent outcome, obesity was clearly a significant predictor of cardiovascular disease, independent of age, cholesterol level, systolic blood pressure, cigarette smoking, left ventricular hypertrophy, and glucose tolerance (Hubert et al., 1983).

A simple classification of three types of obesity, based on the degree of overweight for use in clinical practice, has been proposed by Stunkard (1984): (1) mild obesity—20% to 40% overweight, (2) moderate obesity—41% to 100% overweight, and (3) severe obesity—greater than 100% (Table 11-7).

Almost 91% of all obese women are mildly obese. For these persons the recommended treatment is moderate caloric restriction, along with nutrition education, behavior therapy, and increased activity. This program should provide a safe, comfortable, and reasonable rate of weight loss. Commercial weight-loss programs that use group treatment, such as Weight Watchers, are readily available at the community level. Among the elderly, failure to reduce caloric intake in relation to lowered energy expenditures is the primary cause of increased obesity.

For the special purpose of resolving the pressing questions relating to the health implications of obesity, the NIH Office of Medical Applications of Research, the National Institute of Arthritis, Diabetes, and Digestive and Kidney Diseases, and the National Heart, Lung, and Blood Institute convened a consensus development conference on the health implications of obesity (NIH Consensus Development Conference, Feb. 1985). The objectives were to define obesity, to cite evidence that obesity has adverse effects on health, to cite evidence that obesity affects longevity, to review appropriate uses and limitations of existing height-weight tables, to recommend medical conditions for which weight reduction should be recommended, and to outline directions for future research.

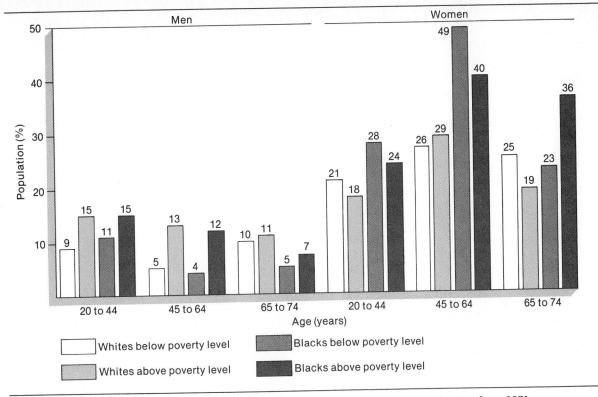

Figure 11-3. Obesity of adults by age, sex, race, and income in the United States from 1971 to 1974.
Redrawn from Lowenstein, F.W.: J. Am. Coll. Nutr. 1:165, 1982.

Table 11-7. Classification of obesity

	Type		
	Mild	Moderate	Severe
Percentage overweight	20% to 40%	41% to 100%	>100%
Prevalence (among obese women)	90.5%	9.0%	0.5%
Pathology	Hypertrophic	Hypertrophic, hyperplastic	Hypertrophic, hyperplastic
Complications	Uncertain	Conditional	Severe
Treatment	Behavior therapy (lay)	Diet and behavior therapy (medical)	Surgical

From Stunkard, A.J.: Treatment for obesity. In Stunkard, A.J., and Stellari, E., editors: Eating and its disorders, New York, 1984, Raven Press.

Table 11-8. Mean values for the distribution of calories in published diet plans

Diet	Energy (kcal)	Percent of Calories		
		Protein	Fat	Carbohydrate
Atkins	2136	23	72	5
Beverly Hills	1058	7	12	81
Carbohydrate Craver's Basic	1145	27	22	51
Carbohydrate Craver's Dense	1190	21	19	60
California (1200 kcal)	1240	27	26	47
California (2000 kcal)	1965	19	28	53
F-Plan	1256	20	24	56
I Love America	1256	25	29	46
I Love New York	1490	25	31	44
Pritikin (700 kcal)	748	30	11	59
Pritikin (1200 kcal)	1304	25	10	65
Richard Simmons*	915	25	28	47
Richard Simmons†	888	28	26	46
Scarsdale	1014	27	28	45
Stillman	1304	45	48	7

From Fischer, M.C., and Lachance, P.A.: Nutrition evaluation of published weight-reducing diets. Copyright The American Dietetic Association. Reprinted with permission from Journal of the American Dietetic Association, Vol. 85, p. 450, 1985.
*Selections made by person not having nutrition knowledge.
†Selections made by person having nutrition knowledge.

Analyses of the data from NHANES II showed a strong association between the prevalence of obesity and cardiovascular risk factors. Intervention studies cited at this consensus meeting confirmed that blood pressure levels and serum cholesterol can be reduced by weight reduction. Likewise, studies clearly show that weight reduction can reverse the abnormal biochemical characteristics of non-insulin-dependent diabetes mellitus.

In addition to the health-related aspects of obesity American society has such a preoccupation with thinness that dieting has become a national obsession. This preoccupation with dieting supports a lucrative business—the publication of diet books. Fisher and Lachance (1985) evaluated 11 published weight-reducing diets. Table 11-8 lists the mean caloric levels and the percentage of calories derived from protein, fat, and carbohydrate; Tables 11-9 and 11-10 list the vitamin and mineral content of the published diet plans expressed as percent of the U.S. RDA. The diversity of the types of diets shows that there is great variation in the nutritional adequacy and health risks of these diets.

Atherosclerosis and Coronary Heart Disease

Atherosclerosis is the most common age-related disorder in Western populations. The atherogenic process in humans begins early in life and develops progressively over the years. This change has been seen in the arteries of American males as early as the second decade of life, as documented by autopsies of American Korean and Vietnam War victims. In the United States there is a fivefold increase in the incidence of atherosclerosis from age 30 to age 65; more than 80% of cases are found in persons over age 65.

Clearly atherosclerosis is not simply the result of an unmodified intrinsic biological aging process, but rather it is a multifactorial disease. Thus an interaction of both the intrinsic aging process and environmental factors (such as diet) operates over many years and is superimposed on unknown genetic factors to produce the disorder.

Of the major factors involved in atherosclerotic risk, three are not reversible (male gender, intrinsic aging, and genetic factors); three are reversible (smoking, hypertension, and obesity) and, when reversed, the risk is reduced. Three

Table 11-9. Vitamin content of published diet plans expressed as percent of U.S. Recommended Daily Allowances

				U.S. RDAs (%)				
Diet	Vitamin A	Vitamin C	Thiamin	Riboflavin	Niacin	Vitamin B$_6$	Folacin	Vitamin B$_{12}$
Atkins	117	118	73	106	115	80	71	145
Beverly Hills	460	610	60	53	45	65	360	0
Carbohydrate Craver's Basic	283	360	93	106	115	70	82	63
Carbohydrate Craver's Dense	289	432	107	106	110	70	90	45
California (1200 kcal)	181	267	87	118	125	80	91	70
California (2000 kcal)	290	367	133	159	150	100	127	75
F-Plan	285	305	153	182	180	145	250	58
I Love America	159	380	87	112	110	60	82	55
I Love New York	316	515	93	135	145	80	106	177
Pritikin (700 kcal)	304	702	73	100	90	75	151	30
Pritikin (1200 kcal)	328	890	120	141	125	110	194	40
Richard Simmons*	68	158	67	82	105	50	58	45
Richard Simmons†	238	362	60	100	105	55	75	108
Scarsdale	228	555	60	71	115	65	84	37
Stillman	50	32	40	88	185	65	32	753

From Fischer, M.C., and Lachance, P.A.: Nutrition evaluation of published weight-reducing diets. Copyright The American Dietetic Association. Reprinted with permission from Journal of the American Dietetic Association, Vol. 85, p. 450, 1985.

*Selections made by person not having nutrition knowledge.

†Selections made by person having nutrition knowledge.

Table 11-10. Mineral content of published diet plans expressed as percent of the U.S. Recommended Daily Allowances

	U.S. RDAs (%)				
Diet	Calcium	Phosphorus	Magnesium	Iron	Zinc
Atkins	80	149	53	69	92
Beverly Hills	33	34	72	64	25
Carbohydrate Craver's Basic	97	127	87	76	71
Carbohydrate Craver's Dense	97	114	90	77	65
California (1200 kcal)	105	150	81	92	89
California (2000 kcal)	120	180	118	125	112
F-Plan	85	179	160	146	138
I Love America	93	129	77	70	75
I Love New York	100	145	108	102	93
Pritikin (700 kcal)	80	91	80	79	52
Pritikin (1200 kcal)	112	142	126	114	86
Richard Simmons*	54	85	53	47	50
Richard Simmons†	67	96	56	57	53
Scarsdale	52	90	74	56	52
Stillman	45	150	55	84	117

From Fischer, M.C., and Lachance, P.A.: Nutrition evaluation of published weight-reducing diets. Copyright The American Dietetic Association. Reprinted with permission from Journal of the American Dietetic Association, Vol. 85, p. 450, 1985.

*Selections made by person not having nutrition knowledge.

†Selections made by person having nutrition knowledge.

are related to abnormal carbohydrate and lipid metabolism (hyperglycemia, hypercholesterolemia, and hypertriglyceridemia) and are potentially reversible. Five major risk factors for the development of atherosclerosis are directly related to aging—hypertension, obesity, hyperglycemia, hypercholesterolemia, and hypertriglyceridemia.

Blood pressure levels also appear to increase inexorably with age, and the risk of atherosclerosis appears to increase progressively with increased blood pressure and can be diminished by therapeutic reduction of blood pressure.

Of the diseases related to nutritional excess, atherosclerosis is the most important in terms of severity and frequency. The relationship of atherosclerosis to diet is mediated largely by the blood lipids and their associated lipid proteins. Although there has been a decrease in the incidence of atherosclerosis over the past 2 decades, specific dietary recommendations have been outlined to achieve a greater decline in this disorder, which still accounts for about 50% of the deaths in the United States and is a leading health problem. Recent U.S. data based on very large sample sizes demonstrate unequivocally that the relationship between baseline serum cholesterol level and future risk of coronary heart disease is a continuous, graded, curvilinear relationship (Multiple Risk Factor Intervention Trial, 1982; Lipid Research Clinics Program, 1984). Increased coronary heart disease resulting from higher levels of serum cholesterol remains widely distributed in the U.S. population. This relationship is independent of age, race, blood pressure, cigarette use, and clinical diabetes (Stamler, 1984).

An expert panel, concurring with the 1978 Dietary Goals and the 1980 Dietary Guidelines, made specific recommendations in 1984. The Consensus Development Panel called on all Americans to adopt a diet that derives a maximum of 30% of its calories from fat, with no more than 10% from saturated fat, and provides a daily maximum of 300 mg of cholesterol (NIH Consensus Development Conference, Dec. 1984). The desirable cholesterol goal is a blood level of less than 180 mg/dl of blood serum for adults aged 20 to 29 and less than 200 mg for those 30 years and older. The typical middle-aged American has a cholesterol reading of 220 to 260 mg, which is considered too high by the Expert Committee.

Similar recommendations regarding hypercholesterolemia were made earlier in 1984 at an American Heart Association (AHA) news conference. A three-phase program with a progressive decrease in the intake of total fat, saturated fatty acids, and cholesterol was suggested. This progressive reduction occurs in the following phases (AHA, 1984):

Phase I	30% of total calories as fat (approximately equal amounts of saturated, mono-unsaturated, and polyunsaturated fatty acids; that is, each should contribute about 10% of total calories), 55% as carbohydrate (complex carbohydrates should constitute the major source), and 15% as protein; 300 mg/day of cholesterol
Phase II	15% of total calories as fat (with equal amounts of the three types of fatty acids), 60% as carbohydrate, and 15% as protein; 200 to 250 mg/day of cholesterol
Phase III	20% of total calories as fat (with equal amounts of the three types of fatty acids), 65% as carbohydrate, and 15% as protein; 100 to 150 mg/day of cholesterol

The rationale for using a low-fat, low-cholesterol diet for treatment of hypercholesterolemia is based on the following principles. It represents a reasonable extension of the diet recommended for the general public. It progressively decreases the major cholesterol-raising constituents in the diet (i.e., saturated fats and cholesterol). It precludes large intakes of polyunsaturated fats, and it facilitates weight reduction by removing foods of high caloric density.

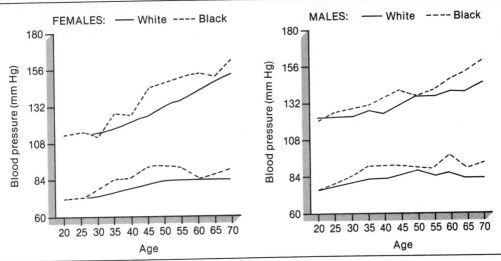

Figure 11-4. Blood pressure by age for white and black males and females in the United States from 1971 to 1975.
Redrawn from Harlan, W.R., et al.: Am. J. Epidemiol. **120**:1, 1984.

Hypertension

One of the most prevalent chronic conditions in the United States—hypertension—affects an estimated 23 to 60 million persons; the number depends on the criteria used to define the condition and the age-groups included. Hypertension of any degree is a major risk factor for the development of various diseases, including coronary heart disease, stroke, peripheral vascular disease, and chronic renal failure. The risk of death increases in direct proportion to blood pressure elevation. Labeled as the "silent killer," the condition is often asymptomatic and can go undetected.

Blood pressure, the pressure exerted by blood on the walls of blood vessels (especially arteries), generally is expressed as systolic (maximal) and/or diastolic (lowest) and is reported in units of millimeters of mercury (mm Hg). Arbitrary standards have been established. A blood pressure measurement consistently over 160 mm Hg systolic/90 mm Hg diastolic is usually considered abnormal, and adults with pressures exceeding 160/90 mm Hg are considered to have hypertension that would benefit from treatment. (The WHO value is 160/95.)

Although many factors have been associated with the development of hypertension, for more than 90% of patients, the actual cause is unknown. Today the most widely accepted view is that interacting factors, when occurring together, give rise to hypertension. These components include age, race, body weight, heredity, salt intake, kidney mass and function, hormonal activity, sympathetic nervous system activity (involuntary nervous system control of circulation) and associated medical problems, and environmental determinants such as psychological stress and nutrition.

Systolic and diastolic blood pressures were found to be progressively higher at successively older ages for U.S. males and females through age 55 based on NHANES-1 data (1971 to 1975) (Harlan et al., 1984) (Figure 11-4). Although systolic pressure was higher after this age, the relationship of diastolic pressure changed. For all men and for black women, the mean diastolic pressure plateaued, and for white men diastolic pressure was lower in the 65- to 75-year-old age-group. For white women, diastolic pressure was higher in the older groups, but the slope was less. Body mass index (weight/height^2) was the nutritional factor most strongly and consistently related to blood pressure.

There is a close relationship between obesity and hypertension. This association is found in adults, adolescents, and children. Hypertension is the most frequent cardiovascular risk factor in obesity. The black population shows higher blood pressure levels than the white population within the same relative weight group. Excessive consumption of sodium and obesity are the major determinants of high blood pressure in genetically susceptible persons. Alcohol abuse and diets deficient in potassium also tend to elevate blood pressure. Part of the confusion about the relationship between sodium intake (or output) and blood pressure results from the interplay of other determinants such as genetics, family history, weight, body mass index, sodium/potassium ratio, and possible role of calcium intake.

The 1984 recommendations of an expert committee of the National High Blood Pressure Education Program (NHBPEP) convened by the National Heart, Lung, and Blood Institute (NHLBI) were that nondrug therapies such as weight loss and life-style changes should be used as adjuncts in prevention and treatment of even the more severe cases of high blood pressure (National Heart, Lung, and Blood Institute, 1984). Although ideal body weight may not be achieved, there is a substantial decrease in blood pressure with even small increments of weight loss.

Other NHLBI recommendations were (1) to restrict dietary sodium to about 2 gm (5 gm salt) per day, with the acknowledgment that some hypertensive persons may not respond but the practice involves no risk; (2) to restrict alcohol intake to the equivalent of 4 ounces (120 ml) of hard liquor per day; (3) to embark on a daily exercise program; and (4) to reduce blood lipids. The

Table 11-11. Provider involvement in phases of high blood pressure control

Level of Participation and Steps in Control	Disciplines and Providers Involved
Detection	
Measure blood pressure Ascertain if elevated If elevated, refer to diagnosis	Dentistry, health education, medicine, nursing, optometry, pharmacy, physician assistants, podiatry
Evaluation, diagnosis, and initial therapy	
History taking, physical examination, laboratory tests Evaluate and correctly diagnose Refer to therapy Select correct therapy	Medicine; nurses and physician's assistants (within specified limits)
Long-term maintenance	
Fill prescription Follow prescribed therapy Monitor therapy Adjust therapy Continue above maintenance	Dentistry, health education, medicine, nursing, nutrition, optometry, pharmacy, physician assistants

From National Heart, Lung, and Blood Institute: Ann. Int. Med. 101:393, 1984.

1984 recommendations represent an increased emphasis on nondrug therapies since the last set of recommendations were issued in 1980.

The Coordinating Committee of the National High Blood Pressure Education Program has indicated that blood pressure control can be improved if patients, in their interactions with physicians and other professionals, are more active participants in their care (National Heart, Lung, and Blood Institute, 1984). It is now recognized that the quality of patient-provider interaction influences patient satisfaction and successful outcome. Important elements are patient and provider understanding of the expectations for each encounter, the quality of the interaction, and the degree to which expectations are met. Provider involvement in various phases of high blood pressure control is shown in Table 11-11. Although most patients see one physician and a pharmacist, some may see providers from many other disciplines such as nurses, nurse practitioners, nutritionists, health educators, and physician assistants.

Two critical ingredients for successful collaboration are the use of existing networks and resources and the creation of new ones. The NHBPEP Committee suggests that at the local, state, and national levels, professionals can increase their knowledge and gain mutual respect of each other's competence by establishing effective collaborative efforts (National Heart, Lung, and Blood Institute, 1984).

Diabetes

Diabetes is a serious health problem at all ages, but it is an especially grave problem among older persons. An estimated 17% of 65 year olds and 26% of 85 year olds have been diagnosed as having diabetes. At this time there is no agreement about whether decreased glucose tolerance is a characteristic of normal aging or a pathological change. This decreased glucose tolerance with aging has been related to many factors: (1) decreased lean body mass: muscle is the main tissue that uses glucose, and muscle mass is known to decrease with aging; (2) obesity: insulin receptor activity is known to be lower in obese persons, and body weight tends to increase up to age 70 and then declines; (3) poor diet; (4) physical inactivity: regular exercise maintains muscle mass and improves glucose tolerance in acute and chronic conditions; (5) decreased insulin secretion: this is possibly a result of senescence of the beta cells of the pancreas; hyperglycemia may accelerate beta-cell senescence; and (6) decreased response of peripheral tissues to insulin. Based on these assumptions, it is possible that regular exercise, avoidance of obesity, and proper nutrition can prevent, in part, the deterioration of glucose tolerance.

Diabetes mellitus represents both an inherited and an acquired disorder characterized by elevated circulating blood glucose levels. Nutrition management is preferred for both insulin-dependent (IDD, usually juvenile onset) and non-insulin-dependent (NIDD, usually adult onset) diabetes.

Epidemiological studies of world distribution of diabetes indicate that it is more common in countries with a high standard of living and a high prevalence of obesity. Diabetic persons have more severe atherosclerosis, twice as many heart attacks, and about twice as many strokes as nondiabetic persons of the same age. For diabetic women the risk of atherosclerotic disease is five times greater than for nondiabetic women. Community programs designed to administer to the needs of the diabetic patient will help reduce the morbidity and mortality from this disease.

Of the diabetic persons in the United States, 80% are non-insulin-dependent; 85% of these persons are obese. Obesity, long associated with abnormal carbohydrate metabolism, may be part of a complex disease or a primary factor responsible for abnormalities in insulin secretion and carbohydrate metabolism. An improvement in hyperinsulinemia and a resulting improvement in glucose metabolism are often seen with weight loss in the obese patient.

Treatment of diabetes requires a careful balancing of diet, insulin levels, and exercise in the dynamic context of a diabetic person's life-style. Thus an ongoing relationship with the health care system is essential. Individualization of the diabetes care plan requires continual assessment of the patient's educational needs in addition to evaluation of pertinent laboratory and physical parameters and diet history. A comprehensive approach to patient education strategy is one that incorporates the sociological approach of the health belief model, a psychological approach, and an educational approach based on patient-specific data (Wylie-Rosett, 1982). Treatment strategies differ with the two major classifications of diabetes: Type I (insulin-dependent) and Type II (non-insulin-dependent). Table 11-12 compares the two major forms of diabetes.

Table 11-12. Comparison of insulin-dependent diabetes mellitus (IDDM) and non-insulin-dependent diabetes mellitus (NIDDM)

Item	IDDM (Type I)	NIDDM (Type II)
Age	Usually under 40	Usually over 40
Sex	No difference	No difference
Race	No difference	No difference
Weight	Normal	60% to 90% obese
Insulin need	Dependent (ketosis without insulin)	May require to control hyperglycemia (no ketosis unless stress)
Diet	Adequate kilocalories to maintain weight	Restrict kilocalories
Plasma glucose	Variable	Stable
Plasma insulin	Low or absent	Low, normal, or high
Insulin receptors	Normal	Low or normal
HLA	B8, B15, Dw3/DR3, Dw4/DR4	No correlation
Islet cell antibodies	50% to 80% positive at diagnosis	Less than 5% positive at diagnosis
Associated autoimmune disease	Present	Absent
Vascular complications	Present	Present
Incidence	10% of diabetes	90% of diabetes
Clinical remission	Short-lived	May be prolonged (if weight loss successful)

From Whitehouse, F.W.: Classification and pathogenesis of the diabetes syndrome: a historical perspective. Copyright The American Dietetic Association. Reprinted by permission from Journal of the American Dietetic Association, Vol. 81, p. 243, 1982.

Specific guidelines have been issued for the treatment and prevention of non-insulin-dependent diabetes:

Energy	Maintain normal weight
Protein	12% to 20% of calories
Fat	30% to 38% of calories
Carbohydrate (complex)	50% to 60%
Sodium	Moderate use
Fiber	From food sources
Alcohol	Limited use (physician's approval)
Artificial sweetners	Moderate use

These guidelines, which are representative of the U.S. Dietary Guidelines, should be promoted with special attention to the maintenance of normal weight as a means to prevent non-insulin-dependent diabetes.

Cancer

Cancer is the second leading cause of death in the United States. More than one third of cancer deaths occur in the middle years (ages 35 to 64). The most common fatal cancers are lung, intestine, and breast cancer in adults and cancers of the intestine, lung, prostate, and uterus in the elderly. Epidemiologists have attempted to demonstrate a correlation between diet in modern affluent societies and the incidence of breast, colon, and uterine cancer. But it has proved to be difficult to establish causal relationships and to determine which, if any, of the dietary components is responsible.

Nutrition, in general, may be related to the development of cancer in three ways: (1) food additives or contaminants may act as carcinogens, cocarcinogens, or both; (2) nutrient deficiencies may lead to biochemical alterations that promote neoplastic processes; and (3) changes in the intake of selected macronutrients may produce metabolic and biochemical abnormalities, either directly or indirectly, which increase the risk for cancer (Reddy et al., 1980).

Excessive fat intake seems to be the most im-

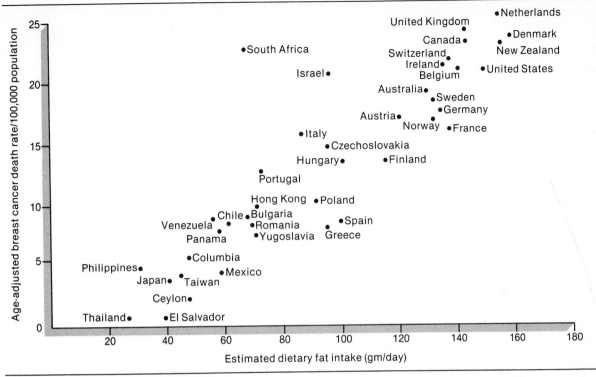

Figure 11-5. Correlation between age-adjusted death rates from female breast cancer and per capita consumption of fat.
Redrawn from Carroll, K.K., and Khor, H.T.: Prog. Biochem. Pharmacol. 10:308, 1975.

portant known environmental determinant of breast cancer. A positive correlation between breast cancer mortality and daily per capita consumption of fat has been demonstrated by a number of researchers (Figure 11-5).

Other epidemiological evidence seems to correlate high fat intake with colon cancer. Wynder and Reddy proposed that dietary fat influences the metabolic activity of the fecal microflora and thus may be involved in the pathogenesis of cancer of the colon (Reddy et al., 1980).

A review of epidemiological data with geographical representations does suggest that high fat intake and lack of fiber in the diet may be involved in the genesis of the disease. However, information about specific dietary factors in general are inconsistent or incomplete.

After an exhaustive study of dietary patterns, components of food, total caloric intake, lipids (fats and cholesterol), protein, carbohydrates, dietary fiber, vitamins (particularly vitamins A, C, and E), minerals (selenium, iron, copper, zinc, molybdenum, iodine, arsenic, cadmium, and lead), and known carcinogens, dietary recommendations have been made by the National Cancer Institute and the American Cancer Society (American Cancer Society, 1984):

- Avoid obesity.
- Cut down on total fat.
- Eat more high-fiber foods, such as whole-grain cereals, fruits, and vegetables.
- Include foods rich in vitamins A and C in the daily diet. Citrus fruits and members of the cabbage family are particularly stressed

here because of their capability of preventing gastrointestinal and respiratory cancers.

- Be moderate in consumption of alcoholic beverages.
- Be moderate in consumption of salt-cured, smoked, and nitrite-cured foods.

Osteoporosis

Osteoporosis, a metabolic bone disease characterized by decreased bone mass, is a major cause of spontaneous fractures and disability among the elderly. Each year in the United States as many as 200,000 persons age 60 or older suffer broken hips. Perhaps one sixth of these persons die of ensuing complications, and many of the survivors are incapacitated. About 25% of all white women have had one or more bone fractures by the age of 65. These fractures include, in addition to broken hips, about 100,000 broken wrists every year. Vertebral fractures, another major feature of osteoporosis, are usually "crush fractures," in which the vertebrae collapse simply from carrying the weight of the body. This type of fracture causes height loss and hump back that are often seen in the elderly. It has been estimated that acute medical care for elderly patients with broken hips is more than $1 billion a year, not including such indirect or long-term costs as lost income and fees for nursing homes, which amounts to $3.8 billion a year.

The acceleration of bone loss with menopause has been generally attributed to the deprivation of the hormone estrogen that occurs when the ovaries stop functioning. Osteoporosis can be caused by increased bone resorption without a counterbalancing increase in deposition, by impaired deposition, or by some combination of the two. Many investigators found that bone resorption in postmenopausal women with osteoporosis is abnormally high; after treatment with estrogen, the resorption decreases.

It is encouraging that in a group of elderly women with osteoporosis, bone density was increased by a combination of calcium-rich foods and a calcium supplement during a 6-month period (Rivlin, 1981). Thus the recommendation

is made that after menopause women may need to ingest approximately 1500 mg of calcium (as opposed to 800 mg per day before menopause). The ratio of calcium to phosphorus is another consideration. A diet high in calcium with consideration of phosphorous intake and adequate vitamin D and fluoride should be recommended.

The NIH Consensus Development Panel on Osteoporosis made a three-part recommendation for prevention (1984):

- Estrogen replacement in postmenopausal women
- Adequate nutrition, including an elemental calcium intake of 1000 to 1500 mg a day
- Regular weight-bearing exercise such as walking

Although the etiology of osteoporosis is complex and includes involvement of the parathyroid hormone, calcitonin, and other humoral agents, vitamin D inactivity, genetics, drug-nutrient interactors, and other factors, appropriate attention to nutritional factors is an important step toward prevention and treatment.

In terms of prevention, a significant contribution can be made by teaching young people the value of making physical activity and balanced nutrition with adequate calcium intake a lifelong habit. Prevention of bone mass loss in future generations may come from today's increased attention to physical fitness. For the older person with established osteoporosis, a therapeutic regimen that emphasizes a healthful life-style may prevent or reverse serious consequences.

Alcoholism

After heart disease and cancer, alcoholism is America's third largest health problem. It affects 10 million people, costs $60 billion per year, and is implicated in 200,000 deaths annually. Although preventive efforts are lower in the elderly than in the middle-aged population, the elderly are vulnerable to greater harm as a result of pharmacokinetic factors and increased tissue sensitivity.

A paper prepared for the White House Conference on Aging (1981) on the subject of alcoholism indicated that alcohol abuse is not the biggest problem in gerontology and aging is not the major concern of alcohol abuse workers. However, it was stated that there should be a thoughtful awareness that a problem does exist and should be of concern to those in the fields of alcoholism treatment and gerontology. Thus an opportunity exists for tangible and timely progress in research, preventive strategies, and active interventions.

Approximately two of every three adults in the United States use alcoholic beverages to some extent. A Harris survey (1974) found that approximately 73% of the men and 49% of the women surveyed identified themselves as drinkers, but only 45% of the adults over 65 years of age identified themselves as drinkers. This supports findings which claim that persons over 50 years of age drink less than when they were younger.

A number of researchers agree there are basically two types of elderly alcoholics: those who began alcohol abuse in their youth and those whose minimal drinking habits increased in old age because of the numerous problems that elderly persons encounter. Common conditions in later life that may lead to alcoholism include (1) retirement, with its attendant boredom, change of role status, and loss of income, (2) deaths among relatives and friends and awareness that more deaths are imminent, (3) poor health and discomfort, and (4) loneliness, particularly among elderly women (Brody, 1982). Consumption of alcohol may lead to a reduction in the intake of more nutrient-dense foods, which in turn may affect the nutritional status of the individual.

Demographic information suggests that the problems of alcohol abuse among the elderly increase in proportion to the population growth of that sector. About 10% to 15% of the elderly who seek medical attention for any reason have alcohol-related problems. Because treatment is relatively easy, detection during health-seeking sessions could have great potential value. It is likely that preventive efforts would find a much more responsive audience in the adult years than

during the teens or early twenties. A major prevention and education program would be of great interest to unions, management, the government, and anyone paying pensions or involved in health insurance. Many who have alcohol-related problems will seek help through medical sources, Alcoholics Anonymous, and other community resources when encouraged to do so.

The identification of nutrition and health-related risks and problems along with intervention and treatment strategies can prevent and delay or alleviate chronic diseases in adults and the elderly. Such a break in the sequence of disease will benefit society as a whole. Economic benefits are realized in the reduction of all components of health care costs. Concurrently personal, psychological, and social benefits will occur, with decreased disability and increased productivity and overall well-being, particularly as one gets older.

ASSESSMENT OF NUTRITIONAL STATUS

Nutritional assessment is an important part of providing nutrition services and has been discussed in Chapter 8. Dietary intake data, anthropometric measurements, biochemical analyses, and clinical evaluation are approaches commonly used to provide an adequate appraisal of an individual's nutritional status. Guidelines for assessing nutritional status along with intervention strategies for the adult appear in Table 11-13; those for the elderly are shown in Table 11-14.

Dietary Assessment

Data from major nutrition surveys—the Ten-State Nutrition Survey, the National Health and Nutrition Examination Surveys (NHANES), and USDA Food Consumption Studies, as well as data from studies by individual investigators—are used to assess the nutritional status of adults and elderly in the United States.

In 1982 an American Society of Clinical Nutrition Symposium examined specific nutrients as they relate to health issues of importance to the elderly (Rivlin and Young, 1982). In a summary statement it was suggested that when the nutritional intake of the population in general and the

Table 11-13. Nutrition assessment and intervention guidelines in community nutrition for adults

Nutritional Assessment Component	Methods	Risk and Problem Indicated	Intervention Guidelines	Referral Sources
Anthropometric 　Height 　Weight 　Skinfold thickness 　Arm circumference	Use standardized equipment for measuring—balanced scales, steel or nonstretch measuring tapes and calipers Use standardized height and weight tables (Metropolitan Life Insurance, 1983, and HANES weight by height by age for adults 18-74 years [U.S. 1971-74]) to determine weight status For skinfold thickness use measurements according to Durnin-Womersley procedure for triceps, biceps, subscapular and suprailiac skinfolds to determine body fat Use mid-arm muscle circumference measurement to indicate total lean body mass Use age- and sex-specific American standards—HANES	Moderate to severe underweight Moderate overweight to obesity	Adjust recommended weight to higher than average for underweight and lower than average for overweight/obesity If weight loss of more than 10 pounds in a year or below the lowest weight for height standard, determine reason for recent weight loss Adjust nutrient density of diet to compensate for increased or decreased energy requirement	Reputable physical fitness program and recreational facilities Worksite health promotion program Senior centers
Biochemical 　Hemoglobin 　Hematocrit 　Serum cholesterol and 　　other lipids 　Blood glucose	Use standardized laboratory equipment and laboratory quality control procedures Compare biochemical values to (1) Centers for Disease Control standards for hemoglobin and hematocrit adjusted for age, sex, and altitude, (2) North American Prevalence Study Reference Lipid, (3) National Diabetes Data Group, National Institutes of Health	Anemia Elevated cholesterol (>200 mg/dl) Hyperlipidemias, types I to V Diabetes	Adjust diet modifications to increase number of foods that are high in iron sources Adjust diet modifications for a moderately low total fat, particularly in saturated fats, and low in cholesterol content and adequate in protein Adjust personal diet modifications using diabetes exchange list	Public, private, and voluntary agencies State/local health departments State/local heart associations State/local diabetes associations Community hospitals
Clinical 　Medical history 　Blood pressure 　Cardiovascular disease 　　risk factor questionnaire—family history, diabetes, and stress 　Physical fitness 　Smoking 　Dental 　Socioeconomic status	Use clinical assessment and physical examination data to determine if there are one or more signs indicative of nutrition-related diseases Use questionnaire to determine risk factors for cardiovascular disease Use a sphygmomanometer and blood pressure procedures established by the Joint National	Hypertension (blood pressure >140/90 mm Hg) Risk of heart attack, stroke, and certain cancers (lung, esophagus, bladder) increases with number and severity of risk factors such as overweight, fat intake, hypertension, elevated cholesterol, smoking, inactivity, and stress	Encourage adherence to drug and diet modifications Develop personalized intervention plan on desirable life-style modifications that include diet and exercise	Stop-smoking clinics Food Stamp Program Cooperative extension services Emergency food programs

From Lee, S.L.: Clin. Nutr. 3:115, May/June 1984.

Table 11-13. Nutrition assessment and intervention guidelines in community nutrition for adults—cont'd

Nutritional Assessment Component	Methods	Risk and Problem Indicated	Intervention Guidelines	Referral Sources
	Committee on Detection, Evaluation and Treatment of High Blood Pressure Use treadmill test for physical fitness Use lung function test for smoking and other respiratory problems Examine oral cavity, condition of teeth and gums, and oral hygiene			
Dietary Evaluation 3-day food record 24-hour recall Food frequency	Determine quantity and quality of diet with special consideration given to alcohol, caffeine, fat, sodium, sugar, and fiber intakes	Alcoholism Drug abuse Marginal intakes of essential nutrients, which could lead to nutritional deficiencies Excessive intakes of foods/nutrients, which could lead to future nutritional problems	Investigate causal factors in substance abuse and suggest coping mechanism Adjust diet modifications in relation to other indicators that contribute to dietary amelioration	Alcoholics Anonymous Public, private, or voluntary behavioral health agencies/programs Consulting registered dietitians or public health nutritionists

elderly in particular is studied, each nutrient must be considered individually. The panel determined that some nutrients, such as iron, folate, and thiamin, generally appear to be consumed adequately by the healthy older population, whereas other nutrients, such as calcium and possibly zinc, are frequently consumed in inadequate amounts.

It is difficult to make comparisons among studies of the nutritional status of adults and the elderly or even to categorize findings of studies reported in the literature over time because the RDAs have been revised nine times since their inception in 1941. In addition, some investigators used 100% of the RDA as their standard of adequate intake, while others have used various levels of the RDA as standards (Garry et al., 1982). Differences in dietary methodology have also resulted in some inconsistencies in reported intake among similar population groups. Most frequently, dietary intake data are collected using the 24-hour recall, food records, or dietary

histories. Dietary methods have some limitations when used with the elderly. First, the 24-hour recall method, which is most frequently used, tends to underestimate energy intake; decreased short-term memory, hearing loss, and poor communication skills may also affect the validity and reliability of information elicited by this method. Also, not all surveys consider the contribution of alcohol to energy intake. Because each method has its advantages and disadvantages, it has yet to be determined which is the best to use with older subjects.

A review of the literature over the past 25 years reveals numerous national and regional studies performed to assess the nutritional status of both institutionalized and noninstitutionalized elderly by examining their dietary habits. The factors that have influenced findings in each of these studies are the region of study, age, sex, body size, and types of illnesses, as well as social and economic conditions and life-style—independent living versus institutionalized living.

Table 11-14. Nutrition assessment and intervention guidelines in community nutrition for the elderly

Nutritional Assessment Components	Methods	Risk and Problem Indicated	Intervention Guidelines	Referral Sources
Anthropometric Height Weight Skinfold thickness Arm circumference	Use standardized equipment for measuring—balanced scales, steel or nonstretch measuring tapes and calipers Use standardized height and weight tables (Metropolitan Life Insurance, 1983, and HANES weight by height by age for adults 18-74 years [U.S. 1971-74]) to determine weight status For skinfold thickness use measurements according to Durnin-Womersley procedure for triceps, biceps, subscapular and suprailiac skinfolds to determine body fat Use mid-arm muscle circumference measurement to indicate total lean body mass Use age- and sex-specific America standards—HANES	Moderate to severe underweight Moderate to overweight to obesity	Adjust recommended weight to higher than average for underweight and lower than average for overweight/obesity If weight loss of more than 10 pounds in a year or below the lowest weight for height standard, determine reason for recent weight loss Adjust nutrient density of diet to compensate for increased or decreased energy requirement	Weight Watchers International, Overeaters Anonymous, TOPS Reputable physical fitness program and recreational facilities Worksite health promotion program Senior centers
Biochemical Hemoglobin Hematocrit Serum cholesterol and other lipids Blood glucose	Use standardized laboratory equipment and laboratory quality control procedures Compare biochemical values to (1) Centers for Disease Control Standards for hemoglobin and hematocrit adjusted for age, sex, and altitude, (2) North American Prevalence Study Reference Lipid, (3) National Diabetes Data Group, National Institutes of Health	Anemia Elevated cholesterol (>250 mg/dl) with elevated proportion of low-density to high-density lipoproteins Hyperlipidemias, types I to V Diabetes	Adjust diet modifications to increase number of foods that are high in iron sources Adjust diet modifications for a moderately low total fat, particularly in saturated fats, low cholesterol content and adequate protein Adjust personal diet modifications using diabetes exchange list	Public, private, and voluntary agencies State/local health departments State/local heart associations State/local diabetes associations Community hospitals
Clinical Medical history Blood pressure Cardiovascular disease risk factor questionnaire—family history, diabetes, and stress	Use clinical assessment and physical examination data to determine if there are one or more signs indicative of nutrition-related diseases Use questionnaire to de-	Hypertension (blood pressure >140/90 mm Hg) Risk of heart attack, stroke, and certain cancers (lung, esophagus, bladder) increases with number and	Encourage adherence to drug and diet modifications Develop personalized intervention plan on desirable life-style modifications that include diet and exercise	Stop-smoking clinics Food Stamp Program Cooperative extension services Emergency food programs Title III congregate meal sites

From Lee, S.L.: Clin. Nutr. 3:115-116, May/June 1984.

Table 11-14. Nutrition assessment and intervention guidelines in community nutrition for the elderly—cont'd

Nutritional Assessment Components	Methods	Risk and Problem Indicated	Intervention Guidelines	Referral Sources
Physical fitness Smoking Dental Socioeconomic status	termine the number of risk factors for cardiovascular disease Use a sphygmomanometer and blood pressure procedures established by the Joint National Committee on Detection, Evaluation, and Treatment of High Blood Pressure Use treadmill test for physical fitness Use lung function test for smoking and other respiratory problems Examine oral cavity, condition of teeth and gums, and oral hygiene	severity of risk factors such as overweight, fat intake, hypertension, elevated cholesterol, smoking, inactivity, and stress Osteoporosis	Adjust dietary intakes higher than average recommendation for calcium and vitamin D	State welfare and social services programs
Dietary Evaluation 3-day food record 24-hour recall Food frequency	Determine quantity and quality of diet with special consideration given to alcohol, caffeine, fat, sodium, sugar, and fiber intakes Determine quantity of multiple drugs or chronic drug therapy with possible food-related side effects or nutrient deficiencies or complications related to alcohol consumption Determine quantity of vitamin and mineral supplementation	Alcoholism Drug abuse and non-compliance with prescribed drug regimen Added self-medication increases the possibility of drug-drug and drug-nutrient interactions Possible therapeutic failure due to inappropriate timing of drug ingestion Possible nutrient deficiencies due to chronic drug use Possible toxic reaction due to alcohol ingestion Marginal intakes of essential nutrients, which could lead to nutritional deficiencies Excessive intakes of nutrients or vitamins/minerals, which could lead to future nutritional problems	Investigate causal factors in substance abuse and suggest coping mechanisms Adjust prescribed drug regime and work on dietary and drug compliance Adjust diet modifications in relation to other indicators of risk that contribute to dietary ameloriation	Alcoholics Anonymous Public, private, or voluntary behavioral health agencies/programs Consulting registered dietitians or public health nutritionists

Table 11-15. Response rates of elderly in nutrition and health research studies

Researchers	Location of Study	Study Description				Number Approached	Positive Response Rate (%)		
		Sample Age	Length of Commitment	Demands	Method of Contact		Total	Male	Female
Krondl et al., 1977	Toronto, Canada	65 to 77	3 years overall	Two interviews—food frequency and food perceptions, demographic information; nutrition intervention program (7 weeks)	Flyer followed by personal visit or telephone call by nutritionist	942 (502 men, 440 women)	21	15	25
Akhtar, 1972	Scotland	65 +	2 appointments	Medical, social, psychiatric and dietary survey	Personal visit by health officer	286 (177 men, 169 women)	70	84	60
Grotkowski and Sims, 1977	United States	62 +	1 week	Knowledge and attitude questionnaire and 3-day food record; group meeting; home visit	Through senior citizen's group	64 (15 men, 49 women)	62	—	—
Leichter et al., 1978	Vancouver, Canada	60 +	Not known	24-hour food record; blood and urine analyses	Letter followed by personal visit by nutritionist to public housing units	201 (111 men, 90 women)	28	29	27
Milne et al., 1971	Scotland	62 +	2 appointments	Physical and psychiatric examination	Home visit by personal physician	748 (285 men, 463 women)	65	76	59
Morgan et al., 1971 —	New Orleans, Louisiana	Not reported; low-income families	2 appointments	Nutritional/health survey—dental, physical examination; blood, urine, fecal analyses; anthropometric diet history	1. Personal visit by inexperienced interviewer 2. Personal visit by competent interviewer	228 families 140 families	20 40	— —	— —
Nutrition Canada 1973	All Canadian	65 +	2 appointments	Clinical anthropometric and dental examination; blood and urine analyses; 24-hour dietary recall	Letter followed by personal visit by advance team	4277 (2146 men, 2131 women)	42	43	40
Nutrition Canada 1973	Ontario, Canada	65 +	As above	As above	As above	828 (404 men, 424 women)	32	31	32

From Coleman, P., and Krondl, M.: J. Can. Diet. Assoc. **42**:352, 1981.

Nutrient intake and nutritional status of the elderly are influenced by four basic factors (Guthrie, 1986):

1. Physical: decreased activity, physical weakness, loss of neuromotor coordination, loss of teeth
2. Physiological: depressed kidney function, decreased taste sensitivity, use of drugs, decreased digestive efficiency, constipation, lactose intolerance
3. Psychological: depression, amnesia, food preferences, long-standing food habits
4. Social: income, living facilities, food beliefs, susceptibility to food fads, and loneliness

In addition to the many variables mentioned, there are other conditions to be considered. Factors such as travel, moving, illness, and death make it difficult to recruit a sample among the elderly. Seniors with few health problems may feel little need to become involved, whereas others apparently fear the discovery of disease. Some consider health surveys an intrusion on privacy. A comparison of response rates of elderly in nutrition and health research studies is shown in Table 11-15.

Anthropometric Variables

The selection of anthropometric variables for the determination of nutritional status in the elderly must be based on validity, the availability of standardized measurement techniques and reference data, and practicality (Roche, 1982). The two groups of anthropometric variables are (1) weight, relative weight (i.e., weight for stature or age, usually expressed as a percentage of the median for a reference population), and weight for stature on a percentile basis and (2) triceps and subscapular skinfold thickness and upper arm circumference, with or without correction for fat. With aging, usually there is not only a decrease in body weight, but also a change in body composition. There is a decrease in lean body mass and a relative increase in body weight as a result of fat. Weight measurements are easily ob-

tained from adults and are useful if no edema is present.

Biochemical and Clinical Assessment

Medical history, routine blood analyses, blood pressure measurement, cardiovascular disease-risk questionnaire, family history, stress factors, physical fitness, smoking history, dental evaluation, and socioeconomic factors are reviewed with the client.

For the most part (as with dietary standards) the biochemical standards that are used to judge nutritional status in the elderly are essentially an extrapolation of data derived from younger populations. In NHANES anemia was seen in a large proportion of the elderly, particularly among blacks. This was represented by a high percentage of low hemoglobin levels (less than 14 gm/dl in men and less than 12 gm/dl in women). However, the usual nutritional factors that cause anemia when deficient (iron, folate, vitamin B_{12}, and pyridoxine) could not account for the high prevalence of anemia in the elderly NHANES population. Of the biochemical nutrient values measured in NHANES, the highest prevalence of low values found among the elderly were serum folic acid, urinary riboflavin, and thiamin. Although other biochemical indicators are reported (amino acids, protein, serum albumin, urea, and creatinine), the exact interpretation based on available data is somewhat limited. Research is needed to set standards.

After assessment of the client's nutritional status, the nutritionist is ready to counsel the adult or geriatric client about normal nutrition with a modified diet (Chapter 12). The practitioner needs to be aware of the economic, social, and homemaking support available to tailor the counseling session to specific needs.

ASSURING QUALITY OF HEALTH CARE FOR ADULTS AND ELDERLY

Specific guidelines for patient management have emerged that incorporate specific expected health outcomes in a health promotion/disease prevention model. These guidelines are recommendations for evaluating the quality of care that provide quality assurance standards.

- Client maintains acceptable weight and height based on the Metropolitan weight tables.
- Client does not deviate more than 25 percentile points from established pattern of weight.
- Client maintains normal blood sugar: 90 to 100 mg/dl.
- Client maintains blood pressure of less than 140/90 mm Hg.
- Client maintains plasma cholesterol levels less than 200 mg/dl.
- Client does not smoke.
- Client consumes adequate amount of nutrients, fiber, and water with caloric intake to maintain acceptable weight.
- Client maintains hemoglobin level between 12 to 15 gm.
- Client reviews appropriate types and amounts of food as defined by Dietary Guidelines.

NUTRITION SERVICES AT THE COMMUNITY LEVEL

A comprehensive network of services to meet the needs of clients is often available at the community level (Figure 11-6). The two most widely used food assistance programs available to adults and the elderly at the community level are the Congregate Meals Program and the Food Stamp Program. A description of federally sponsored food assistance programs for adults and the elderly appears in Table 11-16.

Congregate Meals Program (Title III)

The Nutrition Program for Older Americans, mandated in 1972 through Title VII, appropriated monies to establish a feeding program for the elderly on a national basis. It is known today as the Congregate Meals Program or Title III.*

*For further information, see McCool, A.C., and Posner, B.M.: Nutrition services for older Americans: foodservice systems and technology, Chicago, 1982, The American Dietetic Association.

Congregate meals, which constitute most of the meals served, are available at senior citizen centers, religious facilities, schools, community centers, public housing projects, and restaurants. The five major goals of the Title III program are:

1. To establish nutrition projects that serve at least one hot meal a day 5 days a week at either the congregate meal setting or by home delivery; this meal is to provide at least one third of the RDAs
2. To encourage participation of target groups for social interaction
3. To make available nutrition and homemaker education and shopping assistance when necessary
4. To counsel and refer to other social and rehabilitative services
5. To offer transportation services

An Administration on Aging evaluation carried out in 1982 indicated that the nutrition program was a major instrument in the 1980s to successfully eliminate malnutrition among the elderly, especially the poor and disadvantaged. One concern in the study was the slackening of outreach activities in recent years (CNI, Sept. 1983). Other program evaluations have shown that the major positive effects are increased socialization and improved life satisfaction of participants.

Food Stamp Program

An innovative program, introduced in mid-1984, for use of food stamps by the elderly and disabled includes eating meals at certain restaurants in the state of New York. Sixty-six restaurants have been certified, and approval is pending for 200 more if they meet the requirements set by the USDA. The restaurants must offer nutritionally balanced meals at a minimum discount of 5%. The program was designed particularly to meet the needs of people over the age of 60 who are either incapacitated and unable to prepare meals or who live in accommodations without cooking facilities.

Food stamp allotment levels for fiscal year 1985 reflect a 3% increase for a four-person household compared with 1984. The increase re-

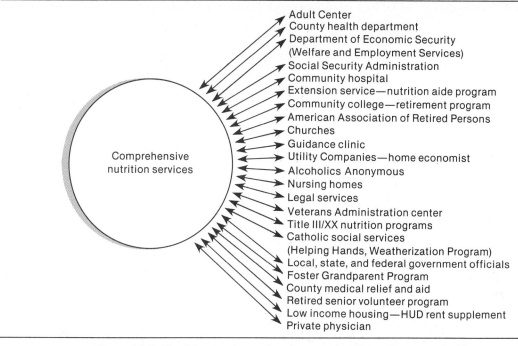

Figure 11-6. Nutrition services referral system for those 60 years and older.

Table 11-16. Federally sponsored food assistance programs for adults and elderly

Program	Purpose of Program	Administering Agencies
Food Stamp Program	Assist families in providing nutritious meals	USDA Food and Nutrition Service (FNS) and state welfare agencies
Food Donation/Commodity Distribution Programs	Encourage and maintain the domestic consumption of commodities; prevent the waste of commodities	USDA Food and Nutrition Service (FNS)
Department of Health and Human Services (DHHS): Title III Nutrition Services	Provide low-cost nutritious meals to the elderly who cannot afford to eat adequately, lack meal preparation skills, have limited mobility, or are lonely	DHHS Human Development Services Office of Administration on Aging and state agencies on aging

From Lee, S.L.: Clin. Nutr. 3(3):119, May/June 1984; modified from Owen, A.L., Owen, G.M., and Lanns, G.: Health and nutritional benefits of federal food assistance programs. In Costs and benefits of nutritional care: phase I, Chicago, 1979, The American Dietetic Association, and Budget of the U.S. government, 1984, Appendix, Washington, D.C., 1984, Executive Office of the President, Office of Management and Budget.

Table 11-17. A day's food as served for four individuals: 1983 Thrifty Food Plan

Food	Unit	Child 6 to 8 Years	Child 9 to 11 Years	Woman 20 to 50 Years	Man 20 to 50 Years
		Number of Units			
Vegetables, fruit	½ cup	3.4	4.0	4.9	4.3
Cereal, pasta (dry)	1 oz	2.7	2.9	2.6	2.7
Bread	1 slice	6.2	6.7	5.8	8.4
Bakery products	1 slice	0.9	1.2	0.3	1.2
Milk, yogurt	1 cup	1.7	2.1	1.1	0.9
Cheese (per week)	1 oz	1.2	1.6	4.4	2.0
Meat, poultry, fish, boned	1 oz	2.1	2.4	4.1	4.0
Eggs (per week)	no.	1.8	2.4	4.2	3.9
Cooked dry beans, peas, nuts	½ cup	0.3	0.4	0.7	0.7
Fats, oils	1 tbsp	2.3	2.7	0.9	3.1
Sugar, sweets	1 tbsp	3.7	4.2	0.7	4.9
Soft drinks, punches, ades	1 cup	0.2	0.2	0.1	0.3

From U.S. Department of Agriculture: Fam. Econ. Rev. 1:23, 1984.

flects the delay in cost of living increases, which are legislated to lag significantly behind the actual impact of higher food costs. The figures are adjusted to reflect the cost of food in the Thrifty Food Plan for June of the preceding year.

The Thrifty Food Plan

The Thrifty Food Plan is the least costly of the four food plans developed by the Human Nutrition Information Service/USDA. Like the more costly plans, this plan specifies the quantities of different types of foods (food groups) that households might use to provide nutritious diets for household members. The Thrifty Food Plan was revised in 1983 to reflect the 1980 RDAs and to use new information on the content of nutrients in food that has become available since the previous update in 1975. Also, recent data on food eaten by men, women, and children of different ages on a nationwide basis have become available with USDA's Nationwide Food Consumption Survey, which gathered data on food intake of individuals in households eligible to receive food stamps. Data from this study were used to estimate the quantities of foods used to prepare meals and snacks; these data were used as starting points in developing the new Thrifty Food Plan.

A summary of the daily quantities of foods in units from 12 groups in the food consumption patterns for a four-person household are shown in Table 11-17.

Sample meals, with recipes and lists of foods used in their preparation, have been developed for families of four persons following the revised Thrifty Food Plan. Copies of the meal plans, *Making Food Dollars Count—Nutritious Meals at Low Cost*, USDA HG-240, are available for 50¢ from the Consumer Information Center, Pueblo, CO 81009.

Long-Term Care Services

Long-term care refers to the support services needed by persons who have functional limitations resulting from or in conjunction with chronic illness or other conditions that make them frail and dependent (White House Conference on Aging, Vol. 1, 1981). It is an area of particular concern to the elderly. There is widespread agreement that a long-term care system should promote independence in making decisions and in performing everyday activities. It should encourage support services in the least restrictive environment, preferably at home or in other community settings. In addition, it should try to make available appropriate, cost-effective, accessible and humane care to all persons who need it while supporting the care provided by family and friends. For those chronically impaired persons in nursing homes and institutional settings, long-term care should ensure the quality of care and seek to maximize the quality of life.

Long-term care needs are financed by a variety of federal, state, local, and private programs and expenditures. The principal federal programs that provide resources for long-term care needs are Medicaid, Medicare, the Social Services Block Grant, Supplemental Security Income, Title III of the Older Americans Act, Veterans Administration programs for disabled veterans and their families, and Department of Housing and Urban Development housing construction and assistance programs.

Prevention Programs in the Workplace

Cardiovascular disease costs American industry and its workers billions of dollars and a reduced quality of life. Industry pays for cardiovascular disease through escalating insurance costs, which are based on the health care experience of its employees, and through absenteeism, decreased productivity, employee replacement and training costs, disability claims, and death benefits. The total cost to the nation from cardiovascular disease is estimated at about $80 billion annually. This $80 billion separates into $26 billion in medical care spending (direct costs) and $54 billion in indirect costs (morbidity and mortality).

The health care costs associated with hypertensive disease total approximately $4 to $5 billion, with a similar figure for indirect costs. The full impact of hypertensive disease, however, must include the cost of its sequelae or complications—heart disease, stroke, and arterial disease.

Corporate costs are rising. Cardiovascular disease–related medical care costs and insurance coverage increases have led to a 10% to 20% per year increase in employers' costs during the last 20 years. A typical corporation in the United States is estimated to spend $1000 to $1500 per year in medical care for each worker and his or her family. With 30 years of research into heart diseases,

the NHLBI has been consulting with industry to undertake joint efforts to reduce major risk factors that contribute to cardiovascular disease.

Some health education and disease intervention programs have already influenced these costs in terms of fewer lost work days, decreased turnover, and decreased insurance costs. Industry is interested in these cost savings. General Motors, Ford Motor Company, Campbell Soups, Johnson & Johnson, Pepsico, and Xerox Corporation are only a few of the many companies investing in health promotion and disease prevention among workers. To meet the demand for weight control in the workplace, Weight Watchers International has developed a special program—Weight Watchers at Work—which is available in communities across the country. Programs in the workplace have become increasingly popular and offer an opportunity for innovative community efforts by the community dietitian/nutritionist.

Innovative Strategies at the Local, Regional, and State Levels

Community dietitians/nutritionists must develop innovative programs for nutrition intervention for adults and the elderly at the local, regional, and state levels. Following are some examples of creative programs that community dietitians/nutritionists have successfully implemented.

PRIVATE PRACTICE
The Expanding Role of the Community Nutritionist
Maria Muesler, R.D., Nutrition Consultant, Suffolk County, Long Island

As the director of INTAKE, Nutrition Counseling Services in Suffolk County, Muesler has developed an innovative approach to serving her community. In a renal dialysis center she accepted the title of "nutritionist" rather than "dietitian" at the request of the physician-in-charge who saw "total" nutrition of the patient as far more encompassing than "diet" alone. Based on clinical and laboratory findings, the diet/nutrition prescription is designed by the nutritionist, who works closely with the nurse and other members of the team in assessing the needs of the patient and designing the health care plan with the family.

As a consultant to group homes for the mentally retarded and day treatment centers, she expands the team concept even further to include the goals that the multidisciplinary team has for the patient. Here the psychiatrist, physical therapist, speech therapist, psychologist, nutritionist, nurse, physician, and pharmacist establish the priorities to be considered; each person must compromise if necessary.

PRIVATE PRACTICE
Private Practice/Nutrition Counseling
Kathy King Helm, R.D., Sports Nutrition

Using the tools of business management allows Kathy King Helm to take nutrition to the consumer, which has resulted in a lucrative and successful practice. Her secret is marketing of her professional skills. A survey conducted for ADA on how heads of households view dietitians found that 65% to 70% would probably consult with a dietitian if their physician, dentist, or child's teacher made such a referral. The market does exist! Helm suggests a market survey be conducted to assess nutritional needs in the community; then the community dietitian/nutritionist must know what to "sell" to the consumer.

The steps Helm recommends in such a survey include the following (King, 1982):

1. Decide what you have to sell—skills, expertise, knowledge—so you can narrow your questioning if necessary.
2. Know where and to whom can you "sell" your skills. Talk to your potential "buyers" and find out what they want and what would they be willing to pay.
3. Know your competition and how well they are doing. Determine how strong they are in the market. Decide if you can improve on what they offer or do it better.
4. Develop what your research has shown will "sell." Brochures, handouts, nutrition consultations, slide presentations, nutrient analysis programs, books or articles, along with your improved image, could eventu-

ally increase your effectiveness, influence, and income. Decide if you need to improve your expertise, experience, or education.

The six market outlets or tools that Helm recommends include:

1. Media. Use television, radio, newspapers, and magazines (public service information, press releases, articles, guest spots, and paid advertisements). Keep reprints or video or audio copies for future promotional use.
2. Public speaking. Many groups are willing to pay $25 to $150 for a local speaker. Make your calling cards and brochures available to pass around.
3. Direct mail. Mailing an announcement, survey, or brochure to physicians and clinics may increase their awareness of available nutrition services, but immediate response may be 2% or less. A personal visit should probably follow a mail-out for best results.
4. Publishing in journals or books. If your skills are weak in this area but you do have good, timely information and a publisher, work with an editor or writer.
5. Other resources. Use local, accessible outlets such as bulletin boards, newsletters, medical or dietetic meetings, letters to the editor, health fairs, "point of sale" educational material in your cafeteria, and community and volunteer organizations.
6. Image. Improve your effectiveness by improving your personal and professional image.

Persons who are well want to stay that way. Because more people are in good health than in ill health, marketing nutrition services should change to recognize this fact. The public, both ill and well, is very excited about nutrition and what it can do. "I feel strongly that people want accurate information from qualified nutritionists, and we should reach out to them now. Improved 'packaging' of ourselves as well as our 'products' will make us more competitive in the marketplace" (King, 1982).

Helm's research indicated strong consumer interest in sports. This led her to take a graduate course in exercise physiology and in turn to work with athletes and trainers. She has been invited to speak on sports nutrition at coaches' conferences and medical seminars. The Denver Broncos football team, the Denver soccer team, and karate competitors seek her advice.

PRIVATE PRACTICE
New Models for Dietetic Practice
Mary Abbott Hess, R.D., Hess & Hunt, Inc.

In late 1979 Hess & Hunt, Inc., Nutrition Education/Communication was formed to meet the growing need for a dependable and professional nutrition support service for business, industry, and government.

This firm brought together the technical expertise of Mary Abbott Hess, a registered dietitian and nutrition educator, and Anne Hunt, a home economist with a background in food journalism and public relations. Their skills, together with a support staff of specialists in nutrition education, food service, human development, marketing, and design, offer nutrition communications that are both creative and accurate.

Hess & Hunt, Inc., has found their clients in four major areas:

1. *Government and social service agencies.* One of their first clients was Chicago's Nutrition, Education, and Training program. The Office for Senior Citizens and Handicapped emerged as a major client when the firm developed food specifications and cycle menus for their congregate and home-delivered meals. The firm also monitors food service contractors and provides food safety and sanitation workshops for workers. To meet the nutrition education requirement of federally funded programs, a "miniposter" series that addresses the special needs of the urban elderly was developed. This series has received national attention.

2. *The food industry and their public relations firms.* Pamphlets, scripts, videotapes, and other informational materials were developed for consumers. Hess & Hunt acted as spokespersons for selected products that contribute to healthful diets.

3. *The food service industry.* Menu items, recipes, and training materials were developed for a major restaurant chain to meet the public's demand for light, fresh, healthful menu choices. Posters, place mats, and quizzes have been produced for employee cafeterias, hospitals, and nursing home food services.

4. *Print and electronic media.* In response to the need for information about the relationship of diet to pregnancy, Hess and Hunt wrote *Pickles and Ice Cream: The Complete Guide to Nutrition During Pregnancy* (1982). This book won the Fishbein Award for excellence in medical writing from the American Medical Writers Association. Numerous appearances on radio and television talk shows, participation in the American Dietetic Association, a satellite program on nutrition misinformation, presentations to professional groups, and frequent consultations and quotes for newspaper reporters and editors have added to the firm's visibility.

Hess and Hunt emphasize that, in addition to being skilled nutrition communication and education practitioners, community dietitians/nutritionists must also be skilled in business techniques. Involvement in professional and community organizations and networks is a priority. Management of a business requires continuing education for the best possible decisions and actions. A considerable amount of time and energy is put into marketing the firm's ability to develop innovative, accurate nutrition materials and programs that help meet the needs of today's society.

REGIONAL NUTRITION SERVICES
Regional Health Center/Nutrition Services
Elvira J. Johnson, R.D., Nutrition Services Coordinator

Here, too, a survey gave direction to nutrition services for a community. A random survey of five middle-income communities north of Boston indicated that residents were especially interested in nutrition being available at the Regional Health Center in Wilmington (RHCW), a modern ambulatory health care facility.

Because RHCW serves a middle-income population, it is not eligible for any state or federal nutrition monies. But today, thanks to Johnson, income has been generated by fees for individual nutrition counseling, weight control groups, and local corporate support. As a hospital-based facility, RHCW is eligible for third-party reimbursement for nutrition services (with physician referrals) from certain insurance companies, which cover 62% of the population.

Reaching out to meet the needs of the community has caused services to become diversified—community health education services, a diabetes service, parenting and fitness courses, speaker's bureaus, and programs for industries. Local supermarkets and industries provide food items and personnel for cooking demonstrations and new product tasting by clients.

Direct income for RHCW is generated from weight control groups, industry programs, and some community health education programs. Indirect income for RHCW is also generated; statistics show that 60% to 75% of nutrition program participants had never used RHCW and many of these new clients often go on to use other RHCW services.

STATE NUTRITION SERVICES
Massachusetts Nutrition Resource Center—A Telephone Hot Line and Mail Service
Johanna Dwyer, Principal Investigator

The Massachusetts Nutrition Resource Center, which originated in 1979, is funded by the Massachusetts Department of Public Health, Division of Preventive Medicine, and staffed by the Frances Stern Nutrition Center of Tufts University New England Medical Center. Their nutrition hot line provides consumers and health professionals with reliable nutrition information. A toll-free number makes the center's services

available throughout the state on Monday through Friday, 9:00 AM to 3:00 PM.

The center has up-to-date nutrition files, a reference library, and extensive directories of nutrition services throughout the state. Consumers, about 80% of the hot line callers, most often ask about the nutritional content of foods, from the best source of calcium to the sodium content of a dill pickle. Questions on diets and weight loss are next in popularity. Many callers look for ways to implement therapeutic diets. The staff also answers questions and provides information through the mail. The center staff has developed more than 50 fact sheets on various nutrition topics.

The various projects undertaken by this innovative group and the growth in mail and phone inquiries are listed below:

1979 to 1980	Establish the Massachusetts Nutrition Resource Center: protocols, filing system, resource directory, advisory board, collection of materials
1980 to 1981	Senior citizen campaign National Nutrition Month activities Adolescent Pregnancy Conference Food additives awareness
1981 to 1982	Heart Health Project (target: low-income Boston area population) Education materials developed on fat, sodium, and weight control
1982 to 1983	Day-Care Newsletter (bimonthly nutrition newsletter for day-care providers) Toll-free hot line—Statewide outreach of Massachusetts Nutrition Resource Center services
1983 to 1984	Day-Care Newsletter (continued) Statewide outreach of Massachusetts Nutrition Resource Center services Low-income project

A summary of the total mail requests and nutrition hot line calls answered by the Resource Center are:

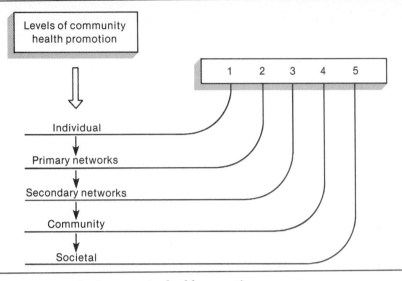

Figure 11-7. Levels of community health promotion.
Courtesy R. Mullis, C. Perry, and P. Pierie, Division of Epidemiology, School of Public Health,
University of Minnesota, 1985.

	Mail Requests	Hot Line Calls
1979 to 1980	406	2640
1980 to 1981	497	3461
1981 to 1982	1330	4232
1982 to 1983	2037	6520
1983 to 1984	2057	7987
1984 to 1985	2348	8201

STATE NUTRITION SERVICES
**Levels of Community Health Promotion: A System Model for
Nutrition Education**
Minnesota Heart Health Program, Rebecca M. Mullis, R.D.,
University of Minnesota

The Minnesota Heart Health Program is a systems approach to community nutrition education that uses a variety of support systems and networks in a multiplicity of settings as seen in Figure 11-7.

The *individual* is the one who eventually must choose behavior patterns and whose health ultimately will be affected by these choices. The individual's awareness of appropriate food behavior and knowledge and attitudes about food and its value for personal health promotion contribute to the adoption or rejection of that behavior.

Food-related decisions are also influenced by *primary networks* such as personal support, close communication, and mutual responsibility and generally involve family and close friends.

Secondary networks are characterized by mutual support, external incentives, individual feedback, and formalized structures, which also influence food choices.

The *community* provides opportunities for individuals to make healthful or unhealthful food decisions because grocery stores, restaurants, educational institutions, and regulations all reflect community values.

At the *societal* level information about food and nutrition comes to individuals through product marketing, mass media, the government, and legislative bodies.

The Minnesota Heart Health Program adopted a model such as the one described earlier in their efforts to develop a nutrition education program. A research and demonstration project, it has been designed to reduce risk of cardiovascular diseases by direct education, external motivation, skills training, and communitywide promotion and reinforcement.

Hospital: Changing Nutrition Services in the Hospital*

HOSPITAL SERVICES
United Hospitals, Inc., St. Paul, Minnesota
Paul Deignan, R.D., Director, Nutrition Services

Financial and regulatory pressures are causing hospitals to reexamine the way they conduct business and their role in the health care industry. As a result, many changes are occurring in the organization of hospitals and in the ways hospitals deal with the complexities of technology, government regulations, fiscal affairs, and competition in the health care market.

United Hospitals, Inc., held a forum, Successful Business Applications in Nutrition Services, to share the strengths of their program in dealing with these increased pressures. Although the patient mix, operating procedures, and role of the dietary department vary widely among hospitals, United Hospitals' experience offers valuable insights to other hospitals and dietitians in this era of rapid change.

One of the changes was a fee-for-service system for which planning began 1½ years before implementation. There were six steps involved in the planning phase: (1) documenting the need for such a system, (2) getting staff commitment to the plan, (3) getting hospital administrative commitment, (4) involving financial/business personnel, (5) explaining the new system to other members of the health care team, and (6) training staff members.

Documentation of the clinical dietitian's activities gathered through time studies, task lists, and ongoing record logs provided the necessary data to justify the need for and to establish a fee-for-service system.

*Modified from Business applications in clinical dietetics, Ross Timesaver Dietetic Currents 11:3, May-June 1984.

Many programs initiated since this reorganization of United Hospitals have contributed to a high level of staff commitment. Through a technical exchange with the University of Cleveland, the business systems unit has introduced a computerized nutrient analysis system and hand-held computers that supply formulary computation. The data base also supplies information for recipe development and scaling, food production scheduling, and meal forecasting. The computerized business department system handles ordering of food and supplies from primary vendors, manages inventory control, and tracks patient admission, discharge, and billing.

Advances in food technology enabled patient services teams to provide better meals to patients. Introduction of a cook/chill system resulted in a 500% increase in hot food production over conventional methods. A tunnel microwave, used to reheat chilled foods, produces a maximum of six hot meals per minute.

Further success was made possible by a dynamic marketing strategy that made announcements of the range of services that the Nutrition Services Department could offer to the public both inside and outside the hospital.

Industry: Reach out for Health

INDUSTRIAL NUTRITION SERVICES
Southern New England Telephone (SNET)
Rosann Ippolito, R.D., Nutrition Consultant

In addition to instituting a nutrition education program for all SNET cafeterias throughout Connecticut, other nutrition enterprises have become available to SNET employees in a health promotion program. Five courses are offered in the areas of nutrition and weight control: Nutrition Awareness Program (a comprehensive look at contemporary nutrition issues); Keep It Off Program (a skills-oriented behavior modification approach to weight control); The Pressure Cooker (a two-class series that examines the relationship between sodium intake and health); Nutrition Potpourri (a three-class series of diverse topics such as nutritional needs of the athlete and the pros and cons of vitamin supplementation);

and Nutrition Nonsense in America (a four-class series that addresses the needs and concerns of the consumer). Each course has a specific built-in evaluation. Within the first year of the program, 2320 employees participated in orientation, health screening, and counseling; 37% enrolled in health education and fitness classes, with 20% of the 37% participating in the various nutrition programs available.

SUMMARY

This chapter has considered those issues that relate to nutrition, the nutritional needs of adults and the elderly, and nutrition-related diseases of this age-group with specific guidelines for treatment and prevention. Programs that are examples of innovative approaches have been reviewed. It is possible to pass through adulthood and enjoy an active, productive, and involved life in the later years if attention is given to preventive health measures.

REFERENCES

American Cancer Society: Nutrition and cancer: care and prevention, Report CA-A, Cancer J. Clin. 34:121, 1984.

American Heart Association: Special report: recommendations for treating hypercholesterolemia in adults, News Conference, May 15, 1984.

Belloc, N.B., and Breslow, L.: The relation of physical health status and health practices, Prev. Med. 1:409, 1972.

Brody, J.A.: Aging and alcohol abuse, J. Am. Geriatr. Soc. 30(2):123, 1982.

Carroll, K.K., and Khor, H.T.: Dietary fat in relation to tumorigenesis, Prog. Biochem. Pharmacol. 10:308, 1975.

Coleman, P., and Krondl, M.: Recruitment of free-living elderly for nutrition research, J. Can. Diet. Assoc. 42:4, 1981.

Community Nutrition Institute (CNI): Elderly nutrition programs poised for change, Washington, D.C., Sept. 22, 1983.

Community Nutrition Institute (CNI): ADA: nutrition major health concern for aging, Washington, D.C., Aug. 23, 1984.

Community Nutrition Institute (CNI): Poverty among elderly tightens grip on women, Washington, D.C., Sept. 13, 1984.

Community Nutrition Institute (CNI): Healthy diets equal lower food budgets, Washington, D.C., Dec. 6, 1984.

Deignan, P.: Business applications in clinical dietetics, Ross Timesaver Dietetic Currents 11:3, May-June 1984.

Fischer, M.C., and Lachance, P.A.: Nutrition evaluation of published weight reducing diets, J. Am. Diet. Assoc. 85(4):450, 1985.

Food and Nutrition Board, National Research Council: Recommended dietary allowances, ed. 9, Washington, D.C., 1980, National Academy of Science.

Garry, P.J., et al.: Nutritional status in a healthy elderly population: dietary and supplemental intakes, Am. J. Clin. Nutr. 36(2):319, 1982.

Guthrie, H.: Introductory nutrition, ed. 6, St. Louis, 1986, Times Mirror/Mosby College Publishing.

Harlan, W.R., et al.: Blood pressure and nutrition in adults: The National Health and Nutrition Examination Survey, Am. J. Epidemiol. 120(1):17, 1984.

Harris, J., and Associates, Inc.: Public awareness and the NIAAA advertising campaign and public attitudes toward drinking abuse (PB-244147), Springfield, Va., 1974, National Technical Information Service.

Hess, M.A., and Hunt, A.: Pickles and ice cream: the complete guide to nutrition during pregnancy, New York, 1982, McGraw-Hill, Inc.

Hubert, H.B., et al.: Obesity as an independent risk factor for cardiovascular disease: a 26-year follow-up of participants in the Framingham Heart Study, Circulation 67:968, 1983.

Kane, R.L., and Kane, R.A.: Long-term care: can our society meet the needs of its elderly? Am. Rev. Pub. Health 1:227, 1980.

King (Helm), K.: Marketing your services, Comm. Nutr. 1(3):16, 1982.

Lee, S.: Nutrition services for adults and elderly, Clin. Nutr. 3(3):115, 1984.

Lipid Research Clinics Program: The Lipid Research Clinics Coronary Primary Prevention Trial Results. II. The relationship of reduction in incidence of coronary heart disease to cholesterol lowering, J.A.M.A. 251(3):365, 1984.

Lowenstein, F.W.: Nutritional status of the elderly in the United States, 1971-74, J. Am. Coll. Nutr. 1:165, 1982.

Monteith, M.: Role of nutritionists in community based long-term care. Paper presented at American Dietetic Association, Anaheim Calif., Sept. 15, 1983.

Multiple risk factor intervention trial, J.A.M.A. 248:1465, 1982.

National Heart, Lung, and Blood Institute: Collaboration in high blood pressure control among professionals and with the patient: National High Blood Pressure Education Program, Am. Int. Med. 101:393, 1984.

National Institute of Health Consensus Development Conference: Osteoporosis, Bethesda, Md., April 2-4, 1984.

National Institute of Health Consensus Development Conference: Lowering blood cholesterol to prevent heart disease, Bethesda, Md., Dec. 10-12, 1984.

National Institute of Health Consensus Development Conference: Health implications of obesity, Bethesda, Md., Feb. 11-13, 1985.

Reddy, B.S., et al.: Nutrition and its relationship to cancer. In Klein, G., and Weinhouse, S., editors: Advances in cancer research, vol. 32, New York, 1980, Academic Press, Inc.

Rivlin, R.S.: Nutrition and aging: some unanswered questions, Am. J. Med. 71:337, 1981.

Rivlin, R.S., and Young, E.A., editors: Symposium on evidence relating selected vitamins and minerals to health and disease in the elderly populations in the United States, Am. J. Clin. Nutr. (Suppl.) 36:5, Nov. 1982.

Roche, A.F.: Anthropometric variables: effectiveness and limitations. In Assessing the nutritional status of the elderly—state of the art, Report of Third Ross Roundtable on Medical Issues, Columbus, Ohio, 1982, Ross Laboratories.

Roe, D.A.: Drug-induced nutritional deficiencies, Westport, Conn., 1976, AVI Publishing Co.

Roe, D.A.: Geriatric nutrition, Englewood Cliffs, N.J., 1983, Prentice-Hall, Inc.

Shock, N.W.: Physiologic aspects of aging, J. Am. Diet. Assoc. 56:491, 1970.

Shock, N.W.: The role of nutrition in aging, J. Am. Coll. Nutr. 1:3, 1982.

Simopoulos, A.P.: The role of the federal government in research on nutrition and aging, J. Am. Coll. Nutr. 1:11, 1982.

Simopoulos, A.P., and Van Itallie, T.B.: Body weight and longevity, Ann. Int. Med. 100(2):285, 1984.

Stamler, J.: Evidence from prospective and other epidemiologic studies. In NIH Consensus Abstract: Lowering blood cholesterol to prevent heart disease, Bethesda, Md., Dec. 10, 1984.

Stunkard, A.J.: Treatment for obesity. In Stunkard, A.J., and Stellari, E., editors: Eating and its disorders, New York, 1984, Raven Press.

United States Department of Agriculture: Thrifty Food Plan, Family Econ. Rev. 1:23, 1984.

United States Department of Commerce, United States Bureau of the Census: Current population reports, Series P-25, No. 929, Washington, D.C., 1983, U.S. Government Printing Office.

United States Department of Health and Human Services: Healthy people: the Surgeon General's report on health promotion and disease prevention, Washington, D.C., 1979, U.S. Government Printing Office.

United States Department of Health and Human Services, Public Health Service: Promoting health preventing disease: objectives for the nation, Washington, D.C., 1980, U.S. Government Printing Office.

White House Conference on Aging: Vol. 1: A national policy on aging; Vol. 2: Program proceedings; Vol. 3: Recommendations, Nov. 30-Dec. 3, 1981.

Whitehouse, F.W.: Classification and pathogenesis of the diabetes syndrome: a historical perspective, J. Am. Diet. Assoc. 81(3):243, 1982.

Wylie-Rosett, J.: Development of new educational strategies for the person with diabetes, J. Am. Diet. Assoc. 81(3):268, 1982.

P·A·R·T III

Tools for Developing Effective Community Nutrition Services

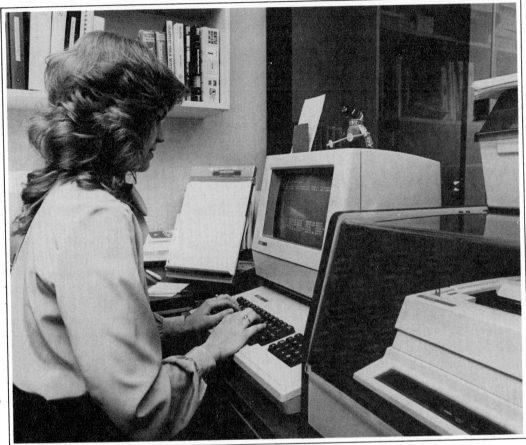

H. Armstrong Roberts

Analytical Skills: Tools of Nutrition Science

GENERAL CONCEPT

The early 1980s were years of rapid growth of knowledge and technological advancement. To keep abreast of this expansion, practitioners in the art of delivering nutrition services must acquire essential basic skills related to computer science, epidemiology, and statistics.

When you finish this chapter, you should be able to

- Discuss the potentials and limitations of the computer
- Cite examples of use of computers in nutrition
- Understand, evaluate, and adapt a classification system for professional use
- Understand how epidemiological studies influence public policy
- Review basic principles of statistical analysis used to evaluate scientific studies

NUTRITION: RELATED DISCIPLINES IN THE DELIVERY OF NUTRITION SERVICES

A career in nutrition and public health in the 1980s means living in an environment of conflict, change, crisis, challenge, and gratification. The word *crisis* has been defined as "the decisive moment," or, as indicated in the Chinese script, "the time of opportunity." As leaders in the health care industry, the scientific base of our profession and its interface with other disciplines, as shown in Figure 12-1, should be reviewed from time to time. For any selected discipline, the intellectual advice of "basic to" and "applied from" is an interfacing of circles beginning with one discipline and eventually overlapping with all the others. Such an overlapping arrangement is shown in Figure 12-1.

Continuing education—an assessment of resources and a critical review of the literature—should be an on-going process of highest priority. If the community dietitian/nutritionist is to seize the opportunity to create more productive experiences, certain skills and knowledge, such as biostatistics, epidemiology, computer science, and clinical judgment, must be acquired and practiced. This may necessitate self-assessment, enrollment in a semester refresher course

in biochemistry every 3 years, or a review of statistics. Continuing education must be attended to in this age of knowledge explosion and technological revolution.

This chapter includes discussions of computer science, epidemiology, statistics, and clinical judgment. We believe that readers of scientific literature should be able to identify the study design; to detect and identify flaws in the epidemiological reasons stated in conclusions drawn from the study; to distinguish between statistical association and causal relationship; to distinguish between incidence and prevalence; and to understand the concept of relative risk and the meaning of the "*p*-value" associated with a test of significance. This chapter will not provide answers to these concepts; it is not a "how-to" chapter. Instead it outlines principles and perhaps leads the reader to a review if necessary.

Computer science, epidemiology, and statistics and clinical judgment were purposely and thoughtfully chosen. The intellectual perception of analytical judgment—the methods of acquiring evidence and organizing thought—has not received the same attention in nutrition as in other contemporary analytical sciences. The basic sciences such as chemistry, physics, and laboratory methodology demand preciseness. How to analyze and classify is a fundamental aspect of statistical analysis in nutrition/dietetics and community nutrition. In a thoughtful approach to the evaluation process, data are collected for problem solving and decision making. Tools are available, and most persons have the intellectual capacity to reason and make critical judgments. Epidemiology, biostatistics, and computer sciences will sharpen critical and analytical judgment.

Computer science allows one to process data and perform analytical tasks quickly and with accuracy; it allows a broad access to computerized data bases for food and nutrition as shown in Table 12-1 (Frank, 1982). Being without a computer skill is "like wandering around a collection the size of the Library of Congress with all the

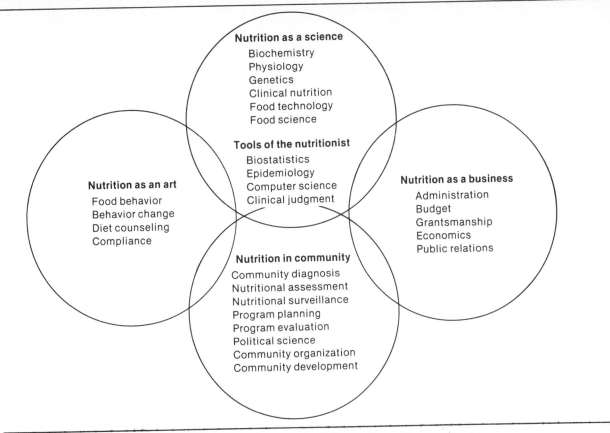

Figure 12-1. Related disciplines in the delivery of nutrition services.

books arranged at random with no Dewey Decimal system, no card catalogue—and of course, no friendly librarian to serve your information needs" (Naisbitt, 1982).

Epidemiology is the study of health and disease in populations rather than individuals and is concerned primarily with the etiology, treatment, and prevention of disease at the community level. *Biostatistics* is a major tool used in epidemiology to form and analyze estimates of disease risk and other pertinent data. Community dietitians/nutritionists need not be epidemiologists, biostatisticians, nor computer scientists but should understand the conceptual framework.

COMPUTERS AND COMPUTER SCIENCE

If every computer in the world were to suddenly go dead, planes would not fly, trains would not run, traffic lights would not change, banks would have to close, space projects would be aborted, and department stores and grocery stores would not be able to sell. . . . if computers were suddenly silenced the world would be thrown into instant chaos (Shelly and Cashman, 1980).

Recently numerous references have appeared in the periodical literature relating to computer applications in nutrition, dietetics, and food service management. A bibliography is available that provides a single source to identify references

Table 12-1. Data bases for food and nutrition

Bibliographic				
Major Emphasis on Food and Nutrition	In-Depth Coverage of Selected Food and Nutrition Areas	Minor Emphasis on Food and Nutrition	Referral	Numeric
Agricultural Online Access	BIOSIS Previews	Comprehensive Dissertation Abstracts	Current Research Information Service	USDA Nutrient Data Bank
Commonwealth Agricultural Bureaux Abstracts	Chemical Abstracts	Conference Papers Index	Smithsonian Science Information Exchange	USDA Nationwide Food Consumption Survey
Food Science and Technology Abstracts	Computerized Engineering Index	Environmental Periodicals Bibliography		Health and Nutrition Examination Survey
Foods Adlibra	Excerpta Medica	Educational Resources Information Center		
	Medlars Online	National Technical Information Service		
		Population Bibliography		
		Psychological Abstracts		
		SCISEARCH		
		Social SCISEARCH		
		Toxicology Information Online		

From Frank, R.C.: Information resources for food and human nutrition, J. Am. Diet. Assoc. 80:4, 1982.

highlighting the use of the computer in health care, human nutrition, business/industry, and college and school food service (Hoover, 1981).

A review of the literature reveals the technological feasibility of using the computer in a variety of ways: nutrition surveillance, dietary assessment tool (nutrient analysis of food intake and recipes), client education, client care with treatment, evaluation, and follow-up plans, food service management, student education, and research. A data base for organizing computer resources to be considered when seeking information in food and human nutrition is outlined in Table 12-1 (Frank, 1982).

It is hard to imagine that 45 years ago no one had heard of a computer. Indeed, when Dr. Geroge Stibitz, one of the early leaders in the development of modern computing devices, approached the management of the prestigious Bell Laboratories in 1937 and advised them that he had designed a calculator that could perform any general calculation, he was told, "Who wants to spend $50,000 just to do calculations" (Shelly and Cashman, 1980).

What Is It? What Does It Do? What Are Its Parts?

What is a computer? The computer is merely a device that can perform computations, including arithmetic and logic operations, without intervention by humans.

A *mainframe* (the central processing unit) can cost anywhere from several hundred thousand dollars to several million. The *microcomputer* is the generic term for a small computer based on microprocess technology. Microcomputers go under several names, which tend to denote how much they cost and where they are kept. A home computer costs between $300 and $2000. A desktop or small business system costs between $2000 and $6000 and is usually found in offices. The *minicomputer* is smaller than a mainframe but larger than a microcomputer and costs $25,000 to several hundred thousand dollars.

What does a computer do? Although the results of computer processing can control a lunar module landing on the surface of the moon or monitor vital signs in a coronary care unit, a computer is capable of performing only a relatively few number of operations:

1. Arithmetic operations, such as the addition, subtraction, multiplication, and division of data
2. Logical operations, such as determining whether one number is greater than another
3. Input/output operations, such as accepting data for processing or causing data to be printed on a report

The common thread in all three operations is the processing of data. Data are representations of facts, concepts, or instructions in a formalized manner suitable for communication, interpretation, and processing by humans or automatic machines. It is the task of the computer system to accept and process data; as a result of the processing, it produces output in the form of useful information. Important terms in computer science are (1) *data base*, a body of information stored by the computer, (2) *input*, a piece of information that the user gives the computer, (3) *output*, data that the computer gives the user, and (4) *program*, a set of instructions that tells the computer how to perform a task (Youngwirth, 1983).

The three primary units of the computer system, the input unit, the processor unit, and the output unit, are controlled by a computer program. A *computer program* is a series of instructions that are stored in main computer storage and specify which processing operations are to occur in the computer system. Each of the instructions that cause the computer system to process data must be arranged in the proper sequence so that correct processing will occur. Computer programmers write these instructions. Any computer system has two basic components: (1) the *software*, programs and tables that direct the performance of the desired task and (2) the *hardware*, the computer equipment necessary to perform the task.

The computer is totally the servant of humans. It reflects the data base, knowledge, criteria, judgments, and values of the persons who wrote its program. It has neither the capacity to design a treatment plan, the versatility to execute the plan, nor the ability to extract conclusions from a hypothesis-research design. If properly used, the computer will improve the practice of any profession by providing data to make better management decisions, thus enhancing the quality of practice.

Computers and Nutrition

The evolution of the use of computers in nutrition, dietetics, and food service has been documented in Hoover's bibliography (1981), which is arranged chronologically from 1958 to 1981. The pioneer work was that of Balintfy, whose 1964 publications describe both inventory control and the use of hospital menu planning by computer. The number of literature reviews of computer applications in dietetics and nutrition has been expanding at a rapid rate (J. Nutr. Educ., 1984; Youngwirth, 1983).

Analysis of Dietary Data

The use of the computer for storing food tables and calculating nutrient data is a logical application of the technology and has allowed for larger studies, storage of nutrient data, and an array of statistical correlations.

The variety of services and microcomputer programs available for the dietitian differs widely in content of data bases, cost, ease of use, reporting of results, and flexibility. Dwyer and Suitor (1984), in an evaluation of 12 programs (7 diet analyses from service vendors and 5 microcomputer programs), advise the user to compare systems and services and to consider carefully whether mechanized dietary analysis is of sufficient benefit in the delivery of high-quality nutrition care to offset its cost.

The largest computerized data base, data on 65 nutrients, is the USDA's Nutrient Data Bank (NDB), which acts as an international repository for any research reports on the composition of food. The NDB includes reports on analyses from the scientific literature in the United States and other countries, as well as unpublished materials from research by state agricultural experiment stations, universities, government-sponsored programs, and food companies.

Nutrient Data Bank Conference

The annual Nutrient Data Bank (NDB) Conference addresses the issue of accurate nutrient data bases and the development of reliable computer programs to use with the data bases. Following the first conference in 1976, several data base developers analyzed a common 1-day menu to test the comparability of their systems. The results indicated the need for a diagnostic tool for both the contents of the data base and the computational routines used in the computer programs. A review model was developed to provide the methodology for the systematic appraisal of a nutrient data base system (Hoover and Perloff, 1981). The NDB Directory facilitates communication between developers and users of nutrient data bank systems by providing a listing of systems and software available (Hoover, 1984). Access to computerized nutrient storage and retrieval systems should help nutritionists to assess nutrient intake and to place and implement dietary changes with their clients.

Quick Input Program

An example of an interactive retrieval method for the analysis of dietary data, the Quick Input Program (QIP), was developed for direct use by nutritionists for their clients (Witschi et al., 1981). By using primarily the NDB, a nutrient data base was constructed initially for use in hyperlipidemia counseling. It lists values for kilocalories, protein, carbohydrate, total fat, saturated, monounsaturated, and polyunsaturated fatty acids, and cholesterol. Approximately 500 line items, representing about 1200 foods, are included in the table. A sample of a breakfast menu that lists totals and averages for all nutrients as well as dietary evaluation for cholesterol, P/S ra-

CALCULATION AND EVALUATION OF NUTRIENTS BY THE QUICK INPUT PROGRAM

Foods: .5 × 1 cup fruit juice (Unsw), 1 × 1 English muffin, 2 × 1 tsp soft margarine, 1 × 1 fried egg, .73 × 1 cup low-fat milk.

	Total	Average/Day
Calories	431.1	431.1
Protein/gm	17.0	17.0
Cho/gm	48.8	48.8
Fat/gm	19.1	19.1
Sat fat/gm	6.0	6.0
Mono fat/gm	7.4	7.4
Poly fat/gm	4.1	4.1
Chol/mg	289.2	289.2
		(—GO—)

Dietary Evaluation

	Actual	Recommended
P/S Ratio	.68	1.0
Cholesterol	289 mg	<300
Caloric distribution (431 calories):		
Protein	15.7%	12–15%
Fat	39.8%	<35%
Polyunsaturated fat	8.5%	>10%
Saturated fat	12.5%	<10%
Carbohydrates	44.5%	50–53%
		(—GO—)

From Witschi, J., et al.: Analysis of dietary data: an interactive computer method for storage and retrieval. Copyright The American Dietetic Association. Reprinted by permission from Journal of the American Dietetic Association, Vol. 78, p. 609, 1981.

tio, and caloric distribution is shown in the box above.

Used to evaluate nutrient intake in research projects, QIP saves times, gives immediate results, helps to improve dietary interviewing skills, and provides knowledge of food composition. Users have commented favorably on the fact that the system is easy to learn, that access does not require coding, and that the program is flexible in providing information relative to amounts of food consumed, and thus is useful to both counselor and client.

Computer Application in Food Service Management

Another area of computer application in dietetics is food service management: inventory control/purchasing systems, forecasting food and labor needs, recipe adjustment, production control, tray assembly delivery, and menu planning and printing (Youngwirth, 1983).

The computerization of diet orders offers instant communication from the patient care unit to the floor diet office. Up-to-date management reports such as diet lists and diet censuses are available on demand (Dunphy and Bratton, 1983). The dietary order entry system shown in Figure 12-2 begins with the patient's admission to an inpatient unit and is followed through to the meal delivery.

Some food service directors claim that the computer is revolutionizing their operations (Schuster, 1981). The University of Wisconsin-Stout has trimmed its inventory by almost 75% and its annual food bill by approximately $92,000 in a food service operation that serves 3300 meals per day. The Memphis school system employed five supervisors in its 30,000-meals-a-day food service operation in 1968. Today the operation has grown to 96,000 meals per day, but it still employs only five supervisors. Five residential institutions run by New Jersey's Department of Human Services are spending 13% less for food than other institutions in the same system. The food service director for a 1150-bed Houston hospital complex has solved the problem of extremely limited storage facilities by getting his vendors to carry his inventory via the computer.

Computer Application in Clinical Care

Computer Menu Planning Program (CMPP) has been described by Wheeler and Wheeler (1980) to help patients with diabetes. Using the patient's diet prescription, usual daily eating pattern, food preferences, stored food characteristics, and menu planning rules, the computer is able to plan any number of days or weeks of menus along with weekly shopping lists (Table 12-2).

In addition, it provides the health care team

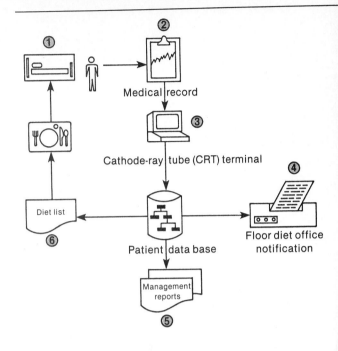

1   The patient is admitted to an in-patient unit.

2   The attending physician writes the diet order in the patient's medical record.

3   Using the online Dietary Order Entry System, nursing personnel enter the diet order into the patient data base via CRTs located on the patient unit.

4   A copy of each order is immediately printed in the appropriate floor diet office for follow-up by a dietitian.

5   Management reports, such as diet census counts and diet lists, are produced from the patient data base.

6   Prior to meal service, the nursing personnel use the CRTs to verify the diet orders for patients on their unit. As a result of this verification activity, a diet list is printed to assist in tray delivery.

Figure 12-2. Overview of dietary order entry system.
Redrawn from Dunphy, M.K., and Bratton, B.D.: A computerized dietary order entry system. Copyright The American Dietetic Association. Reprinted by permission from Journal of the American Dietetic Association, Vol. 82, p. 68, 1983.

with an extensive nutrient analysis of the menu. Thus the CMPP performs a repetitive, complicated task that is useful in diabetic nutritional education but is too time consuming to be per-

Table 12-2. Computer-planned shopping list

Food	Amount to Buy	Cost	Number of Exchanges Not Used
Milk, 2%	1.00 1 gal ctn	$1.88	9
Carrots	0.43 pound	0.40	0
Celery	1.00 whole stalk	0.80	3
Green pepper	3.00 pepper	1.02	0
Spinach	2.00 15 oz can	0.64	1
Mushrooms, fresh	0.50 pound, raw	0.52	0
Tomatoes, canned/fresh	1.00 1-pound can	1.14	1
Vegetable juice	1.00 46 oz can	0.53	5
Lettuce	1.00 medium head	0.69	3
Apple	0.10 3-pound bag	0.16	0
Apple juice	1.00 46 oz can	0.70	13
Banana	1.45 pound	0.57	0
Cantaloupe	1.00 1 small	0.79	2
Orange juice	1.00 46 oz can	0.72	3
Pineapple	1.00 1¼-pound can	0.59	4
Bread, whole wheat	2.00 20 oz loaf	1.03	17
English muffin	1.00 12 oz pkg	0.59	6
Shredded wheat	1.00 18 oz box	0.87	15
Oatmeal	1.00 18 oz box	0.53	27
Graham crackers	1.00 1-pound pkg	0.69	18
Corn, whole kernel	2.00 1-pound can	0.50	2
Peas, green	3.00 1-pound can	0.86	1
Potato, white	0.16 5-pound bag	0.19	0
Sirloin steak/roast	0.43 pound	1.26	0
Chicken	0.80 pound	0.62	0
Salmon, canned	2.00 7¾ oz can	3.42	1
Tuna, canned, water	2.00 6½ oz can	1.20	2
Hamburger, lean	0.38 pound	0.60	0
Pork loin, lean	1.00 pound	1.68	0
Margarine	1.00 pound	0.39	72
Bacon	1.00 pound	1.79	14
Salad dressing	1.00 32 oz jar	0.75	79
TOTAL COST		$28.12	

From Wheeler, M.L., and Wheeler, L.A.: Diabetes Care 3:6, Nov./Dec. 1981. Reproduced with permission from the American Diabetes Association, Inc.

formed routinely by health care professionals. Wheeler and Wheeler emphasize that the CMPP is only a tool; to serve a useful purpose, it must be integrated into a comprehensive program of diabetic nutritional education, including organized nutritional follow-up on an outpatient basis.

The Computer in Education

In the dietetic internship program at Emory University in Atlanta the computer functions as an in-structional management tool (Argo, Watson, and Lee, 1981). Because the computer scores, records, monitors, and reports information on student performance, the computer-managed system lends itself well to a competency-based curriculum. Evaluation becomes an integral part of the learning process because of immediate feedback. Computer-simulation of case studies for nutritional care has been developed and implemented in a coordinated undergraduate dietetic program at

NUTRITION RESEARCH CLASSIFICATION SYSTEM

I. Biomedical and behavioral sciences
  A. Normal nutritional requirements throughout the life cycle:
    1. Maternal nutrition
    2. Infant and child nutrition (0-12 years) (includes the low-birth-weight infant)
    3. Adolescent nutrition (13-18 years)
    4. Adult nutrition (19-65 years)
    5. Nutrition of the elderly (65 + years)
  B. Diseases and conditions—research on the role of nutrition in the prevention, amelioration, and treatment of diseases and conditions:
    6. Cardiovascular disease and nutrition
    7. Cancer and nutrition
    8. Other diseases and nutrition (e.g., osteoporosis, diabetes, etc.)
    9. Trauma (including burns) and nutrition
    10. Infection—immunology and nutrition
    11. Obesity, anorexia, and appetite control
    12. Genetics and nutrition
    13. Nutrition and function (includes mental, psychomotor, and work performance; environmental stress)
    14. Nutrient interactions (includes nutrient–nutrient drug interactions, nutrient-toxicant interactions, and nutrient toxicity)
    15. Other conditions and nutrition
    16. Nutritional status (includes research on methods for the determination of nutritional status and surveillance: dietary history and food consumption, biochemical determinants, anthropometry, and clinical examination)
  C. Nutrient metabolism and metabolic mechanisms at the cellular and subcellular levels—these categories classify biochemical, subcellular, cellular, and animal research, such as studies of nutrient mechanisms and metabolism not related to specific diseases, conditions, or stages of the life cycle:
    17. Carbohydrates
    18. Lipids (fats and oils) (includes essential fatty acids, lipoproteins and apoproteins)
    19. Alcohols (includes ethanol, sorbitol, and other alcohols used as components in synthetic foods and semisynthetic foods)
    20. Proteins and amino acids (includes essential as well as nonessential amino acids such as taurine and carnitine)
    21. Vitamins (includes vitamin A, C, B_6, B_{12}, D, E, K, thiamin, riboflavin, niacin, folacin, biotin, and pantothenic acid)
    22. Minerals and essential trace elements (includes calcium, phosphorus, magnesium, iron, zinc, iodine, copper, maganese, fluoride, chromium, selenium, and molybdenum)
    23. Water and electrolytes (includes sodium, potassium, and chloride)
    24. Fiber
    25. Other nutrients in food (such as cobalt, nickel, vanadium, silicon, tin, arsenic, cadmium, choline, lecithin, and various growth factors)
II. Categories for research in the nutritional aspects of food sciences
    26. Food composition (includes nutritional quality, nutrient content, and research on methods of analysis for nutrients and fiber)
    27. Bioavailability of nutrients (includes methods for the determination of bioavailability of nutrients)
    28. Effects of technology on acceptability and nutritional characteristics of foods and diets (includes the beneficial and adverse effects of varietal and species differences, harvest and postharvest technology, retail food practices, food processing, handling, preservation, and home cooking)
    29. Other research in food sciences
III. Nutrition monitoring and surveillance of populations
    30. Food consumption surveys (includes research on methods for determination of food consumption and its trends, and research utilizing data derived from such surveys)
    31. Studies of dietary practices, food consumption patterns, and their determinants
    16. Nutritional status (See no. B-16)
IV. Nutrition education (encompasses research in nutrition education)
    32. Studies on methods for informing and educating the public about nutrition, health, and dietary practices and for countering nutrition misinformation
    33. Other research in nutrition education
V. The effects of government policy and socioeconomic factors on food consumption and human nutrition
    34. Effects of government policy and socioeconomic factors on food consumption and human nutrition

From NIH Nutrition Coordinating Committee, Bethesda, Md., 1980, National Institute of Health.

Ohio State University (Breese, Welch, and Schimpfhauser, 1977).

Computer in Nutrition Data Retrieval System

A review article of computerized data bases separates them into three types: bibliographic, referral, and numeric as shown in Table 12-1 (Frank, 1982). *Bibliographic data bases* are primarily concerned with citations of published journal articles, books, and audiovisual materials. *Referral data bases* refer to current research at various locations in the United States. *Numeric data bases* are primarily numbers and codes that cite statistical data or other types of information.

A basic classification system was designed in 1980 by NIH's Nutrition Coordinating Committee in an effort to comply with a 1977 Congressional mandate to develop a common human nutrition information management system. By 1983 a HHS-USDA task force had completed work on 5 basic categories and 34 subgroups (box, p. 355). Specifications were also developed for a computer data system that is currently undergoing a trial period to become accessible to the public in 1986. It is now currently available on the DIALOG System for federal employees only.

• • •

In summary, the digital computer brings with it the capacities for facilitating dietary assessment, for making multiple analytical correlations rapidly and accurately, and for devising a systematic treatment plan. In addition, various computer systems allow for statistical analyses of data, word processing, management information, decision making, and, of course, playing games such as Space Invaders and backgammon.

This new therapeutic technology enables the dietitian to perform extraordinary tasks. The human mind is unsurpassed in the ability to perceive, think, analyze, imagine, and create, but it is greatly limited in its ability to store large numbers of facts permanently and to recall the data precisely. It is hoped that the computer will free the dietitian for patient/client contact to maintain the humanness in the profession.

Feinstein's philosophical view of the computer is worthy of thought:

> A computer is a beast of intellect. It cannot produce new forms of movement, like an automobile, an elevator, or an airplane. It cannot produce new materials or transform tangible substances, like the equipment used in a steel mill, an oil refinery, or a chemistry laboratory. It cannot generate new types of observation and data, like an x-ray, an electrocardiograph, an electrophoresis apparatus, a chemical test, or a person. It is simply a "brain" and nothing else. . . . And it is not a very good "brain," either; it can only do three things. It can coordinate the action of its appendages; it can transform the information it receives; and it can store the information (Feinstein, 1976).

EPIDEMIOLOGY

Public policy related to changes in established lifestyle patterns is made by government officials guided by scientific information. Hearings of the Senate Select Committee on Nutrition and Human Needs document the background epidemiological data that led to the Dietary Goals. Further evidence relating six dietary factors to the nation's health (cholesterol, dietary fat, sugar, alcohol, excess calories, and sodium) (Ahrens, 1979) and the Food and Nutrition Board/National Research Council report *Toward Healthful Diets* (FNB, 1980) provided background data for the Dietary Guidelines for Americans. The Food and Nutrition Board believes that advice should be given to the public when the strength, extent, consistency, coherence, and plausibility of the evidence from lines of investigation ranging from epidemiology to molecular biology converge to indicate that certain dietary practices or other aspects of life-style promote health benefits without incurring risks.

More recently consensus statements have appeared on calcium and osteoporosis, cholesterol, and heart disease and obesity in Americans (NIH, 1984a, b, 1985). Each consensus statement considers a dietary factor and its relationship to disease by looking at the kinds of evidence, the quality and strength of evidence, and the risks and benefits of changing the intake of the factor being considered. Evidence is reviewed from epidemiological, animal, and human studies. The quality and strength of the evidence primarily depends on consistency among various population groups and individuals within a population. This evidence, evaluated for its quality and strength, is then assessed in terms of possible harm or benefit of recommending the increase, reduction, or removal of a dietary constituent. Everything relies on epidemiological evidence.

In its simplest application, epidemiology compares the mortality and/or morbidity experience for a specific disease in different population groups to determine whether the observed differences can be related to specific agents (environment, personal living habits, genetics) (Nutritional Epidemiology, 1982).

Types of Studies

Epidemiologists, using mostly observational designs, seek to identify disease risk factors and explain the biological and social mechanisms of causation. For purposes of classification, population study designs can be divided into two broad types: (1) observational (e.g., retrospective and prospective), where the risk factor or treatment is randomly allocated by the investigator; and (2) experimental (e.g., clinical and community trials), where the risk factor or treatment is randomly allocated by the investigator. There is also the quasiexperimental study design, where the risk factor or treatment is manipulated without randomization(Kleinbaum,Kupper,andMorganstern, 1982).

A *retrospective study* is one where the investigator begins at the end of the cause-effect pathway by collecting cases or persons with disease and looks retrospectively or back in time to identify any distinctive (suspected) precursor characteristic. Controls are selected from persons who do not have the disease but who are as much like the cases in other respects as possible.

In *prospective studies* one starts not with a specific disease, as in retrospective studies, but with a suspected disease precursor. Specific characteristics of a group of individuals or cohort free of disease are recorded, and the cohort is followed up over time to observe the subsequent outcome (e.g., development of disease). Individuals exposed to a suspected cause of disease and those not exposed are compared according to whether the disease developed. Examples of prospective studies that have been in progress for many years include the Tecumseh Community Health Study in Tecumseh, Michigan (Nichols et al., 1976), the Framingham Study in Framingham, Massachusetts (Kannel et al., 1971), and, the Seven Countries Heart Study (Keyes, 1980).

In *experimental studies*, which consist of clinical and community trials (field experimentation), the investigator has direct control over the conditions of the study such as the assignment of individuals to groups exposed and not exposed to a preventive measure. Experimental studies provide more definite proof of causation of disease than observational studies.

Table 12-3 summarizes the major characteristics of retrospective and prospective study designs.

Incidence Versus Prevalence

Distinction should be made between two rates of measure. *Incidence* refers to the number of new cases of a disease during a specified period of time; *prevalence* refers to the number of existing cases of a disease at a particular time. The incidence rate is a measure of risk; it is a dynamic concept that tells the rate at which new cases of disease occur in a given population over a period of time. By combining information on incidence rates with other variables, factors that may affect the risk of acquiring diseases can be determined. In contrast, the prevalence rate is a static concept; it provides an indication of the amount of disease prevailing in a given population at a given point and allows the assessment of the burden of a particular disease in the community. Prevalence is an essential measure for planning, monitoring, and evaluating health care programs.

Table 12-3. Summary of the characteristics of prospective and retrospective epidemiological studies

	Prospective	Retrospective
Method of data collection	Usually specifically designed for the study	Usually exploits data collected for other purposes
Principal bias	Knowledge of exposure influences diagnosis	Knowledge of disease influences report of exposure
Respondent bias	Response precedes illness	Response following illness may be biased by the illness
Estimates of risk	Measures the risk of disease in persons with and without a stated characteristic	Measures the risk of a stated characteristic in persons with and without disease
Duration of study	Usually long	Usually brief
Uncommon disease	Requires large population and long period of study	May discover and use aggregation of cases
Cost	Relatively expensive	Relatively less expensive
Sampling	Usually easier to select a probability sample	Usually more difficult to select a probability sample
Sample size dependent on	Disease frequencies	Exposure frequencies

From Course syllabus, Department of Preventive Medicine, University of Texas Medical Branch at Galveston, 1980.

Table 12-4. Some commonly used indices of community health*

Name of Index and Definition	Rate for United States with Units (1979)	Remarks
Annual crude death rate: Number of deaths occurring in a defined population during a given year / Number in that population at midyear of the same year	8.7 deaths per 1000 population per year	A very crude measure of risk because of the great variation with age; useful as measure of population decrement due to natural causes
Annual age-adjusted death rate: Number of deaths that would occur in the standard population / Number in the standard population	6.0 deaths per 1000 population per year	Based on the 1940 U.S. population as the standard; lower than the crude rate because there was a smaller proportion of old people in 1940 than in 1977
Annual age-specific death rate: Number of deaths in a specified age group occurring in a defined population during a given year / Number in the specified age group in that population at midyear of the same year	29.7 deaths at ages 65-74 per 1000 population aged 65-74 per year	Approaches a measure of risk especially if also specific for sex
Annual cause-specific death rate: Number of deaths from a specified cause occurring in a defined population during a given year / Number in that population at midyear of the same year	334.0 deaths from disease of the heart per 100,000 population per year	100,000 is used here as a base simply to avoid awkward decimals, especially for less important causes of death

From National Center for Health Statistics: Monthly Vital Statistics Report 28:12, March 1980.
*All indices refer to residents of a specified locality, observed for 1 year unless otherwise stated.

Table 12-4. Some commonly used indices of community health—cont'd

Name of Index and Definition	Rate for United States with Units (1979)	Remarks
Proportionate mortality from a specified cause: Number of deaths from a specified cause occurring in a defined population during a given year ─────────── Total number of deaths occurring in that population during the same year	38 deaths from diseases of the heart per 100 deaths from all causes	A useful but potentially misleading measure of mortality because changes in the frequency of other causes can change the total and thereby change the proportion for a specific cause
Annual infant mortality rate: Number of deaths under 1 year of age occurring in a defined population during a given year ─────────── Number of live births occurring in that population during the same year	13.2 infant deaths per 1000 live births	Approximate measures of risk: Not all infants dying in 1 calendar year were born in the same calendar year (i.e., denominator of rate does not completely include numerator, but accurate when the number of births is fairly constant from one year to the next)
Annual neonatal mortality rate: Number of deaths of children under 28 days of age occurring in defined population during a given year ─────────── Number of live births occurring in that population during the same year	8.8 neonatal deaths per 1000 live births	
Annual postneonatal mortality rate: Number of deaths of children at ages 28 days through 12 months occurring in a defined population during given year ─────────── Number of live births occurring in that population during the same year	4.4 postneonatal deaths per 1000 live births	Also used with live births minus neonatal deaths in denominator; when this is done infant mortality rate will not equal neonatal mortality rate plus postneonatal mortality rate
Annual fetal death rate (also called stillbirth rate): Number of fetal deaths of 20 weeks or more gestation occurring in a defined population during a given year ─────────── Number of live births plus fetal deaths of 20 weeks or more occurring in that population during the same year	10.6 fetal deaths per 1000 live births plus fetal deaths of 20 weeks or more	Subject to large errors in reporting
Annual perinatal mortality rate: Number of fetal deaths 28 weeks or more and infant deaths 7 days of age occurring in a defined population during a given year ─────────── Number of live births and fetal deaths 28 weeks or more occurring in same population during the same year	16.8 perinatal deaths per 1000 live births and fetal deaths	Perinatal mortality is designed to include fetal and infant deaths near the time of birth to avoid problems of misclassification of stillbirth and infant death; many causes of death are similar for late fetal and early infant death

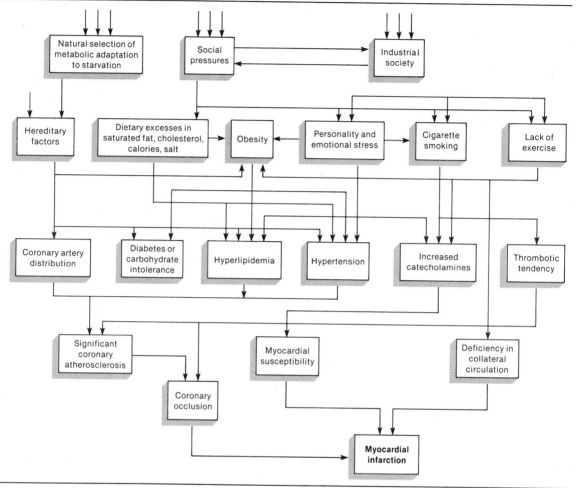

Figure 12-3. Web of causation for coronary heart disease.
Redrawn from Friedman, G.: Primer of epidemiology, New York, 1980, McGraw-Hill, Inc.
Reproduced with permission.

Indices of Health Status in Community

Commonly used indices of health status in a community are summarized in Table 12-4. Among these are the widely employed crude birth and crude death rates. These are called "crude" because they are summary rates. As summary indices, however, they are useful in assessing population change or growth.

Association and Causality

After completing data analysis, the researcher is ready to form inferences from the data. If no association is found between a factor and a disease, the conclusion is that the factor does not appear to cause the disease. However, when an association is found, statistical tests are available to help resolve the dilemma of whether or not the

NATURAL HISTORY OF DISEASE IN HUMANS

Prepathogenesis ─────────────────────────────────→ Pathogenesis

Stages of Disease

Predisease Stage	**Preclinical**	**Clinical**	**Chronic**
Interaction of following before disease: Disease agent Human host Environmental factors	Inapparent disease	Manifest early clinical disease	Advanced disease, leading to: Recovery No change Worsening Complications Disability Death

Levels of Prevention

Primary	**Secondary**	**Tertiary**
Health education Specific protection (immunization) Environmental control measures Nutrition Genetic counseling	Screening Early diagnosis Minimize disability	Rehabilitation Palliative therapy Minimize disability

From Leavell, H.R., and Clark, E.G.: Preventive medicine for the doctor in his community: an epidemiological approach, New York, 1965, McGraw-Hill, Inc. Reproduced with permission.

finding is a chance phenomenon. A consideration of the multiple factors that are actually involved in the causation of a complex disease entity such as coronary heart disease indicates the need to evaluate the many associations with the criteria for consistency. This web of causation for coronary heart disease and the multiple factors involved are shown in Figure 12-3.

Inferring an etiological relationship from epidemiological studies of diet and chronic degenerative diseases is particularly difficult. Nutrients seldom act independently but are more likely to interact with other nutrients, as well as with nondietary components. Diseases such as coronary heart disease, cancer, and hypertension are of multifactorial etiology. Diet is only one of the several components of life-style that may influence risk of developing disease. When sufficient information has been accummulated regarding the natural history and etiology of a particular disease, it is then possible to develop programs for the prevention or control of this disease or to alter the course of the disease by therapeutic intervention. There still remains the necessity, however, of determining whether or not the intervention strategies are effective.

Prevention

Prevention depends on knowledge of the underlying disease process and the level of technology available. Leavell and Clark (1965) outlined three levels of prevention: primary, secondary and tertiary as shown in the box above.

Primary prevention, designed to reduce exposure or susceptibility, is characterized by immunizations, nutrition, genetic counseling, and environmental control measures. *Secondary prevention* is directed at early detection and is represented by screening programs and prompt treatment of identified disease. *Tertiary prevention* is directed toward alleviation of disability resulting from the disease and includes efforts to restore function and productivity of the patient; renal dialysis programs represent this level of care.

During the past decade a "new perspective on health" has emerged (or reemerged) in several nations that have sought to assess the health status and the provision of health care in their populations. In the United States widespread interest in primary prevention has resulted partly from the escalating cost of health services. On the basis of results from epidemiological studies, it is possible to identify certain parameters regarding the distribution of the risk factor that is to be modified in the population, the magnitude of the association between the risk factor and disease, and the total risk of disease in the population. Using epidemiological data, health planners and researchers are able to make cost-effective analyses to determine the impact preventive measures may have on expected gains in years of life.

Six basic questions can summarize the role of epidemiology in health care (Dobbins and Buffler, 1980):

1. What is the diagnosis?
2. What is the prognosis?
3. Who gets the disease?
4. Why do they get the disease?
5. What treatment is best for the disease?
6. How can the disease be prevented?

The answers to the first two questions are based on a comparison of signs and symptoms to "normal" or "expected" values of these signs and symptoms. This comparison is the essence of epidemiology as applied to individuals. The answers to the third and fourth questions form the basis of epidemiology in dealing with population data. The answer to the fifth question lies in an application of epidemiological methods to clinical medicine in the form of clinical trials. And, finally, the answer to the last question is the focus of the study of preventive medicine and community health.

As stated earlier, epidemiology is the study of health and disease in populations rather than in individuals and is concerned primarily with the etiology, treatment, and prevention of disease.

Biostatistics is a major tool used in epidemiology to form and analyze estimates of disease risk.

STATISTICS

Although Florence Nightingale is remembered as a pioneer in nursing and a reformer of hospitals, an equally important contribution that is less well known is her use of statistical analysis in her efforts to reform the British military health care system during the Crimean War (1854-1856) (Cohen, 1984). Nightingale demonstrated that improved sanitary conditions in military hospitals and barracks could sharply cut the death rate and save thousands of lives. This she accomplished by observation and record keeping, the statistical method. Thus she helped pioneer the revolutionary idea that social phenomena could be objectively measured and subjected to mathematical analysis.

The founder of this science, which is simply the collection of numerical data, was Adolphe Jacques Quételet. In 1841 Quételet organized Belgium's statistical bureau. He showed that "whereas there are no laws determining individual behavior, there are regularities in the attributes and behavior of groups, and that these regularities could be characterized mathematically by the laws of probability" (Cohen, 1984). Today the most widely used ratio for height and weight to determine body mass index (weight in kilograms divided by height in centimeters squared—wt/ht^2) bears his name, the Quételet index. (Overweight is a body mass index between 24 and 30, and obesity is a body mass index above 30.)

The scientific method is an intellectual concept. It refers to the quality with which an experiment is designed, executed, and appraised. It demands a working knowledge of statistics. Almost anyone can make some plans, carry them out, and see what happens. The scientific quality of the activity depends on the methods used for making and consummating the plans and for observing and interpreting what happens.

For its reasoning and conclusions to be valid,

an investigation must fulfill the following principles *after* it begins (Feinstein, 1976):

1. The observation period must be long enough for pertinent events to be noted.
2. The data of both sides of a correlation must be appropriate and clearly specified.
3. Important correlations must be analyzed to determine to what extent their numerical distinctions are significant or possibly attributable to chance.
4. The features or events held responsible for significant relationships must be evaluated as direct or indirect, causal or coexistent.
5. The experimental results must be established as having come from a valid sampling of the "universe" they supposedly represent or to which the conclusions will be extrapolated.

These principles—adequate duration, specificity of correlation, statistical significance, identification of cause, and valid extrapolation—are basic to scientific reasoning.

This section is included for the person who needs to be a knowledgeable reader of quantitative research in the field of nutrition but who lacks the necessary statistical background. In other words, this is not a how-to-do-it section on statistics but rather a how-they-do-it section; it is a review of the practical logic and application of statistical methods. Today's biomedical literature is replete with statistical analyses and interpretation of numerical data. Improper statistical treatment of numerical information may often lead to improper conclusions. The ability to critically evaluate the statistical treatment of numerical information is of utmost importance in evaluating the overall quality and accuracy of the conclusions presented in a journal article.

The nutritionist of today is often faced with collection, organization, analysis and interpretation of numerical information. Too often researchers believe that their data are sufficient to support their conclusions when, in fact, they are not. There is need for an objective approach to the collection and analysis of quantitative experimental data. This approach requires a study of statistical methodology.

Basic Concepts

Research procedures may be broken down into three critical steps: (1) researchers must clearly specify *what* it is they are observing; (2) they must indicate precisely *how* they go about observing it; and (3) they must describe the *group* about which these observations are made. In the jargon of empirical research, these three steps have special names. When researchers specify *what* it is they are observing, they are defining the *variable* (or variables) *of interest*. When they indicate exactly *how* they will be observing this variable, they are defining the *measurement process*. And when they describe the group about which their observations are made, they are defining the *population of interest*. Thus statistics is a branch of applied mathematics that provides the tools that help in conducting scientific research. The research plan will state the problem, method, results, and conclusions. The researcher's report of the variables comprises the data.

Descriptive Versus Inferential Statistics

The statistical treatment of such data may be descriptive or inferential. *Descriptive statistics* involves the process of organizing and summarizing the important aspects of a data set. It includes the condensation of data in the form of tables, their graphic presentation, and the computation of numerical indicators of central tendency (e.g., mean, median, mode) or variability (e.g., range, standard, deviation). Examples are readership surveys, studies of message content of television commercials, the measurement of fiber intake of various family members, an assessment of continuing education needs of dietitians, and consumption of caffeine. The key feature is that some existing situation is being studied.

Inferential statistics consists of a series of techniques (univariate and multivariate) that allow conclusions to extend beyond an immediate data set. Given some information regarding a small subset of a population, the methods of inferential statistics can be used to make probability statements about the entire population. The two most important types of inference are parameter estimation and hypothesis testing. The parameter of interest is that attribute or characteristic of a population being estimated.

In the descriptive method the variables are described based on the observation of them, but there is no direct control of variables. In addition, in descriptive problems an entire population is measured in terms of a relevant parameter, such as its mean or standard deviation. When only a subset of a particular population is measured, an inferential approach is used. The subset is called a sample, and the role of inferential statistics is to use information derived from the sample to make a statement about the population as a whole. The most frequently employed inferential approach is hypothesis testing. The usual intent is to test a hypothesis of cause and effect. Does the manipulation of one variable lead to consequences in another? For example, will a diet high in saturated fat raise plasma cholesterol?

Hypotheses

Hypotheses can be predictions of relationships or differences. A research hypothesis is stated as a prediction. For statistical purposes, *a null hypothesis* states that whatever difference is observed between samples is a result of sampling error. Sampling statistics provides a basis for estimating the probability that some observed difference between samples would be expected on the terms of the null hypothesis because of sampling error. If this obtained value of probability is equal to or less than some value preset as a rejection region (significance level), the null hypothesis is rejected in favor of its logical alternative, the research hypothesis. (Examples of significance levels can be stated as $p < .001$ or $p < .005$.)

Variables

The variable is a characteristic that may have different values from individual to individual or from observation to observation. Each variable has a name and associated set of values:

1. *Nominal variables* include categorical data where the categories have no special order. Examples are race, marital status, cause of death, and type of patient (inpatient or outpatient).
2. *Rank-order variables* are also known as *ordinal scale variables.* There are no fixed categories into which observations may fall. Observations are compared with each other and put in order, perhaps from the best to the worst. Examples are state of disease (1 to 4 for breast cancer) and self-perceived state of health (poor, fair, or excellent).
3. *Numerical discrete variables* include data with numerical integer values. Some examples are the number of transient ischemic attacks in 1 year in a stroke patient and the number of nutrition clinic visits for a given patient.
4. *Numerical continuous variables* include data for which there are underlying continuous scales. Examples are diastolic blood pressure, age, and plasma cholesterol level.

Because different types of variables call for different statistical techniques, it is important to be able to examine a set of data and determine which of these types of variables is involved.

Classification matrices for organizing and presenting empirical data and for descriptive and inferential problems, developed by Twaite and Monroe (1979), are shown in Figures 12-4 to 12-6.

Each matrix summarizes the level of measurement of variable(s) of interest and the various types of problems. To use the matrix and to locate the specific cell of relevance, the following questions need to be answered:

1. Is the problem descriptive or inferential?
2. Is the problem univariate (a single variable) or bivariate (two or more variables)?
3. If the problem is bivariate, into which of these three categories may it be placed?

LEVEL OF MEASUREMENT OF VARIABLE(S) OF INTEREST

	Categorical: nominal or ordered categories	Rank-order	Interval scale (or ratio-scale)
Univariate problems	Frequency distribution, relative frequency distribution Bar graph, pictograph, circle graph	Set of ranks	Frequency distribution, grouped frequency distribution, cumulative frequency distribution *Graphs for discrete interval data:* discrete graph, step function *Graphs for continuous interval data:* histogram, frequency polygon, cumulative frequency graph
Bivariate problems — Correlational problems	Bivariate frequency distribution: the crosstabulation table	Two set of ranks	Scatterdiagram
Bivariate problems — Experimental and pseudo-experimental problems: independent groups	*Independent and dependent variable categorical:* the crosstabulation table		*Independent variable categorical, dependent variable interval:* paired frequency polygons, paired cumulative frequency graphs *Independent and dependent variable interval:* scatterdiagram
Bivariate problems — Dependent measures: pretest and posttest or matched groups	Crosstabulation table		Paired cumulative frequency graphs, paired frequency polygons

TYPE OF PROBLEM

Figure 12-4. Classification matrix: techniques for organizing and presenting empirical data.

Redrawn from Introductory Statistics by James A. Twaite and Jane A. Monroe. Copyright © 1979 by Scott, Foresman & Co. Reprinted by permission.

LEVEL OF MEASUREMENT OF VARIABLE(S) OF INTEREST

	Categorical: nominal or ordered categories	Rank-order	Interval scale (or ratio-scale)
Univariate problems	Modal category Proportion of observations falling outside modal category *With ordered categories:* Median category	Percentile rank	Mode, median, mean Range, interquartile range, standard deviation Percentile rank, standard score
Correlational problems	Cramer's index of contingency	Spearman rank-order correlation	Pearson product-moment correlation
Experimental and pseudo-experimental problems: independent groups	Compare modes in different groups	Rank all scores in all groups taken together, then compare the overall rankings of the middle score in each group	Compare mode, median, mean Compare range, interquartile range, standard deviation
Dependent measures: pretest and posttest or matched groups	Compare modes (either pretest and posttest modes or modes in the two groups)	Use ranking method described in the cell above this one	Use methods described in the cell above this one

TYPE OF PROBLEM — Bivariate problems

Figure 12-5. Classification matrix: descriptive statistics.

Redrawn from Introductory Statistics by James A. Twaite and Jane A. Monroe. Copyright © 1979 by Scott, Foresman & Co. Reprinted by permission.

LEVEL OF MEASUREMENT OF VARIABLE(S) OF INTEREST

TYPE OF PROBLEM		Categorical: nominal or ordered categories	Rank-order	Interval scale (or ratio-scale)
Univariate problems		Binominal test Normal approximation to binominal χ^2 one-variable test *With ordered categories:* Kolmogorov-Smirnov one-variable test		One-sample z-test One-sample t-test Confidence interval for population mean (z- or t-method)
Bivariate problems	Correlational problems	χ^2 test of association	Test for significance of Spearman r_S	t-Test for significance of Pearson r Fisher z_r transformation for testing significance of Pearson r Confidence interval for ρ
	Experimental and pseudo-experimental problems: independent groups	Fisher exact probability test χ^2 test of homogeneity	Mann-Whitney U-test Kruskal-Wallis analysis of variance by ranks	t-Test for independent samples One-way analysis of variance Scheffé contrast
	Dependent measures: pretest and posttest or matched groups	McNemar test	Wilcoxon signed-ranks test	t-Test for dependent samples

Figure 12-6. Classification matrix: inferential statistics.

Redrawn from Introductory Statistics by James A. Twaite and Jane A. Monroe. Copyright © 1979 by Scott, Foresman & Co. Reprinted by permission.

    a. Is it a correlational problem, in which a single group is measured on two variables at one point in time?

    b. Is it an experimental or pseudoexperimental problem, in which two or more independent groups are formed and then compared on some variable of interest?

    c. Is it a problem involving two sets of dependent measures, such as a pretest and posttest problem or a matched group's experimental problem?

4. What is the level of measurement of the variable(s) of interest?

Although there are more complicated statistical problems that may not fit into the matrix, such as multivariate problems involving more than two variables, the matrix allows an introduction to the range of problems. Relationship analysis (correlation, regression, and multiple regression) and multivariate analysis (factor analysis, canonical classifications, and multiple discriminate analysis) are briefly reviewed later in this chapter.

Measurement

The determination of the value of a particular variable in a particular subject or at a particular point in time is the measurement of that variable. The process may be simple or complex, depending on what the variable is and which group it is being measured. Unless a true measure of the variable of interest is obtained, none of the statistical techniques mean anything. In empirical research it is a truism that "You can't get good results without good data." What exactly are good data? Typically, good data mean that the measurement procedure is reliable and valid.

Reliability. Reliability of a particular measurement process is the consistency or repeatability of its results. A measurement process as objective as the measurement of temperature may not be totally reliable. The thermometer may have some imperfection that results in different readings at different times for the same true air temperature.

Validity. Validity is concerned with the extent to which the process is measuring what is actually meant to be measured rather than some other variable.

Operational definition. The method by which the variable is measured is known as the *operational definition* of the variable of interest and it gives the reader of a research report the information needed to judge whether the research has achieved a reliable and valid measure of the variable of interest. For example, when age is the variable of interest, one subject may lie about his age. Another might give her age in terms of years at the time of her last birthday. Another might look ahead and round off the age to the nearest year. Thus the article stating "age was given to the nearest whole year" would enable the reader to have more confidence in the consistency of measurement of this variable.

Population of Interest

When a research study is completed and a conclusion is drawn, there are two questions to ask. The first has to do with *internal validity* and whether differences between two experimental groups are real. Has the investigator shown that the control group performed differently from the experimental group? The second question is related to *external validity.* Can a generalization be made from the study to a larger population of subjects? For the reader to judge the external validity of a particular study, the research must provide a complete description of the population of interest, the group to which the results of the study are to be applied.

Procedures

As stated at the beginning, this discussion is not intended to be a how-to-do-it section but rather to tell how they do it. In the remainder of this chapter, various statistical procedures used in tests of difference and relationship analysis are reviewed.

Difference Analysis

The *t* test is a statistical method that can be used for testing the significance between the means of two different populations. The *t* test is actually a ratio between the sample mean difference and the standard error of that difference. Given a calculated value of *t*, this value is interpreted for its probability of occurrence in testing a null hypothesis against an alternative research hypothesis. If this probability value is equal to less than the level set for significance, the null hypothesis is rejected in favor of the research hypothesis. In a study assessing family similarities in food preferences the *t* test was used to compare child-mother and child-father food choices with those of pseudo-parents (parents of another child in the sample) (Pliner, 1983).

Analysis of variance. Whereas the *t* test is usually used in testing the difference between two population means based on differences found between them based on differences found between sample means, analysis of variance is used when the research hypothesis incorporates two or more sample means. Thus when more than two groups on a dependent variable are to be compared, the technique used is the analysis of variance. There are techniques for the single-factor analysis of variance (a single independent variable or factor) and multiple-factor analysis of variance (more than one factor).

In Pliner (1983) the analysis of variance revealed a highly significant effect of the relationship ($p < .0001$), indicating that the food preference of students resembled those of their real parents to a much greater degree than they resembled those of their pseudoparents.

Single-factor analysis of variance is a statistical model used for testing the significance of difference among two or more means when these means reflect the consequences of different levels of a single independent variable. The statistical logic of analysis of variance is incorporated in the *F* ratio, a ratio of between-groups variance to within-groups variance. Given a calculated value of *F*, this value is interpreted in a sampling distribution for its probability under the terms of the null hypothesis, which states that there is no difference among the means of the sampled populations. If this probability is equal to or less than the criterion set for statistical significance, the null hypothesis is rejected in favor of the research hypothesis, which states that there is a difference between at least one group of means. Analysis of covariance is a method by which known pretreatment intergroup variations can be mathematically removed from measures of posttreatment intergroup variations before conducting an *F* test.

Multiple-factor analysis of variance is a statistical model for testing the consequences of manipulating two or more independent variables in a single research design. Each independent variable (factor) will have two or more levels. The *F* ratios are also used to conduct the appropriate hypothesis tests in multiple-factor designs. Significance tests among different levels of each factor are known as *main effects*. Whatever effects are solely the result of the combination of factors are known as *interaction effects*.

Nonparametric tests. In addition to the three tests just described, there are tests that do not directly incorporate estimates pertaining to population characteristics. These are called *nonparametric tests*. The most common such test is *chi square*. Nonparametric statistical models are generally used when the researcher is faced with the use of nominal or ordinal scaling or when particular assumptions cannot be made about the nature of populations being studied. With nominal scaling, a commonly used statistic is chi square. It applies in tests centering on how observations in a sample distribute into different categories, as well as how two samples may differ in terms of their distributions. There are additional nonparametric tests for comparing more than two groups, as well as tests of relationships among sets of measures. Generally speaking, nonparametric tests are considered less powerful than their parametric counterparts, yet nonparametric tests were created to deal with data that could not be analyzed using parametric measurements.

Relationship Analysis

Correlation. Correlation characterizes the relationship between variables, that is, the degree to which two variables vary together (positive correlation) or vary inversely (negative correlation). The Pearson product-moment correlation coefficient, r, has a range of values from $+1.0$ (perfect positive correlation) through -1.0 (perfect negative correlation). In the study of family similarities of food preferences mentioned earlier, to determine the degree of child-parent similarity in food preference a Pearson product-moment correlation was adopted (Pliner, 1983). A Pearson product-moment correlation was computed between the food preference ratings of each student and his or her mother and father. Thus for each child-mother and child-father pair, there was a correlation computed for the ratings of 47 foods on the questionnaire. These correlations represent a measure of the degree of resemblance between members of each pair.

Regression. In addition to indexing the relationship between variables discussed above, the relationship can be further used as a basis for prediction. Given values of one variable, what are the best estimates of related values of another variable? The basis for such prediction is found in the logic of regression analysis. The predictive relationship can be shown in terms of a *line of best fit*, or in terms of the mathematical definition of this line, called a *regression equation*. A range of probable error for predictions can be calculated; this is known as the *standard error of the estimate*. Predicted variance can be further tested to see if the variance exceeds a chance occurrence by use of the F test (the same essentially as in analysis of variance).

Multiple regression analysis provides for the prediction of values of a variable given the values of two or more variables. The equation describes the mathematical combinations of the predictors for the best estimate of the predicted variable. Here, too, an F test can be used. The equation

for multiple linear regression is an extension of the two-variable simple regression equation. Much of the focus in multiple regression analysis is centered on predictor variables—their statistical significance in regression equations, effects of adding or deleting variables, and their practical interpretation. An example of the use of multiple regression is reported in a study of food intake frequencies of food co-op shoppers (Fjeld et al., 1984). Shoppers were surveyed in one co-op store and one commercial supermarket in each city studied to determine whether food intake of shoppers differed according to the market in which they shopped. Multiple regression analysis was used to determine if the frequency of intake of each food differed according to whether respondents were co-op or supermarket shoppers. For each of 28 food products, frequency of consumption scores served as the dependent variable, and type of shopper (co-op or supermarket), educational level, age (indices), gender, and city were the independent variables. Results indicated that co-op shoppers consumed the following foods more frequently than did supermarket shoppers: tofu, brown rice, alfalfa sprouts, honey, dry beans, yogurt, granola, and squash. Supermarket shoppers consumed significantly more franks, beef, poultry, pork, white bread, white rice, and candy bars than the co-op shoppers.

Multivariate Analysis

Factor analysis describes relations among a relatively large number of variables with relatively fewer hypothetical variables called *factors*. Factor analysis begins with a matrix of intercorrelations and estimates of the measurement error involved in each variable. The solution itself redefines the correlation matrix in terms of a *factor matrix*. There are different procedures for rotating the factor matrix according to such criteria as simple structure or psychological fit. Given a rotated factor matrix, the researcher then attempts a subjective interpretation of the factors that have been obtained. Sources of variation in factor analysis include definition of common factor variance (variance attributable to the factors extracted), specific variance (nonerror variance not included in the factor structure), and error variance.

Canonical correlation is the correlation of one cluster of variables with another. Its basis is the calculation of the linear combinations of two sets of variables that are maximally correlated. Each combination is a pair of canonical variates that yield a canonical correlation coefficient and a set of coefficients that describe the weighing of each variable in the two sets on canonical variates. Successive variants attempt new maximum linear correlations; hence for a particular analysis there may be more than one correlation coefficient and several sets of variable weights. Canonical correlation has much in common with factor analysis and multiple regression analysis.

Multiple discriminant analysis provides for the differentiation of single-variable groups or categories on the basis of relationships with an array of discriminating variables. Calculation seeks to identify maximum multiple linear relations of discriminating variables with the groups. Each set of relationships is called a *discriminant function*. Multiple discriminant analysis is used to describe the differentiation of groups, based on discriminating variables, as well as a basis for classifying new cases into likely groups. Such analyses are part of a family of multivariate methods, all of which involve assessments of relationships within, among, or between groups of variables. Discriminant function scores are standardized and are thus interpretable in terms of distributional probabilities.

SUMMARY

This chapter is designed to help community dietitian/nutritionist students learn to perform more effectively whether they are engaged in providing services, teaching, or research. With the advancement of science there is an explosion of knowledge and the introduction of new technology. There are analytical techniques that are tools for the dietitian/nutritionist—computer science, epidemiology, and statistics. The application of these tools can enhance the role of the community dietitian/nutritionist.

REFERENCES

Ahrens, E.H., Jr.: Introduction: the evidence relating six dietary factors to the nation's health, Am. J. Clin. Nutr. 32(12):2627, 1979.

Argo, J.K., Watson, D.R., and Lee, E.C.: A computer-managed instruction system applied to dietetic education, J. Am. Diet. Assoc. 79:5, 1981.

Balintfy, J.L.: On a basic class of multi-item inventory problems, Management Sci. 10(2):287, 1964.

Breese, M.S., Welch, A.C., and Schimpfhauser, F.: Computer-simulated clinical encounters. I. Development, utilization and evaluation of a program, J. Am. Diet. Assoc. 70(4):382, 1977.

Cohen, S.B.: Florence Nightingale, Sci. Am. 250:128, 1984.

Computers in nutrition education, J. Nutr. Educ. 16:2, June 1984.

Dobbins, J.G., and Buffler, P.A.: Epidemiology. In Course syllabus, Galveston, 1980, University of Texas Medical Branch.

Dunphy, M.K., and Bratton, B.D.: A computerized dietary order entry system, J. Am. Diet. Assoc. 82(1):68, 1983.

Dwyer, J., and Suitor, C.W.: Caveat emptor: assessing needs, evaluating computer options, J. Am. Diet. Assoc. 84(3):302, 1984.

Feinstein, A.R.: Clinical judgment, Melbourne, Fla., 1976, R.E. Krieger Publishing Co., Inc.

Fjeld, C.R., et al.: Food intake frequencies of food co-op shoppers, J. Nutr. Ed. 16(3):142, 1984.

Food and Nutrition Board: Toward healthful diets, Washington, D.C., 1980, National Academy of Science.

Frank, R.C.: Information resources for food and human nutrition, J. Am. Diet. Assoc. 80:4, 1982.

Hoover, L.W.: Computers in nutrition, dietetics, and food service management: a bibliography (1958–1981), Columbia, 1981, University of Missouri Press.

Hoover, L.W.: The Nutrient Data Bank Directory, ed. 4, Columbia, 1984, University of Missouri Press.

Hoover, L.W., and Perloff, B.P.: Model for review of nutrient data base system capabilities, Columbia, 1981, University of Missouri Press.

Kannel, W.E., et al.: Serum cholesterol, lipoproteins, and the risk of coronary heart disease: The Framingham Study, Ann. Intern. Med. 74:1, 1971.

Keyes, A.: Seven countries: a multivariate analysis of death and coronary heart disease, Cambridge, Mass., 1980, Harvard University Press.

Kleinbaum, D.G., Kupper, L.L., and Morganstern, H.: Epidemiologic research: principles and quantitative methods, Blemont, Calif., 1982, Lifetime Learning Publications.

Leavell, H.R., and Clark, E.G.: Preventive medicine for the doctor in his community: an epidemiologic approach, New York, 1965, McGraw-Hill, Inc.

Naisbitt, J.: Megatrends: ten new directions transforming our lives, New York, 1982, Warner Books, Inc.

National Institute of Health Consensus Development Conference, Osteoporosis, Bethesda, Md., April 2-4, 1984.

National Institute of Health Consensus Development Conference, Lowering blood cholesterol to prevent heart disease, Bethesda, Md., Dec. 10-12, 1984.

National Institute of Health Consensus Development Conference, Health implications of obesity, Bethesda, Md., Feb. 11-13, 1985.

Nichols, A.B., et al.: Daily nutritional intake and serum lipid levels: The Tecumseh Study, Am. J. Clin. Nutr. **29**:1384, 1976.

Nutritional epidemiology, Dairy Council Dig. **53**:4, July–August 1982.

Pliner, P.: Family resemblance in food preferences, J. Nutr. Ed. **15**(4):137, 1983.

Schuster, K.: The choice: computers in food service, Food Man. **16**:43, August 1981.

Shelly, G.B., and Cashman, T.J.: Introduction to computers and data processing, Belmont, Calif., 1980, Anaheim Publishing Co.

Twaite, J.A., and Monroe, J.A.: Introductory statistics, Glenview, Ill., 1979, Scott, Foresman & Co.

Wheeler, M.L., and Wheeler, L.A.: Computer-planned menus for patients with diabetes mellitus, Diabetes Care **3**:6, Nov./Dec. 1980.

Witschi, J., et al.: Analysis of dietary data: an interactive computer method for storage and retrieval, J. Am. Diet. Assoc. **78**(6):609, 1981.

Youngwirth, J.: The evolution of computers in dietetics: a review, J. Am. Diet. Assoc. **82**(1):62, 1983.

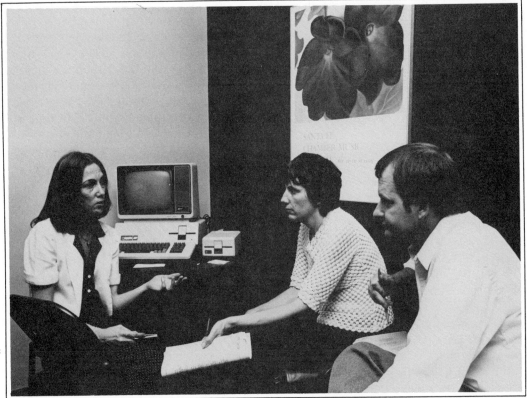

H. Armstrong Roberts

Developing Behavioral Change Skills

GENERAL CONCEPT

Over the past two decades an impressive change has occurred in the life-styles of many persons in the United States and other parts of the world. The evidence clearly demonstrates that large-scale interventions at the community level based on diet counseling techniques are feasible and effective. To change the eating behavior of the client, the community dietitian/nutritionist is most effective when working to facilitate the client's understanding of his or her behavior. Learning involves change. Learning is concerned with the acquisition of habits, knowledge, and attitudes. Thus the community dietitian/nutritionist assumes the role of change agent, which requires special client-focused skills.

When you finish this chapter, you should be able to
- Define and cite examples of how life-style affects health
- Relate learning theory to behavior change
- Design nutrition counseling plans for specific nutrition-related diseases
- Cite an example of a community program that has effected behavioral change in the population treated

LIFE-STYLE BEHAVIOR

Healthy People, the Surgeon General's Report on Health Promotion and Disease Prevention (USDHEW, 1979) has called for a renewed national commitment to both societal prevention (e.g., reducing environmental risks) and individual prevention (e.g., changing unhealthy behavior or life-style). The report estimates "that perhaps as much as half of the United States mortality in 1976 was due to unhealthy behavior or life-style: 20% to environmental factors; 20% to human biological factors; and only 20% to inadequacies in health care." A similar finding was announced by the Canadian Department of Health Promotion and prompted the issuance of a life-style poster (box, p. 375) that was displayed throughout Canada (Lalonde, 1974).

Studies by Breslow and Enstrom (1980) of almost 7000 adults followed for 5½ years showed that life expectancy and health are significantly related to basic habits: three meals a day at regular times, breakfast every day, moderate exercise two or three times a week, adequate sleep, no smoking, moderate weight, and alcohol in moderation. Health is determined by life-style, including dietary habits, food intake, and the nature of the environment.

Many health promotion studies have documented the correlation between personal health practices and subsequent morbidity and mortality. The goal of nutrition counseling is to help the client to select and implement more desirable nutrition and life-style behaviors. Behavior change is conveyed to the client by the nutrition counselor, who has the specific skills required for the process. Thus the community dietitian/nutritionist employed by community agencies often serves as a change agent with clients.

The question arises: How do clients learn and adapt new life-style behaviors? A review of learning theories seems appropriate.

LEARNING THEORIES: HOW IS BEHAVIOR CHANGED?

Learning involves change. Learning is concerned with the acquisition of habits, knowledge, and attitudes. Learning enables the individual to make both personal and social adjustments. Because the concept of change is inherent in the concept of learning, any change in behavior implies that learning is taking place or has taken place. Learning that occurs during the process of change can be referred to as the *learning process*. Learning theorists see learning as a process by which behavior is changed, shaped, or controlled. Knowles (1978) defines learning in terms of growth, development of competency, and fulfillment of potential. Other therapists believe that learning entails personal involvement of the whole person and includes both feelings and cognitive aspects; it is self-initiated and pervasive.

The Rogers-Shoemaker Change Process

The adoption of new ideas or practices is seen as the result of a sequence of events by Rogers and Shoemaker (1971), who describe this sequence as the *innovation-decision process*. The process consists of the following stages: *knowledge*—the individual is exposed to the innovation's existence and learns about it; *persuasion*—the individual forms a favorable or unfavorable attitude toward the innovation; *decision*—the individual engages in activities that lead to a choice to adopt or reject the innovation; *confirmation*—the individu-

LIFE-STYLE

Life-style is the unique pattern of your daily life. It is neither sickness nor health. It is the food you eat, the weight problem, the malnutrition, the balanced diet.

Life-style is the cars you drive and the seat belts you don't wear. It's speeding or taking it easy. It's the alcohol you drink. . . . it's the deadly "one more for the road." It's moderation and alcoholism. It's knowing when to get treatment . . . and getting it. It's protecting your loved ones or letting them down.

Life-style is the drugs you take, the cigarettes you smoke, the alcohol you drink. It is addiction and moderation . . . it's abuse of over-the-counter drugs, use of illegal drugs, and it's intelligent use of medication.

Life-style is staying in shape or getting fit through regular physical activity, or it's going to seed. It's participating in sports or being an observer. It's pursuing a hobby or sitting for hours watching television . . . it's getting out and doing something enjoyable or being bored.

Life-style is how you handle stress, tension, and loneliness . . . it's knowing how to relax. It's how you feel about yourself, your life, job, family, and friends. It's being able to change some things in your life and living with those you can't. It's contentment or despair.

Life-style is using safeguards or taking needless risks with your health, on the job, at home, at school, or when playing sports.

Life-style is learning how to deal with emergencies or being helpless. It's learning to swim, practicing water safety, and being able to give first aid. It's common sense or foolhardiness.

Your *life-style*, at this moment, whether good or bad, is distinctly your own; it will change according to your attitude and ability to change. Your life-style reflects with reasonable accuracy what your health may be in the future . . . unless changes are made for the better.

From A new perspective on the health of Canadians: a working document, 1974; with permission from Health and Welfare Canada, Ottawa, Canada.

---

al continues with the innovation or may reverse the previous decision if exposed to conflicting messages. Rogers and Shoemaker stress the significance of the confirmation stage because it underlines that desired changes in dietary practices may not be maintained without follow-up support and counseling.

The Health Belief Model

The health belief model suggests that people are likely to follow health recommendations if they are motivated and if they believe (1) that they are susceptible to illness; (2) that the occurrence of this condition will have a serious impact on their lives; (3) that following a particular set of health recommendations will be beneficial; and (4) that the health recommendations will provide psychological benefits (Rosenstock, 1982). This theory of learning when related to efforts to modify eating practices has five axioms:

1. Clients bring to any situation their own sets of beliefs, attitudes, motives, experiences, knowledge, and expectations.

2. Learning proceeds best when it is incremental, that is, when the learner acquires a little knowledge at a time.

3. Behaviors that are reinforced or rewarded tend to be learned and repeated, whereas behaviors that are not rewarded tend to be extinguished and not repeated.

4. Many of the behavior patterns that may affect health represent habits learned early in life, and these patterns are difficult to change.

5. Learning has both a cognitive and a skill component.

These axioms demonstrate the following: prior beliefs and attitudes influence interpretations; effective learning is incremental; reinforcement is of great value; much behavior is habitual; and learning includes both cognition and skills. With identification of a person's status on each variable in the health belief model an educational diagnosis may be made that will lead to the formulation of an educational plan, which is directed toward modifying beliefs.

Stewart's Behavioral Change Plan

Sequential, incremental learning may be the only process needed for those clients who are able to see the steps needed to reach their objectives sequentially. Stewart suggests the following plan to promote learning and to minimize failure: (1) divide nutrition information into small, manageable steps arranged in sequence; (2) arrange for the first step to be easy; (3) sequence the steps that follow; (4) attempt to make each step small but not trivial; (5) involve the client in planning changes in nutrition behavior; and (6) state each step within a total nutrition instruction plan (Stewart et al., 1978).

Knowles' Adult Learning Concepts

Knowles (1978) introduces the concept of a unified theory of adult learning for which the label *androgogy* has been coined to differentiate it from the theory of youth learning (*pedagogy*). Androgogical theory is based on four major assumptions that are different from those of pedagogy:

1. Changes in self-concept. It is assumed that as a person grows and matures the individual's self-concept moves from one of total dependency to one of increasing self-directedness. For example, a student entering a professional school has made a step toward seeing himself as essentially self-directed. Likewise, adults joining a community weight loss program exhibit self-directedness.
2. The role of experience. As persons mature, they accumulate an expanding reservoir of experience that causes them to become increasingly rich resources for learning. At the same time they are provided with a broadening base to which to relate new learnings. In adult learning lectures, pre-recorded audiovisual presentations, and assigned readings are not as successful as discussions, laboratory and field experiences, team projects, and other action-learning techniques.
3. Readiness to learn. It is assumed that as an individual matures, readiness to learn is decreasingly the product of biological development and academic pressure and is increasingly the product of developmental tasks required for performance of evolving social roles. A community nutrition student needs to have direct experience with patients, community programs, and agency exposure to make classroom learning of nutrition surveillance and public health programming seem relevant.
4. Orientation to learning. Children have been conditioned to have a subject-centered orientation to most learning, whereas adults tend to have a problem-centered orientation. New management skills to address an eating problem will enhance the learning process.

HOW TO CHANGE BEHAVIOR: NUTRITION COUNSELING

The goal of nutrition counseling is to help the client select and implement more desirable nutrition behaviors. Snetselaar (1983) suggests a model that provides a sequenced path for counselors to follow by listing essential components in each step of the process (Figure 13-1).

In this model the counselor (1) prepares for the interview by reviewing all available data; (2) explains the counseling relationship so the client knows precisely what will take place; (3) evaluates the client's nutritional status and relates food intake data to behavioral indicators; (4) monitors the client's performance; (5) ends the program and perhaps allows for periodic follow-up; and (6) does a self-evaluation of his or her performance.

Dietary change may involve modifications in intake of calories, fat and cholesterol, carbohydrates, protein, sodium, and bland foods. Snetselaar outlines specific objectives for each counseling situation: low-calorie, low-fat and low-cholesterol, low-carbohydrate, low-protein, or low-sodium eating patterns and liberal bland diets. Each situation is approached with the following considerations:

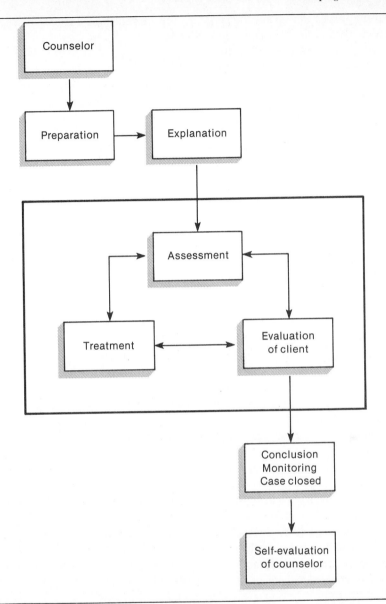

Figure 13-1. Model for nutrition counseling.
Redrawn from Snetselaar, L.C.: Nutrition counseling skills: assessment, treatment, and evaluation. Reprinted with permission of Aspen Systems Corporation, © 1983.

1. What are the inappropriate eating behaviors associated with the diet?
2. What assessment has been made of individual eating behaviors?
3. Which treatment strategies are appropriate to combat inappropriate eating behaviors? Behavioral strategies? Cueing devices? Nutrition basics?
4. How is new appropriate eating behavior evaluated? Monitoring devices? Checklists of evaluation criteria for client and counselor?

In addition to counseling objectives, examples of dietary adherence tools and reading lists for each dietary modification are provided (Snetselaar, 1983).

Cormier and Cormier (1979) suggest that it is important that before the task of counseling practitioners seek to examine their own behavior—to acquire self-knowledge. The way in which nutrition counselors view themselves and their priorities, values, and expectations will determine how the interview proceeds. Potential self-image traits that can result in negative consequences during an interview are competence, power, and intimacy. The counselor who lacks self-confidence may project a sense of inadequacy and fear and may avoid positive interactions by negating positive feedback and making self-deprecating or apologetic comments. The overpowerful counselor may assume a role of authority and may project an overbearing presence to the client, whereas the underpowerful counselor loses control of the interviewing process and can be easily manipulated by the client. Feelings of intimacy can range from affection and concern to lack of interest and rejection. To determine whether a counselor's characteristics are conducive to effective counseling, practitioners should ask of themselves "Who am I?" and "What is important to me?"

Four Basic Elements in Nutrition Counseling

The basic elements in nutrition counseling are (1) nutritional assessment, (2) the treatment plan, (3) intervention leading to change, and (4) evaluation.*

Assessment

Assessment consists of the initial interview, the process of data gathering, and the analysis of these data for nutritional adequacy and food and life-style habits.

The interview, the initial point of contact, is of vital importance because it is the structure within which the client and the practitioner develop a trusting, nonjudgmental relationship. Rogers (1951) has identified three characteristics essential for relationship-building skills: the counselor's empathy, genuineness, and unconditional positive regard for the client. Danish (1975) has expanded this approach into a six-stage program: (1) understanding the dietitian's need to be a helper; (2) using effective nonverbal behavior, (3) using effective verbal behavior, (4) using effective self-involving behavior, (5) understanding the other's communications; and (6) establishing effective helping relationships. Snetselaar (1983) lists nutrition interviewing skills as listening, verbal communication, nonverbal communication, teaching responses, sharing, and action responses (Figure 13-2).

Active listening, or sensitive listening, is an effective agent for individual change and development. Listening by a concerned person brings about changes in individuals' attitudes toward themselves and others. It also effects change in basic values and personal philosophy. Listening says "I care." The verbal communication skills used in an interview and counseling session include (1) explanatory responses (passive, nondirective, directive), (2) clarification, (3) empathy, (4) self-decisions, (5) confrontation, and (6) information giving.

*Refer to Baird, S.C., and Sylvester, J.: Role delineation and verification for entry-level positions in community dietetics, Chicago, 1983, The American Dietetic Association, which summarizes comprehensive nutrition care in a variety of settings for individual clients.

Explanatory responses are part of the art of listening. In passive listening the counselor makes a brief verbal intervention such as "Um-huh" or "Really." Nondirective responses encourage the client to continue discussing the problem and to explore it further ("Please tell me more" or "Go on"). Directive responses encourage clients to explore various aspects of a topic that they seem to be avoiding ("When that happened, what did you feel?").

Clarification merely allows for a restatement of the situation. Empathy, a skill that can be learned and used effectively, sets the stage for achieving the desired goals of the relationship. Self-disclosure is a sharing response that allows counselors to interject some information about themselves that may strengthen the relationship.

Confrontation is an invitation to examine and possibly change some form of behavior that seems to be self-defeating or harmful. Confrontation helps individuals see more clearly what is happening, what the consequences are, and how they can assume responsibility for taking action to change in ways that can lead to a more effective life-style.

Information giving is the final verbal communication skill. Here the counselor is able to deliver a part of the treatment plan that evolves from the information gathered during the interview and assessment session.

After the interview, the next task in the assessment process is to gather reliable data about food intake patterns, eating behavior, feelings, and attitudes—both past and present—that will provide insight to allow for effective counseling. Then the goal of nutrition counseling, which is to facilitate behavior change, can be achieved using a more realistic approach.

There are essentially four kinds of data collected throughout the assessment phase (Mason, Wenberg, and Welch, 1982). *Environmental* data include factors in the client's personal life that play a role in food choices (employment, family status, community, education). *Biological* data are descriptive of physiological elements in

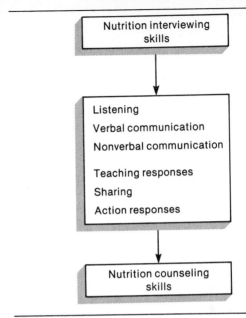

Figure 13-2. Interviewing skills as a foundation for counseling.
Redrawn from Snetselaar, L.C.: Nutrition counseling skills: assessment, treatment, and evaluation. Reprinted with permission of Aspen Systems Corporation, © 1983.

the client's health history (laboratory evaluations, anthropometric measurements, physical findings). *Food intake* data describe the client's food and food supplement consumption. *Behavioral* data encompass the client's behavior, thoughts, and feelings that affect eating behavior. Specific instruments such as Initial Data Schedules, Food Frequency Schedule, Food Practices Schedule have been designed by Mason.

There are two factors to be considered when dietary intake data are assessed: (1) types of nutrients consumed and (2) appropriate quantities. Two methods commonly used are comparison with the USDA Daily Food Guide, wherein servings from each food group are evaluated, and most recently computerization of diet history resulting in figuring amounts of specific nutrients based on food composition tables.

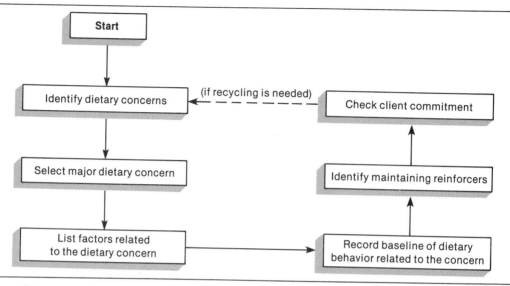

Figure 13-3. Setting up a process for dealing with client concerns.
Redrawn from Norman R. Stewart et al., Systematic Counseling, © 1978. Adapted by permission of
Prentice-Hall, Inc., Englewood Cliffs, N.J.

These four types of data—dietary, biological, environmental, and behavioral—are usually collected simultaneously and are compiled to enable the counselor to design a treatment plan. A statement of needs based on the analysis of the collected data is the route to the development of client objectives.

The Treatment Plan

The treatment plan, the second major step in counseling, is designed with consideration for the following major steps (Cormier and Cormier, 1979; Snetselaar, 1983):

1. *Goal setting/objectives.* A hypothetical patient's data might reveal the following needs assessment, which would determine specific patient objectives. For example, *biological* data reveal an elevated serum cholesterol level; *food intake data* reveal low intake of fruits and vegetables and high fat intake; *environmental* data show the need for financial assistance; and *be-*

havioral data indicate erratic meal times, lack of menu planning, and impulsive buying habits. (See Chapter 3 for further discussion of objectives.)

2. *Identification of dietary concerns.* Once goals are established, dietary concerns are identified as a joint responsibility of the client and counselor. Dietary concerns may be related to a specific food group, a family situation, or portion sizes. Here priority is established and immediate concerns are dealt with. Stewart et al. have outlined a process for dealing with client concerns (Figure 13-3).

3. *Helping strategies.* Helping strategies are plans of action designed to meet specific goals for each client. They focus on goals and objectives.

4. *Factors influencing diet adherence.* The client and the counselor both play a role in diet adherence. Too much information at one time tends to decrease recall because it

overloads the client. Adherence is increased when there is satisfaction with both the counselor and the care being received.

5. *Adherence predictions.* Adherence predictions include the attitudes of the client, the clinical judgment of the counselor, and self-prediction.

Counseling techniques that assess client behavior change and involve the client in the counseling process tend to have positive outcomes that increase dietary adherence. Familiarity with the following deterrents to dietary adherence will alert the counselor to anticipate negative outcomes: restrictiveness of dietary patterns, required changes in life-style and behavior, lack of meaningful relief once change is made, increased cost of foods, unavailability of foods, and change in food preparation techniques (Glanz, 1979).

Documentation of the nutrition care plan in the client's record is the responsibility of the community dietitian/nutritionist. By rendering meaningful observations and information on food habits, food acceptance, and dietary treatment, the nutrition staff establishes communication with the physician and other professionals participating in the client's total care.

Professional Standards Review Organizations (PSROs), created under PL 92-603 in 1972, are required to include nonphysician health care practices, such as charting by the community dietitian/nutritionist, in the review of care provided by their peers to recipients of Medicare, Medicaid, Maternal and Child Health Services, and Crippled Children's Services. This involvement includes development of standards and criteria for use by peers in reviewing the quality of services delivered by practitioners in their own discipline.

Intervention/Behavior Change

Intervention, the application of the treatment plan, focuses on behavior. Whether a particular eating pattern or a general life-style that is being examined with recommendation for change, at the end of the visit the client should be planning to do something different.

Behavior modification related to dietary behavior had its origins in the treatment of obesity. Ineffectiveness in the treatment of obesity before 1959 was summarized in an often cited paper by Stunkard and McLaren-Hume (1959):

> Most obese persons will not remain in treatment. Of those who do remain in treatment, most will not lose much weight, and of those who do lose weight, most will regain it.

The situation was radically changed with the appearance of Stuart's landmark paper "Behavioral Control of Overeating" in 1967. Most studies that report application of behavior therapy for obesity use Stuart's program with slight modifications. His method is based on principles of social psychology, which demonstrate that eating patterns are a function of environmental controls and that often eating behavior is determined by the presence of different things in the environment, particularly food cues.

Most behavioral programs have employed one or more of the following components: (1) self-monitoring of body weight and/or food intake, (2) implicit or explicit goal setting, (3) nutrition, exercise, and health counseling, (4) tangible operant consequences (reward and punishment), (5) aversion therapy, (6) social reinforcement in the form of a support system such as therapist, group, or family (7) covert conditioning and cognitive restructuring strategies, (8) self-presented consequences (self-reward, self-punishment), and (9) stimulus control procedures.

Stuart (1967), in what has been called the classic study on the behavioral control of obesity, used these stimulus control procedures with eight obese women. His results were unprecedented in the obesity literature. Stuart's least successful subject lost 11.7 kg (26 pounds); the remaining seven ranged up to a 21.2 kg (47-pound) loss at the end of the year. These impressive results stimulated a host of studies and became the basic

BEHAVIORAL STRATEGIES AND TECHNIQUES

I. Techniques for increasing awareness
  A. Daily recording of eating behavior
  B. Sitting down while eating
  C. Eating more slowly
  D. Avoid distracting activities while eating
  E. Limit eating to fewer places

II. Techniques for decreasing exposure
  A. Rearranging food supplies
  B. Adjust packaging and storage
  C. Keep food out of rooms other than kitchen or pantry
  D. Have children make their own snacks
  E. Ask family and friends not to use food for gifts
  F. Avoid passing by particular store or vending machine if problem
  G. Keep extra food away from the table
  H. Clear table immediately after eating
  I. Prepare snacks in small quantities
  J. At parties position yourself away from source of food

III. Techniques for altering susceptibility
  A. Write food intake in advance
  B. Plan in advance for preferred foods
  C. Preplan food intake for each day

D. Set up a time schedule each day for meals and snacks
E. Decide beforehand what you will order in a restaurant
F. Avoid long periods of deprivation prior to a party or restaurant meal
G. Prepare a complete shopping list
H. Shop when not hungry

IV. Techniques for altering response
  A. Changing the way you eat
    1. Plan a short delay before you eat
    2. Slow down eating
    3. Eat preferred foods first
    4. Leave a small amount of food on your plate
    5. At restaurant make special requests
  B. Alternative activities
    1. Make a list of chores to be done
       5 min (e.g., watering plants)
       10 min (e.g., write a letter)
       20 min (e.g., paying bills)
       30 min (e.g., straighten a closet)
    2. Make hobbies and recreation available and ready
    3. Use physical activity (e.g., walking, running in place, etc.) instead of eating

structure for the behavior modification series in the successful Weight Watchers program.

The standard behavioral treatment program is usually based on record keeping, stimulus control for restricting the external cues that set the occasion for eating, cognitive restructuring, changing eating patterns, and reinforcement of the altered eating behavior. Record keeping, or self-monitoring of specific behavior, thoughts, or feelings in relation to eating (and exercise), is a vitally important component of a successful treatment program. Not only is self-monitoring the mainstay of behavior assessment of eating patterns, it is also part of the behavior change process.

Cue elimination, the elimination of environmental stimuli, involves two steps. The first step is to identify eating cues, or stimuli, in the environment that induce eating when not hungry or continuation of eating when satisfied. The second step in cue elimination is restructuring the environment to avoid these cues. Cognitive restructuring involves using positive thoughts to replace negative or self-defeating ones. Here it is the individual's attitudes, perceptions, and beliefs that determine food intake.

Social skills training can assist clients in coping more constructively with interpersonal problem situations that often trigger inappropriate eating. Eating in restaurants, peer pressure, and

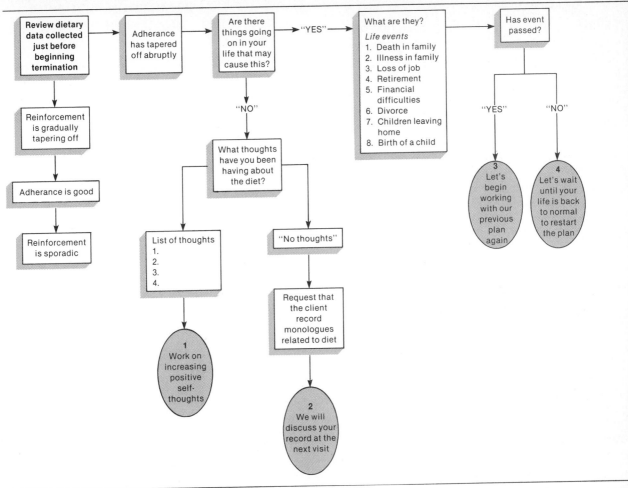

Figure 13-4. Algorithm for nutrition counseling termination.
Redrawn from Snetselaar, L.C.: Nutrition Counseling skills: assessment, treatment, and evaluation.
Reprinted with permission of Aspen Systems Corporation, © 1983.

social situations involving foods can be met with rational behavior as a result of social skills training. Storlie (1984) outlines four major behavioral strategies and techniques: (1) developing the client's awareness of both eating and physical activity patterns; (2) helping the client reduce exposure to situations that cause excessive eating or that allow energy expenditure to be limited; (3) building resistance to those determinants which cause maladaptive eating or limit physical activity; and (4) altering the person's response to problematic situations. These strategies and the techniques are summarized in the box on p. 382.

There comes a time in the process of nutrition counseling when a client is ready to end the sessions. Provision of a planned follow-up is often overlooked. A comprehensive step-by-step procedure for termination is seen in Figure 13-4.

Evaluation

Evaluation is an ongoing process that takes place in all stages of the counseling process. The client's record of eating behavior is compared with objectives. The degree of adherence can be measured by client interviews, biochemical analysis, and daily food records. The counselor, too, should make a self-assessment: Did I help the client meet the objectives? How effective were my counseling techniques, the physical setting, and the follow-up plan?

Following is a six-step procedure for evaluating or assessing the outcomes of nutrition care interventions (Baird and Sylvester, 1983):

1. Monitor each client's progress in attaining nutrition objectives.
2. Evaluate each client's progress in attaining short- and long-term nutrition objectives.
3. Revise the individual client's nutritional care plan.
4. Document the assessment of nutrition care interventions and follow-up for every client.
5. Provide data for the analysis of costs and benefits of nutrition intervention for the client.
6. Apply quality assurance criteria to delivery of nutrition care to individual client.

Thus far the four basic elements of the nutrition counseling process—assessment, treatment, intervention, evaluation—have been discussed with reference to theories of learning. The successful facilitation of the four basic elements is incumbent on the counselor as stated by Mason, Wenberg, and Welch (1982):

This implies that the clinician provides a support system for the achievement of client independence. That is, the clinician shows the client how to remove the obstacles that render a behavior difficult to change; he does not coerce or do for the client anything the client can do for himself. Other synonyms most often substituted for facilitator are counselor and helper. The best counselor or helper works himself out of a job with each client by facilitating client independence.

PRACTICAL APPLICATION: BEHAVIOR CHANGE AT THE COMMUNITY LEVEL
Process Guides

Process guides that incorporate dietary assessment into the multiplicity of steps involved in the delivery of nutrition care can be developed. The purpose of process guides is to guide community health professionals through appropriate nutritional assessment techniques, intervention strategies, follow-up documentation, and referral. Mullis and Bowen (1985) describe the development of process guides by selecting target groups identified by the nutrition section of the Virginia Department of Health. These groups include pregnant women, infants from birth to age 2, children 2 to 18 years old, clients from family planning clinics, home health clients, and older adults. The process guide for adults 60 years of age and older includes a specific criterion, an attribute the client might single out, such as weight loss or underweight, poor dentures, poor appetite, changes in digestion, diminished physical and human resources affecting nutritional status, prescribed diet, self-imposed restricted diet, and drug therapy. Then specific strategies are designed for the nutrition counselor or health professional to deal with screening (How do I decide?), assessment (What judgments do I make?), intervention (What do I do?), reporting (What do I note in the client's chart?), and follow-up and referral (What do I do next?).

National Heart, Lung, and Blood Institute

Adopting healthy dietary habits to help control at least four of the treatable cardiovascular risk factors—high serum cholesterol, high blood pressure, obesity, and diabetes—has long been a concern of the National Heart, Lung, and Blood Institute (NHLBI) and the American Heart Association. To learn how to encourage persons to assume responsibility for their health behavior, especially eating habits, NHLBI has supported a number of research efforts and conferences toward this end. Some recommended readings that can be used to encourage behavior change include:

Heart to Heart: A Manual on Nutrition Counseling for the Reduction of Cardiovascular Disease Risk Factors (NHLBI, 1983)

Proceedings of the Nutrition Behavioral Research Conference (Tillotson, 1975)

Model Workshop on Nutrition Counseling in Hyperlipidemia (USDHHS/NIH, 1980)

Applying Behavioral Science to Cardiovascular Risk (Enelow and Henderson, 1975)

A federal initiative in 1973, called the National High Blood Pressure Education Program, has led to the detection and treatment of persons with hypertension. Public awareness of the dangers of high blood pressure has increased substantially. The value of intervention has been demonstrated by the Hypertension Detection and Follow-Up Program, which is supported by NHLBI. More than 150,000 people in 14 communities across the United States were screened for hypertension, and nearly 11,000 participated in the study (Hypertension Detection, 1979).

The Working Group identified 10 steps the patient must take in making dietary changes for hypertension control (USDHHS, 1981). The steps apply to two therapeutic dietary approaches—sodium reduction and weight management:

Step 1 Acknowledge disease.
Step 2 Consider effectiveness of dietary measures.
Step 3 Assess current dietary influences.
Step 4 Acknowledge that change is long term.
Step 5 Develop a strategy and set goals.
Step 6 Plan for each change.
Step 7 Act to change.
Step 8 Assess success of each change.
Step 9 Assess attainment of blood pressure goal.
Step 10 Maintain diet changes.

An in-depth discussion of these steps in the Working Group Report focuses primarily on the ways behavior can be changed. Specific information about concepts, knowledge, and skills necessary for dietary management and dietary counseling for both the client and the counselor is discussed. The premises on which the 10 client steps were formulated clarify for health professionals an approach to facilitating permanent change in client eating habits. The premises relate to diet management and counseling considerations: aspects of short- and long-term dietary change, patient responsibility and motivation, dietary plan, and environmental changes.

Community Weight Control Programs

Communities can exert a powerful influence on the health of their constituents. Some communities are far better able to supply the cues and consequences of human behavior than is a therapist. Community programs, often delivered by lay members via self-help groups, have met the needs of community members to control obesity. One of the largest and most successful is Weight Watchers International with programs in the United States, Canada, and 23 other countries. Other such groups are TOPS (Take Off Pounds Sensibly), Diet Centers, and Diet Workshop with chapters throughout the United States.

When behavioral modification techniques are added to a positive group environment and nutritionally balanced food program, weight loss results are improved. A 1976 study contrasted the outcome of the traditional Weight Watchers International program with and without the addition of behavior modification methods in a total of 7623 members over a 12-week period (Stuart and Guire, 1979). Those persons participating in the traditional program lost an average of 0.51 kg (1.1 pounds) per week. In contrast, those in the behavioral program lost an average of 0.73 kg (1.6 pounds) per week. When the population tested was restricted to those who attended 8 to 12 meetings during the 12-week test period, the weight loss was improved as much as 24%. Similar findings carried over into a maintenance study. Fifteen months after reaching their goal weights about 70% were within 10% of their goal weights (Stuart and Guire, 1979).

The Weight Watchers International program is four pronged in its approach: a food plan (nutrition), an exercise plan, a self-management plan (behavior modification), and a group support system. The self-management plan consists of 52 skill builders—one for each week of the year. A

WEIGHT WATCHERS
HOW TO MANAGE WEEKEND EATING

Because we have more unstructured time on weekends, our moods and behaviors tend to drift in some often problematic ways. It is important to schedule specific activities on weekends because we are very likely to overeat during unstructured hours.

Steps You Can Take

1. Know your times of weakness. Identify the weekend hours when you are least likely to structure time and most likely to overeat.

2. Develop an activity schedule for the entire weekend, with particular stress on these high-risk hours.
3. Devote some time every weekend to each of the following:
   a. An activity that helps someone else.
   b. An activity that brings you special pleasure.
   c. An activity that helps you complete some important self-care, home maintenance, or work task.
4. Follow through on every planned activity.

A Weekend Activity Planner

Plan activities for this coming weekend. Be sure to devote some time to each category of activity, although you will probably not do all three each day. Write down *exactly* what you will do.

Day	Time	To Help Others	My Special Pleasure	A Chore
Friday evening				
Saturday				
Sunday				

skill builder describes a problem situation that may present a weight loss challenge and offers specific steps to meet the challenge. An example of a skill builder dealing with the problem of weekend eating and steps to be taken is shown in the box above.

Stanford University Study

A university-sponsored program to reduce coronary risk factors was carried out for 2 years by Stanford University in two communities; each had a population of 14,000 (Farquhar, 1978). A massive media campaign—radio, television, newspaper articles, billboard posters, and direct mailings—eliciting a change in behavior was the major intervention in the experimental community. By the end of the second year the risk of coronary heart disease had decreased by 17% in the treatment communities with a 6% increase in the control community. Similar positive findings from community-based programs have been reported from Finland and Sweden.

Programs at Work Sites

Over recent years many major corporations have become aware of losses in dollars and employees as a result of cardiovascular disease. Consequently these corporations have started their own health promotion and disease intervention programs. Among those companies offering comprehensive worksite programs are Campbell Soup Company, Food Motor Company, Kimberly-Clark Corporation, Metropolitan Life Insurance Company, and Johnson & Johnson Products, Inc.

The North Karelia Project

The North Karelia (Finland) Project, in contrast to the university-initiated Stanford Program with its strong research focus, was the result of active community members. In 1971 people in North Karelia asked their government for help in reducing the community's rate of morbidity and mortality from cardiovascular disease, which was among the highest in the world. The project was initiated with specific behavioral objectives: to reduce the incidence of smoking, to change dietary habits to lower intake of saturated fats, and to increase use of vegetables and low-fat products. The successful results of these multiple, behaviorally oriented interventions have been reported by Puska, Neittaanmaki, and Tuomilehto (1980).

The Swedish Diet and Exercise Program

The Swedish Diet and Exercise Program is a landmark in the efforts of an entire nation in the interest of health promotion (Isaksson, 1978). It has become a model for large-scale efforts to improve health behavior. Health professionals, primarily nutritionists, concerned about the high fat content and the decrease in the consumption of cereals and grains in the Swedish diet, joined forces to launch this program. Within the government, the agency responsible for diet and the agency responsible for exercise combined efforts to design and deliver the program. The program recommended specific dietary changes such as lower fat intake, along with planned increase in physical activity. Practical suggestions such as using stairs rather than taking the elevator were adapted.

SUMMARY

To develop effective behavioral strategies that lead to life-style changes, the community dietitian/nutritionist should understand human behavior and how people learn. The goal of nutrition counseling is to help the client adopt more desirable nutrition behavior. This process involves four steps: nutritional assessment, the treatment plan, intervention leading to change, and evaluation. Communities can exert a powerful influence on the health of their constituents through well-designed programs.

REFERENCES

Baird, S.C., and Sylvester, J.: Role delineation and verification for entry-level positions in community dietetics, Chicago, 1983, American Dietetic Association.

Breslow, L., and Enstrom, J.E.: Persistence of health habits and their relationship to health practices and mortality, Prev. Med. 9:469, 1980.

Cormier, W.H., and Cormier, L.S.: Interviewing strategies for helpers: a guide to assessment, treatment, and evaluation, Monterey, Calif., 1979, Brooks/Cole Publishing Co.

Danish, S.J.: Developing helping relationships in dietetic counseling. J. Am. Diet. Assoc. 67:107, 1975.

Enelow, A.J., and Henderson, J.B.: Applying behavioral science to cardiovascular risk, Dallas, 1975, American Heart Association.

Farquhar, J.W.: The American way of life need not be hazardous to your health, New York, 1978, W.W. Norton & Company, Inc.

Glonz, K.: Strategies for nutritional counseling, J. Am. Diet. Assoc. 74:431, 1979.

Hypertension detection and follow-up program cooperative group: 5-year findings of the Hypertension Detection and Follow-Up Program. I. Reduction in mortality of persons with high blood pressure including mild hypertension, J. Am. Med. Assoc. 242:2562, 1979.

Isaksson, B.: Diet and exercise assessment of the Swedith Program. In Bray, G., editor: Recent advances in obesity research. London, 1978, Neuman.

Knowles, M.: The adult learner: a neglected species, ed. 2, Houston, 1978, Gulf Publishing Co., Book Div.

Mason, M., Wenberg, B.G., and Welch, P.K.: The dynamics of clinical dietetics, New York, 1982, John Wiley & Sons, Inc.

Mullis, R.M., and Bowen, P.E.: Process guides for nutrition care in community health, J. Am. Diet. Assoc. 85:1, 1985.

National Heart, Lung, and Blood Institute: Heart to heart: a manual on nutrition counseling for the reduction of cardiovascular disease risk factors, NIH Pub. No. 83-1528, Washington, D.C., 1983, U.S. Government Printing Office.

National Heart, Lung, and Blood Institute: Multiple risk factor intervention trial: risk factor changes and mortality results, J. Am. Med. Assoc. **248**:12, 1982.

A new perspective on the health of Canadians: a working document, Ottowa, 1974, Health and Welfare.

Puska, P., Neittaanmaki, L., and Tuomilehto, J.A.: A survey of local health personnel and decision-makers concerning the North Carolina Project: a community program for control of cardiovascular disease, Prev. Med. **10**:402, 1981.

Rogers, C.R.: Client-centered therapy, Boston, 1951, Houghton Mifflin Co.

Rogers, E.M., and Shoemaker, F.F.: Communication of innovations: a cross-cultural approach, New York, 1971, Free Press.

Rosenstock, I.M.: The health belief model and nutrition education, J. Can. Diet. Assoc. **43**:184, 1982.

Snetselaar, L.G.: Nutrition counseling skills: assessment, treatment, and evaluation, Rockville, Md., 1983, Aspen Systems Corp.

Stewart, N.R., et al.: Systematic counseling, Englewood Cliffs, N.J., 1978, Prentice-Hall, Inc.

Storlie, J., and Jordan, H.A., editors: Behavioral management of obesity, New York, 1984, Spectrum Publications, Inc.

Stuart, R.B.: Behavioral control of overeating, Behav. Res. Ther. **5**:357, 1967.

Stuart, R.B., and Guire, K.: Some correlates of the maintenance of weight loss through behavior modification. In Brace, G., editor: Obesity, London, 1979, John Libby & Co., Ltd.

Stunkard, A.J., and McLaren-Hume, M.: The results of treatment of obesity: a review of the literature and report of a series, Arch. Int. Med. **103**:79, 1959.

Tillotson, J.L.: Proceedings of the Nutrition Behavioral Research Conference, DHEW Publication No. (NIH) 76-978, Bethesda, Md., 1975.

U.S. Department of Health, Education, and Welfare: Healthy people, the Surgeon General's Report on Health Promotion and Disease Prevention, DHEW (PHS) Pub. No. 79-55071, Washington, D.C., 1979, U.S. Government Printing Office.

U.S. Department of Health and Human Services/National Institute of Health: Model workshop on nutrition counseling in hyperlipidemia, NIH Publication No. 80-1666, Washington, D.C., 1980, U.S. Government Printing Office.

U.S. Department of Health and Human Services/National Institute of Health: Report of the Working Group on Critical Patient Behaviors in the Dietary Management of High Blood Pressure, NIH Publication No. 81-2269, Washington, D.C., 1981, U.S. Government Printing Office.

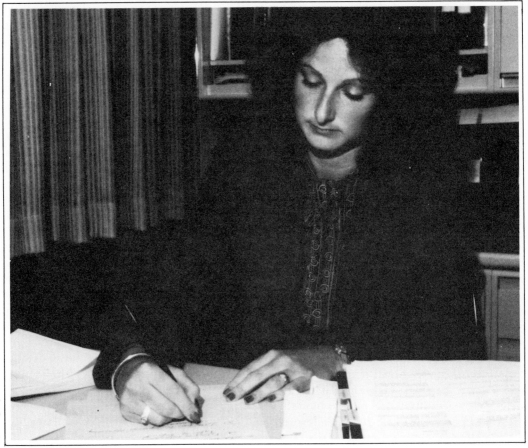

SLOTS: Jacqueline Durand

Grants and Grantsmanship

GENERAL CONCEPT

Grants, a form of financial assistance, from federal, state, voluntary, and private agencies and industry provide extra monies for service, training, and research for nutrition programs.

When you finish this chapter, you should be able to
- Trace the development of federally funded health care programs
- List the sources of funding from federal, state, voluntary, and private sectors
- Define how extra funding can enhance service, research, or training that will improve nutritional status of population groups
- Identify the parts of a proposal for a grant
- List reasons that grants are denied

With increasing competition for tax funds and with the uncertainties of the future role of federal grants-in-aid, financing is currently less stable than in the past. The community dietitian/nutritionist as a leader in agency health planning would benefit from seeking extra funds for service, training, and research for health programs. The financing of local and state health services has always been a critical matter in developing community health programs. In most state health agencies nutrition is funded by state legislatures as part of the total state health program.

In a 1974 study of 50 states and the District of Columbia, Guam, Trust Territories of the Pacific Islands, Puerto Rico, and the Virgin Islands, Nichaman and Collins reported that 496 nutrition-related positions were budgeted, including 32 part-time positions. However, the support for almost all health and medical research at teaching and research centers comes from government agencies, with additional aid from organizations and private foundations. The provision of community health services in the United States today is a cooperative project with responsibility shared by federal, state, and local government.

It should be stated at the outset of this chapter that financing of nutrition services is an integral part of the agency budget. Every health care program should include nutrition as an item in its budget. There may be instances, such as in the case of single-provider sites or in projects offering limited services, that it may not be feasible to identify a separate budget item for nutrition; however, this should be the exception and not the rule.

The budget for nutrition services should include salaries, expenses, and fringe benefits of nutrition personnel; supportive services (clerical, secretarial, etc.); space and facilities; equipment including laboratory supplies and educational materials and manuals; office supplies; computer and data processing costs; overhead and operating costs; travel costs; expenses for staff development; and communication and mass media. Funds for consultant services will contribute to the efficient functioning of the unit.

Grants and grantsmanship, or how to obtain funding, is concerned with monies from federal, state, voluntary, and private agencies and industry foundations in addition to the hard monies provided by the agency budget line for nutrition personnel to expand nutrition programming in the community.

The fiscal climate of the federal government determines monies and funding sources available for nutrition services. Government agencies at federal, state, and local levels have been the basic sources of funding, followed by voluntary health organizations and private foundations. Through the years the system of grant awards has evolved as the most satisfactory mechanism for distributing funds available from these agencies.

Grants-in-aid represent a form of transfer of public funds for the purpose of equalizing revenue among several levels of government and among states and areas within the state. They are intended to improve the quality and expand the quantity of government programs in less affluent areas and areas of special need by augmenting revenue with legal transfers of funds from more wealthy regions. A second justification for the increasing use of grants-in-aid is to help local government units, which are more restricted as to types of revenues available for health programming. A third purpose is to provide some measure of supervision or control over the activities of the lower units of government. Related to this is a fourth purpose of grants-in-aid: the enforcement of minimum standards on the recipient of the grant. As Hanlon and Pickett (1983) point out, few things have been as influential in promoting the employment of qualified public health personnel as have been the conditions attached to grants by both state and federal health agencies.

HISTORY OF GRANTS AND GRANT LEGISLATION

The idea of grants-in-aid is by no means new, having been first applied in the United States for the improvement of schools in the poorer parts of the nation, particularly the rural areas. The support of constitutional law, legislation, contract law, accountancy, management, and administration related to funding has long been with us. Even the inaugural address of George Washington referred to the "promotion of science and literature" as a function of government (Bledsoe and Ravitz, 1957). The United States Commission on Intergovernmental Relations has characterized the history of grants-in-aid in terms of three periods: from 1785 to 1918 education and agriculture were dominant; from 1918 to 1930 highway construction predominated; and from 1930 to the present social welfare has been dominant.

Morrill Act of 1862 and Hatch Act of 1887

Congressional interest in research was manifested during the agriculturally dominated nineteenth century by the passage of the Morrill Act in 1862 and the Hatch Act in 1887. The Morrill Act entitled each state to a grant of public lands based on the total number of members in Congress. States not containing public land were given scrip. The only condition was that not less than 90% of the gross proceeds was to be used for the establishment, endowment, and maintenance of agricultural and mechanical colleges.

The Hatch Act provided $15,000 per year to each state for the establishment of agricultural experimental stations. With this act there was instituted the condition of submission of an annual financial report, to be followed 8 years later by provision for a federal audit. This established a pattern that has not since been altered. These legislative acts established land grant colleges and agricultural stations as adjuncts to schools. The oldest continuous support of research by the federal government is thus in the fields of agriculture and nutrition.

Sheppard-Towner Act of 1921

The first federal health grants to states were instituted in 1918 for the control of venereal disease through the Public Health Service. Grants-in-aid specifically for mothers and children to improve their health were provided by the Children's Bureau through the Sheppard-Towner Act of 1921, which operated through 1925. Maternal and child health and expanded public health programs were reinstituted in 1935 through special and general grants provided by the Social Security Act.

Social Security Act of 1935

The Social Security Act of 1935 provided for federal and state cooperation in public health matters on a permanent basis. It provided for annual grants "to assist states, counties, health districts, and other political subdivisions of states in establishing and maintaining adequate public health services" (Smolensky and Haar, 1972). Under this act state-supported services included maternal and child health, child welfare, crippled children's care, and some grants to pay for the foster care of children. The annual appropriation was to be distributed among the states by the Surgeon General of the U.S. Public Health Service on the basis of three factors: population, special health problems, and financial need. Since the initial Social Security Act, grants have been extended to include hospitals, nursing homes, and other types of health centers, primarily through the Hospital and Construction (Hill-Burton) Act of 1946.

These federal funds are matched by one third to two thirds in state and local funding.

National Cancer Institute (1937) and National Institutes of Health (1944)

Of further historical interest in the issuance of grants was the creation of the National Cancer Institute by Congress in 1937. This grant was used as the instrument to advance and promote cancer research. In 1944, with the creation of the National Institutes of Health, Congress extended the right to use research grants to all components of the National Institutes of Health. This was followed in 1950 with the establishment of the National Science Foundation, to which Congress gave general grant authority (Willner and Hendricks, 1972).

The Great Society

With the Korean War came relative economic prosperity. After it ended, the cities were decaying; there was racial unrest; and an antiwar movement was gathering. By the time John F. Kennedy was assassinated, the federal government was geared to include the poor in grants programs. In 1953 grants amounted to $17 per capita. By 1964 the figure had soared to $51.30 per capita. The total spent increased from $2.3 billion in 1950 to $7 billion in 1960 and $11 billion in 1965.

In 1965 War on Poverty programs were thriving, but money was also being appropriated to combat heart disease and cancer. That same year, the Office of Economic Opportunity (OEO) created Project Head Start. Then came VISTA (Volunteers in Service in America), the domestic counterpart of the Peace Corps; next the Community Action Program (CAP) was funded in 500 locations at a cost of $237 million, which was later increased to $628 million in 1966. Block grants (sums of monies given to states) had their birth during the Great Society when they were used to bypass reluctant local politicians and to supplement categorical grants that had too many stipulations to meet the urgent needs of the tumultuous mid-1960s.

Comprehensive Health Planning Law of 1967

The Comprehensive Health Planning and Public Health Service Amendments of 1967 (PL 89-749) provided for comprehensive planning for health services, health manpower, and health facilities on the state and local levels. This law broadened and increased the flexibility of support services in the community and provided for the interchange of federal, state, and local health personnel.

Changes in agency organization at the federal and state levels were an outcome of the PL 89-749. An office of comprehensive health planning was established in the Public Health Service, and a major reorganization of the regional office structure of the Public Health Service became necessary. Applications for grants under the law passed through the appropriate regional office. Each regional health director was provided assistance through an Advisory and Review Council, the membership of which had to be representative of wide interests, including industry, the medical profession, and universities (Cavanaugh and McHisack, 1967).

The great increase in the numbers and types of grant-in-aid programs in the health and health-related fields in the mid-1960s created serious management problems. Over 170 federal aid programs existed, financed by over 400 appropriations, 21 federal departments, 150 Washington D.C. bureaus, and 400 regional offices.

The New Federalism

Richard Nixon laid out the agenda for New Federalism during his 1968 campaign. At that time middle-class Americans and business interests were fed up with poverty programs, riots, street demonstrations, and programs that took huge wage deductions. Federalism had traditionally provided for a strong central government. Nixon promised to decentralize its power by restoring a rightful balance between state capitals and the national capital; to share federal tax revenues with state and local governments; and to eliminate categorical grant programs in favor of block grants.

The National Health Planning and Resources Development Act of 1974

In 1976 the U.S. health system was large and expensive. It employed about 4.5 million people—double the number it employed 25 years earlier. Spending for health care in the United States was in excess of $100 billion annually, or about 8% of the gross national product, and health expenditures were still rising. New developments in the health field—in financing and delivery of health care and in training—and the need for effective health resources planning led to PL 93-641, the National Health Planning and Resources Development Act of 1974, which combined the responsibilities of the former Comprehensive Health Planning, Regional Medical Program, and the Health Facilities Assistance Program (Hill-Burton).

Health Systems Agencies

PL 93-641 established Health Systems Agencies across the country that were responsible for designing and implementing plans to improve the health of the residents of its health service area; to increase the accessibility, acceptability, continuity, and quality of health services in the area; to restrain increases in the cost of providing health services; and to prevent unnecessary duplication of health resources. Under the Health Systems Agencies, funds become available for grants or contracts for health service development projects that advance the goals specified in the law. The funds are not to be used for actual delivery of health services (Public Health Service, 1974).

The Omnibus Budget Reconciliation Act of 1981: Block Grants

The Omnibus Budget Reconciliation Act of 1981 (PL 97-35) amended Title V of the Social Security Act and consolidated 27 separate programs. It converted federal categorical health grant programs to state-controlled block grants in four areas to be administered by the Department of Health and Human Services (DHHS). This act reorganized the amount and type of federal health care expenditures in the states and had two distinct effects. First, traditional federal categorical grant programs were converted into state-controlled block grant programs. Second, the overall authorized fundings for these newly consolidated traditional public health programs decreased by approximately 25%.

The term *grant* has been defined by the Director of Institutional Relations of the Division of Research Grants, National Institutes of Health, as a "conditional gift" (Chalkley, 1970). Chalkley states "that there is no 'the Grant Philosophy.' It varies from agency to agency, and it varies within agencies. It undergoes evolutional changes from year to year. The evolutional pressures are many; they are budgetary, they are legislative, they are bureaucratic, and they produce changes that affect the way grants are used and the purposes to which grants are put." These points are important to remember because the areas of granting and funding are ever changing.

GRANT VERSUS CONTRACT

A constantly repeated source of grievance in the use of government grants has been that "there is not a formal statement of public policy setting criteria for using the grant or the contract" (Grossbaum, 1971). A continuous source of confusion is the difference between a grant and a contract, and there are fundamental distinctions between the two. A *grant* is an award of financial or direct assistance to an eligible recipient under programs that provide for such assistance, based on review and approval of an application, plan, or other documents setting forth a proposed activity or program. A *contract* is a promise or set of promises for the procurement of future monies. Whereas the grant is an agreement to support research, a contract is an instrument to procure research or services. Grants entail ideas originated and defined by the grantee; contracts contain work requirements specified by the government.

Grant investigators do not conduct research for the government agency supplying the funds; rather, they explore ideas of their own choosing in health areas in which there is a high degree of public interest. Grant applications are approved and funded based on considerations of merit and relevance to the grantor organization's program objectives. Grants are supportive in character; their objective is to strengthen the investigators' opportunities for making valuable contributions to the government granting agency's mission. Grants are made to educational and nonprofit institutions to the exclusion of commercial organizations.

Contracts, on the other hand, offer more universal competitive opportunities to all types of scientific sources and are used by the awarding agency as a means of fulfilling *its* programs objectives. Government offerors compete for a commonly understood requirement, and contract proposals received are evaluated within the framework of technical evaluation criteria that are announced to all competing sources.

Although the dividing line between grants and contracts is not always apparent, Congress has used the two terms to describe essentially different transactions (Wilcox, 1968). A grant is an award of funds, included in a written instrument executed by the head of a government agency or a duly authorized representative. The grant is usually made for a stated purpose and contains few limiting conditions.

The grant is distinguished from the contract in that it does not constitute the procurement of goods and services. A grant is a unilateral act. The primary concern in the grant award is the identification of the public value to be gained through the grant and the capability of the grantee to advance such a value. The grant period then follows.

In the grant system responsible investigators are asked to define their goals, analyze their previous achievements, and give evidence of the scientific value of their ideas. The ability to interest an impartial, usually unknown group of scientists in any investigative effort, large or small, ultimately determines the amount of success a person will enjoy in the highly competitive field of gaining financial backing.

The usual grant instrument contains a number along with the name and address of the grantee institution; the grant title is descriptive and sum-marizes the research and effort described in the proposal. It names the principal investigator— the individual under whose direction the work is carried out. However, it should be emphasized that grants are generally made to institutions.

Almost every federal agency includes language in its regulations and literature to the effect that once a grant is made, the principal investigator, operating with the policies of the grantee institution, is in the best position to determine the means by which the research may be conducted most effectively. Accordingly, the primary responsibility for performance under any grant is shared by the grantee institution and the principal investigator.

TYPES OF GRANTS

Grants are classified in several ways such as on the basis of purpose (research, training, service, etc.) or on the basis of the method of award (formula or discretionary). A brief glossary of commonly used designations has been designed by the Public Health Service, Department of Health and Human Services, without regard to classification systems. Therefore these designations are not mutually exclusive. In the *Grants Policy Statement*, a specific grant might be described by more than one of the following terms (Public Health Service, 1976).

Biochemical research support. This grant is to assist an eligible institution to maintain, develop, and advance its biomedical research capabilities. An eligible institution must have received a minimum number of PHS research project grant funds within a given period of time to qualify.

Capitation. A capitation grant is awarded to an eligible institution to provide, maintain, or improve its educational program in areas such as nursing, allied health, and health-professional education. The amount of the award is based on enrollment factors, including the number of full-time students and the potential for increased enrollment.

Conference. A conference grant is awarded to support the costs of meetings clearly within the areas of PHS program interests.

Consortium. Consortium grants are made to one institution in support of a research project in which the program is being carried out through a cooperative arrangement between or among the grantee institution and one or more participating institutions.

Construction. This is a type of facilities assistance grant made to provide support for building, expanding, and modernizing health facilities. (See Facilities Assistance later.)

Consultation and education. These grants are awarded to develop and coordinate the effective provision of health services and to increase public awareness of the nature of particular health problems and of the types of service available.

Continuing education. Continuing education grants are usually short term and are made to provide support for additional or updated training for professionals, paraprofessionals, or non-professionals working in a given health field.

Demonstration. A demonstration grant is generally of limited duration. It is made to establish or demonstrate the feasibility of a theory or approach.

Discretionary or project. This grant supports an individual project in accordance with legislation that permits Public Health Service to exercise judgment in selecting the project, the grantee, and the amount of the award.

Facilities assistance. A facilities assistance grant is made for the acquisition, remodeling, expansion, or leasing of existing facilities or the construction of new facilities. It can be used for initial equipping such facilities.

Fellowship. A fellowship is given in behalf of an individual to support specific training that will enhance that individual's level of competence in a particular area of health. Under certain programs, fellowship recipients may be subject to service and payback requirements.

Financial distress. The financial distress grant is awarded to an eligible institution that is in serious financial difficulty to meet operational costs required to maintain a certain level, quality, or type of health services or educational program. Also eligible are institutions that have a special need for financial assistance to meet accreditation requirements.

Formula. A formula grant is one in which funds are provided to specified grantees on the basis of a specific formula, which is prescribed in legislation or regulations. The formula is usually based on factors such as population, per capita income, enrollment, mortality, and morbidity. In some cases, such as formula grants to states, these grants are mandatory.

Planning. A planning grant supports planning, developing, designing, and establishing the means for performing research, delivering health services, or accomplishing other approved objectives.

Research. Research grants are made in support of investigation or experimentation aimed at the discovery and interpretation of facts, revision of accepted theories in the light of new facts, or the application of such new or revised theories.

Service. A grant made to support costs for the purpose of organizing, establishing, providing, or expanding the delivery of health services to a specified community or area is called a service grant.

Study and development. These grants are awarded to study and develop innovative and experimental programs leading to an established health services delivery component.

Training. Training grants are awarded to organizations to support costs of training students, personnel, or prospective employees in research or in the techniques or practices pertinent to the delivery of health services in the particular area of concern. Under some programs, student trainees may be subject to service and payback requirements.

SOURCES OF FUNDING

The alert administrator-nutritionist will be aware of the federal and private sources of extra monies for nutrition-related projects. Funds may be highlighted for alcoholism, drug abuse, cancer, services to mothers, infants, and children, training paraprofessionals; any of these might include a nutritional component. Also, there may be a need within an agency for gathering baseline data for a specific design for an innovative approach to examine nutritional practices.

Catalog of Federal Domestic Assistance

The Federal Program Information Act, PL 95-220, mandates that the Office of Management and Budget (OMB) disseminate information on federal domestic assistance programs through the Federal Assistance Program Retrieval System (FAPRS) and the Catalog of Federal Domestic Assistance (CFDA). The most comprehensive and authoritative compilation of grant proposals, the CFDA is the best place to begin a search for funds.

The CFDA is a government-wide compendium of federal programs, projects, services, and activities that provide assistance or benefits to the Americans. It contains financial and nonfinancial assistance programs administered by departments of the federal government. The primary purpose of the CFDA is to aid potential beneficiaries in identifying and obtaining available assistance. It is also intended to improve coordination and communication in federal program activities among federal, state, and local governments as well as to coordinate programs within the federal government.

Published annually and available on a subscription basis, the basic edition of the CFDA is published in June; fall and winter updates are available from the Superintendent of Documents. The June edition reflects completed congressional action on program legislation. The update, normally published in December, reflects completed congressional action on the President's budget proposals and on substantive legislation as of the date of compilation. It is suggested that the update be used along with the basic edition to obtain the most current information on program revision. The OMB distributes a limited number of free copies to members of Congress and federal offices of the U.S. government. At the state level, copies are provided to directors of State Planning Agencies, Director of State Agricultural Extension, and Chief State School Officer. At the local level, copies are provided to mayors, county chairmen, and city planners.

The 1983 edition of the CFDA ($32.00) lists 976 programs administered by 51 federal agencies. Examples of these programs are education, community development, consumer protection, food and nutrition, income security, and social services. Under "food and nutrition" the subject index indicates the following areas for which financial assistance is available: children (14 different programs), individuals and families (10), food inspection (8), nutrition research (8), and food and drug (17), (CFDA, 1983).

The types of assistance listed in the CFDA include the following:

1. *Formula grants.* Allocations of money to states or their subdivisions in accordance with a distribution formula prescribed by law or administrative regulation, for activities of a continuing nature not confined to a specific project.
2. *Project grants.* The funding, for fixed or known periods, of specific projects or the delivery of specific services or products without liability for damages for failure to perform. Project grants include fellowships, scholarships, research grants, training grants, traineeships, experimental and demonstration grants, evaluation grants, planning grants, technical assistance grants, survey grants, construction grants, and unsolicited contractual agreements.
3. *Direct payments for specified use.* Financial assistance from the federal government provided directly to individuals, private firms, and other private institutions to encourage or subsidize a particular activity by conditioning the receipt of the assistance on a particular performance by the recipient. This does not include solicited contracts for the procurement of goods and services for the federal government.
4. *Direct payments for unrestricted use.* Financial assistance from the federal government provided directly to beneficiaries

who satisfy federal eligibility requirements with no restrictions being imposed on the recipient as to how the money is spent. Included are payments under retirement, pension, and compensation programs.

5. *Direct loans.* Financial assistance provided through the lending of federal monies for a specific period of time, with a reasonable expectation of repayment. Such loans may or may not require the payment of interest.

6. *Guaranteed/insured loans.* Programs in which the federal government makes an arrangement to indemnify a lender against part or all of any defaults by those responsible for repayment of loans.

7. *Insurance.* Financial assistance provided to assure reimbursement for losses sustained under specified conditions. Coverage may be provided directly by the federal government or through private carriers and may or may not involve the payment of premiums.

8. *Sale, exchange, or donation of property and goods.* Programs that provide for the sale, exchange, or donation of federal real property, personal property, commodities, and other goods including land, buildings, equipment, food and drugs. This does not include the loan of, use of, or access to federal facilities or property.

9. *Use property, facilities, and equipment.* Programs that provide for the loan of, use of, or access to federal facilities or property wherein the federally owned facilities or property does not remain in the possession of the recipient of the assistance.

10. *Provision of specialized services.* Programs that provide federal personnel to directly perform certain tasks for the benefit of communities or individuals. These services may be performed in conjunction with nonfederal personnel, but they involve more than consultation, advice, or counseling.

11. *Advisory service and counseling.* Programs that provide federal specialists to consult, advise, or counsel communities or individuals including conferences, workshops, or personal contacts.

12. *Dissemination of technical information.* Programs that provide for publication and distribution of information or data of a specialized technical nature frequently through clearinghouses or libraries.

13. *Training.* Programs that provide instructional activities conducted directly by federal agencies for individuals not employed in the federal government.

Even with two annual updates, the CFDA often does not provide all the information grant applicants need. For this reason, the Federal Program Information Act transferred into the OMB an experimental program that began about 1975 in the Department of Agriculture to make constantly updated catalog information available through computer terminals. This program is called the Federal Assistance Program Retrieval System (FAPRS). Containing a data base with 20 categories and 178 subcategories, the FAPRS has been developed with information on federal grants and contracts. It permits computer searches for data on federal domestic assistance. For information on how to use this service, write to the Rural Development Service, Department of Agriculture, 14th and Independence Avenues, Washington, DC 20250.

To provide dissemination of biomedical information, the National Library of Medicine has developed a network arrangement through which interlibrary loan activities and computerized bibliographic retrieval capabilities (MEDLINE and other on-line services) can be shared more effectively by medical libraries around the nation (box, p. 398).

Two publications supplement the basic information found in the CFDA—*The Federal Register* and the *Commerce Business Daily. The Federal Register* is published every day (Monday through Friday) and presents proposed and final rules and regulations developed by all federal

REGIONAL MEDICAL LIBRARIES

The Regional Medical Library Program is intended to provide health science practitioners, investigators, educators, and administrators in the United States with timely, convenient access to health care and biomedical information resources. The Program is coordinated by the National Library of Medicine and carried out through a nationwide network of more than 3000 health science libraries and information centers. The Network includes seven Regional Medical Libraries, or RMLs. These are major institutions designated by NLM to administer and provide backup services in

each of seven geographical regions. Services offered through the Network include document delivery, reference service, basic library training, consultation, and on-line access to more than 20 data bases on the NLM Medical Literature Analysis and Retrieval System (MEDLARS). Some 1800 Network libraries, including medical schools, hospitals, public health, and other institutions currently have access to MEDLARS. For information about MEDLARS centers in a specific area, write the RML for the region.

1   Greater Northeastern Regional Medical Library
        Program
    The New York Academy of Medicine
    2 East 103rd Street
    New York, NY 10029
    Phone: 212-876-8763
    States served: CT, DE, MA, ME, NH, NJ, NY,
        PA, RI, VT, and Puerto Rico
    TWX: 710-581-6131

2   Southeastern/Atlantic Regional Medical Library
        Services
    University of Maryland
    Health Sciences Library
    111 South Greene Street
    Baltimore, MD 21201
    Phone: 301-528-2855
                800-638-6093
    States served: AL, FL, GA, MD, MS, NC, SC,
        TN, VA, WV, and the District of Columbia
    TWX: 710-234-1610

3   Region 3—Regional Medical Library
    University of Illinois at Chicago
    Library of the Health Sciences
    Health Sciences Center
    P.O. Box 7509
    Chicago, IL 60680
    Phone: 312-996-2464
    States served: IA, IL, IN, KY, MI, MN, ND, OH,
        SD, WI
    TELEX: 206243

4   Midcontinental Regional Medical Library Program
    University of Nebraska
    Medical Center Library
    42nd and Dewey Avenue
    Omaha, NE 68105
    Phone: 402-559-4326
    States served: CO, KS, MO, NE, UT, WY
    TWX: 910-622-8353

5   South Central Regional Medical Library Program
    University of Texas
    Health Science Center at Dallas
    5323 Harry Hines Blvd.
    Dallas, TX 75235
    Phone: 214-688-2085
    States served: AR, LA, NM, OK, TX
    TWX: 910-861-4946

6   Pacific Northwest Regional Health Sciences
        Library Services
    Health Sciences Library
    University of Washington
    Seattle, WA 98195
    Phone: 206-543-8262
    States served: AK, ID, MT, OR, WA
    TWX: 910-444-1385

7   Pacific Southwest Regional Medical Library
        Service
    UCLA Biomedical Library
    Center for the Health Sciences
    Los Angeles, CA 90024
    Phone: 213-825-1200
    States served: AZ, CA, HI, NV
    TWX: 910-342-6897

From U.S. Department of Health and Human Services, Public Health Service, National Institutes of Health, Bethesda, Md., 1983, U.S. Government Printing Office.

agencies as well as information about program deadlines and applications. Each issue has a highlights page that can be skimmed for pertinent material. *Commerce Business Daily* has information on federal contracts up for bid. In addition, requests for proposals (RFPs) can be made from federal agencies that are likely to have a nutrition component in their program.

Public Health Service

The Public Health Service (PHS) is the principal health component of the Department of Health and Human Services. The basic purpose of the Public Health Services, as a whole, is to protect and advance the nation's health. According to the *Grants Policy Statement* (PHS, 1976), one important activity that PHS carries out is awarding grants in support of efforts that help PHS and the recipient institutions to achieve mutually beneficial goals.

The PHS administers an array of grant programs that are concerned with the whole spectrum of health concerns. These are reflected in the goals of its six agencies.

1. The Alcohol, Drug Abuse, and Mental Health Administration is responsible for developing knowledge, manpower, and services to prevent mental illness, to treat and rehabilitate the mentally ill, to prevent the abuses of drugs and alcohol, and to treat and rehabilitate drug and alcohol abusers.

2. The Centers for Disease Control is responsible for the national program of prevention and control of communicable and vector-borne diseases and for the control of certain other noninfectious conditions.

3. The Food and Drug Administration, the nation's first consumer protection agency, is concerned with research and regulations in such areas as food, drugs, cosmetics, and medical devices.

4. The Health Resources Administration is responsible for health planning, research, evaluation and development of health resources and needs, including manpower and

health facilities, and the collection and dissemination of health data.

5. The Health Services Administration is responsible for the improvement of the delivery of health services to the American people.

6. The National Institute of Health seeks to improve the nation's health by increasing knowledge related to health and disease through the conduct and support of research, research training, and biomedical communications.

These 6 PHS agencies (Figure 14-1) and the 10 PHS regional offices (Figure 14-2) are responsible for the award, administration, and monitoring of grant programs under a variety of legislative authorities, governing regulations, policies, and procedures.

The Health Services Administration (HSA) is the focal point for programs and health services for specific population groups in the United States and is concerned with the availability, efficiency, and quality of health care.

The Bureau of Community Health Services (BCHS), also part of PHS, administers programs designed to provide high quality health services primarily to those who are underserved—or unserved—by the nation's health service systems. The following are some examples of project and formula grant programs supported by BCHS.

The Appalachian Health Demonstration Program (ADHP) involves a partnership between the Department of Health and Human Services and the Appalachian Regional Commission. This grant program authorizes support for health planning, construction, equipment, and operation of multicounty demonstration, health, nutrition, and child-care projects which will show the value of adequate health facilities and services to the economic development of the region.

Community Health Centers (CHC) is a program of project grants (Community Health Center and Family Health Center project grants) to provide primary health care and arrange for specialty and inpatient care, primarily for people living in medically underserved areas.

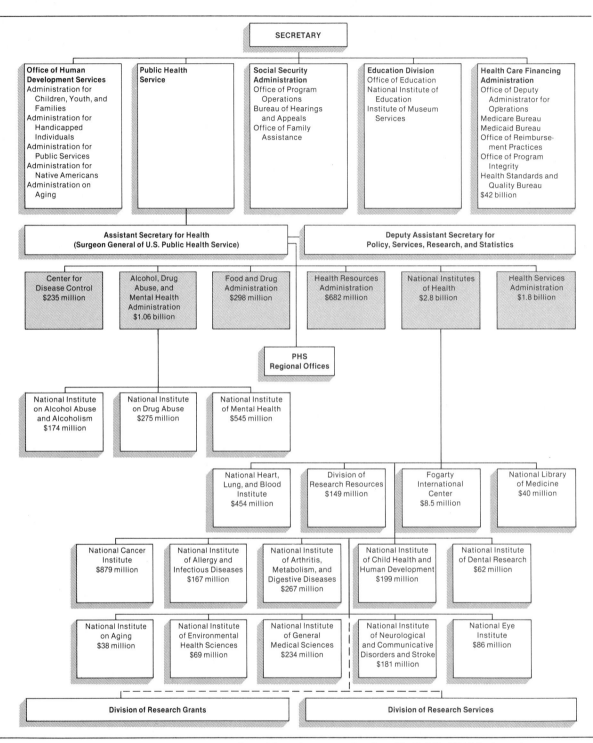

Figure 14-1. The Department of Health and Human Services Six Public Health Agencies, USHHS 1979. Figures are from President's proposed budget for fiscal year 1979.

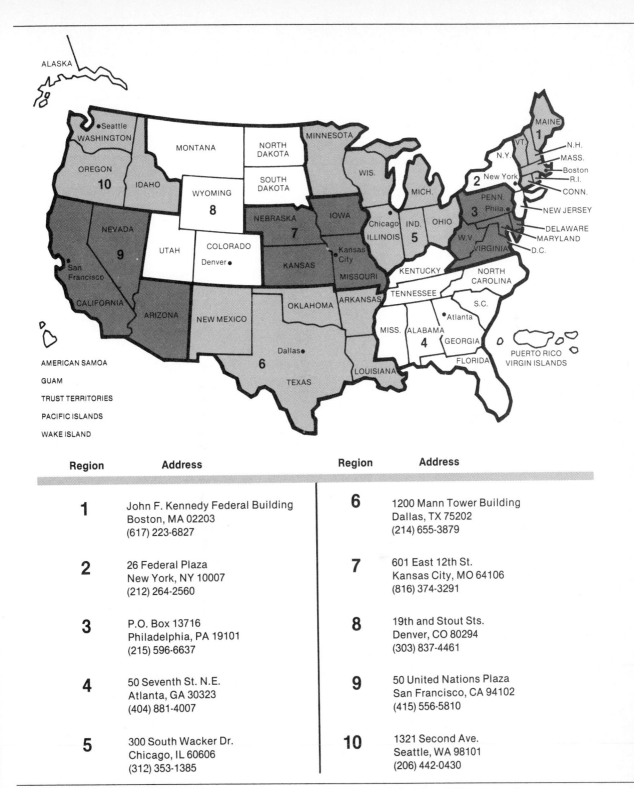

Region	Address	Region	Address
1	John F. Kennedy Federal Building Boston, MA 02203 (617) 223-6827	6	1200 Mann Tower Building Dallas, TX 75202 (214) 655-3879
2	26 Federal Plaza New York, NY 10007 (212) 264-2560	7	601 East 12th St. Kansas City, MO 64106 (816) 374-3291
3	P.O. Box 13716 Philadelphia, PA 19101 (215) 596-6637	8	19th and Stout Sts. Denver, CO 80294 (303) 837-4461
4	50 Seventh St. N.E. Atlanta, GA 30323 (404) 881-4007	9	50 United Nations Plaza San Francisco, CA 94102 (415) 556-5810
5	300 South Wacker Dr. Chicago, IL 60606 (312) 353-1385	10	1321 Second Ave. Seattle, WA 98101 (206) 442-0430

Figure 14-2. Public health regional offices, U.S. Department of Health and Human Services, Public Health Service.

Comprehensive Public Health Services provides for formula grants to assist states in establishing and maintaining adequate community, mental, and environmental public health services, including training of personnel for state and local public health work.

Family Planning (FP) provides for project grants to give families full opportunity to exercise freedom of choice to determine the number and spacing of their children through access to family planning information, educational materials, and adequate medical services.

Maternal and Child Health (MCH) provides for formula grants to the states to improve and extend services for reducing infant mortality, promoting the health of mothers and children, and locating and providing medical, surgical, and other services and care for crippled children or those suffering from conditions that lead to a crippling condition. In addition, it provides for a program of projects including Maternity and Infant Care, Children and Youth, Dental Health, and Intensive Care of Infants and special services such as Pediatric Pulmonary Care Centers, Child Abuse Services, Sudden Infant Death Syndrome programs, and others. Funds for research and training projects are also included.

Migrant Health (MH) provides for project grants to improve the health status and the environment of migrant agricultural workers and seasonal farm workers and their families through the provision of comprehensive health services that are accessible to people as they migrate to work.

National Health Service Corps (NHSC) provides for the assignment of commissioned officers and civil service personnel of the PHS to areas of the United States to improve the delivery of health care in areas where health services are inadequate because of critical shortages of health personnel.

Block Grants

A block grant is a funding mechanism by which the federal government supports state or local government public services. Normally a block grant is a lump sum given by the federal government to a state government unit. The federal government may spell out certain broad restrictions in the use of block grants, but the receiving state retains much discretion as to how it will finance various activities within the block grant functional area. Like block grants, categorical grants make federal funds available for state and local public programs, but categorical grants can be used only for specifically designated programs. Categorical funds are usually limited to activities narrowly defined by federal statute and allow less flexibility in their use than block grants.

According to the philosophy of the Reagan administration, state-controlled block grants result in improved services at lower costs by allowing for the development of health care programs more responsible to local needs, consolidating duplicative or similar programs, and having fewer restrictive federal regulatory requirements. Unfortunately the block grant programs could also harm local health programs that already exist by terminating federally established program allocation criteria, decreasing program evaluation and monitoring, setting up unclear new state administrative procedures, and using funds for political rather than public health concerns. For the first time, the state legislative and executive branches are mandated by the block grant to have an active role in deciding how federal health care programs shall be conducted in their states.

The explosive growth in the federal grants-in-aid system between 1960 and 1980 has produced dissatisfaction with the administration of categorical grants and the federal grant system as a whole. The number of federal aid programs increased from just 50 in 1960 to approximately 500 in 1980 (Stanfield, 1981).

Problems in the categorical grant system have been attributed to the disproportionate distribution of power, authority, and responsibility among the federal, state, and local levels of government. Most of the attention has been focused on the growth in size of the federal bureaucracy and the centralization of power and authority at the federal level. This dilemma created roadblocks in the federal grant system such as fragmentation, overcentralization, overregulation, confrontation and crisis-only negotiation, state and local tensions, and aid to places rather than aid to people (Kraatz and Shields, 1981).

The efforts of former Presidents Carter and Nixon to change the federal system of fiscal aid produced limited results. However, the experiences and learnings from previous block grants and proposals assessed in terms of the roles and responsibilities carried out at the federal, state, and local levels are helpful for future planning. Such a study, which was performed by the Advisory Commission on Intergovernmental Relations (ACIR) and published in 1977, does provide the following information on assessment.

There have been five block grant programs enacted in the last 15 years: Health Incentive Grants (Section 314 [d] of the Public Health Service Act) in 1966, Omnibus Crime Control and Safe Streets Act of 1968 (often referenced by the administrating agency initials LEAA), Comprehensive Employment and Training Act (CETA) in 1973, Community Development Block Grant (CDBG) in 1974, and Title XX of the Social Services Act in 1975. Although there has been some evidence that these blocks are considered less intrusive than categorical grants, they all have mixed records on achieving state and local flexibility in operating programs (ACIR, 1977).

The problem of determining what is and what is not a block grant further complicates any attempt to assess the advantages of block grants versus categorical programs. Block grants have been described as the "middle ground" between the idea of no strings attached (general revenue sharing) and the conditional framework of categorical programs. ACIR identified five distinguishing characteristics of a block grant:

1. Federal aid is authorized for a wide range of activities within a broadly defined functional area.
2. Recipients have substantial discretion in identifying problems, designing programs, and allocating resources to deal with them.
3. Administrative, fiscal reporting, planning and other federally imposed requirements are kept to the minimum amount necessary to ensure that national goals are being accomplished.
4. Federal aid is distributed on the basis of a statutory formula, which results in narrowing federal administrators' discretion and providing a sense of fiscal certainty to recipients.
5. Eligibility provisions are statutorily specified and favor general purpose governmental units as recipients and elected officials and administrative generalists as decision makers.

Based on their review and assessment of the block grants mentioned earlier, the ACIR has concluded that the role of the federal government in block grants should be as follows (ACIR, 1977):

1. To serve as a middleman between Congress and interest groups on one side and recipient jurisdictions on the other.
2. To provide national leadership and direction, while allowing recipients maximum latitude in exercising discretion.
3. To take proper steps to ensure that the statute's intent is being carried out and that federal funds are being used effectively and efficiently.
4. To ensure recipients of genuine flexibility in tailoring funds to their needs.
5. To provide required technical assistance and guidance to recipients and regional offices in the conversion from categorical to block grants.

Public health nutritionists and nutrition educators have provided specific areas for nutrition services to receive monies from block grants to the states (Kaufman, 1982). This is summarized in the box on p. 404.

An example of a block grant created by the Omnibus Budget Reconciliation Act is Title V Maternal and Child Health (MCH) Services

BLOCK GRANTS: IMPLICATIONS FOR NUTRITION SERVICES

Programs in each block grant include the following.

Community Services

Community action/local initiative
Senior opportunities and services
Community food and nutrition

Social Services

Title XX social services program

Preventive Health and Health Services

Rodent control
Risk reduction/health
  education
Health incentive
Emergency medical services
High blood pressure
Fluoridation
Home health
Rape crisis

Maternal and Child Health Services

Maternal and child health
Crippled children's service
Sudden infant death
  syndrome
Lead-based paint poisoning
  prevention
SSI disabled children
Hemophilia
Genetic diseases
Adolescent pregnancy

Alcohol and Drug Abuse and Mental Health

Alcoholism state formula grants
Alcohol abuse and alcoholism project grants and
  contracts
Special grants for Uniform Alcoholism Intoxication and
  Treatment Act
Drug abuse state formula grants and contracts
Drug abuse project grants
Mental health services

Primary Care

Community health centers
Primary care research and demonstrations

Summarized by Mary Egan, Office of Maternal and Child Health, DHHS; Mildred Kaufman, University of North Carolina; ASTPHND representatives Harriet Duncan (South Carolina); Molly Graber (Michigan); Barbara Ann Hughes (North Carolina); Martha Kjentvet (Wisconsin); Alyn Park-Potter (Colorado); Eileen Peck (California).

block grant. The purpose of this block grant is to enable the states:

1. To ensure that mothers and children, especially those with low income or limited availability of health services, have access to quality health services.
2. To emphasize preventive measures, such as those to reduce infant mortality and prevent handicapping conditions, and to promote health of mothers and children.
3. To provide rehabilitative services to blind and disabled children eligible for Supplemental Security Income (SSI) under Social Security.
4. To provide comprehensive services to handicapped children.

This block grant specified the transmittal of a Report of Intended Expenditures (RIE), which includes needs assessment data, a statement of goals and objectives for meeting those needs, information on services to be provided, and population to be served. Thus the block grant provides a clear mandate to the states to distribute resources according to an assessment of the need for these MCH services (Guyer et al., 1984).

By changing the way tax dollars are spent for some health and social services, the block grant approach is envisioned as doing the following:

1. Placing decision making closer to the local level and encouraging states and localities to define and resolve their own problems and issues.
2. Allowing more flexibility in the use of federal funds and giving more discretion to the states.
3. Reducing federal regulations and reporting requirements and fostering the state's accountability to its citizens.
4. Providing for more public input in program development and implementation.
5. Promoting more efficient use of tax dollars through consolidation and integration.

Officials of each state—governors and/or legislators—determine which state agency will administer each of the block grants. The exception is the Maternal and Child Health Services block grant. The new law provides for the state health agency to administer it with the exception that other agencies administering the Crippled Children's Services program before July 1, 1967, can continue to do so.

It is important to remember that for block grants the state "is where the action is." Nutritionists, both individually and collectively, will need to take the following appropriate actions:

- Identify and interpret nutritional needs and problems within the state for state officials, agency administrators, and program directors responsible for administering the block grants. Using their knowledge and skills, nutritionists should participate in the development of the descriptions of intended use of funds (RIE), which must contain a needs assessment, goals and objectives to meet needs, information about services to be provided, categories of people to be served, and criteria and methods for distributing funds within the state.
- Ensure that the views and suggestions of the nutrition community are included and considered in the public input provided for the block grants (i.e., public hearings, comments on plans published in the media, etc.).
- Promulgate sound criteria and standards that will ensure high-quality nutrition services provided under block grants.
- Participate in the preparation of required reports and audits to support accountability for expenditures for nutrition services.

Community dietitians/nutritionists should be willing to take some initiative in the block grant process, to move ahead, and to become informed, involved, and committed to effective and efficient nutrition services as an integral component of all block grants.

Foundation Grants

Each year nearly 1 million requests for funding are made to the approximately 22,000 active foundations in the United States. Of these requests, perhaps no more than 6% or 7% of those who apply eventually obtain the support they seek. Many applications fail because they represent programs or projects that do not match the interests of the foundations approached. Still others are declined because they appear to be of lower quality than those few programs that are funded. Although it is impossible to eliminate these kinds of rejections entirely, grantseekers can increase their chances for success by understanding the priorities of individual foundations and by relating directly to these interests (Kurzig, 1981).

What Is a Foundation?

A private foundation is generally a nongovernmental, nonprofit organization with funds and programs managed by its own trustees or directors; it is established to maintain or aid social, educational, charitable, religious, or other activities serving the common welfare, primarily through the making of grants.

Company-sponsored foundations obtain their funds from profit-making companies but are legally independent entities. They are often used as conduits for corporate giving. Companies often make grants to organizations that serve company employees or to communities where the company has operations. Grants can be used to conduct research in related fields or to improve the company's public image.

Most private foundations are independent. The assets of an independent foundation are received from an individual or a family functioning under the direction of family members, which is often called the *family foundation*. The Ford Foundation bears a family name but has an independent board of trustees and professional staff.

Community foundations generally make grants only in their metropolitan area and are governed by boards broadly representative of their community.

The federal government operates programs similar to foundations, such as the National Science Foundation and the National Endowment for the Arts. These are grant-making bodies operated with tax money appropriated by Congress and function as government agencies rather than private foundations.

Corporate Grants

Corporations give in two ways: through separately established foundations and through corporate contribution programs operated within their companies. Usually annual reports are issued that list the recipients of monies and their research areas. This is a good guide for assessing past corporate funding. Inquiries should be directed to the corporate contribution officer by name, which can be found in the company's annual report.

Preparations for Funding Request

The actual grant-making universe is a good deal smaller than the 22,000 foundations mentioned because many of these foundations have endowments of less than $1 million, have no professional staff, and mainly tend to support organizations relating to their own interests. For this reason, Kurzig (1981) suggests that, to compete effectively in the grants market, the following questions should be answered before applying for foundation funding:

1. Are you convinced that the program for which you seek support meets a real need and, furthermore, that it provides a convincing solution to the problem you have identified?
2. Does the scope of the proposed solution or program relate directly to the scale of the problem you have defined?
3. Is it clear that the program actually needs foundation support?
4. Are you approaching those foundations that you have firm reasons to believe will be interested in your proposal?
5. What do you do if, after reviewing all available information about a particular foundation, you are still uncertain whether to approach with your request?
6. Is your group structured so that it may receive foundation grants?

7. Do you understand the foundation review and administrative processes?

After these questions are answered, the first step in the grant-writing process then becomes the search for available funding sources. This step is important because many foundations or corporations award grants only in certain geographical areas. In addition, these funding sources may have their own priorities that determine the kinds of projects or organizations they will support. Last, some will support only projects that seek specific information in certain areas, such as trends in the health industry or the range of salaries in a particular profession. An innovative and promising project that requires "seed" money to get started may also be favored.

The Foundation Center

The Foundation Center has a nationwide network of references for free public use. The following four libraries designated as "Reference Collections Operated by the Foundation Center" offer the widest variety of service and the most comprehensive collections of information pertaining to private foundations and other grantors:

The Foundation Center
79 Fifth Ave.
New York, NY 10003
212-620-4230

The Foundation Center
Kent H. Smith Library
1442 Hanna Building
1422 Euclid Ave.
Cleveland, OH 44115
216-861-1933

The Foundation Center
1001 Connecticut Ave., NW
Washington, DC 20036
202-331-1400

The Foundation Center
312 Sutter St.
San Francisco, CA 94108
415-397-0902

Among the reference collections are Foundation Center publications; books, services, and magazines pertaining to philanthropy; IRS returns; and foundation annual reports, newsletters, and press clippings. Special orientations and basic grant workshops are also part of the service provided. In addition, there are cooperating collections at many public libraries across the country. Information about local resources can be obtained from the four Foundation Centers.

Two reference books published by the Foundation Center provide vital information for grant seekers. The 1984 Foundation Directory, ninth edition, is the standard reference work for information about nongovernmental, grant-making foundations in the United States. The Directory provides the address of each foundation, a statement of its purposes and activities, and financial data. The Foundation Grants Index is the most current source of specific information about the kinds of grants funded by the various foundations.

A special supplement to the Foundation Directory contains complete entries for 1923 foundation, which are listed alphabetically by state. Edition nine lists names, staff, officers, addresses, telephone numbers, funding deadlines, grant-making interests, and application procedures for each foundation.

Other Sources

Another excellent publication is *The Complete Grants Sourcebook for Higher Education,* which was published in 1984 and is available from The American Council on Education, 1 Du Pont Circle, Washington, DC 20036. This document details the grant-writing process and includes worksheets for use in the development of proposals, a directory of funding sources, and an index to the sources by type, areas of interest, and state/region.

After an appropriate funding source has been selected, the next step is to make a personal contact with the chief staff officer to discuss the foundation, its current priorities, and the possibility of a favorable response to a specific proposal. A personal visit and contact with the right person are extremely important because of the stiff competition the grant writer faces in seeking funds from foundations and corporations. This contact can be invaluable in the development of an ongoing relationship with the organization (Clayton, 1982). If personal contact is not possible, a letter should be sent. Sometimes the letter becomes the proposal. It should be brief—usually no more than three to four pages.

THE PROPOSAL

In the world of grants, the perspective grantee, a representative of the agency, known as the principal investigator, is the person who submits the proposal to the granting/funding agency. In the past it has been customary procedure for grants to be awarded to persons well known in the field, those whose past performance has made a contribution to the knowledge and practice of sound nutrition principles. Too often monies were awarded to the country's top medical centers. Today, with more competitive entries, monies are being more widely dispersed. Much depends on the strength of the proposal submitted. For this reason, it is essential to know the how's and why's of proposal writing.

A proposal writing guide is a useful tool for the grant administrator. It will not solve all the problems nor provide answers to all the questions, but it is an excellent starting point and a help in creating a frame of reference. Two guides that may be useful to the person writing the proposal are those of Wilner and Hendricks (1972) and Crawford and Kieslmeier (1970).

The Wilner guide, *Grants Administration,* evolved from instructional material prepared for a number of institutes and courses in grants and contracts given by the National Graduate University in the early 1970s. Among the subjects presented are the rise and fall of grants, the grant instrument, role of the grant administrator, organizing the grant office, and proposal assistance.

The Crawford guide, *Proposal Writing: A Manual and Workbook,* contains a text and several appendices. The text is an overall view of proposal writing, which is accompanied by a workbook section. The text tells what should be done; the workbook activities help develop skills in doing. Suggested guidelines for evaluating proposals are presented in the last section; it provides insight into what grant reviewers consider important.

The Grantsmanship Center's *Program Planning and Proposal Writing* booklet is a good basic guide (Kiritz, 1979). Two other excellent books extensively discuss how to prepare research proposals: Krathwol's *How to Prepare a Research Proposal* (1966) and Kurzig's *Foundation Fundamentals: A Guide for Grantseekers* (1981).

The objective of a proposal is the award of a grant or contract that will result in a successful research, training, service, or other kind of project that will make a contribution to the improvement or advancement of society. It is most unlikely that a grant or contract would ever be awarded without a proposal. The proposal document, therefore, assumes a great deal of importance, magnified in recent years by the increase in competition for grant awards. Although there is no set form for proposal preparation, one approach will be presented later.

A dialogue between the grantee and the grant administrator should precede the actual writing of the proposal. The purpose of this early dialogue is to ensure that the author of the grant is "in tune" with the program for which the proposal is to be submitted. Although the grant writer should recruit help on the technical aspects of the proposal from peers, the grant administrator can be of considerable service by advising the seeker of funds on the probable reaction of the government review process to the proposal.

An early dialogue between the grantee and the fiscal officer of the agency is also a vital step. The purpose of this dialogue is to alert the fiscal officer of the pending project and the application for funds. This will determine in the early stages whether such funding is acceptable within the confines of the agency's policy. Important questions can be answered at this stage also. What are the institution's indirect costs? Who will control the monies if the grant is approved? What flexibility is there in the use of funds? What are the various categories for which monies can be used?

The groups that review and evaluate project grant proposals deal only with the information submitted by perspective grantees. Whereas the grant is the award, the proposal is the act of putting forward a plan or stating a scheme for consideration. Therefore the project proposal should include sufficient information to enable the reviewers to determine accurately what is to be done, why it is to be done, how it is to be accomplished, the anticipated results, and the ability to carry out the project proposal submitted.

Major Parts of the Proposal

Reviewing groups are assisted in their evaluations when statements in the application are arranged under a uniform pattern of captions as shown in Crawford's example on p. 409 (top), which indicates the major components of the proposal. Another example is Kiritz's program planning and proposal writing (PP&PW) as shown on p. 409 (bottom).

In the introduction it is important to state the title concisely and accurately so that it clearly indicates to an unfamiliar reader the nature and intent of the project. In stating the problem, the reason the project is being proposed should be indicated, as well as what questions are to be solved and their need to be answered. Information should be supplied that will orient the reader to the setting in which the questions or problem occurs. A description of the situation, events, and characteristics in a specific setting that led to the subject of inquiry will help the reviewers with specific data and pertinent factual information that can support and justify the significance of the project. A review of work already done in the setting that relates to the question or project will establish credibility to the logic of pursuing the study further. A review of the literature of related work is helpful. If the project has wider implications, such as for other disciplines, it is helpful to state these. The objectives should be concise and clear. A statement of specific testable goals and

MAJOR PARTS OF A PROPOSAL

Topic	Function in terms of general questions answered
Introduction	
Statement of the problem	What needs to be done and why?
Review of the literature	What has been done that is relevant?
Objectives	What are the specific testable goals?
Procedures	
Design	What is the structural plan?
	What control will it afford?
Sampling	What population will be sampled?
	What size sample and how drawn?
Measurement and data	What will be measured? How?
Analysis and evaluation	How will the data from the measures be examined?
Time schedule	How much time will be needed to complete each portion of the study?
Product and use	What will be the end-product of the study? What contribution can it make?
(dissemination)	How?
Personnel and facilities	Who will do the study? What is their relevant competence?
Budget	What will each part of the study cost?

From Crawford, J., and Kielsmeier, C.: Proposal writing: a manual and workbook, A Continuing Education Book, Oregon State System of Higher Education, Corvallis, 1970, Oregon State University.

COMPONENTS OF PROGRAM PLANNING AND PROPOSAL WRITING

Summary	Clearly and concisely summarizes the request	V. Evaluation	Presents a plan for determining the degree to which objectives are met and methods are followed
I. Introduction	Describes the agency's qualifications or "credibility"	VI. Future or other necessary funding	Describes a plan for continuation beyond the grant period and/or the availability of other resources necessary to implement the grant
II. Problem statement or needs assessment	Documents the needs to be met or problems to be solved by the proposed funding		
III. Objectives	Establishes the benefits of the funding in measurable terms	VII. Budget	Clearly delineates costs to be met by the funding source and those to be provided by the applicant or other parties
IV. Methods	Describes the activities to be employed to achieve the desired results		

From Kiritz, N.J.: Grantsmanship Center News, May/June 1979, p. 1. © The Grantsmanship Center, 1031 S. Grand Ave., Los Angeles, CA 90015.

how achievement of these goals will relate to the stated questions or problem is essential.

In the procedure or methodology, the plan that will help achieve the specific objectives of the study must be presented. What is the plan? How will the plan be carried out? That is, how will it be implemented and in what time schedule? How will the population be sampled?

A built-in evaluation that allows for data collection and decision making is essential and impressive. Which methods and measuring devices will be used? How will the status at the beginning of the project period, progress made during the project, and the outcome of the project be determined? This outline for periodic assessment should be consistent with the project proposal and be a reasonable period for accomplishing the work. If evaluation tools are to be developed by project personnel as part of the project, the plans for construction of these tools should be included in the discussion of methodology.

The reviewing committee will ask who will carry out the work of the project and who will assume responsibility for its fulfillment. The program director should be the person available and committed to undertake the work if the grant is awarded. The director should be available for an amount of time sufficient to accomplish the proposed project. The education and experience of the project director must be appropriate or at least applicable to the problem with which the project is concerned and to the methods used to carry it out. The application should describe the program director's educational background and prior work in the area with which the project is concerned. Other pertinent experiences and information in sufficient detail to permit evaluation of anticipated direction of the plans proposed will highlight the proposal.

There are some instances when it may not be possible to have the project director under firm commitment to undertake the direction of the project at the time the proposal is submitted. In this instance, information should be included to indicate how the project director will be recruited, how successful the search will be, and

TYPICAL BUDGET CATEGORIES

I. Direct costs
  A. Personnel
    1. Research
    2. Support
    3. Secretarial/clerical
    4. Consultants
  B. Employee benefits
  C. Travel
  D. Supplies and materials
    1. Project and/or instructional materials
    2. Office supplies
    3. Books and journals
  E. Communications
  F. Services
  G. Final report
  H. Equipment and/or equipment rental
  I. Other direct costs
  J. Subtotal direct costs
II. Indirect costs
III. Total costs

what the educational background and experience are that are being sought. Specific identification of all personnel who will be carrying out various parts of the work planned (faculty, project staff, technical assistants, consultants) will strengthen the proposal.

Another major question that the reviewing committee will have in mind is which facilities and supporting services will be used in carrying out the work of the project? A description of the facilities available, such as special equipment, laboratory space, and communications center, should be included. In addition, a list of the supporting services on hand such as technical assistance, consultation, testing services, and maintenance of equipment will add to the reviewers' understanding of the nature of the project. Are there any factors in the institutional environment that will support the project and thereby contribute to its success? Are there any plans to collaborate with other institutions or agencies that are not directly affiliated with the institution where the project is to be carried out? If so, a de-

Table 14-1. Shortcomings found in 605 disapproved research grant applications

Area of Application Found Deficient	Frequency	Shortcoming
The problem (the question which the proposed research seeks to answer)	58%	Problem is of insufficient importance; is more complex than the investigator realizes; warrants only a pilot study; research proposed is overly involved; description of research is without clear research aim
The approach (the means by which the answer is to be sought)	73%	Proposed methods and procedures are unsuited to the objective; are too unclear to permit adequate evaluation; overall design not carefully thought out; statistical aspects not given sufficient consideration; controls inadequate; material proposed for research is unsuitable
The person (the scientific and technical competence proposed toward pursuit of the research)	55%	The investigator does not have adequate experience or training; appears to be unfamiliar with recent pertinent literature or methods in his area; the investigator's previously published work in *this field* does not inspire confidence; investigator proposes to rely too heavily on insufficiently experienced associates; investigator is spread too thin; needs more liaison with colleagues
Miscellaneous (nonscientific aspects)	16%	Equipment and/or personnel proposed are unrealistic; other responsibilities would prevent devoting sufficient attention to the proposed project; there is an unfavorable institutional setting for the proposed research

From Allen, E.M.: Science **132**:1533, 1960. Copyright 1960 by the American Association for Advancement of Science.

scription of the organizational structure of that institution that shows the lines of authority and the working relationships that will be used to carry out the project with other agencies is necessary. A letter of agreement signed by a responsible officer of each of the associated organizations should be included.

Budget

The reviewing committee will want to know the plans for continuing the project at the end of the grant period and how findings can be disseminated to other interested persons. The budget is all too often a source of confusion. The easiest way to get a feel for proper budget allowance is to peruse some budgets approved by that agency. The agency will probably include as part of the application form a rather detailed budget schedule. It is useful to construct a sample budget and review it with an experienced researcher or the fiscal officer of the institution. Omission and underestimation are the chief areas of concern to reviewers. The typical budget consists of three

categories: direct costs, indirect costs, and total costs, as shown on p. 410.

SHORTCOMINGS FOUND IN DISAPPROVED GRANT APPLICATIONS

Allen (1960), an NIH official, performed an extensive study as to why research grant applications are often disapproved. Based on a review of 605 disapproved research grant applications during the period of April to May 1959, a breakdown of the shortcomings (Table 14-1) occurred as follows: the problem, 58%; the approach, 73%; personnel, 55%; miscellaneous, 16%.

Although a great deal of flexibility in the preparation of grant requests is generally allowed, almost all major sources insist on the presentation of similar information in one form or another. The reviewer should be convinced as to the scientific merit of the study and the competence of the investigator. Remember, it is in the formulation and offering of the specific proposal plan that the conscience and imagination of the reviewer of the grant are captured.

SUMMARY

Although the sources for funding for grants may swing from public to private agencies and back, the basic fundamentals remain the same. A good proposal is essential and should consist of a summary statement, introduction, needs assessment, objectives, methods, evaluation, and budget. The grant seeker should become familiar with funding resources whether these be catalogs, libraries, branches of NIH and USDA, block grant agencies within the state or local government, or foundations and corporate sources.

REFERENCES

Advisory Commission on Intergovernmental Relations: Block grants: a comparative analysis, A-60, Washington, D.C., October 1977, U.S. Government Printing Office.

Allen, E.M.: Why are research grant applications disapproved? Science 132:1533, 1960.

Bledsoe, E.P., and Ravitz, H.I.: The evolution of research and development as a procurement function of the federal government, Fed. Bar J. 17:189, July-Sept. 1957.

Catalog of federal domestic assistance, Executive Office of the President, Office of Management and Budget, Washington, D.C., 1983, U.S. Government Printing Office.

Cavanaugh, J., and McHisock, J.: Comprehensive Health Planning and Public Health Service Act of 1966 (PL 89-749), Health, Education and Welfare Indicators, Jan. 1967.

Chalkley, D.T.: The grant philosophy: Federal Grants Management Proceedings, Bethesda, Md., 1970, National Graduate University Press.

Clayton, K.: Obtaining grants from foundations and corporations, J. Home Econ. 74:1, Spring 1982.

Crawford, J., and Kieslmeier, C.: Proposal writing: a manual and workbook, Corvallis, 1970, Oregon State University.

Grossbaum, J.J.: Choosing between research project grants and contracts in mission agencies, Natl. Contract Man. J. 5:40, Spring 1971.

Guyer, B., et al.: Needs assessment under the Maternal and Child Health Services block grant: Massachusetts, amen, J. Pub. Health 74:9. 1984.

Hanlon, J.J., and Pickett, G.E.: Public health: administration and practice, ed. 8, St. Louis, 1983, The C.V. Mosby Co.

Kaufman, M., et al.: Highlights of block grants—implications for nutrition services, Members Association State and Territorial Public Health Nutrition, Jan. 12, 1982.

Kiritz, N.J.: Program planning and proposal writing, Grantsmanship Center News, May/June 1979.

Kraatz, R., and Shields, M.: Federal roles under block grants, Washington Public Affairs Center, Nov. 13, 1981.

Krathwol, D.R.: How to prepare a research proposal, Syracuse, N.Y., 1966, Syracuse University Press.

Kurzig, C.M.: Foundation fundamentals: a guide for grant-seekers, New York, 1981, The Foundation Center.

Nichaman, M.Z., and Collins, G.E.: Nutrition programs in state health agencies, Nutr. Rev. 32:65, 1974.

Public Health Service: Profiles of grant programs, HEW Pub. No. (OS) 75-50, 002, Washington, D.C., 1974, U.S. Government Printing Office.

Public Health Service: Grants policy statement, HEW Pub. No. (OS) 77-50,000, Washington, D.C., 1976, U.S. Government Printing Office.

Smolensky, J., and Haar, F.B.: Principles of community health, Philadelphia, 1972, W.B. Saunders Co.

Stanfield, R.L.: What has 500 parts, costs $83 billion and is condemned by almost everybody? Washington, D.C., Jan. 3, 1981, Federalism Report, National Journal.

Wilcox, A.W., General Counsel, U.S. Department Health, Education and Welfare: Letter to M. Wesker, Assistant Solicitor, U.S. Department of Interior, December 20, 1968.

Willner, W., and Hendricks, P.B., Jr.: Grants administration, Washington, D.C., 1972, National Graduate University.

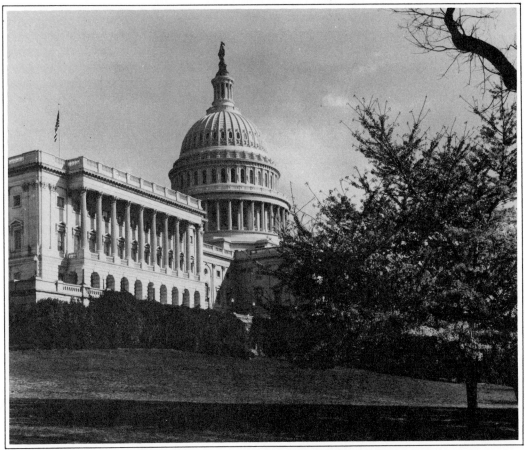

Developing Public Policy Skills and Legislation

GENERAL CONCEPT

Public policy, the political process, and legislation determine the nature of the health care system and, in turn, the practice of the health professional. Therefore legislative issues pertaining to health and nutrition that give direction to nutrition practice and nutrition programs are the responsibility of the community dietitian/nutritionist.

When you finish this chapter, you should be able to

- Give an example of how public policy shapes legislation
- Review past and current federal legislation related to nutrition
- Understand the legislative process and congressional standing committees
- Recognize the need for advocacy skills on the part of the health care professional
- Become involved in lobbying for a nutrition issue
- Evaluate the strength of professional organizations in legislative matters

PUBLIC POLICY

Public policy is the culmination of activities initiated by individuals or groups that affect the lives of other individuals or groups in society. Public policies are adopted and implemented through public laws, programs, or institutions. Before any desired activity can become a public law or program, however, it must go through a political process. In a real sense public policy is determined by legislators who make decisions within a framework of personal priorities, limited funds, constituent concerns, and political compromise. As voters and as representatives of an organized group, community dietitians/nutritionists can influence and help shape public policy by communicating their concerns, directly and emphatically, to their legislators.

Knowledge and understanding of the legal process and the political system are essential for the public health worker, particularly the community dietitian/nutritionist who may be in charge of planning, initiating, and maintaining a comprehensive program. The importance of nutrition in maintaining health and preventing disease and also the vital role of nutrition care during illness have been established. Now it is necessary that these concerns be communicated to those empowered to enact health legislation so that provision can be made for including nutrition as a significant component in health and consumer legislation. Legislation and related public policies will determine the future of health programs, the conditions under which health professionals will practice, and, indeed, whether professionals will practice at all. The government is becoming increasingly involved in the delivery, cost containment, and evaluation of health services.

Awareness of current and proposed health legislation and policies at every level—national, state, and local—in addition to an understanding of the mechanisms of the political process will enable community dietitians/nutritionists to become involved in the legislative arena. This involvement should take place early when legislation is being formulated, as well as in the active lobbying stage. Community dietitians/nutritionists should advise legislators how nutrition services, nutrition education, and nutrition research improve the quality of life and reduce the cost of health services. Such accountability looms uppermost in the minds of legislators.

NUTRITION POLICY

In the United States there have been a number of attempts to formulate a national nutrition policy: the White House Conference on Food, Nutrition, and Health (1969), the U.S. Senate Select Committee on Nutrition and Human Needs (1974 and 1975), the National Nutrition Consortium (1974), and more recently the USDA/USHHS *Dietary Guidelines* (1980) and the *Diet, Nutrition, and Cancer Prevention: Guide to Food Choices* (1984).

The Food and Agriculture Act of 1977 (PL 95-113) designated USDA as the agency responsible for human nutrition: to provide the public with information about what to eat and how food intake is linked to health outcomes. This act also created human nutrition centers to combine various nutrition activities such as research and dietary guidance.

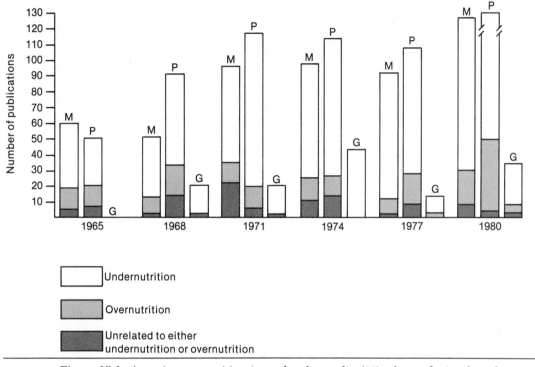

Figure 15-1. Attention to nutrition issues by the media (*M*), the professional-academic publications (*P*), and the government (*G*) from 1965 to 1980.

From Sims, L.S.: The ebb and flow of nutrition as a public policy issue, J. Nutr. Ed. 15:4, 1983.

The interest of the popular press, the government, and academic-professional publications in nutrition issues varied from 1965 to 1980 (Figure 15-1) (Sims, 1983). All three sources of interest peaked from 1971 to 1974 and again concurrent with the publication of *Dietary Goals for the United States* in 1977 and the subsequently released *Nutrition and Your Health: Dietary Guidelines for Americans* in 1980. A similar peak occurred in 1982 with the publication of the National Academy of Sciences report *Diet and Cancer* which linked diet to certain forms of cancer.

In a review of the ebb and flow of nutrition as a public policy issue, Sims (1983) makes a plea to nutrition practitioners:

As Nutrition educators interested in public policy, I urge us to not let nutrition issues fade from the public's attention and thus from the agenda-setting cycle. Only by the constant vigilance of those of us in the field will nutrition again be cast onto the public agenda and regarded by policy makers as a legitimate area of concern and action.

FEDERAL LEGISLATION SUPPORTING NUTRITION SERVICES

The activities of the U.S. Senate Select Committee on Nutrition and Human Needs served as a catalyst for federal legislation that is concerned with the nutritional status of high-risk Americans. However, the nutritional well-being of the nation's children has been a continuing concern of the federal government. Egan (1977) reminds us that "this concern has evoked a variety of responses depending upon the interest and commitment of the leadership, the advances of science and technology, as well as the problems, pressures, priorities, and fashions of the times."

Legislation with nutritional implications began as early as 1915 to 1920, when the Children's Bureau, then a part of the U.S. Department of Labor, issued technical bulletins on aspects of nutrition to help health and welfare workers and teachers in their work with children and families. The bureau initiated a nutrition survey of children from low-income families in the mountainous area of Kentucky. This was one of the first of many such studies on the prevalence of malnutrition.

The Social Security Act of 1935 authorized grants-in-aid to the states for health services for mothers and children. The School Lunch Act of 1946 made grants-in-aid available to the states to assist them in providing an adequate supply of food and other facilities for the establishment, maintenance, operation, and expansion of not-for-profit school lunch programs.

In the 1950s there was increasing recognition that appropriate dietary treatment could prevent mental retardation by correcting inborn metabolic errors. This recognition gave impetus to community mental health programs with a nutrition component. In the 1960s the number of nutritionists in health care programs increased as a result of support from the Maternal and Child Health and Mental Retardation Planning Amendments of 1963.

The 1963 amendment to Title V of the Social Security Act provided a new program of grants for maternity and infant care, especially for low-income families, and children and youth programs. Nutrition service and dietary counseling became integral parts of these projects. In the 1970s child nutrition programs were extended to residential programs and brought the benefits of food service to family day-care homes and licensed not-for-profit, private, residential institutions such as homes for the mentally retarded, orphanages, and temporary shelters.

In 1972 Congress passed legislation that authorized the Special Supplemental Food Program for Women, Infants and Children (WIC) to improve the outcome of pregnancy. The program is funded and administered by USDA through state health departments and Native American tribes, bands, or groups.

In 1974 the Food Stamp Program became a nationwide program operating throughout the United States and territories based on a uniform set of federal rules.

Two major nutrition programs designed especially for the elderly, the Congregate Meals Program and the Home Delivered Meals Program, were established by an act of Congress in 1972 as an amendment to the Older Americans Act of 1965. All persons who are over age 60 are eligible to receive meals from one of these programs, regardless of their income level.

CURRENT PUBLIC POLICY AND LEGISLATIVE ISSUES THAT RELATE TO NUTRITION
Third-Party Reimbursement

Third-party reimbursement refers to payment by a third party for services rendered by a health care provider to a patient. Payment is made by the government through Medicare and Medicaid and in the private sector through Blue Cross and Blue Shield, several large commercial carriers, workers' compensation, and the Veterans Administration. Dietitians do receive indirect reimbursement, but few receive direct payment. Other allied health professionals (e.g., occupational therapists) do receive direct payment. The prognosis for third-party reimbursement is uncertain at this time because of budget cuts.

The American Dietetic Association (ADA) supports third-party payment for nutrition care services, which are vital to the health care delivery system, and calls on its membership to educate insurers, physicians, clients, and administrators about its importance (ADA Third-party Payment, 1984):

> Nutrition care services are vital to the health care delivery system, and it is your responsibility to publicize and promote that fact. Each of you must work at the local level with the insurance companies covering your clients, your local Blue Cross/Blue Shield plan, and the commercial carriers in your area. You must anticipate some resistance, questions, and possible first-round rejection—but persist and be helpful so that all patients may profit from affordable, reimbursable nutrition care services.

Licensure

Although dietetic registration (RD) has gained considerable acceptance as a recognized professional certification in the health community, it does not provide legal recognition for dietitians or define a scope of practice. Many state dietetic associations are working to enact state licensure laws as the only effective legal recourse for consumer protection from incompetent nutrition practitioners.

In 1982 the California legislature passed a law that allows use of the titles "dietitian" and "registered dietitian" by qualified individuals. Louisiana and Montana have passed similar laws since then. In 1983 the governor of Texas signed the Licensed Dietitian Act, which protects the titles "licensed dietitian" and "licensed registered dietitian" from fraudulent use. The law established a state board to ensure that licensed dietitians adhere to a strict code of professional standards and to provide a mechanism for local enforcement.

Georgia and Oklahoma have also passed voluntary licensure laws. Governor George Wallace of Alabama signed a law to regulate the use of the title "nutritionist," as well as "dietitian" and "RD." The act forbids untrained, self-styled "nutritionists" and those with mail-order degrees from diploma mills to use the "nutritionist" title.

More important, the Alabama law protects the rights of appropriately educated individuals who are not ADA members or RDs to use the "nutritionist" title. Those nutritionists must have an advanced degree with a nutrition major from an accredited college or university. Thus the public can be assured that an Alabama nutritionist does indeed have the appropriate educational background in nutrition.

The current political climate is deregulatory, and many states are reluctant to license unless the threat to public health is real. The fact that seven states have passed laws to regulate nutrition counselors in just 2 years shows that those state legislators are convinced that such a threat exists (Mathieu, 1984c).

From home health care provided through a home health agency, nutrition care services are covered and reimbursed to the extent that such services are medically necessary in the course of providing explicitly covered home health services under Part A of the Medicare program. Such services include the following:

- Part-time or intermittent nursing care provided by or under the supervision of a registered professional nurse and physical, occupational, or speech therapy.
- Medical social services under the direction of a physician
- Part-time or intermittent services of a home health aide who has successfully completed an approved training program
- Medical supplies other than drugs and biologicals and the use of medical appliances
- Any of those services which are provided on an outpatient basis under arrangements made by the home health agency at a hospital, skilled nursing facility, or rehabilitation center

As long as nutrition care services are required in conjunction with one or more of these services, the cost of the nutrition care services will be incorporated in the home health agency overhead costs and will not be billed separately. Presently, the only nutrition-related services that are billable under Part B in a home setting are home parenteral and enteral nutrition (ADA Home Health Care, 1984).

Prospective Payment System and Diagnosis-Related Groups (Social Security Act Amendment of 1983)

USDHHS released data which confirmed that the rise in health care costs were "well above the rate of inflation": $287 billion spent in 1981, an increase of 15.1%, with Medicare costs rising 21.5%. Future estimates indicate that health care costs could reach $850 billion by 1990. Medicare and Medicaid alone will account for $158 billion by 1989. The first step toward controlling these spiraling costs was to create financial incentives for hospitals to provide efficient care. Thus the most significant legislative development of 1983 was the passage of the bill (Social Security Act Amendment of 1983) that created the Medicare prospective payment system (PPS) based on 470 diagnosis-related groups (DRGs). Attached to the law to ensure solvency of the Social Security system for the next 75 years was a provision to fundamentally change the way the government pays hospitals for treating Medicare patients.

The Health Insurance Association of America confirmed that Medicare DRGs will change the rules for all payers and that a PPS for everybody is the key to saving money nationally.

The DRG system pays a hospital a regionally adjusted, fixed sum for each patient, depending on diagnosis, regardless of length of stay. Benefits include incentives for hospital economy, federal cost savings, and more uniform payments among hospitals. Drawbacks include the possibility that hospitals and physicians could be pressed to treat those with "profitable" versus "unprofitable" diagnoses and bring undue strain on the relationship between the physician and the hospital.

Of the 10 conditions most likely to be seen in hospitals, dietitians should know that for 6 of these, nutrition intervention is indicated (Mathieu, 1984a):

DRG 127—Heart failure plus shock; mean length of stay; MLOS 7.8 days

DRG 182—Esophagitis, gastroenteritis, plus miscellaneous digestive disorders, patient older than age 69, plus/or complicating condition; MLOS 5.4 days

DRG 132—Atherosclerosis, patient older than age 69, and/or complicating condition; MLOS 6.7 days

DRG 88—Chronic obstructive pulmonary disease; MLOS 7.5 days

DRG 14—Specific cerebrovascular disorders, except transient ischemic attacks; MLOS 9.9 days

DRG 294—Diabetes, patient age 36 or older; MLOS 7.7 days

Initial effects of Medicare's based on DRGs are being reported:

The Health Care Financing Administration indicates that average length of stay per discharge was 7 days for PPS hospitals but 8.7 days for other short-stay hospitals for the 4-month period of October 1983 to January 1984.

The American Hospital Association reported that hospital admissions, occupancy rates, and Medicare patient stays declined toward the end of 1983. The rate of increase in inpatient expenses was contained at 9.6% in 1982. Growth in hospital employment slowed from 3.7% in 1982 to 1.4% in 1983.

Medicaid expenditures increased only 9.9% in 1983, compared with the 15% annual average. Home-based and community-based care waivers requested and received by many states may account for the savings (Mathieu, 1984b).

Three-year phase-in for implementation will allow payment based on 75% of each hospital's costs and 25% based on DRG rates in 1984, a 50%/50% mix in 1985, a 25% cost/75% DRG payment schedule in 1986, and 100% of payments based on DRGs in 1987.

Maternal and Child Health Services Block Grant

The MCH Block Grant has mandated states to review historical patterns and to introduce new methods for reaching populations in need. The Massachusetts Maternal and Child Health Agency has developed a needs assessment process that includes four components: a statistical measure of need based on indirect, proxy health and social indicators; clinical standards for services to be provided; an advisory process that guides decision making and involves constituency groups; and a management system for implementing funds distribution, namely open competitive bidding in response to a Request for Proposals (Guyer et al., 1984).

Nutrition Labeling

Food industries, supermarket chains, and voluntary agencies are providing point-of-purchase information that helps consumers locate products that are lower in fat, cholesterol, and salt or higher in polyunsaturated fat and fiber than conventional products. In the legislative arena the disclosure of amount of sodium is actually being regulated. The Food and Drug Administration (FDA) has effected its first major change in the nutrition labeling panel on processed food products since the panel was introduced in 1974. Effective July 1, 1985, FDA will require processors to disclose the sodium content of products when nutrition claims are made.

A *low-sodium* product is defined as containing 140 mg of sodium or less per serving; a *very low sodium* product contains 25 mg or less; and a *sodium-free* product contains less than 5 mg. If a product claim is made for "reduced sodium," the manufacturer must show that it is processed to reduce the normal levels of sodium by 75%. *Unsalted* will describe products that are processed without salt when salt is normally used.

FDA assumes that approximately 3500 food manufacturers will be affected, incurring total start-up costs of up to $20.3 million and annual costs of $700,000 to comply with the rule. The phased-in shift from voluntary to mandatory sodium labeling allows manufacturers more than a year to design new labels and use up old label inventories. Among the commenting organizations that encourage all Americans to reduce sodium intake are ADA, the American Heart Association, the American Public Health Association, and the American College of Cardiology.

Nutrition Education and Training Program

The Nutrition Education and Training Program (NET) came into being as an amendment to the Child Nutrition Act of 1966. The intent of the legislation establishing NET was to teach children through a positive daily lunchroom experience and appropriate classroom reinforcement the value of a nutritionally balanced diet, to develop curricula and materials, and to train teachers and school food service personnel to carry out this task (Maretzki, 1979).

With a budget of $15 million per year, by 1980 NET was operating in 52 states and territories and had reached over 5.7 million students, 212,000 teachers, and 104,000 food service personnel with nutrition education information. Efforts to eliminate the program by the federal administration succeeded in reducing the funding for the program by 67% in fiscal year 1982. The Society for Nutrition Education has a long history of involvement in NET and through legislative efforts has established bipartisan support for NET among both senators and representatives.

Nutrition Monitoring Bill (HR 4684)

Legislation authorizing a national monitoring program on the nutritional status of the American people fell 18 votes short of the two-thirds majority it needed in the 1984 Congress. This bill would authorize a 10-year program to gather continuous data on the dietary and nutritional status of the American population, sponsor research, maintain a nutritional status data bank, and assist state and local agencies to develop monitoring capabilities. The bill would coordinate the NHANES, now conducted intermittently by USDHHS, and the Food Consumption Survey prepared each decade by USDA.

LOBBYING: WHY AND HOW NUTRITIONISTS SHOULD BE INVOLVED

There are some cardinal rules for working effectively with legislators and other public officials, either when testifying at a public hearing or at a less formal meeting. The first step is to be informed. It would be unwise to meet with public officials to advocate a position without first studying the facts and the arguments for and against. Second, there is a need to be realistic. The advocacy of controversial legislation and regulations usually results in compromise. This has always been so and will continue in a democracy. A third principle is candidness and openness. Views should be stated along with supportive data, and there should be a willingness to listen to the problems that a particular position may create for the public official. A fourth point is to evaluate and weigh issues, thus establishing priorities in one's own mind and for the public official.

Communication is always a good way to start. Involve and inform your state legislators between their legislative sessions and give them a chance to meet your group. One nutritionist who was successful in getting state support invited legislators to have lunch and dinner with her staff and community groups. Kits were prepared for their perusal. It was an opportunity to present problems and needs and to point out how new legislation could help to meet these needs. The nutritionist's request for progress reports from the legislators at regular intervals impressed the officials regarding the sincerity of the health profession.

The Pennsylvania Dietetic Association (PDA) staged a continental breakfast for members of the Pennsylvania Senate and House of Representatives in the main Capitol building in Harrisburgh; it was held in conjunction with the PDA annual meeting. The invitation noted that a dietitian from the congressman's district would contact him or her. Informal contacts resulted in a foundation for a working relationship (ADA Legislative Newsletter, 1982).

How does one present the case or cause to a public official? Schlossberg (1973), former Staff Director, U.S. Select Committee on Nutrition and Human Needs, recommends that many people should present the case. First, you need a good cause; second, you need a good case to promote that cause; and finally, you need a good campaign to put your case across the Congressional goal line. The first step in any campaign is to reach out and build a coalition with as many groups around the country as you can reach. There is no question that Congress responds to organizations, not individuals. Thus it is important to engage many national organizations concerned about children, education, and health in the effort and to have them engage their local chapters around the country.

As concerned citizens of the United States and as the principal providers of nutrition care, nutritionists must play a pivotal role in the legislative and policy arena. Most nutrition-related programs are initiated in state and federal legislatures. Nutritionists have responsibility to seek to influence the content of laws when they are being formulated. Nutritionists and dietitians traditionally have not played a very active role in influencing the legislative process on behalf of health and nutrition concerns. There is often a feeling that "one voice won't make a difference."

As citizens, nutritionists should act to develop an environment conducive to change for the betterment of society and the groups of which they are a part or which they serve. As members of a major group of health care providers in the nation, nutritionists should act to shape health policies, rather than react after they are made, and to be influential in community, state, and national affairs. Professional responsibility and accountability are closely aligned with the amount and level of one's input into the decision-making process. The survival of the profession depends on the involvement of nutritionists in legislation and policies affecting practical, educational, and research components of nutrition.

The growth of those nutrition programs designed to protect the health of children and low-income citizens has been very encouraging to anyone committed to improving the quality of life in the United States today. Probably the single most encouraging aspect of this growth has been the critical and absolutely fundamental contribution of concerned citizens at the local, state, and federal levels. Progress without this kind of community energy would not have been possible.

WHAT IT TAKES TO PASS LEGISLATION

After having specified why nutritionists should be active in decision-making involving nutrition and health-related policies and legislation, we now turn to the means by which nutritionists can become actively involved. Fisher (1974) outlines the role of the dietitian in the legislative arena:

> Every dietitian has responsibility for action in two major areas relating to legislation and public policy: (1) to know what legislation is being considered and to show when and how nutrition services may enhance its effectiveness and (2) to practice so that nutrition services are, and therefore, can be presented to the public as an effective part of other available health services. Action in these two areas is closely related and both are essential for an effective legislative program.

The legislative process, in the simplest analysis, consists of the interaction between the legislative, executive, and judiciary branches, which are interlocked by a system of checks and balances. The *executive* branch may veto legislation or sign it into law; the *legislature* may introduce and enact a law and can override a veto by the executive branch; and the *judiciary* branch may discard a law if it considers it in violation of a person's basic freedoms and rights. To these three branches may be added the operating or enforcement agencies that are responsible for carrying out the intent of the legislation. Some examples of operating or enforcement agencies follow:

Federal Trade Commission (FTC) (founded in 1914). Five commissioners enforce some antitrust laws, protect businesses from unfair competition, and enforce truth-in-lending and truth-in-labeling laws.

Food and Drug Administration (FDA) (founded in 1931). A commissioner in USDHHS sets standards for certain foods and drugs and issues licenses for the manufacture and distribution of drugs.

Federal Communications Commission (FCC) (founded in 1934). Radio and television stations are licensed, and interstate and international telephone and telegraph operations are monitored.

A bill passes through three stages before becoming reality. The first stage is for the proposed legislation to be passed by Congress and approved by the President. Following this stage, an appropriations bill must be passed to provide the funding to implement the bill. The final stage is the formulation of the regulations that interpret and operationalize the law. Each law that is passed is assigned to a federal agency within the executive branch of the government, such as USDA or USDHHS. It is the responsibility of the agency to establish procedures that will be necessary to implement the legislation—that is, the regulations. Regulations define such laws as specifications of qualifying local, state, and regional agencies (procedures for applying for funding), parameters of use of funds, and procedures for reporting use of funds. Before the federal regulations become final and are transmitted to appropriate regional, state, or local agencies for implementation, there is an opportunity for hearings and public commentary. Then, regulations become law (Little and Sims, 1981).

Congressional Standing Committees

Among the many standing committees that deal with food and nutrition policy are Agriculture, Nutrition, Forestry, and Labor and Human Resources in the Senate and Aging, Agriculture, and Education and Labor in the House of Representatives.

A *select committee* is one established by the House or Senate, usually for a limited period and generally for a strictly temporary purpose. An example of a select committee that gave impetus to nutrition programs was the Select Committee on Nutrition and Human Needs chaired by Senator George McGovern.

When a committee decides to consider action on a bill, it usually schedules a public hearing. Here testimony is taken from the bill's sponsors, administration officials, outside experts, and any special interest groups that want to be heard. At this point the nutrition profession begins to take action. However, early in the planning stage, before a bill becomes legislation, groups such as the ADA, the Society for Nutrition Education, the American Home Economics Association, the American Public Health Association, and State and Territorial Public Health Nutrition Directors should meet and make their combined views known to senators and representatives. There is strength in combined actions. Then these legislators can actually help in the formulation of bills and even present them to other legislators in advance. Meanwhile, it should be kept in mind that all legislators are subject to pressures from lobbyists, the Administration, and their constituents.

Professional associations, such as the ADA, the American Public Health Association, and the Society for Nutrition Education, are important to members, to government, and to society. In a broad sense, associations serve to improve the economic and social well-being of the entire nation when they are successful in improving the well-being of their members. Some of the earliest functions of U.S. associations included influencing legislation, and the overwhelming majority of modern associations are involved in government relations activities. Assisting the government in taking informed and equitable action on behalf of members and citizens is but one of the tasks of government relations staff. The communication of government affairs to members is another major component. An increased focus on government activities has produced a growing social awareness among the profession (ADA, Sept. 1983).

Coalitions are becoming an important and effective means for various groups, organizations, or associations to join forces for a common cause and reflect a united voice on a particular issue. Coalitions can be formed by bringing together any group, organization, or association, church members, parents, advocates, local organizations, or locally based national organizations who are interested in working together to pro-

mote a common cause. By combining resources and dividing the work, a coalition is often more likely to be successful in promoting a specific cause or concern than a single organization.

To form a coalition in your community, you may want to consult the following national groups and their state and local affiliates:

The American Dietetic Association
630 North Michigan Ave.
Chicago, IL 60611

American Public Health Association
1015 Fifteenth Street
Washington, DC 20005

Children's Foundation
1420 New York Ave., NW, Suite 800
Washington, DC 20005

Food Research and Action Center
1319 F St., NW
Washington, DC 20004

Society for Nutrition Education
1736 Franklin St.
Oakland, CA 94612

THE FEDERAL BUDGET

The federal budget today is the result of two separate processes: the presidential and congressional budgets. In 1984 Congress passed the Congressional Budget and Impoundment Control Act, which established a process and timetable by which Congress itself developed an overall federal budget. This act established the House and Senate Budget Committees, which recommend budget resolutions for spending and revenue goals. It also established the Congressional Budget Office to provide technical information to congressional members. This office is the legislative branch's counterpart to the Office of Management and Budget in the executive branch. The functional difference between these two offices is that the Office of Management and Budget may actually recommend budgetary policies, whereas the Congressional Budget Office does not (SNE, 1983). The federal budget timetables for both the congressional and executive budget are summarized in Figure 15-2.

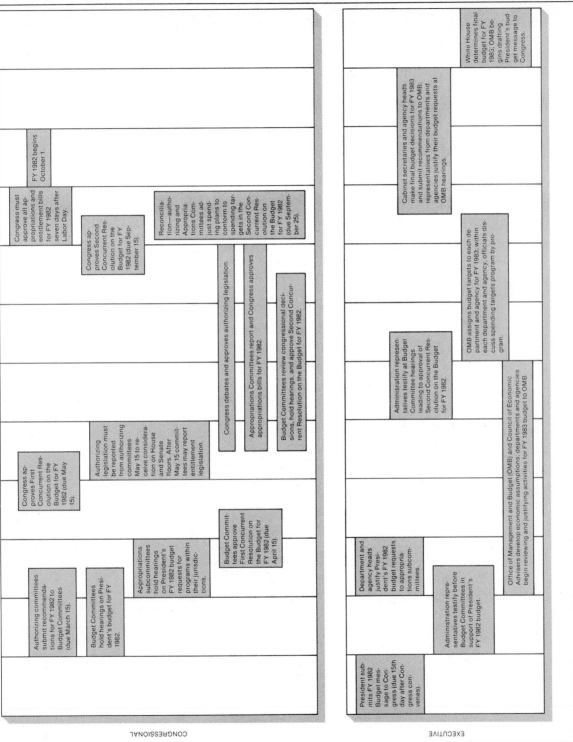

Figure 15-2. The federal budget timetables for 1981.

From Children's Defense Fund: Children and the federal budget/how to influence the budget process, Washington, D.C., 1980, Children's Defense Fund.

An excellent reference for the public health nutritionist and the dietitian who plan to get involved in the legislative arena is "A Nutritionist's Guide to Washington," which is found in the appendix to this chapter.*

SUMMARY

Translation of scientific knowledge of nutrition into public policy is a legislative process. Federal legislation supporting nutrition services has been reviewed. Current public policy and legislative issues such as third-party reimbursement, the prospective payment system, and diagnosis-related groups affect nutrition policy. The community dietitian/nutritionist and the combined strengths of professional agencies can play an important role in lobbying and the legislative process.

*See *A Brief Guide to Becoming A Nutrition Advocate*, Society for Nutrition Education, 1736 Franklin Street, Oakland, CA 94612 (415-444-7133).

REFERENCES

American Dietetic Association: Legislative newsletter, Chicago, 1982, The American Dietetic Association.

American Dietetic Association: Beneficiaries of ADA's legislative and public policy program, Chicago, 1983, The American Dietetic Association.

American Dietetic Association: Home health care, J. Am. Diet. Assoc. 84:6, 1984.

American Dietetic Association: Third party payment for nutrition care services, J. Am. Diet. Assoc. 84:6, 1984.

Egan, M.S.: Federal nutrition support programs for children, Pediatr. Clin. North Am. 24:229, 1977.

Fisher, F.E.: The dietitian in the legislative arena, J. Am. Diet. Assoc. 64:621, 1974.

Guyer, B., et al.: Needs assessment under the Maternal and Child Health Services Block Grant: Massachusetts, Am. J. Pub. Health 74(9):1014, 1984.

Little, L., and Sims, L.S.: Let's get involved in the legislative process. In Wright, H.S., and Sims, L.S., editors: People, policies, and programs, Belmont, Calif., 1981, Wadsworth, Inc.

Maretzki, A.N.: A perspective on nutrition education and training, J. Nutr. Ed. 11:176, 1979.

Mathieu, M.: Legislative highlights: six of top 10 DRGs involve nutrition intervention, J. Am. Diet. Assoc. 84(1):88, 1984a.

Mathieu, M.: Legislative highlights: DRGs reduce hospital costs, J. Am. Diet. Assoc. 84(6):692, 1984b.

Mathieu, M.: Legislative highlights: licensure of nutrition professionals, J. Am. Diet. Assoc. 84(10):1228, 1984c.

Schlossberg, K.: What it takes to pass nutrition legislation, J. Nutr. Ed. 5:228, 1973.

Sims, L.S.: The ebb and flow of nutrition as a public policy issue, J. Nutr. Ed. 15:4, 1983.

Society for Nutrition Education: A brief guide to becoming a nutrition advocate, Oakland, Calif., 1983, The Society.

APPENDIX 15-1

A NUTRITIONIST'S GUIDE TO WASHINGTON

Agencies

Administration on Aging (AoA)
(elderly feeding program)
330 Independence Ave., S.W.
Room 4760, North Building
Washington, DC 20201
202-245-0724

Agency for International Development
(world hunger)
320 21st St., N.W.
Washington, DC 20523
202-632-1850

Agricultural Research Service (ARS)/USDA
(nutrition research)
302-A Administration Building
Beltsville, MD 20705
301-344-3355

Consumer Nutrition Center/USDA
6505 Bellcrest Rd.
(consumer research)
Hyattsville, MD 20782
301-431-8470

Federal Trade Commission (FTD)
(food advertising)
6th and Pennsylvania
Washington, DC 20580
202-523-3830

Food and Drug Administration (FDA)
(food safety)
200 C. St., S.W.
Washington, DC 20204
202-443-1544

National Institutes of Health (NIH)
(nutrition research)
9000 Rockville Pike
Bethesda, MD 20205
301-496-4000

Office of Consumer Affairs (OCA)
(consumer issues)
1009 Premier Building
Washington, DC 20201
202-634-4140

U.S. Department of Agriculture (USDA)
Food and Nutrition Service (FNS)
(food program administration)
3101 Park Center Dr.
Alexandria, VA 22302
703-756-3062

Congress

Capitol Hill Switchboard
(information)
202-224-3121

General Accounting Office
(program evaluation)
441 G St.
Washington, DC 20548
202-275-5525

House Agriculture Committee
(farm and food stamp programs)
1301 Longworth Building
Washington, DC 20515
202-225-2171

House Appropriations Committee
(money bills)
H218, The Capitol
Washington, DC 20515
202-225-2771

House Committee on Health and the Environment
(food safety)
2415 Rayburn Building
Washington, DC 20515
202-225-4952

House Education and Labor Committee
(nutrition programs except food stamps)
2181 Rayburn Building
Washington, DC 20515
202-225-4527

House Science Committee
(nutrition research)
2321 Rayburn Building
Washington, DC 20515
202-225-6371

Continued.

A NUTRITIONIST'S GUIDE TO WASHINGTON—cont'd

Congress—cont'd

Office of Technology Assessment
(special projects)
Congress of the United States
Washington, DC 20510
202-224-8711

Select Committee on Aging
(aging)
712 H.O.B. Annex #1
Washington, DC 20515
202-226-3375

Senate Agriculture Committee
(farm and food programs)
322 Russell Building
Washington, DC 20510
202-224-2035

Senate Appropriations Committee
(money bills)
S-128, The Capitol
Washington, DC 20515
202-224-7282

Senate Human Resources Committee
(aging, community nutrition programs, nutrition
  research, food safety)
4230 Dirksen Building
Washington, DC 20510
202-224-5375

Senate Special Aging Committee
(aging oversight)
G-233 Dirksen Building
Washington, DC 20510
202-224-5364

Private Organizations

American Institute of Nutrition
(nutrition research)
9650 Rockville Pike
Bethesda, MD 20814
301-530-7050

Center for Science in the Public Interest
(food advocacy)
1501 16th St., N.W.
Washington, DC 20036
202-332-9110

Children's Foundation
(child care food program)
815 15th St., N.W., #928
Washington, DC 20005
202-347-3300

Community Nutrition Institute
(nutrition program and policy issues)
2001 S St., N.W.
Washington, DC 20009
202-462-4700

Congress Watch
(consumer issues)
215 Pennsylvania Ave., S.E.
Washington, DC 20003
202-546-4996

Consumer Federation of America
(consumer issues)
1314 14th St., N.W.
Washington, DC 20004
202-387-0121

Federation of American Societies for Experimental
  Biology
(nutrition research)
9650 Rockville Pike
Bethesda, MD 20814
301-530-7000

Food Research and Action Center
(feeding programs and advocacy)
1319 F St., N.W.
Washington, DC 20004
202-393-5060

Institute for Local Self-Reliance
(food co-ops and urban gardens)
2425 18th St., N.W.
Washington, DC 20009
202-232-4108

International Life Sciences Institute-Nutrition
  Foundation
1126 16th St., N.W., #100
Washington, DC 20036
202-872-0778

A NUTRITIONIST'S GUIDE TO WASHINGTON—cont'd

National Consumers League
(consumer issues)
600 Maryland Ave., S.W.
202 West Wing
Washington, DC 20024
202-554-1600

National Nutrition Consortium
(nutrition policy)
24 3rd St., N.E.
Washington, DC 20003
202-547-4819

Worldwatch Institute
(world hunger)
1776 Massachusetts Ave., N.W.
Washington, DC 20036
202-452-1999

Glossary

abstracting Process of collecting concise data from patient records.

action planning An element of program planning that addresses itself to presenting the steps involved in achieving program objectives.

action plans (also, **work statements or methods**) Plans that state the means by which objectives are to be achieved.

activity The performance of a function by an organizational unit, directed toward the achievement of a stated objective.

adequacy The extent to which a problem can be eliminated by a particular program.

administration The planning, facilitation, execution, evaluation, and control of services.

advocacy The act or process of pleading in favor of; support for.

ambulatory care Preventive, therapeutic, and/or rehabilitative personal health services provided to a patient/client who is not confined to a health care facility.

ambulatory health care center A public or private organizational unit (free standing or institution based) that provides health care services, directly or through contractual arrangements, to meet the needs of noninstitutionalized patients.

American Dietetic Association A professional organization responsible for establishing educational and supervised clinical experience requirements and standards of practice in the profession of dietetics.

anthropometric assessment Measurement of the physical dimensions and gross composition of the body at different age levels and degrees of nutrition.

appropriateness The extent to which programs are directed toward those problems that are believed to have the greatest importance.

at-risk clients Those clients whose indicators of nutrition status, as determined by nutrition assessment, deviate from the norm, therefore potentially jeopardizing health status.

audit Formal study or examination of the documentation of outcomes/processes of health care to determine if criteria are being met.

autocratic leadership In the continuum of leader authority, autocratic leadership is illustrated by the manager who makes decisions and then announces them to the group.

baseline data Data on health indicators and/or level of health care delivery, collected as the initiating step; precedes the implementation of a quality assurance program.

behavioral Describes an action by an individual or group in response to a given situation.

biographic data bases, computerized These data bases are primarily concerned with citations of published journal articles, books, and materials.

biostatistics A major tool used in epidemiology to form and analyze estimates of disease risk and other pertinent data.

block grant (MCH) A grant that is a principal source of support to states, assisting them in their efforts to maintain and strengthen their leadership in planning, promoting, and coordinating health care, including nutrition services, for mothers and children.

budget Formal statements of the financial resources set aside for carrying out specific activities in a given period of time.

budgeting A plan expressed in monetary terms.

certification The act of documenting the fulfillment of requirements.

clients Health care consumers who are either patients, potential patients, or others with legal/family/personal responsibilities and/or concern for the health and well-being of an individual or a consumer unit.

communication Creation or exchange of understanding between a sender and receiver.

community A group of individuals or families living together in a defined geographical area.

community assessment (community diagnosis) Process of identifying and describing a community, its ecology, and the factors influencing the way its people live. Health problems of the community with nutrition implications and available resources for nutrition services can be identified by this process.

community dietetic technician A person who has completed a 2-year approved dietetic technician program; also, one who has completed more than 2 years of education in dietetics but less than is necessary for a B.S. degree, or one who has a B.S. degree but is not a registered dietitian.

community dietetics The delivery of nutrition care services, with a focus on community health, to promote and maintain health, prevent disease, continue rehabilitative efforts, and initiate health care.

community dietitian/nutritionist An individual who provides direct nutrition care and nutrition education to patients/clients and to the public. This is the entry-level position for professional public health nutrition personnel. The community dietitian provides nutrition assessment and implementation, including education and referral, for patients and clients and evaluates the nutrition component of patient care.

community nutrition Academic discipline that deals with identification and solution of health problems with nutritional implications in communities or human population groups.

community nutrition program services The food- and nutrition-related activities performed as part of the organization/agency's plan for the promotion of health of a given population, for example, services such as clinical care, group education, consultation/technical assistance to community organizations, training, and nutrition surveillance.

community nutrition support personnel Those members of the community dietetics team who possess less than a B.S. degree or who possess a B.S. but are not registered dietitians.

completeness The extent to which a phenomenon of interest (for example, a program) is assessed in totality rather than in part.

computer A device that can perform computations, including arithmetic and logic operations, without intervention by humans.

computer program A series of instructions in a main computer's storage that specify which processing operations are to occur in the computer system.

computer science Science that allows one to process data and perform analytical tasks quickly and accurately; it allows a broad access to computerized data bases.

computer system A computer system has two basic components: (1) *software*, or programs and tables that direct the performance of the desired task; and (2) *hardware*, or the computer equipment necessary to perform the task.

conflict, organizational A disagreement between two or more organization members or groups arising from such problems as sharing scarce resources or work activities or having different status, goals, values, or perceptions.

consultation The act of giving professional guidance or services; the act of conferring on a case or its treatment.

consultative leadership In this style of leadership, the manager "sells" a decision, presents ideas and invites questions from subordinates, or both.

consumer Individual who is a recipient or potential recipient of health care.

contract A promise or set of promises that acts as an instrument to procure research or services.

control The process through which managers ensure that actual activities conform to planned activities.

controlling The process that ensures that plans are being followed.

coordination The essence of managership; the achievement of harmony of individual efforts toward the accomplishment of group goals.

cost-benefit analysis (CBA) All costs and all benefits of a program, valued in monetary terms.

cost-effective analysis (CEA) The health-related effects of programs or techniques, not valued in monetary terms but measured in some other unit (such as years of life gained).

coverage The extent to which measurements are applied to each client or to clients.

criteria Predetermined elements of health care services used for quality assessment; professionally developed statements of desirable health care processes or desired outcomes.

critical time Specified period of time to which a criterion applies; identification of a specified time period during which a practice, service, or behavior occurred.

cross-sectional data Data collected over a short interval describing given parameters in groups of various ages.

data base A body of information stored by the computer.

decision making The process through which a course of action is selected as the solution to a specific problem.

deficiency diseases Disorders or disease conditions with characteristic clinical signs caused by dietary deficiencies of nutrients; they can be cured or prevented by supplying the nutrients that are lacking.

Delbecq technique A group technique for eliciting ideas from every participant. It can be divided into the following steps: (1) individuals silently record all ideas; (2) "round robin," during which each participant states one of his or her ideas, which is recorded on a flip chart; this is continued around the room until all participants have all of their ideas recorded; no evaluation is allowed during this process; (3) period of discussion of each recorded idea; and (4) participants rank ideas in order of priority.

delegation The assignment to a person of formal authority and responsibility for carrying out specific activities.

democratic leadership In this style of leadership, the manager defines the limits of the situation and the problem to be solved and asks the group to make the decision.

demography The statistical study of human populations, especially with reference to size and density distribution and vital statistics.

departmentalization The grouping together of similar or logically related work activities.

determinants of change Factors that can be identified by study and research as being responsible for change in the attitudes, beliefs, or behavior of individuals or groups, especially with regard to the acceptance of new food products and new methods for food preparation.

diagnosis-related groups (DRGs) Insurance groups that pay a hospital a regionally adjusted fixed sum for each patient depending on diagnosis, regardless of length of stay.

diet counseling The provision of individualized professional guidance to assist people in adjusting daily food consumption to meet health needs. This process actually involves three components: interviewing, counseling, and consulting. Success depends on one's ability to explain the nutrition plan in simplest language, considering the patient's background, socioeconomic needs, and personal preference.

dietary history A detailed account of the kinds, estimated amounts, and preparation methods of the usual daily food intake and variations for an individual, obtained in an interview by a professional worker; should include socioeconomic factors.

dietary study methodology Methods of obtaining dietary information include the following. For individuals: (1) estimation by recall, with the client or client's parent recalling food intake of previous 24 hours or longer; (2) food intake record, which is a listing of all foods eaten (including between-meal intakes) for varying lengths of time, usually 3 to 7 days; (3) dietary history taken by recall, repeated food records, or both to discover the usual food pattern over relatively long periods of time; (4) weighed food intake of the client, or weighing the client him-

self/herself. For groups: (1) food account or running reports of food purchased or produced for household use; (2) food list or recall of estimated amounts of various foods consumed during the previous days, usually the previous 7 days; (3) food record or weighed inventory of foods at the beginning and end of the study, with or without records of kitchen and plate wastes.

dietary study (survey) Method of determining or evaluating the dietary intake of an individual, group, or population at large. The adequacy of a given diet is determined by qualitative comparison with the basic food groups or by quantitative comparison with the recommended dietary standard of a particular country. A dietary study is used to detect adequacy or inadequacy of diets to give valuable information concerning food habits; menu preparation; and food procurement, availability, and distribution.

dietetic practice Performance of activities in fulfilling a professional position in nutritional care.

dietetics Profession concerned with the science and art of human nutritional care, an essential component of health science. Dietetics includes the extending and imparting of knowledge concerning foods that will provide nutrients sufficient to health, foods to be used during disease, diet throughout the life cycle, and the management of group feeding.

direct service provider In the field of nutrition, a professional or paraprofessional whose interaction involves nutrition counseling and education on a one-to-one or group basis.

documentation Written notation of health care provided as found in a health or medical record.

double-blind technique A method that eliminates much of the conscious or unconscious bias of both subject and investigator by keeping them unaware of who is getting what specific treatment. Classically, this involves the use of the look-alike placebo in intervention studies.

draft criteria Criteria developed by an audit committee or audit task force that have not been ratified and that are subject to change by those whose practice will be audited.

effectiveness A measure of the actual accomplishment of a program compared with the amount intended or planned, which may be less than total eradication or prevention. The effectiveness of a prophylactic measure is the percentage of cases prevented by the measure that are expected in a population.

efficiency A measure of the cost in resources necessary to accomplish the program's objectives or the ratio between an output (net attainment of program objectives) and an input (program resources expended).

entry level In each level of practice, the position requiring the minimum level of training and experience; operationally defined as position that can be filled by a person with 3 years' or less experience.

environmental analysis In marketing, the attempt to analyze the environment in which the organization operates; trying to identify the leading trends and their implications for the organization.

epidemiology The study of health and disease in populations rather than individuals; concerned primarily with the etiology, treatment, and prevention of disease at the community level.

evaluation The process of determining the value or amount of success in achieving a predetermined objective. It includes at least the following steps: formulation of the objective, identification of the proper criteria to be used in measuring success, determination and explanation of the degree of success, and recommendations for further program activity.

exceptions Circumstances or situations that may prevent the achievement of an outcome because of conditions beyond the control of the practitioner or client.

expected level of performance Percentage of achievement developed for each criterion, below which corrective action is indicated.

experimental design The essential requirement for a true experiment is the randomized assignment of people to programs. The classic design uses both experimental and control groups.

experimental mortality (evaluation) The differential loss of respondents from comparison groups.

explicit criteria Predetermined elements of health care services that specify the exact method(s) to be used for verification.

extinction Lack of response designed to reduce undesired behavior; absence of reinforcement.

Food and Nutrition Board, NAS/NRC This board, established in 1940 under the Division of Biology and Agriculture of the National Academy of Sciences/National Research Council, serves as an advisory body in the field of food and preparation. Its earliest activity was the preparation of Recommended Dietary Allowances (RDAs), which are revised periodically.

food patterns The kinds of foods customarily used by people in a given area, region, or ethnic group and the way those foods are prepared and served.

food scientist or technologist The food scientist uses the disciplines of biology and chemistry to understand the nature of food, its composition and properties, and the chemical reactions that take place therein. The food technologist is concerned with the application of the laws and processes of biology, physics, chemistry, and engineering in the preparation, preservation, and analysis of food products that, in the interest of public health, are of high nutritional quality, are safe, and can be stored for reasonable periods of time to allow for maximum distribution. Professional qualifications vary depending on the place of employment and responsibilities involved. High-level positions in industry usually require training beyond a Bachelor's degree. Academic positions either in teaching or research or a combination of the two almost always require a Ph.D. Food scientists and technologists often come into the field through related areas such as microbiology, chemistry, physics, or engineering.

force field analysis Identification of the environment that may help or hinder in carrying out a strategy.

forecasting The difference in accuracy between a predicted outcome that is based on sound information and one that is not.

format to complete objectives A format with the following composition: "To" / action verb / desired result / time frame / resources required. For example: "To reduce the prevalence of anemia in 1- to 2-year-olds by 30% in 1 year, using the nutrition staff."

function An area of responsibility whose discharge is required to meet program objectives.

Gantt scheduling A technique using a bar chart to reflect completion dates and activities in developing an action plan.

generic criteria Predetermined elements of health care services that are common to all programs or to the care of all clients or patients.

geriatrics The branch of medicine dedicated to the care of the aged.

gerontology The study of the psychological, sociological, economic, physiological, and medical aspects of aging.

goal Statement of broad direction, general purpose, or interest. It may be somewhat unreachable, and it is often not quantifiable.

government (local) A unit of government below the state level, specifically including a county, municipality, city, town, township, school district, council of governments, sponsor group, representative organization, or other regional or interstate government entity or any agency or instrumentality of a local government, exclusive of institutions of higher education and hospitals. This term also includes federally recognized Indian tribal governments.

government (state) Any governing body of the several states of the United States, the District of Columbia, the Commonwealth of Puerto Rico, any territory or possession of the United States, or any agency or instrumentality of a state, exclusive of state institutions of higher education and hospitals.

grant An award of financial or direct assistance to an eligible recipient under programs that provide for such assistance based on review and approval of an application, plan, or other document(s) setting forth a proposed activity or program.

grantee The institution, public or private corporation, organization, agency, or other legally accountable entity that receives a grant and assumes legal and financial responsibility and accountability both for the awarded funds and for the performance of the grant-supported activity. In certain cases, a grantee may be an individual.

guideline Statement prepared to direct future action.

health A positive state of physical, mental, and social well-being and not merely the absence of disease.

health care Combined service components delivered to consumers to promote wellness and/or to prevent and treat disease.

health care/medical audit Retrospective examination of the medical record to assess the quality and appropriateness of health care provided to an individual.

health care practitioners Health professionals or paraprofessionals—qualified by education, experience, and/or registration, licensure, or certification to practice their profession—who are involved in delivery of direct patient care in ambulatory or institutional care settings.

health care team A group of health care professionals who provide coordinated services to achieve optimal health care for the client.

health maintenance Preventive, diagnostic, curative, and restorative health services available to a client, group, or community.

Health Maintenance Organization (HMO) An organized system of health care that accepts the responsibility to provide or otherwise ensure the delivery of an agreed-on set of comprehensive health maintenance and treatment services for a voluntarily enrolled group of persons in a geographic area. It is reimbursed through a prenegotiated and fixed periodic payment made by or on behalf of each person or family unit enrolled in the plan. The HMO provides comprehensive care with major emphasis on prevention, care continuity, and maximum health service at a reasonable cost.

health (medical) care evaluation A program of an organized health care staff designed to measure the quality of care in a health care institution.

health promotion Unlike traditional curative medicine, health promotion is directed toward people who are basically healthy and fosters the development of lifestyles to monitor and enhance a state of health and well-being.

health status An individual's relative condition of wellness or illness.

Health Systems Agency (HSA) Authorized in PL 93-641, the HSA is responsible for health planning and development throughout the country in health service areas designated by the governor of each state. These agencies are responsible for preparing and implementing plans for the development of health services, manpower, and facilities and for the prevention of unnecessary duplication of health resources or of other inefficiencies in the health care delivery system.

history (evaluation) Events that may occur in addition to experimental treatment and may thus provide alternate explanations of effects.

implementation A phase in the planning process that makes a plan operational; during implementation, definite action is taken to commit resources for the purpose of achieving desired results.

incidence Refers to the number of new cases of a disease during a specified period of time.

infant An individual between the ages of 29 days and 12 months.

infant feeding practices Methods of feeding (such as breast-feeding or bottle-feeding), the kind and amount of supplements given, weaning age, kinds of foods given at weaning, and similar information regarding infant feeding practices.

influence An action that either directly or indirectly causes a change in behavior or attitude of another person or group.

in-kind contributions Contributions that represent the value of noncash contributions provided by the grantee or third parties. In-kind contributions may consist of charges for real property and nonexpendable personal property and the value of goods and services directly benefiting and specifically identifiable to the grant-supported activity.

instrumentation (accuracy) In evaluation, the changes in the calibration of a measuring instrument or changes in the observer's scores may produce changes in the obtained measurement.

Interdepartmental Committee on Nutrition for National Defense (ICNND) A group established to assess, assist in, and learn about the food and nutrition situation in countries to which the United States is giving military support. Local specialists in each country assist personnel from the United States in defining the major nutritional problems.

International Council of Scientific Unions An organization that consists of sixteen unions, one of which is the International Union for Nutritional Sciences. It sponsors international congresses of nutrition every 3 years.

International Union for Nutritional Sciences (IUNS) One of sixteen unions of the International Council of Scientific Unions. Its aim is to provide a means for international cooperation in the study of basic and applied nutrition. Information is exchanged at international congresses.

lactation Milk production; the process of breast feeding results from the interplay of hormones and the instinctive reflexes and learned behavior of the mother and the newborn.

laissez-faire leadership In this style of leadership, subordinates are permitted to function within the limits set by the manager's superior. There is no interference within the group by the manager, who attempts to make decisions with no more influence than any other member of the group.

leadership The process of influencing the activities of an individual or a group in efforts toward goal achievement in a given situation.

leading The process by which managers direct and influence subordinates, motivating others to perform essential tasks. It is the creation of a work environment that both satisfies employees and promotes the organization's objectives.

length of stay The number of days a patient remains in a specific institution, from the day of admission to the day of discharge.

licensure The process by which an agency of government grants permission to an individual to engage in a given occupation, on finding that the applicant has attained the minimal degree of competency necessary to ensure the protection of public health, safety, and welfare.

life-style An individual's mode of living as affected by physiological, psychosocial, environmental, economic, and religious influences.

longitudinal data Data derived from periodic measurements in the same person over a long stretch of time.

longitudinal studies Continuous or repeated experimental observations and measurements carried on for many years with the same group of human subjects or through one or more generations of animals.

malnutrition A state of poor health with symptoms that can be clinically identified as being caused by inadequate intake of one or more essential nutrients over a sustained period of time.

management The art of getting things done through people. It is the process of planning, organizing, leading, and controlling the efforts of an organization's members and of using all other organizational resources to achieve stated organizational goals.

Management by Objectives (MBO) A management tool by which a definition of work objectives for each department, division, and employee within an organization is established. Its basic philosophy is that employers and employees work together to (1) set specific measurable objectives, (2) make dated action plans for their implementation, and (3) periodically review the results of these objectives and plans together. All activities must be related to overall organizational goals.

management theory Includes three well-established schools of management thought—classical, behavioral, and quantitative—which have contributed to managers' understanding of organizations and their ability to manage them.

managerial skills The tools necessary to achieve planning, organizing, leading, and controlling in an organization. Managers need technical, human, and conceptual skills. Technical skills imply an understanding of and proficiency in a specific kind of activity, particularly one involving method processes, procedures, or techniques. Human skills involve the ability to work effectively as a group member and to build cooperative efforts within the team. Conceptual skills involve the ability to see the organization as a whole and include recognizing how the various functions of the organization depend on one another and how changes in one part affect all others.

marasmus A condition occurring mostly in infants 3 to 18 months of age as a result of gross deficiency of calories over a period of time and an accompanying lack of protein and other nutrients. It is frequently accompanied by diarrhea and characterized by low body weight, loss of subcutaneous fat, and wasting of muscle tissue. (Some cases of marasmus show edema and are best described as kwashiorkor rather than marasmic kwashiorkor.)

marketing The analysis, planning, implementation, and control of carefully formulated programs designed to bring about organizational objectives (see Social marketing).

matching A study technique for neutralizing confounding variables; it matches each exposed individual with an unexposed individual who is identical with respect to all confounding factors.

maturation (evaluation) Events within respondents that reflect changes as a function of the passage of time per se, such as growth and secular trends.

meal patterns The kind and amounts of food eaten at the various meals of the day.

Medicaid (Title XIX) The program under federal law that provides payments for medical care services to recipients of categorical public assistance. This program is administered by the individual states, which in turn receive matching federal funds to support it.

medical audit Retrospective review of medical care, in which in-depth assessments of the quality and/or nature of the utilization of medical services are made.

medical care Care provided specifically under the direction of a physician, including the scientifically determined diagnosis, treatment, and patient care management.

Medicare (Title XVIII) An amendment to the Social Security Act, which provides a federal health insurance program to persons over 65 years of age.

microcomputer The generic term for a small computer based on microprocessing technology.

minicomputer Computer that is smaller than a mainframe but larger than a microcomputer.

mission (of an organization) The unique aim that sets the organization apart from others of its type.

monitoring Ongoing measurement of health care quality indicators to identify potential problems.

morbidity ratio A ratio of the sick/well in a given area; expressed in terms of population, usually 100,000.

mortality (death rate) A measure of the frequency of death for a specified period of time, usually a year, in relation to the total population.

motivation That which causes, channels, and sustains people's behavior.

National Academy of Sciences/National Research Council (NAS/NRC) Government group that established the Food and Nutrition Board, which is concerned with nutrition policy and the development of materials for use by professionals. The board also advises national and international groups about nutrition.

National Center for Health Statistics Federal agency established specifically to collect and disseminate data on health in the United States; designs and maintains national data collection systems, conducts research in statistical and survey methodology, and cooperates with other agencies in the United States and in foreign countries in activities to increase the availability and usefulness of health data.

National Health and Nutrition Examination Survey (NHANES) The National Center for Health Statistics is conducting nutritional status surveys of the United States population on a 2-year cycle. The sample consists of persons from 1 through 74 years of age who are not institutionalized. There is an oversampling of groups that are susceptible to nutritional difficulties such as poor children of preschool age, women of childbearing age, and the aged. The survey includes household interviews, questionnaires, physical measurements, physical examinations, tests and procedures, and biochemical determinations on blood and urine samples.

National Institutes of Health (NIH) Research unit of the Public Health Service in the DHHS. It is engaged in clinical research of diseases of public health importance such as allergic, dental, mental, and metabolic diseases.

National Nutrition Survey In 1967, Congress requested that the DHHS survey malnutrition and related health programs in the United States. Kentucky, Louisiana, South Carolina, Texas, West Virginia, California, Massachusetts, Michigan, New York, and Washington were surveyed. From 1968 to 1970, data were collected regarding general demographic, dietary intake, clinical, anthropometric, dental, and biochemical considerations.

National Science Foundation (NSF) A foundation established in 1950 for the purpose of improving scientific research and education in the United States. Grants are awarded to universities and other nonprofit institutions to support research. The foundation also maintains a register of scientific personnel.

need That state or condition in the community that indicates a lack of essential public health protection and well-being.

needs assessment In nutrition, the process of identifying and describing the extent and type of health and nutrition problems observed among individuals and/or target populations in the community.

neonate An individual in the age period between birth and 28 days.

nominal group process (Delbecq process) Structured group process of specific sequential steps used to identify problems or generate information.

nonequivalent control groups The use of available individuals as controls in research or evaluation when there is no random assignment to program and control (as there would be in a true experiment).

nonexperimental designs Those designs that have (1) a before and after study of a single person, (2) an "after only" study of a program participant, and (3) an "after only" study of participants and nonrandom controls.

norms Numerical or statistical measures of most frequently observed performance, derived from aggregate data regarding specific aspects of care provided to patient populations over a statistically significant period of time.

numeric data bases Primarily, numbers and codes that cite statistical data or other types of information.

nutrition The science of food, the nutrients and other substances therein, their action, interaction, and balance in relation to health and disease, and the processes by which the organism ingests, digests, absorbs, transports, utilizes, and excretes food substances. In addition, nutrition must be concerned with social, economic, cultural, and psychological implications of food and eating. Furthermore, it includes an evaluation of nutritional status and the effect on the individual's health of an inadequacy or imbalance of nutrients consumed. In this diverse field of study a number of subspecialties have evolved, which require varying competencies and depths of knowledge in the biological, medical, chemical, and social sciences.

nutrition, public health The theory and practice of nutrition as a science through organized community effort, with the family as the smallest unit under study. The overall aim of public health nutrition is to improve or maintain good health through proper nutrition. Various agencies, governmental or nongovernmental, are concerned with nutrition work at local, national, or international levels.

nutrition assessment Evaluation of the nutritional status of an individual who has been identified by a screening process as being at nutrition risk. The assessment includes a review of socioeconomic, dietary, clinical/medical, anthropometric, and biochemical data.

nutrition care interventions Actions undertaken to alter or maintain nutrition status (for groups or individuals); means of bringing about or maintaining positive nutrition effects—preventive, curative, or rehabilitative.

nutrition care plan A detailed formulation of a program of action to meet the nutrition needs of clients.

nutrition counseling The process by which patients/clients are most effectively helped to acquire more healthful behavior.

nutrition education The process by which beliefs, attitudes, environmental influences, and understanding about food lead to practices that are scientifically sound, practical, and consistent with individuals' needs and available food resources.

Nutrition Education and Training Program (NET) The result of an amendment to the Child Nutrition Act of 1966. The purpose of the program is to teach children, through a positive daily luncheon experience and appropriate classroom reinforcement, the value of a nutritionally balanced diet; and to develop curriculum and materials to train teachers and school food service personnel to carry out this task.

nutrition history An informative and comprehensive description of laboratory and clinical findings, as well as of the dietary history of an individual. (See Dietary history and Nutritional status.)

nutrition program plan Written document that describes the nutrition component of the health services to be provided to a population. It should clearly describe community needs; priorities; objectives; activities, including standards, policies, protocols, and procedures used; resources, including staff and budget; and evaluation methods.

nutrition scientist A trained nutritionist who has undergone studies leading to an advanced degree in nutrition or in allied science; has attained the competencies required for a degree in nutrition; and, in addition, has developed competence in research techniques and methodologies as applied to nutrition such that he or she is capable of independent research in the field.

nutrition surveillance In contrast with "survey," "surveillance" implies continuity, or a frequent and continuous watching over.

nutritional care The application of the science and art of human nutrition in helping people select and obtain food for the primary purpose of nourishing their bodies in health or disease throughout the life cycle. This participation may be in single or combined functions; in food service systems management to groups; in extending knowledge of food and nutrition principles; in teaching these principles for application according to particular situations; and in dietary counseling.

nutritional status State of the body resulting from the consumption and utilization of nutrients. Clinical observations, biochemical analyses, anthropometric measurements, and dietary studies are used to determine this state.

nutritional status assessment An evaluation of one's nutritional state is accomplished by one or more of the following methods: (1) dietary survey (to detect a faulty diet, that is, a primary factor), (2) medical and clinical examination (to detect conditioning factors), (3) biochemical tests (to detect tissue levels), and (4) anthropometric tests (to detect anatomical changes). All of these methods are used in nutrition surveys. Other sources of information helpful in appraising the nutritional status of groups of individuals or populations are vital and health statistics, food balance sheets, and other pertinent data compiled by organizations such as government agencies, hospitals, clinics, and insurance companies.

nutritional survey Study of the nutritional status of a population group in a given area of operation. The population may be homogeneous (for example, teen-aged girls or diabetics) or heterogeneous (for example, hospital patients). Thus the survey may be slanted with respect to various factors such as age, sex, race, or socioeconomic, geographic, physiological, or pathological conditions, depending on the aims of the study. In general, the main objectives of the nutrition survey are to determine the extent of malnutrition and ascertain feeding problems; to provide ways and means of correcting or preventing nutritional problems; and to help in nutrition education, economic planning, and other programs for the improvement of the health status of the population or group.

objective A defined end result of specific public health activity to be achieved in a finite period of time. Objectives are stated as definite aims or goals of action, which should be quantitatively measurable and capable of being reflected in standards performance.

Objectives can be either long range, intermediate, or short range. (See Format to complete objectives.) *Outcome objectives* are those that state the ultimate result, not steps, processes, or actions to achieve that result. *Process objectives* are the steps (action) taken to reach the outcome objective.

Omnibus Budget Reconciliation Act of 1981 (PL 97-35) This act amended Title V of the Social Security Act and consolidated 27 separate programs; it converted federal categorical health grant programs to state-controlled block grants in four areas.

operation A specific task or series of tasks that, when completed, advances work to the next operation.

operational planning Planning that focuses on present operation; its prime concern is efficiency (doing things right) rather than effectiveness (doing the right things).

organizing The development of a work structure—a framework in which the necessary tasks are carried out to reach the organization's objectives.

outcome criteria Predetermined elements demonstrating measurable and observable end results of change in the health status of the patient or client.

parameters of patient population Factors defining the patient population to be audited.

participative leadership In this style of leadership, the manager identifies the purpose, the problems, and the means by which the activities should be carried out; presents a tentative decision already made, or seeks subordinates' opinions; and then makes the final decision.

patient Any recipient, client, or consumer of primary, secondary, or tertiary health care.

patient care All of the services rendered to the person receiving preventive or curative treatment from health professionals.

patient care audit Process of surveillance of the quality of patient care, using predetermined criteria by the team of health care professionals.

peer review Formal process of assessment of the quality, efficiency, and appropriateness of professional practice ordered and/or provided, conducted by members of the same health profession as that of the reviewee.

performance budgeting Document summarizing the program activities performed in terms of the cost of specified accomplishments.

performance deficiency Unacceptable level of performance.

performance discrepancy Result that does not conform to expected norms of performance.

Pert chart A technique used in action planning when it is necessary for many tasks to be accomplished in sequence and in the shortest possible time.

plan An orderly construction of major objectives and the steps needed for their achievement; it includes (1) formulation of objectives, (2) assessment of resources available to realize these objectives, and (3) preparation of a work program to achieve the objectives.

planning A process for determining a future course of action, the purpose of which is to bring about a certain condition or goal. This process involves a series of recurring phases, beginning with goal formulation and proceeding to the development of alternative plans for goal achievement, plan implementation, plan evaluation, and plan updating.

pocket veto In the Constitution, the President is allowed 10 days (exclusive of Sundays) from the date of receiving a bill to give it his approval; if, within 10 days, Congress adjourns and so prevents the return of a bill to which the President objects, that bill does not become law. In many cases, where bills have been sent to him toward the close of a session, the President has taken advantage of this provision, holding (or "pocketing") certain measures until after adjournment. These are often measures of which he disapproves but which for some reason he does not wish to return promptly with objections to Congress for further action. This action is called the pocket veto.

policy Definite course or method of action selected from among alternatives, in light of given conditions, to guide and determine present and future decisions.

positive reinforcement A consequence that encourages repetition of a given behavior.

precision The extent to which a measurement technique can discriminate between differences in magnitude.

preliminary draft criteria Initially selected critical elements of care, tentatively prepared for an audit topic.

prevalence The number of existing cases of a disease at a particular time.

prevention The avoidance of disease and/or its consequences.

primary care Coordinated personal approach to patient care, encompassing the following functions: (1) "first contact" care, serving as the patient's point of entry into the health care system; (2) outreach and follow-up for both the patient and the community; (3) expertise of all relevant major disciplines; (4) continuing responsibility for the patient, both in health and in sickness; and (5) coordinating the care of all the patient's health problems.

priorities The relationship of possible goals and objectives to each other; setting priorities is a means of determining the relative importance of various problems and therefore various activities.

problem Undesirable situation or condition of people or of the environment.

problem analysis Audit procedure used to examine performance gaps critically. It includes description of problem, causes, and alternatives for correction.

problem-oriented medical record Health or medical record that is specifically and sequentially organized to describe each of the patient's problems, with information, discussion, conclusions, and the diagnostic and treatment plan for each respective problem.

procedure Series of steps followed in a regular, prescribed order.

process criteria Predetermined elements of care selected to identify key activities or procedures; used by health professionals in a course of management for a defined health condition in the delivery of patient care.

Professional Standards Review Organizations (PSROs) Organizations empowered by federal law (Public Law 92-603) to monitor health care services paid for wholly or partially under Titles V, XVIII, and XIX of the Social Security Act.

profile A presentation of patterns of health care information during a defined period of time.

program Prescribed sequence of defined activities required to meet a program objective within the framework of the organization and in line with definite policies.

program evaluation That part of the manager's job that calls for measuring outcomes and assessing relative and absolute worth of specific undertakings.

program planning The process of determining the organization's plan of action to be performed within a specified time interval. It includes the delineation of program content, objectives, procedures, criteria for evaluation, timetable of activities, and coordination with related activities.

Project Head Start Program started in 1965 by the Office of Economic Opportunity to help disadvantaged preschool children from poverty areas attain their potential in growth and physical and mental development before entering school. Nutrition is an important part of this project. Meals and snacks are provided at the Head Start centers. In addition, meal planning and preparation classes are held for the parents of these children.

protocol Set of standards used to develop, implement, and evaluate a client's individualized care plan. It designates what screening levels constitute risk, at what point and when to make referrals, when to evaluate for health status change, and what subject matter to cover in client education.

public health nutritionist A member of the public health agency staff with advanced training in nutrition, public health, and related coursework, who manages the nutrition services for the agency. His or her role is to assess community nutrition needs and plan, organize, direct, coordinate, and evaluate nutrition components of the health agency's services.

Public Law 89-749 The Comprehensive Health Planning and Public Health Service Amendments (1966).

Public Law 92-603 The Social Security Act Amendments of 1972 (H.R.I.), passed by the 92nd Congress and signed into law by the President on October 30, 1972; PSROs were established by section 249F(B) of this law and added as sections 1151-1170 of the Social Security Act of 1935.

Public Law 93-641 The National Health Planning and Resources Development Act (1974).

Public Law 94-317 The National Consumer Health Information and Health Promotion Act (1977).

Public Law 95-220 The Federal Program Information Act; mandates that the Office of Management and Budget disseminate information on federal domestic assistance programs through the Federal Assistance Program Retrieval System and the Catalog of Federal Domestic Assistance.

Public Law 97-35 Created Maternal and Child Health Block Grant (1981).

Public Law 98-21 Inaugurated preferred payment organizations (PPOs), which provide a channel through which health care deliverers can bid for the right to serve the health needs of a particular group or organization (1982).

public policy The culmination of activities initiated by individuals or groups that have an effect on the lives of other individuals or groups in society.

public representative An individual who may be a health care consumer or provider, who has distinguished himself or herself by objective scholarship and/or leadership in the health field or a related field, and who is not identified with a single interest or point of view.

purpose A broad aim that applies not only to a given organization but to all organizations of its type in a society.

quality assessment Formal, systematic review of part or all of a health delivery program using criteria established by program personnel who conduct the review, analyze findings, and identify deficiencies and discrepancies.

quality assurance Certification of continuous, optimal, effective, and efficient health and nutrition care.

quality assurance review Review, organized and administered by practitioners, that is designed to certify continuously optimal quality and efficient care provided within a health agency.

quality assurance system System organized and administered by health practitioners and consumers; designed to certify continuous, optimal, effective, and efficient health and nutrition care, with evaluation and feedback of results followed by appropriate corrective action whenever a performance deficiency or discrepancy is identified.

quality circle A small group of employees who meet regularly to identify, analyze, and solve a company's problems.

quasi-experimental design Design that does not meet all the strict requirements of an experimental design but nevertheless can be satisfactory in applied programs.

ratification Process of submitting a proposed set of criteria to those whose practice is to be audited so that they may accept, reject, and/or modify the criteria.

ratified criteria Indicators of care, pertaining to a particular audit topic objective, that have been approved by the whole group whose health care delivery is being audited.

re-audit The procedure that follows remedial action; it consists of applying criteria a second time to a new sample of charts to determine if the remedial action was effective in correcting a problem.

recall A method used in dietary surveys; clients are asked to recall everything they have eaten in the previous 24 hours or other specific period; the reliability of this procedure is highly variable.

Recommended Dietary Allowances (RDAs) The amounts of various nutrients recommended by the Food and Nutrition Board of the National Research Council, as normally desirable objectives toward which to aim in planning practical dietaries in the United States; sufficiently higher than the minimal requirements of people in normal health. Allowances are related to body size and are stated for reference men and women at moderate physical activity, for pregnant and lactating women, and for children and adolescent boys and girls of various age groups.

referral A network of providers used for continuity of care and to maximize the services available from other sources.

referral data bases (computerized) Refers to current research at various locations in the United States.

Registered Dietitian (RD) Individual who has met the standards of and is registered by the Commission on Dietetic Registration of The American Dietetic Association.

regression artifacts (statistical regression) Pseudoshifts occurring when persons or treatment units have been selected on the basis of their extreme scores.

rehabilitation The act or process of restoring to a condition of health.

reliability Consistency with which a measurement yields similar outcomes under the same set of circumstances.

remedial action The action taken to correct a deficiency discovered by an audit.

research, nutrition-related Inquiry or investigation aimed at the discovery and interpretation of facts.

resources Personnel, funds, materials, and facilities available to support the performance of an activity.

retrospective study A study that deals with persons who have already developed a condition and examines the record for the characteristic; often called the case-control study. (See Prospective study.)

review committee Convened group of persons conducting a quality assurance review.

role A configuration of major and specific responsibilities for which a person is held accountable.

role delineation A process for determining the minimum-basis level of major and specific responsibilities that must be performed by personnel in a given generic position.

RUMBA Acronym that represents desirable characteristics of criteria, that is, Relevant, Understandable, Measurable, Behavioral, Achievable.

screening A process in which norms, criteria, and standards are used to process large numbers of items, activities, or transactions to identify a smaller sample for study in detail.

secondary care Care provided by medical specialists, community hospitals, and other such providers who generally do not have first contact with patients.

selection (evaluation) Biases resulting from differential recruitment of comparison groups, producing different mean levels of the measures of effects.

sensitivity (of a predictor or screening test) The proportion of true cases correctly identified. Sensitivity = True positives ÷ (True positives + False negatives).

side effects (evaluation) Effects of a program operation other than attainment of objectives.

skinfold thickness Measurement, with calibrated calipers, of thickness of a fold of skin at a selected body site. These measurements indicate subcutaneous fat and the state of nurture. Commonly selected sites for measurement, particularly in nutrition surveys, are the upper arms or triceps, subscapular region (just below the shoulder blade), and upper abdomen.

social marketing The use of marketing principles and techniques to advance a social cause, idea, or behavior.

span of management The number of subordinates who report directly to a given manager.

specificity (of a predictor or screening test) The percentage of healthy persons (true noncases) correctly assessed by a negative report as healthy. Specificity = True negatives ÷ (True negatives + False positives.)

standards Professionally developed statements indicating the acceptable level of performance for health care delivery.

standards of practice Models or criteria designated to provide effective dietetic service to clients; the American Dietetic Association's statements of the dietetic practitioner's responsibilities for providing nutrition care.

starvation Complete or partial deprivation of food for varying lengths of time; the resulting condition may be classified as mild, moderate, severe, or extreme.

statistics The collection of numerical data; the study of methods and procedures for collecting, classifying, summarizing, and analyzing data and for making scientific inferences from such data. *Descriptive statistics* involve the process of organizing and summarizing the important aspects of a data set. *Inferential statistics* consist of a series of techniques (univariate and multivariate) that allow conclusions to extend beyond an immediate data set.

strategic planning The formalized, long-range planning process used to define and achieve organizational goals. It is also called *comprehensive planning* and *long-range planning*.

surveillance The process of gathering routine data for the purpose of identifying and responding to problems. As contrasted with "survey," "surveillance" implies continuity, or a frequent and continuous "watching over."

target population A grouping of patients with similar conditions or characteristics to be studied in a quality assurance review.

techniques The particular skills required for the performance of a specific operation or function.

terms and conditions All legal requirements imposed on a grant by the federal government, whether by statute, regulations, the grant award document itself, or other documents.

tertiary care Services of highly specialized providers (for example, neurologists, neurosurgeons, thoracic surgeons, and intensive care units). Such services frequently require highly sophisticated technological and support facilities. The development of these services has largely been a function of diagnostic and therapeutic advances attained through basic and clinical biomedical research.

third-party reimbursement Payment by a third party for services rendered by a health care provider to a patient.

threshold for action The point at which, looking at a specific group of patients, a responsible individual would become anxious about the quality of care they are receiving and would be willing to mobilize resources to take major action for change.

Title III (Older Americans Act) Formerly Title VII; provides congregate and home-delivered meals for the elderly through the area or local agencies on aging.

Title V (Social Security Act) This title authorizes health programs for mothers and children, including maternity care, well child services, crippled children's services, training, and research. It is a federally supported, state-operated program in which the state funds match or exceed the federal funds.

Title XVIII (Social Security Act) This title, known as Medicare, authorizes the Social Security health insurance program. It is federally operated with funds contributed through the Social Security tax system.

Title XIX (Social Security Act) This title authorizes a program with a wide range of benefits to needy persons. Among its provisions are a medical assistance program known as Medicaid, which is designed for the indigent, aged, dependent children, and blind and permanently disabled persons. Other medically needy persons can be included. It is a state-operated program that is supported largely by federal funds.

undernutrition Inadequate intake of one or more nutrients or of calories. (The converse term, "overnutrition," is not a recommended term.)

United States Department of Agriculture (USDA) Department of federal government, consisting of a Human Nutrition Research Division, experiment stations, and extension services, all of which are concerned with nutrition. These divisions carry out research and program services such as the Food Stamp Program and publish data on the nutritive value of common foods and information on the eating patterns of people in the United States.

United States Department of Health and Human Services (HHS) Department of the federal government that has several agencies dealing with nutrition, such as the Maternal and Child Health Service, the Office of Education, the Food and Drug Administration, and the National Institute of Health and its Public Health Services agency.

utilization review Examination of efficiency of institutional use and appropriateness of admissions, services ordered and provided, length of stay, and discharge practices on a prospective and concurrent basis.

validity Degree to which measurement represents the phenomenon being measured without undue distortion by other phenomena.

value Relative worth, utility, or importance. Values provide a general "guidance system" for a person's behavior.

variable Qualifier limiting the population; used in writing outcome criteria.

verification Process of establishing the location of the data source to determine whether or not criteria have been met.

veto Of Latin derivation, meaning "I forbid." The President is authorized by the Constitution to refuse his assent, if he so chooses, to any measure presented by Congress for his approval. In such a case, he returns the measure to the House in which it originated, at the same time indicating his objections—the so-called veto message. The veto goes to the entire measure; the President is not authorized, as are the governors of some states, to veto separate items in a bill.

White House Conference on Food, Nutrition, and Health As a result of the concern about hunger and malnutrition in the United States, a conference was held in December of 1969 in Washington, D.C. Its objectives were to advise the President and to create a national nutrition policy. The areas discussed at the conference included methods for continual evaluation of (1) the nutritional status of the American people; (2) nutritional needs of vulnerable groups such as children, pregnant and lactating women, adolescents, and the aged; (3) foods to meet the nutritional needs of the people; (4) nutrition education; and (5) the role of voluntary groups in improving the nutritional state of the people of the United States.

World Health Organization (WHO) International organization whose goal is to eliminate all kinds of diseases. In the field of nutrition, WHO has been involved in developing and testing new protein-rich foods; combating protein-calorie malnutrition, nutritional anemias, vitamin A deficiency, endemic goiter, and rickets; assessing nutritional status; determining nutritional requirements; and developing coordinated applied-nutrition programs and training personnel for them. WHO was created in 1948 and is composed of about 90 member countries, with headquarters in Geneva, Switzerland.

zero-based budgeting Budgeting that enables the organization to look at activities and priorities starting from a base at which there are no debits or credits. The previous year's allocations are not automatically considered as the basis for the present year's allocations. Each request for funds must be justified.

Recommended Resources

ADDITIONAL READINGS

Chapter 1

Ernst, N.D.: NIH consensus development conference on lowering blood cholesterol to prevent heart disease: implications for dietitians, J. Am. Diet. Assoc. 85:586, 1985.

Etzioni, A.: An immodest agenda: rebuilding America before the 21st century, New York, 1982, McGraw-Hill, Inc.

Finn, S.C., and Gussler, J.D.: Women's issues and dietetics: implications for professional development, Diet. Currents 11:1, Jan./Feb. 1984.

Owen, A.L.: Challenges for dietitians in a high tech/high touch society, J. Am. Diet. Assoc. 84:285, 1984.

U.S. Department of Health and Human Services: Prospects for a healthier America: achieving the nation's health promotion objectives (proceedings), Nov. 1984, Office of Disease Prevention and Health Promotion.

Chapter 2

Boettinger, H.M.: Is management really an art? Harvard Bus. Rev., No. 75101, Jan./Feb. 1975.

Koontz, H., and O'Donnell, C.: The functions of the manager. In Koontz, H., and O'Donnell, C.: Principles of management, ed. 8, New York, 1984, McGraw-Hill, Inc.

Livingston, J.S.: Myth of the well-educated manager, Harvard Bus. Rev., No. 71108, May/June 1971.

Quinn, J.B.: Managing innovation—controlled chaos, Harvard Bus. Rev. 85:73, May/June 1985.

Skinner, W., and Sasser, W.E.: Managers with impact: versatile and inconsistent, Harvard Bus. Rev. 55:140, Nov./Dec. 1977.

Chapter 3

Bennis, W., Benne, K.D., and Chen: The planning of change, ed. 3, New York, 1976, Holt, Rinehart & Winston General Book.

Cole, R.E.: Target information for competitive performance, Harvard Bus. Rev. 85:100, May/June 1985.

Gailbraith, A.: Twenty-four carat dietetic practice for the eighties, J. Am. Diet. Assoc. 77:529, 1980.

Loomis, K.: Managing the change process, J. Allied Health 8:172, Aug. 1979.

Rosen, B., and Jerdee, T.H.: Effects of decision permanence on managerial willingness to use participation, Acad. Man. J. 21:722, 1978.

Chapter 4

Gabarro, J.J.: When a new manager takes charge, Harvard Bus. Rev. 85:110, May/June 1985.

Lovestock, C.H., and Weinberg, C.B.: Public and non-profit marketing comes of age: cases in public and non-profit marketing, Palo Alto, Calif., 1977, The Scientific Press.

Schmidt, S.M., and Kochan, T.A.: Conflict: toward conceptual clarity, Admin. Sci. Q. 17:3, Sept. 1972.

Selby, C.C.: Better performance from non-profits, Harvard Bus. Rev. 56:92, Sept./Oct. 1978.

Shaw, M.E.: Group dynamics, ed. 3, New York, 1981, McGraw-Hill, Inc.

Chapter 5

Drucker, P.F.: The discipline of innovation, Harvard Bus. Rev. 85:67, May/June 1985.

Katz, R.L.: Human relation skills can be sharpened, Harvard Bus. Rev., No. 56407, July/Aug. 1956.

Kotter, J.P.: Power, dependence and effective management, Harvard Bus. Rev. 55:125, July/Aug. 1977.

Peters, T., and Austin, N.: A passion for excellence, New York, 1985, Random House, Inc.

Prentice, W.C.H.: Understanding leadership, Harvard Bus. Rev., No. 61511, Sept./Oct. 1961.

Chapter 6

Alkin, M.C.: A guide for evaluation/decision-makers, Beverly Hills, Calif., 1985, Sage Publications, Inc.

Chelimsky, E.: Differing perspectives of evaluation. In Rentz, C.C., and Rentz, R.R., editors: Evaluating federally sponsored programs: new directions for program evaluation, San Francisco, 1978, Jossey-Bass, Inc., Publishers.

Cooley, W.W., and Leinhardt, G.: The instructional dimensions study, Ed. Eval. Pol. Anal. 7:25, 1980.

Deniston, O.L., and Rosenstock, I.M.: Evaluating health programs, Public Health Rep. 85:835, 1970.

Fitz-Gibbon, C.T., and Morris, L.L.: How to design a program evaluation (Center for the Study of Evaluation), Beverly Hills, Calif., 1978, Sage Publications, Inc.

Chapter 7

Avorn, J.: Benefit and cost analysis in geriatric care—turning age discrimination into health policy, N. Engl. J. Med. 310:1294, 1984.

Donabedian, A.: The quality of medical care: methods for assessing and monitoring the quality of care for research and for quality assurance programs, Science **200**:856, 1978.

Egan, M.C., and Kaufman, M.S.: Financing nutrition services in a competitive market, J. Am. Diet. Assoc. **85**:210, 1985.

Joglekar, P.N.: Cost-benefit studies of health care programs, Ed. Health Prof. **7**:285, 1984.

Sweeney, A., and Wisner, J.N.: Budgeting basics: a how-to guide for managers. Part 6. Preparing and presenting a budget plan, Supervis. Man. **20**:7, 1975.

Chapter 8

Hamill, P.V.V., and Moore, W.H.: Contemporary growth charts: needs, concentration and application, Public Health Currents, Special Service edition, 1976.

Kanawate, A.: Assessment of nutritional status in the community. In McLaren, D.S., editor: Nutrition in the community, ed. 2, New York, 1983, John Wiley & Sons, Inc.

Mullis, R.M., and Bowen, P.E.: Process guides for nutrition care in community health, J. Am. Diet. Assoc. **85**:25, 1985.

Pao, E.M., Mickle, S.J., and Burk, M.C.: One-day and 3-day nutrient intakes by individuals, Nationwide Food Consumption Survey findings (Spring 1977), J. Am. Diet. Assoc. **85**:313, 1985.

Woteki, C.E.: Improving estimates of food and nutrient intake: applications to individuals and groups, J. Am. Diet. Assoc. **85**:295, 1985.

Chapter 9

Calloway, D.H.: Nutritional balance during pregnancy. In Winick, M.E., editor: Nutrition and fetal development, ed. 2, New York, 1974, John Wiley & Sons, Inc.

Falkner, F.: Maternal nutrition and fetal growth, Am. J. Clin. Nutr. (suppl.) **34**:769, 1981.

Orstead, C., Arlington, D., Kamath, S.K., Olson, R., and Kohrs, M.B.: Efficacy of prenatal nutrition counseling: weight gain infant birth weight and cost-effectiveness, J. Am. Diet. Assoc. **85**:40, 1985.

Schaefer, L.J., and Kumanjika, S.K.: Maternal variables related to potentially high-sodium infant feeding practices, J. Am. Diet. Assoc. **85**:433, 1985.

U.S. General Accounting Office: Better management and more resources needed to strengthen federal efforts to improve pregnancy outcome, HRD-80-24, Washington, D.C., Jan. 1980, U.S. Government Printing Office.

Chapter 10

American Academy of Pediatrics: Current issues in feeding the normal infant, Pediatrics (suppl.) **75**:1, Jan. 1985.

Brasel, J.A.: Hormonal changes during adolescence: a selected review of the literature. In McKigney, J.I., and Munro, H.N., editors: Nutritional requirements in adolescence, Cambridge, 1976, MIT Press.

Graham, G.C.: Poverty, hunger, malnutrition, prematurity and infant mortality in the U.S., Pediatrics **75**:117, 1985.

Paige, D.M., and Owen, G.M.: Childhood and adolescence. In Paige, D.M., editor: Manual of clinical nutrition, Pleasantville, N.J., 1983, Nutrition Publications, Inc.

Peck, E.B., and Ullrich, H.D.: Children and weight: a changing perspective, Berkeley, Calif., 1985, Nutrition Communications Associates.

Chapter 11

American Heart Association, Committee on Nutrition: Rationale of the diet—heart statement of the American Heart Association, Circulation **65**:839, 1982.

Heaney, R.P., Gallagher, J.C., Johnston, C.C., Neer, R., Parfitt, A.M., and Whedon, G.D.: Calcium nutrition and bone health in the elderly, Am. J. Clin. Nutr. (suppl.) **36**:986, 1982.

National Heart, Lung, and Blood Institute: The lipid research clinic coronary primary prevention trials results. II. The relationship of reduction in incidence of coronary heart disease to cholesterol lowering, J.A.M.A. **25**:365, Jan. 1984.

Palmer, S.: Diet, nutrition and cancer: the future of dietary policy, Cancer Res. **43**:250, May 1983.

Chapter 12

Burch, E.E., and Gooding, C.: Planning for computerization, Manager. Planning **26**:29, March/April 1978.

Burr, M.L.: Epidemiology for nutritionists. I. Some general principles, Hum. Nutr. Appl. Nutr. **37A**:259, 1983.

Kircaldy-Hargreaves, M.: Utility of an on-line computer system in a clinical setting for nutrient intake analysis, J. Can. Diet. Assoc. **41**:112, 1980.

Remington, R.D., and Schork, M.A.: Statistics with applications to the biological and health sciences, ed. 2, Englewood Cliffs, N.J., 1985, Prentice-Hall, Inc.

Russo, J.A.: What to look for in computer-assisted planning systems, Manager. Planning **25**:5, July/Aug. 1976.

Sweetnam, P.M.: Epidemiology for nutritionist, V, some statistical aspects, Hum. Nutr. Appl. Nutr. **38A**:215, 1984.

Williams, C.S., and Burnet, L.W.: Future applications of microcomputer in dietetics, Hum. Nutr. Appl. Nutr. **38A**:99, 1984.

Chapter 13

Aronson, V., and Fitzgerald, B.D.: Guidebook for nutrition counselors, Norwell, Mass., 1980, Christopher Publishing House.

Hackney, H., and Cormier, L.S.: Counseling strategies and objectives, ed. 2, Englewood Cliffs, N.J., 1979, Prentice-Hall, Inc.

Hertzler, A.A., and Owen, C.: Culture, families and the change process, J. Am. Diet. Assoc. **84**:535, 1984.

Mazzeo-Caputo, S.E., Danish, S.J., and Kris-Etherton: Dietary change: prescription vs goal setting, J. Am. Diet. Assoc. **85**:553, 1985.

U.S. Dept. of Health and Human Services, NIH: Building nutrition counseling skills. Vol. I. A guidebook for workshop planning. Vol. II. Workshop resource manual, NIH Pub. No. 84-2661 and 84-2662, Superintendent of Documents, Washington, D.C., 1984, U.S. Government Printing Office.

Chapter 14

Corporate Fund Raising Directory, 1985-1986 edition, Hartsdale, N.Y., 1985, Public Service Materials Center.

Hillman, H.: The art of winning corporate grants, Hartsdale, N.Y., 1984, Public Service Materials Center.

Margolin, J.B.: About foundations: how to find the facts you need to get a grant, Chicago, 1978, The Foundation Center.

Marquis Who's Who, Inc.: Grantsmanship: money and how to get it, ed. 2, Chicago, 1972, Marquis Academic Media.

Proposal Writers' Swipe File: 15 winning fund-raising proposals, Chicago, 1984, Donors Forum.

Chapter 15

Dunlop, D.W.: Benefit-cost analysis: a review of its applicability in policy analysis for delivering health services, Social Sci. Med. **9**:133, 1975.

House, P.W.: The art of public policy analysis, Sage Lib. Social Res. **135**:25, 1982.

Sackett, D.L., and Torrance, G.W.: The utility of different health states as perceived by the general public, J. Chronic Dis. **31**:697, 1975.

Schelling, T.C.: Procedures for valuing lives, Public Pol. **23**:419, 1975.

Tinker, I.: Women in Washington, Sage Yearbook in Women's Policy Studies **7**:300, 1983.

GENERAL HEALTH PROMOTION PUBLICATIONS

The following books are important background reading for anyone involved in health promotion.

Office of Disease Prevention and Health Promotion, Public Health Service, Department of Health and Human Services: Healthy people: the Surgeon General's report on health promotion and disease prevention, U.S. Government Printing Office, Superintendent of Documents, Washington, DC 20402, 1979, 177 pages (Stock No. 017-001-00416-2; $5.00; make check payable to: Superintendent of Documents).

This landmark document sets forth some new priorities for the nation's health and calls for a renewed commitment to prevention. "The report's central theme is that the health of this Nation's citizens can be significantly improved through actions individuals can take themselves, and through actions decision makers in the public and private sectors can take, to promote a safer and healthier environment for all Americans at home, at work, and at play." Specific goals are set forth in 5 stages of human development, and 15 priority areas are identified in the categories of preventive health services, health protection, and health promotion.

Office of Disease Prevention and Health Promotion, Public Health Service, Department of Health and Human Services: Living well: an introduction to health promotion and disease prevention, U.S. Government Printing Office, Superintendent of Documents, Washington, DC 20402, 1980, 36 pages (Stock No. 017-001-00428-6; $4.25; make check payable to: Superintendent of Documents).

Aimed at the individual, the content of this booklet is drawn from *Healthy People* and is designed to introduce the concepts of health promotion and disease prevention, outline health risks that readers face in daily life, and show them how minor changes in the way they live can reduce the risk of disease or disability. An appendix offers suggestions for resources that the individual can use to find additional information on the various topics covered in the text.

Office of Disease Prevention and Health Promotion, Public Health Service, Department of Health and Human Services: Strategies for promoting health for specific populations, U.S. Government Printing Office, Superintendent of Documents, Washington, DC 20402, 1981, 53 pages (Stock No. 017-001-00439-1; $4.25; make check payable to: Superintendent of Documents).

This report presents findings from a series of meetings convened by DHHS to examine the health promotion needs, priorities, and concerns of minorities and special populations and to obtain advice on actions that should be taken to reach them. Included are recommendations on reaching Asian/Pacific Americans, black Americans, Hispanic Americans, elderly Americans, and American Indians.

Public Health Service, Department of Health and Human Services: Promoting health/preventing disease: objectives for the nation, U.S. Government Printing Office, Superintendent of Documents, Washington, DC 20402, 1980, 102 pages (Stock No. 017-001-00435-9; $5.00; make check payable to: Superintendent of Documents).

This document, a companion to the national strategy set forth in *Healthy People*, identifies specific and measurable objectives for 15 priority areas that provide keys to achieving our national health aspirations. Many of these objectives, developed with the help of panels of experts in each area, have direct implications for the workplace.

U.S. Department of Agriculture and U.S. Department of Health and Human Services: Nutrition and your health—dietary guidelines for Americans, National Health Information Clearinghouse, P.O. Box 1133, Washington, DC 20013,

1980, 20 pages (single copy free). Also available from the U.S. Government Printing Office, Superintendent of Documents, Washington, DC 20402 (Stock No. 001-000-00428-3; $2.25 per copy; $27.00 per 100 copies; make check payable to: Superintendent of Documents).

This set of seven dietary recommendations is intended for people who are already healthy and includes information on fat, starch and fiber, sodium, sugar, alcohol, and various aspects of nutrition and health. The recommendations are to eat a variety of foods; maintain ideal weight; avoid too much fat, saturated fat, and cholesterol; eat foods with adequate starch and fiber; avoid too much sugar; avoid too much sodium; and, if you drink alcohol, do so in moderation.

WORKSITE HEALTH PROMOTION PUBLICATIONS (GENERAL)

This annotated list of selected resources was developed by the Office of Disease Prevention and Health Promotion, the Department of Health and Human Services, to assist individuals in planning and implementing health promotion and disease prevention programs at the worksite.

Berry, C.A.: An approach to good health for employees and reduced health care costs for industry, Health Insurance Association of America, 1850 K. St., NW, Washington, DC 20006, 1981, 36 pages (single copy free; additional copies $2.00).

Dr. Berry reviews background information about our nation's health status, emphasizing that the top killers in the 1980s are related in large part to our life-styles. He reviews what companies currently are doing and the cost savings they have estimated from a health promotion program. The book identifies the major health risk factors and their potential impact on employee health and presents a series of steps for developing an employee health program.

Fairfield/Westchester Business Group on Health: Health care—you owe it to yourself, Business Institute for Health, Inc. (ATTN: Mrs. D. Alvater), Box 189, Stanton, NJ 98885, 1983, 14-minute film/tape cassette (\$250 for film; $190 for ¾- or ½-inch tape cassette).

This film—aimed at employees, their dependents, and the general public—discusses the magnitude of the cost problem, the need for everyone to have a better understanding of the problem, and the importance of becoming better users of the health care delivery system. The need for a more responsible attitude from each of us toward health promotion and self care is emphasized.

Goldman, S.K.: A primer on health promotion at the workplace, Alpha Center, 7316 Wisconsin Ave., Suite 400, Bethesda, MD 20814, 1983, 33 pages ($3.75).

This primer was designed to serve as a review or status report on what is known about worksite health promotion and to provide general information on a variety of topics, including the basics of health promotion and disease prevention, their importance to employers, types of program approaches being implemented in the workplace, realistic expectations about the benefits that can be achieved, examples of programs in operation, guidelines for getting started, and additional resources.

Health Insurance Association of America and the American Council of Life Insurance: Health, education and promotion/agenda for the eighties: a summary, Health Insurance Association of America, 919 Third Ave., New York, NY 10022, 1980, 56 pages (single copy free).

This report of an Insurance Industry Conference on Health Education and Promotion contains summaries of papers given by some leading thinkers and practitioners in the field of worksite health promotion. Topics include the effects of health care on health, the case for prevention, health self-appraisal systems, motivating individuals to change behavior, insurance incentives and disincentives, and strategies for marketing health education. In addition, some existing programs are described.

HealthWorks Northwest: Employee health promotion: a guide for starting programs at the workplace, HealthWorks Northwest, Puget Sound Health Systems Agency, 601 Valley St., Seattle, WA 98109, 1983, 92 pages ($15.00).

Step-by-step instructions liberally sprinkled with examples and worksheets make this guide a valuable addition to the library of anyone starting a worksite health promotion program. More than most how-to books, this one focuses on cost containment as management's reason for starting a program. It also places heavy emphasis on the use of members of an employee committee as key planners in the process and identifies key "decision points"—points at which presentations must be made to management and "go, no-go" decisions must be made.

Minnesota Coalition on Health Care Costs and Minnesota Department of Health: Employer's guide to health promotion in the workplace, Minnesota Coalition on Health Care Costs, Suite 440, Health Associations Center, 2221 University Ave. SE, Minneapolis, MN 55414, 1981, 41 pages ($3.00).

The introduction to the publication states, "This guide is the result of a cooperative effort by business and health professionals to clarify the promise of a health activity that is attracting employers' interest in Minnesota. Health promotion and risk reduction programs are defined in theory and in practice. The intent is to display the substantial medical and economic credibility of these programs and to allow decision makers to select between alternative programs." Included are chapters on costs; the promise of health promotion; programs; tools, including assessments, risk appraisals, screening, group education, contracts, and rewards; plus some questions and cautions.

Office of Disease Prevention and Health Promotion, Department of Health and Human Services: National Conference on Health Promotion Programs in Occupational Settings, National Technical Information Service, Port Royal Rd., Springfield, VA 22161, 1979, set of 11 papers (Order No. HRP-00030860; $23.00).

A series of background papers for an invitational conference sponsored by the Office of Disease Prevention and Health Promotion, Department of Health and Human Services. It describes the state of the art of worksite health promotion programs covering such topics as hypertension, weight and nutrition, alcohol and drug abuse, smoking cessation, stress management, physical activity, and cost effectiveness. (Seven of the background papers appeared in *Public Health Reports*, Vol. 95, No. 2 (Mar/Apr 1980), and many also were updated and incorporated into *Managing Health Promotion in the Workplace*.)

A practical planning guide for employee health promotion programs, The Health Planning Council, Inc., 995 Applegate Rd., Madison, WI 53713, 1982, 45 pages ($4.00).

This publication provides a step-by-step approach to the development of employee health promotion programs, with chapters highlighting benefits of a program, getting started, program elements, evaluation, legal and financial considerations, motivation, and some do's and dont's. A list of health risk appraisals and a short bibliography are also included.

Thomas, J.: Promoting health in the worksetting, Institute for Health Planning, 702 N. Blackhawk Ave., Madison, WI 53705, 1981, 18 pages ($3.00; $6.00 for billed orders).

This booklet discusses the cost-saving potential of worksite health promotion programs, the components and keys to a successful worksite program, and ways in which a health planning agency or other group can provide assistance to community businesses in establishing or expanding worksite programs.

WORKSITE HEALTH PROMOTION PUBLICATIONS (SPECIFIC CONTENT AREAS)
Aging

National Institute on Aging: Age pages, National Institute on Aging, Box FL, Building 31, Room 5C35, Bethesda, MD 20205, 1980, 1981, 1982, a continuing series (single set free).

This series of two-page health information flyers is written for older people, their families, and those who work with the elderly. Topics covered include how to find good medical care, accidents, senility, high blood pressure, sexuality, and exercise. The material can be reproduced for distribution or incorporated into a company's regular publication.

Cardiovascular Disease

National Heart, Lung, and Blood Institute, Public Health Service, Department of Health and Human Services: Cardiovascular primer for the workplace, High Blood Pressure Informa-

tion Center, 120/80 National Institutes of Health, Box WS, Bethesda, MD 20205, 1981, 88 pages (single copy free).

Responding to the questions being asked by business leaders, this publication discusses what is known and unknown about cardiovascular disease risk factor reduction and health promotion, factors to consider when deciding on adoption of a worksite health promotion program, and resources available to help get started. The document is liberally sprinkled with examples of business programs and data about the risk factors associated with cardiovascular disease including smoking, high blood pressure, elevated blood cholesterol, and diabetes, as well as related risk factors such as obesity, stress, and physical inactivity.

Evaluation

Institute of Medicine: Evaluating health promotion in the workplace: conference summary, Institute of Medicine, National Academy of Sciences, 2101 Constitution Ave., NW, Washington, DC 20418, 1981, 38 pages ($5.50).

The proceedings from this invitational conference of experts contain brief summaries of a series of background papers on topics including methodologies for data collection and validation; the cost of evaluation; some case examples—lessons learned and issues unresolved; and themes and future directions. The paper "Evaluation of Worksite Health Promotion Programs" is reproduced in its entirety.

Fitness

Fitness in industry, Health Education Center, 200 Ross St., Pittsburgh, PA 15219, 1978, 38 pages ($3.50 plus postage).

Although much of the data and some of the facts in this 1978 publication are out of date, one section, entitled "A Practical Guide to the Organization and Administration of an Industrial Fitness Program," contains enough valuable information to be worth the price. A poster diagramming procedures for the development of an industrial fitness program covers needs assessment, program components, facilities, administration and supervision, and organizational alternatives.

President's Council on Physical Fitness and Sports: Fitness in the workplace: a handbook on employee programs, President's Council on Physical Fitness and Sports, Washington, DC 20201, 14-page pamphlet (single copy free).

This pamphlet provides a look at physical fitness programs in business and industry that includes such useful information as general statistics about the apparent value of fitness programs and some common features of successful employee fitness programs.

Health Risk Appraisals

Center for Health Promotion and Education of the Centers for Disease Control: Health risk appraisal general information packet, Director of Special Projects, Center for Health Promotion and Education, Centers for Disease Control, 1600 Clifton Rd., NE, Atlanta, GA 30333, 1981, various materials (single copy free).

This packet of material contains sample questionnaires and printouts from CDC's version of a health risk appraisal, a general description of CDC's own employee health appraisal program, and a list of other health risk appraisal providers. In addition, two publications are included: an introduction to health risk appraisal and an interpretation guide.

National Health Information Clearinghouse, Office of Disease Prevention and Health Promotion, Public Health Service, Department of Health and Human Services: Health risk appraisals: an inventory, National Health Information Clearinghouse, P.O. Box 1133, Washington, DC 20013, 1981 (single copy free).

This is a handy guide to more than 25 health risk appraisal tools that can be used at the worksite. The name, address, and method of analysis (computer- or self-scored) are included for each.

Hypertension Control

Alderman, M.H.: A handbook for worksite blood pressure programs, Health Education Services, P.O. Box 7126, Albany, NY 12224, 1980, 43 pages ($1.84; payment must accompany order).

Developed under a grant from the New York State Health Department. As stated within the document, "This manual is designed to help individuals from management, personnel, occupational health staff, or labor union officials understand the seriousness of hypertension and ways that it can be managed. The manual will familiarize the reader with the varieties of worksite programs for hypertension detection, treatment, and control and should facilitate the planning and execution of a suitable program for a particular employee group."

Erfurt, J.C., and Foote, A.: Blood pressure control at the worksite: manual of procedures for blood pressure control programs in industrial settings, Institute of Labor and Industrial Relations, c/o Worker Health Program, 401 Fourth St., Ann Arbor, MI 48103, 1979, 83 pages ($5.00).

This publication presents detailed procedures and sample forms for a worksite high blood pressure control program, based on pilot programs developed in a variety of industrial settings. Chapters are devoted to screening, referral, follow-up, employee education, record keeping, and program evaluation.

ADDITIONAL RESOURCES

The following organizations and agencies have additional information or services for specific content areas, which may be useful in developing disease prevention and health promotion programs for the worksite.

National Health Information Clearinghouse, P.O. Box 1133, Washington, DC 20013, (800) 336-4797, (703) 522-2590 (in Virginia)

The National Health Information Clearinghouse offers a one-stop shopping approach to obtaining health information on a wide variety of topics. Often the NHIC can immediately answer your question or provide you with a resource. If not, it will refer your request to one of 2000 groups and organizations that provide health information to the public. So, when you are looking for health-related information, consider calling the NHIC first. Keep in mind, however, that the NHIC staff cannot give medical advice, diagnose, or recommend specific physicians or treatment centers.

Aging

National Institute on Aging, Information Office, Building 31, Room 5C35, Bethesda, MD 20205

Exercise and Physical Fitness

American Alliance for Health, Physical Education, Recreation, and Dance, 1900 Association Dr., Reston, VA 22091

American Association of Fitness Directors in Business and Industry, c/o Xerox Health Management Program, 800 Phillips Rd., Bldg. 337, Webster, NY 14580

American College of Sports Medicine, 1440 Monroe, Madison, WI 53706

Blue Cross and Blue Shield Association, Communications Division, 676 N. St. Clair St., Chicago, IL 60611

Institute for Aerobics Research, 11811 Preston Rd., Dallas, TX 75230

President's Council on Physical Fitness and Sports, Room 7103, Judiciary Plaza, 450 Fifth St., S.W., Washington, DC 20001

High Blood Pressure

American Heart Association, 7320 Greenville Ave., Dallas, TX 75231 (Or your local chapter)

High Blood Pressure Information Center, 120/80 National Institutes of Health, Bethesda, MD 20205

Nutrition

The American Dietetic Association, 430 N. Michigan Ave., Chicago, IL 60611

Food and Drug Administration, Office of Consumer Communications (HFE-88), Room 15B32, Parklawn Building, 5600 Fishers Lane, Rockville, MD 20857

Home Economics and Human Nutrition Extension Service, U.S. Department of Agriculture, Washington, DC 20250 (or your local cooperative extension service office listed under

County or City Government in the white pages of your phone book)

Human Nutrition Information Service, U.S. Department of Agriculture, 6525 Belcrest Rd., Hyattsville, MD 20782

National Dairy Council, 6300 N. River Rd., Rosemont, IL 60018

Nutrition Foundation, Suite 300, 888 Seventh St., N.W., Washington, DC 20006

Society for Nutrition Education (SNE) Resource Center, 1736 Franklin St., 9th floor, Oakland, CA 94612

Prenatal Care

March of Dimes Birth Defects Foundation, 1275 Mamaroneck Ave., White Plains, NY 10605

PROFESSIONAL ASSOCIATIONS

Following are selected sources for nutrition publications for health care providers and consumers.

American Academy of Pediatrics, 1801 Hinman Ave., Evanston, IL 60204

Ask for nutrition reprint and price list. They offer reprints of authoritative position statements on many aspects of infant and child nutrition.

The American College of Obstetricians and Gynecologists, 1 East Wacker Dr., Chicago, IL 60601

Ask for list and prices of publications on pregnancy and maternal nutrition.

American Dental Association, Order Section Catalog CA 176, 211 East Chicago Ave., Chicago, IL 60611

Ask for list of publications and price list. Patient and public information leaflets on diet and dental health, covering such topics as nursing-bottle caries and fluoridation levels, are available.

The American Diabetes Association, 1 West 48th St., New York, NY 10020

Distributes a variety of publications useful for diabetic patients. Consult local association representative or write the national association for list.

The American Dietetic Association, 430 N. Michigan Ave., Chicago, IL 60611

Publications list includes position papers on various aspects of nutrition services, "Guidelines for Nutritional Care in Long-Term Facilities," and many relevant subjects for health providers. All publications for purchase; publications list free.

The American Heart Association (National Center), 7300 Greenville Ave., Dallas, TX 75251

Pamphlets for patients on diet and heart disease, cholesterol/fat, and hypertension; a cookbook is also available. Consult local association representative or write national association for list.

The American Home Economics Association, 2010 Massachusetts Ave., N.W., Washington, DC 20036

Ask for list of publications and price list. Technical and professional brochures on food and nutrition, programs for adolescents, and parent education.

The American Medical Association, Order Department, 535 North Dearborn St., Chicago, IL 60610

Ask for list of publications. Source for pamphlets and reports on additives, allergies, cardiovascular diseases, deficiencies/diseases/special diets, general nutrition information, and obesity.

BIBLIOGRAPHIES AND INDEXES OF NUTRITION PUBLICATIONS

Consumer Information Center, General Services Administration, Pueblo, CO 81009

A dispensing center for selected government publications that are especially suitable for consumer information. Includes several food and nutrition publications. Request a catalog. Single copies of many publications are free.

Food and Nutrition Information and Educational Materials Center, National Agricultural Library Building, Room 304, Beltsville, MD 20705

National Nutrition Education Clearinghouse (NNECH), 2140 Shattuck Ave., Suite 1110, Berkeley, CA 94704

Request the list "Nutrition Information Resources for Professionals" and a descriptive leaflet on the *Nutrition Education Resource Series*. Lists are free. Also publishes the *Journal of Nutrition Education*, which has timely commentaries, features and research articles on nutrition, program ideas, and book reviews. Subscription rate, $16.00.

Office of Education and Public Affairs, The Nutrition Foundation, Inc., 888 Seventeenth St., N.W., Washington, DC 20006

Publishes *Index of Nutrition Education Materials* (237 pages, $8.75), which includes an extensive listing of nutrition publications, teaching aids, and their sources. Includes a brief section of publications in Braille and Spanish.

Index

A

Abilities, 94
Accidents, risk factors for, 16
Accountability, 128-130
  of managers, 27
Accuracy in obtaining measurements, 127
Achievement, McClelland's characteristics indicating high need for, 96
ACIR; *see* Advisory Commission on Intergovernmental Relations
Action
  bias for, 26-27
  and evaluation, 128-130
Action plans for nutrition services
  authority, delegation, and decentralization, 70-74
  basic elements of organizing, 68-70
  for case study on obesity in preschool population, 124
  checklist for, 91
  completing, 87-91
  managing organizational change, 75-76
  managing organizational conflict and creativity, 76-81
  organizing for action, 82-91
  organizing for changing environments, 74-75
  steps in, 87-90
Action programs, problems in, 117
Action settings, evaluation in, 119-120
Acute care settings, quality assurance in, 148
ADA; *see* American Dietetic Association
Adequacy of program in evaluation, 125
ADHP; *see* Appalachian Health Demonstration Program
Adipometer, 274
Administration on Aging, 306, 314, 334
Administrative audit, 149, 151, 153
Adolescents
  energy requirements for, 289
  food assistance programs for, 294-295
  food intake of, factors affecting, 292
  guidelines for patient management, 293
  health objectives for, 250
  hormones in, 288
  local-level strategies for, 295-296

Adolescents—cont'd
  nutrient requirements in, 288-291
  nutrition-related health problems of, 250, 251
  nutritional assessment of, 294
  nutritional risk factors associated with pregnancy during, 225
  protein, carbohydrate, and lipid requirements for, 289
  psychological and environmental influences on, 291-293
  quality assurance of health and nutrition care for, 294
  recommended dietary allowances for, 288, 289
  referral for nutritional care, 294-295
  vitamin and mineral requirements for, 289-291
  weight control project for, 296
Adult learning concepts of Knowles, 376
Adults and elderly
  alcoholism in, 326-327
  assessment of nutritional status in, 327-333
  atherosclerosis and coronary heart disease in, 318-320
  cancer in, 324-326
  community-level nutrition services for, 334-343
  diabetes in, 323-326
  diet-drug interactions in, 312-314
  dietary methodology for, 329
  federally sponsored food assistance programs for, 335
  hypertension in, 321-323
  innovative strategies for, 337-343
  nutrition assessment and intervention guidelines for, 328-329
  nutrition-related health problems of, 304-308
  nutritional needs of, 308-311
  obesity in, 316-318
  osteoporosis in, 326
  and physiological changes during aging process, 306, 308, 309
  poverty and other sociological concerns of, 314-315
  and prevention of nutrition-related diseases in, 316-327
  quality assurance of health care for, 333-334
  and supplementation and faddism, 311-312

Advisable intakes, 255-256; *see also* Recommended Daily Dietary Allowances
Advisory and Review Council, 392
Advisory Commission on Intergovernmental Relations, 403
Advisory service and counseling, 397
Affection and social activity needs, 95
Age
  height and weight for, 182
  population distribution by, 307
Aging process, 308
Agreement and negotiation for overcoming resistance to change, 75, 76
AHA; *see* American Heart Association
Aid to Dependent Children, 50
Alcohol, Drug Abuse, and Mental Health Administration, 399
Alcohol ingestion during pregnancy, 222
Alcoholics Anonymous, 327
Alcoholism
  in adults and elderly, 326-327
  as nutritional risk factor, 226
Alternate food patterns as nutritional risk factor, 225-226
Alternative courses of action in decision making, 61-63
AMA; *see* American Management Association
Ambulatory nutrition care
  achieving quality assurance in, 135-137
  characteristics of, 135
  cost-benefits of, 163
  developing quality assurance measures for, 137-138
  model criteria for quality assurance in
    for adolescents, 293, 294
    for children, 284, 285
    for infants, 278
    for obese infants and children, 142, 143
    for pregnant women, 239-240
Amenorrhea, 291
American Academy of Pediatrics, 271, 277
American Cancer Society, dietary recommendations of, 325-326
American Dietetic Association
  Commission on Dietetic Registration, 9

American Dietetic Association—cont'd
  cost-benefits of ambulatory
    nutrition care, 163
  membership census, 18
  Quality Assurance Committee, 134
  Role Delineation and Verification
    Study, 5
  Study Commission on Dietetics, 18
  support for third-party payment for
    nutrition care, 416-417
American health, Public Health
    Service report on, 12-13
American Heart Association, 320, 384
American Hospital Association, 418
American Management Association,
    109-111
American Public Health Association,
    191
American Society of Clinical Nutrition
    Symposium, 327-329
Analysis
  of covariance, 369
  of dietary data, 351-352
  difference, 369-370
  factor, 370
  multiple discriminant, 371
  multivariate, 370-371
  relationship, 370
  of variance, 369
Analytical skills in nutrition science
  computers and computer science,
    349-356
  epidemiology, 356-362
  related disciplines in delivery of
    nutrition services, 348-349
  statistics, 362-371
Androgogy, 376
Anemia
  characterization of, 280
  in children, 280, 284
  in elderly, 333
  of pregnancy, 222, 226
Anorexia nervosa, 291
Antacids, 313
Anthropometric assessment, 191-199
  of adolescents, 294
  of adults and elderly, 333
  of children, 281-284
  clinical, 195-199
  growth charts, 195
    guidelines for, 198-199
  head circumference, 193, 271
    percentiles for, 266-269
  height and length, 191-193, 260,
    262-265
    measuring, 260, 270
    percentiles for, 266-269
  of infants, 260-274
  in nutritional assessment, 197
  of pregnant women, 232-233
  quality control in, 195

Anthropometric assessment—cont'd
  skinfold thickness, 193-195, 271-274
  weight, 191, 260, 262-265
    percentiles for, 266-269
Appalachian Health Demonstration
    Program, 399
Applying Behavioral Science to
    Cardiovascular Risk, 385
Artifacts, regression, 127
Artificial sweeteners, 324
Aspirin, 313
Assessment
  community, 43-60
  need, 122-123
  in nutrition counseling, 378-380;
    see also Nutritional status,
    assessment of
Association of State and Territorial
    Health Officials, 9
Association of State and Territorial
    Public Health Nutrition
    Directors, 9
Atherosclerosis
  in adults and elderly, 318-320
  in infants, 259-260
Audit
  administrative, 149, 151, 153
  dietetic, 148-153
  monodisciplinary nutritional care,
    151-153
  nutritional care, 148, 149
  patient care, 144-148
  quality assurance, 144-148
Audit abstract form, 147
Audit data summary, 148
Audit system, written, 137
Authority, 70-72
  formal, 31, 32, 72
Autocratic leadership style, 100
Autonomy and entrepreneurship, 27
Avoidance as manifestation of
    dominance and suppression, 79
Avoidance learning, 97

B

BCHS; see Bureau of Community
    Health Services
Behavior, organized sets of, 31-33
Behavior change in nutrition
    counseling, 381-383
Behavior modification, 381-383,
    385-386; see also Behavioral
    change skills
  methods for, 97-98
Behavior styles, leadership, 103, 104
Behavioral change plan, Stewart's,
    376
Behavioral change skills
  at community level, 384-387
  learning theories and, 374-376
  and life-style behavior, 374
  in nutrition counseling, 376-384

"Behavioral Control of Overeating,"
    381
Behavioral criteria, 140
Behavioral data, 379
Behavioral objectives, 55
Behavioral scientists, 8
Best fit, line of, 370
BHCDA; see Bureau of Health Care
    Delivery and Assistance
Bias for action, 26-27
Bibliographic data bases, 350, 356
Biochemical assessment, 185, 200-203
  of adolescents, 294
  of adults and elderly, 333
  of children, 284
  of infants, 274
  of pregnant women, 233-237
Biochemical methods, interpretation
    of, 202-203
Biochemical research support, 394
Biochemical tests in nutrition
    assessment, 201
Biochemical variables, dietary intake
    correlated with, 201
Biological data, 379
Biostatistics, 349
Birth, life expectancy at, 12
Birth weight, 220
  evaluation of effect of WIC on, 247
Block grants, 393, 402-405
Blood-forming nutrients, 233
Blood lipids, glucose, and enzymes,
    233-236
Blood pressure, 320, 321-322
Blood volume during pregnancy, 221
Blue Cross/Blue Shield, 163
Bone fractures in elderly, 326
Brainstorming, 61, 80
Breast cancer, death rates from, and
    fat intake, 325
Breast development, stages of, 228
Breast-feeding
  common problems during, 230
  effect of nutrition education on, 247
  immunological benefits of, 257
  management of lactation and,
    228-229
  supplementation with, 274
Breast tissue during pregnancy, 221
Budget
  categories in, 410
  federal, 422-424
  in grant proposal, 411
  justification of, 155
  for nutrition services, 390
  performance, 156-157
  preparation of, 154-155
  purpose of, 154
  zero-based, 157
Budget cycle, 155
Budget requests and expenditures,
    167, 168

Budgeting, 154-157
Bureau of Community Health Services, 399
Bureau of Health Care Delivery and Assistance, 209
Bureau of Training, 195

C

Caffeine ingestion during pregnancy, 222
Calcium intake, 177, 179, 180
Calcium/phosphorus ratio, 326
Calcium supplementation, 326
Calipers, 194, 195, 271, 274
Caloric intake, 179, 180
Canadian Dietary Standard for iron in adolescents, 290
Cancer, 324-326
  and diet, 16-17
Canonical correlation, 371
CAP; *see* Community Action Program
Capitation grants, 394
Carbohydrate requirements
  for adolescents, 289
  for adults and elderly, 310
Cardiovascular disease
  costs associated with, 337
  risk factors for, 10
    obesity, 318
Care services, long-term, 336-337;
    see also Nutritional care
Case study
  of community, 44-45
  of obesity, in preschool population, 120-121
Catalog of Federal Domestic Assistance, 396-399
Categorical grants, 402-403
Cathartics, 313
CBA; *see* Cost-benefit analysis
CDR; *see* Committee on Dietetic Registration
CEA; *see* Cost-effectiveness analysis
Centers for Disease Control, 399
  Bureau of Training, 195
  Nutrition Biochemistry Section, 200
  Nutrition Surveillance System, 181-183
  Pediatric Nutrition Surveillance System, 250-252
  Pregnancy Nutrition Surveillance System, 220-221
Certainty-provisionalism, 108
CFDA; *see* Catalog of Federal Domestic Assistance
Change
  organizational, management of, 75-76
  overcoming resistance to, 76
  for twenty-first century, management and, 33-34

Changing service programs, evaluation in, 119-120
CHC; *see* Community Health Centers
Checklist for action plan, 91
Chi square test, 369
Child Care Food Program, 295
Child Nutrition Act, 9, 10, 294-295, 419
Children
  deficiencies and growth retardation in, 10
  feeding patterns in, 280
  guidelines for patient management of, 281
  health objectives for, 250
  nutrition assessment of, 281-284
  nutrition intervention, counseling, and education for, 284
  nutrition programs for, 294-295
  nutrition-related health problems in, 250, 251, 280
  nutritional requirements for, 279
  preschool, obesity in, 295
  and referral for nutrition care, 284
  school-age, nutrition education for, 296
Children's Bureau, 416
Cholesterol, 259-260
  food groups providing, 178
Cholesterol intake, 177, 178
  for adults and elderly, 311
Cholesterol levels, 10
  and atherosclerosis, 320
  for children, 284
Chronic systemic diseases as nutritional risk factor, 226
Citizens Board of Inquiry into Hunger and Malnutrition, 174-175
Clarification, 379
Classification matrices, 364-368
Client care plan, 206
Client/group audit, general information form for, 146
Clinic personnel, training for, in weighing and measuring, 193
Clinical assessment, 189-191
  of adolescents, 294
  of adults and elderly, 333
  anthropometric, 195-199
  of children, 284
  of infants, 274
Clinical care, computer applications in, 353-354
CMPP; *see* Computer Menu Planning Program
Coalitions, 422
Coercion for overcoming resistance to change, 75, 76
Coercive power, 72
Commerce Business Daily, 397-398
Committee, select, 421

Committee to Develop a Research Study on Cost-Benefit of Ambulatory Nutrition Care, 159
Committee on Dietetic Registration, 9
Committee on Maternal Nutrition, 226, 227
Committee on Nutrition of American Academy of Pediatrics, 271
Commodity Distribution Program, 244
Communication(s), 105
  effective barriers to, 106-107
  effective listening, 107
  good, guidelines for, 110
  humor in, 108
  importance of, 104-106
  moving from defensive to supportive, 108-109
  oral, 105
  in organizations, 109-111
  for overcoming resistance to change, 75, 76
  written, 105-106
Communication process, 105, 106
Community, 43
  case study of, 44-45
Community Action Program, 392
Community assessment
  areas for
    community political organizations, 49
    cultural factors, 49
    demographic information, 47
    dental health, 49
    education, 51
    food programs and resources, 50
    geography and environment, 51
    health statistics resources on morbidity and mortality, 48
    housing, 49-50
    local health resources, 48-49
    occupational data, 51
    school nutrition programs, 50
    social welfare programs, 50-51
    socioeconomic stratification, 47
    surveys and surveillance, 51-52
    transportation, 51
  data collection in, 45-47
  developing goals and objectives in, 54-57
  process for defining need/problem in, 52-54
  setting priorities in, 57-60
Community assessment profile, 46-47
Community-based long-term care, 314
Community diagnosis, 122
Community dietetic technicians, 5-8
Community dietetics, entry-level positions in, 7
Community dietitians, 4-5
  employment areas for, 8-10
  roles of, 5

Community dietitians/nutritionists
  future for, 17-18
  future educational needs for, 18-19
  management and marketing skills
    for, 18-19
  role of, and nutritional screening,
    203
Community health, indices of,
    358-359, 360
Community Health Centers, 399
Community health promotion, 341
Community level, behavior change at,
    384-387
Community-level nutrition services
  for adults and elderly, 334-343
  Congregate Meals Program, 334
  Food Stamp Program, 334-336
  long-term care services, 336-337
  prevention programs in workplace,
    337
  Thrifty Food Plan, 336
Community nutrition, 3-20, 43
  health promotion in, 15-17
  role of managing and managers in,
    21-35
  societal trends affecting
    elderly population, 12
    family, 11-12
    health, 12-13
    health care costs, 14-15
Community political organizations, 49
Community Services Block Grant Act,
    211
Company values, 42
Comparison in evaluation, 125
Competition, 77
Competitive environment, 85
*The Complete Grants Sourcebook for
  Higher Education*, 407
Completeness of measurement, 126
Comprehensive Health Planning Law
    of 1967, 392
Comprehensive Older Americans Act
    Amendments of 1978, 314
Comprehensive planning; see Strategic
    planning
Compromise as conflict resolution
    method, 79
Computer Menu Planning Program,
    353-354
Computer-planned shopping list, 354
Computer program, 351
Computer sciences, 348-356
Computers
  and nutrition, 351-356
    analysis of dietary data, 351-352
    application in clinical care,
      353-354
    application in food service
      management, 353
    in education, 354-356

Computers—cont'd
  and nutrition—cont'd
    Nutrient Data Bank Conference,
      352
    in nutrition data retrieval system,
      356
    Quick Input Program, 352
  parts of, 350-351
Conceptual skill, 30-31
Conference grant, 394
Confirmation, 374-375
Conflict
  changing views of, 77
  managing professionals as type of,
    78-79
  old and current views of, 77
  organizational, 78
  "quiet," 78
  types of, 77-78
Conflict resolution methods, 79-80
Confrontation, 379
Congregate housing, 12
Congregate Meals Program, 334, 416
Congressional Budget Office, 422
Congressional Standing Committees,
    421-422
Consensus Development Panel, 320
Consensus Development Panel on
    Osteoporosis, 326
Consensus statements, 356-357
Consortium grant, 395
Construction grant, 395
Consultation grant, 395
Consultative leadership style, 100
Consumer views on nutrition, 11
Consumption measurement methods,
    187-189
Content in quality assurance, 134
Contingency approaches
  to organizational design, 74-75
  to responding to external
    environment, 34
Continuing education, 348
Continuing education grant, 395
Contracts versus grants, 393-394
Control group, 117
Control-problem orientation, 108
Control process in management of
    nutrition services, 114, 115,
    135; see also Evaluation
Control theories, 94-96
Controlling, 24-25
Cooperation, 77
Co-option and manipulation, 75, 76
Coordination
  in division of work and
    departmentalization, 68, 69
  as essence of management, 25-26
  managerial functions and, 26-28
  and referral system, 206-214
Coronary heart disease in adults and
    elderly, 318-320, 360

Corporate grants, 406
Corrective action, 114
Correlation, 370
Cost-benefit analysis, 133
Cost containment, 14; see also
    Financial control
Cost-effectiveness, 22
Cost-effectiveness/benefit analysis,
    133, 157-163
  definitions of, 157-158
  distinctions between, 158
  factors affecting use of, 159, 160
  and findings of OTA, 158
  models of, 161-163
  in nutritional care, 159-161
  potential users of, 159
  principles of methodology of,
    158-159
*Costs and Benefits of Nutritional
  Care, Phase 1*, 159
Costs of cardiovascular and
    hypertensive diseases, 337
Counseling, advisory services and,
    397; see also Nutrition
    counseling
Country club leadership style, 102,
    103
Covariance, 369
Coverage of measurements, 126
Cow's milk, 257-259
Crash weight control, 312
Creative group decision making, 80
Creativity, 80, 81
Crisis, 348
Criteria
  behavioral, 140
  model; see Model criteria
  for nutritional care of diabetic
    patients, 150-151
  for outcome and/or process, 140-141
Crude measurements, 126
Cue elimination, 382
Cultural factors in community
    assessment, 49
Cultural influences on food practices,
    243
Culture and food intake, 314-315
Customer, closeness with, 27
Customer philosophy, 84

D

Daily Food Guide, USDA, 379
Daily food guide for pregnant women,
    241, 243
Data, good, 367
Data base, 350, 351
Data collection, 379-380
  for assessment of nutritional status,
    185
  methods of, 186-187
  in community assessment, 45-47

Data collection—cont'd
    in dietary methodology, 186
    recall for, 186, 187
Data retrieval system, nutrition,
        computer in, 356
Death, nutritional risk factors
        associated with, 307
Death rates, 13; *see also* Mortality
    from breast cancer, correlation
        between fat intake and, 325
Decentralization, 74
Decision, 374
    health care resource allocation, 158,
        161
    types of, 64
Decision makers, managers as, 28
Decision making
    alternative courses of action in,
        61-63
    creative group, 80
    group, 139-140
    problem identification in, 61
    roles of managers in, 32
    styles of dietitians, 64
    techniques of, 64
    value of forecasting information in,
        60
Decision-making authority, leader,
        continuum of, 99
Decision packages, 157
Defensive communication, 108-109
Deficiencies
    conditions related to, 250-251
    and growth retardation in infants
        and children, 10
    in pregnant women, 10
Degenerative disease, chronic, and
        diet, 361
Delegation, 72-73
Democratic leadership style, 100
Demographic information, 47
Demonstration grant, 395
Dental health, 10-11, 49
Dental hygienists, 8
Dentists, 8
Departmentalization, 69
Descriptive statistics
    classification matrix for, 366
    versus inferential statistics, 363-364
Diabetes in adults and elderly,
        323-326
Diabetic patients, nutritional care of,
        150-151
Diagnosis, community, 122
Diagnosis-related groups, 418
DIALOG System, 356
Diet
    adherence to, 380-381
    relationship of atherosclerosis to,
        320
    relationship of cancer to, 16-17

Diet—cont'd
    relationship of chronic degenerative
        diseases to, 361
Diet and Cancer, 415
Diet, Nutrition, and Cancer
        Prevention: Guide to Food
        Choices, 414
Diet-drug interactions in adults and
        elderly, 312-314
Diet history and analysis of pregnant
        women, 237
Diet plans, 318, 319
Dietary assessment, 185
    of adults and elderly, 327-333
    of children, 284
    of infants, 274, 276
    of pregnant women, 236-237
Dietary change, 376-377
    for hypertension control, 385
Dietary concerns, identification of,
        380
Dietary data, analysis of, 351-352
Dietary deficiencies, 251
Dietary Goals for the United States,
        415
Dietary guidelines, 16-17
Dietary Guidelines for Americans, 10,
        356, 414
Dietary habits of elderly, 329-333
Dietary history, 186, 187
Dietary intake and biochemical
        variables, 201
    of infants, 274, 275
Dietary methodology, 185-187
    for adults and elderly, 329
Dietary order entry system, 353
Dietary overabundance, 9
Dietary recommendations of National
        Cancer Institute and American
        Cancer Society, 325-326; *see*
        also Recommended Daily
        Dietary Allowances
Dietetic audits, 148-153
Dietetic registration, 417
Dietetic technicians, community, 5-8
Dietetics
    community, entry-level positions in,
        7
    professional preparation in, 31
    recommendations for future of, 18
Dieting, 318
Dietitians
    community, 4-5
    decision-making styles of, 64
Difference analysis, 369-370
Digestion in infants, 253-254
Digitalis, 312
Diplomats, managers as, 28
Direct contact, 25
Direct financial assistance, 396-397
Discretionary grant, 395

Discriminant function, 371
Disease
    association and causality, 360-361
    chronic systemic, as nutritional risk
        factor, 226
    natural history of, 361
    quality nutrition services for
        prevention of, 173-217
Disease prevention, 361-362
    in workplace, 337, 386-387
Disseminator role of manager, 32
Diuretics, 313
Documentation for nutrition services,
        139
Documentation/recording of care, 137
Dominance and suppression in conflict
        resolution, 79
DRGs; *see* Diagnosis-related groups
Drug addiction as nutritional risk
        factor, 226
Drug-diet interactions in adults and
        elderly, 312-314
Drugs and intestinal malabsorption,
        312-313

E
Early Periodic Screening, Diagnosis,
        and Treatment, 48
Eating behavior and living situation,
        236-237
Economic benefits of nutritional
        counseling in pregnancy, 162
Economic deprivation as nutritional
        risk factor, 225
Education, 51
    continuing, 348
    nutrition; *see* Nutrition education
    to overcome resistance to change,
        75, 76
Education grant, 395
Educational needs for community
        dietitians/nutritionists, 18-19
Educational plan, 137
Effectiveness of program in
        evaluation, 125
Efficiency, 29
    operational, 84
    of program, in evaluation, 125-126
EFNEP; *see* Expanded Food and
        Nutrition Education Program
Elderly population, 12, 305-306; *see*
        also Adults and elderly
    anemia in, 333
    dietary habits of, 329-333
    nutrients consumed by, 329
    nutrition assessment and
        intervention guidelines for,
        330-331
    response rates of, in nutrition and
        health research studies, 332
Empathy and neutrality, 109

Empirical data, classification matrix for, 365
Employment areas for community dietitians/nutritionists, 8-10
Energy intake, 179, 180
Energy requirements
  of adolescents, 289
  of adults and elderly, 310
  of children, 279
  during lactation, 229
Entrepreneurship and autonomy, 27
Environment, 51
  analysis of, 84-85
  external, for managing and managers, 34-35
  organizing for changing, 74-75
Environmental data, 379
Environmental influences on adolescents, 291-293
Enzymes, measurement of, 233-236
Epidemiology, 348, 356-362
  of cancer, 325
  of diabetes, 323
  dietary history methods in, 187
  disease association and causality in, 360-361
  disease prevention in, 361-362
  incidence versus prevalence in, 357
  and indices of health status in community, 360
  types of studies in, 357
EPSDT; see Early Periodic Screening, Diagnosis, and Treatment
Equality and superiority, 109
Equipment and financial assistance, 397
Esteem and status needs, 95
Estimate, standard error of, 370
Ethnicity, 315
Evaluation, 114-117
  and action, gap between, 128-130
  in action settings, 119-120
  categories of, 125-126
  circular model for, 120, 121
  differentiated from quality assurance, 135, 136
  essential steps in
    identifying and implementing objectives, 123
    measurement and comparison, 125
    needs assessment, 122-123
    objective measuring criteria, 123
    setting objectives, 123
    value formation, 122
  in nutrition counseling, 384
  of quality assurance, 134-135, 137
  in quality nutrition services, 214
  use of results of, 128-130
Evaluation checklist, 128
Evaluation-description, 108

Evaluation design, 117-119
Evaluators, role of, 128
Excesses, conditions related to, 251-252
Executive branch of government, 421
Expanded Food and Nutrition Education Program, 210
Expectancy model, 97
Expenditures and budget requests, 167, 168
Experimental design, 117-118
Experimental model for evaluation design, 117-118
Experimental mortality, 127
Experimental studies, 357
Expert Committee on Medical Assessment of Nutritional Status, 189, 190
Expert power, 72
Explanatory responses, 379
External environment for managing and managers, 34-35
External validity, 368
Extinction and punishment, 97-98

F
F ratio, 369
F test, 370
Facilitation and support to overcome resistance to change, 75, 76
Facilities and financial assistance, 397
Facilities assistance grant, 395
Factor analysis, 370
Factor matrix, 370
Factors, 370
Faddism among adults and elderly, 311-312
Family, 11-12
Family foundation, 405
Family information, 185
Family Planning, 402
FAO; see Food and Agriculture Organization
FAPRS; see Federal Assistance Program Retrieval System
FAS; see Fetal alcohol syndrome
Fast-food, nutritional value of, 290-291, 293
Fat intake, 177, 179, 180
  associated with cancer, 324-325
  program for decrease in, 320
Fat requirements of adults and elderly, 311
Fat stores during pregnancy, 221
Fatty acid intake, program for decrease in, 320
FCC; see Federal Communications Commission
FDA; see Food and Drug Administration
Federal Assistance Program Retrieval System, 396, 397

Federal budget, 422-424
Federal Communications Commission, 421
Federal government and block grants, 403
Federal legislation and nutrition services, 415-416
Federal Program Information Act, 396, 397
Federal programs
  for long-term care services, 337
  and state and local nutrition services, 209-210
The Federal Register, 397
Federal Trade Commission, 421
Federally financed food assistance programs, 210-214; see also Food assistance programs
Fee-for-service system, 342
Feeding guidelines for infants, 274-277
Feeding patterns in children, 280
Feeding practices for infants, 295
  and obesity in preschool children, 295
  recent trends in, 259
Fellowship, 395
Fetal alcohol syndrome, 226
Fiber requirements of adults and elderly, 311
Field test, 142-143
Financial assistance for food and nutrition programs, 396-397
Financial control, 153-157; see also Cost containment
Financial distress grant, 395
Fiscal policy, 154
Fluid needs during pregnancy, 221
Fluoride supplementation
  for infants, 274, 277
  during lactation, 231
FNS programs; see Food and Nutrition Service programs
Folic acid deficiencies in pregnant and lactating women, 10
Folic acid supplementation during pregnancy, 222, 226
Follow-up services, 205-206
Food
  for Child Care Food Program, 277
  data bases for, 350
  included in WIC, 246
  solid, as nutrient source for infants, 259
Food and Agriculture Act of 1977, 414
Food and Agriculture Organization, 8
  and WHO standard for iron in adolescents, 290
Food and Drug Administration, 188, 399, 421
Food and Nutrition Board/National Research Council, 356

Food and Nutrition Board/National Research Council—cont'd
Recommended Daily Dietary Allowances; see Recommended Daily Dietary Allowances
Food and Nutrition Service programs, 214
Food accounts, 186
Food assistance programs, 210-214
 for adults and elderly, 335
 for infants, children, and adolescents, 277, 294-295
 for pregnant women, 243-246
 referral for, 243-246
Food consumption, comparison of RDA with, 187
Food costs, 50
Food Distribution Program, 214
Food frequency questionnaires, 186, 187
Food groups and food intake for good nutrition, 282
Food guide
 daily, for pregnant women, 241, 243
 vegetarian, 241
Food intake
 of adolescents, 292
 and culture, 314-315
 for good nutrition, 282
Food intake data, 379
Food lists, 186
Food patterns, alternate, as nutritional risk factor, 225-226
Food practices, influences on, 243
Food programs, 50
 financial assistance for, 396-397
Food records, 186
Food service management and computers, 353
Food Stamp Act, 9
Food Stamp Program, 211-214, 243, 244, 277, 334-336, 416
Food standards, 50
Force field analysis, 62-63
Forcing as manifestation of dominance and suppression, 79
Forecasting information in decision making, 60
Formal authority, 31, 32, 71
Formula grant, 395, 397
Formulas, prepared, infant, 257-259
Foundation Center, 406-407
Foundation Directory, 407
Foundation Fundamentals: A Guide for Grantseekers, 408
Foundation grants, 405-406
Foundation Grants Index, 407
FP; see Family Planning
Framingham Study, 316
Frequency determination, 187

Frequent pregnancies as nutritional risk factor, 225
The Functions of the Executive, 98
Funders, 83
Funding
 block grants, 393, 402-405
 Catalog of Federal Domestic Assistance, 396-399
 Foundation Center, 406-407
 foundation grants, 405-406
 preparations for request for, 406
 Public Health Service, 399-402

G

Gantt scheduling, 88, 89
Gastrointestinal tract during pregnancy, 221
General information form for client/group audit, 146
Geography, 51
Geriatrics, 305
Gerontology, 305
Glucose, measurement of, 233-236
Glucose tolerance, 323
Goal setting/objectives, 85, 380
Goals
 in community assessment, 54-57
 leading to achieve, 93-112
 role of managers in balancing competing, 28
Good data, 368
Government attention to nutrition issues, 415
Grant proposal writing guide, 407
Grants, 393
 categorical, 402-403
 formula, 397
 foundation, 405-406
 history of, 391-393
 project, 397
 proposal for, 407-411
 shortcomings in disapproved applications for, 411
 sources of funding for, 395-407
 types of, 394-395
 versus contracts, 393-394
Grants-in-aid, 390-391
Grants Administration, 407
Grants Policy Statement, 394-395, 399
Great Society, 392
Group decision making, 139-140
 creative, 80
Growth of infants, 252-255
Growth charts, 195
 guidelines for, 198-199
 Stuart-Meredith, 195
Growth grids, 260, 262-265
Growth percentiles, 260, 266-269
Growth stunting, 250-251, 252
 in infants and children, 10
Guaranteed/insured loans, 397

Guide to Quality Assurance and Ambulatory Nutrition Care, 137, 144
Guidelines for Diet, Nutrition, and Cancer, 10
Guidelines on Dietetic Services, 134, 148
Guidelines for Evaluating Dietetic Practice, 134

H

Hatch Act of 1887, 391
Hawthorne effect, 33, 117
Head circumference, 271
 of children, 281, 283
 of infants, 266-269, 271
 measurement of, 193
 percentiles for, 266-269
Health
 community, indices of, 358-359
 dental, 49
 and nutrition research studies, 332
 nutrition services for promotion of, 173-217
 Public Health Service Report on, 12-13
 redefinition of, 15-17
Health belief model, 375
Health care
 model based on level of, 151-153
 quality assurance of
  for adolescents, 294
  for children, 284, 285
  for infants, 278
Health care costs, 14-15
Health care delivery, nutrition services in, 138-139
Health Care Financing Administration, 418
Health care resource allocation decisions, 158, 161
Health care services and third-party payers, 14
Health care team members, 8
Health consequences of infants at nutritional risk, 259-260
Health Education Branch of Office of Prevention, Education, and Control, 210
Health educators, 8
Health Examination Survey, 176
Health expenditures, national, 14
Health habits and life expectancy, 316
Health Insurance Association of America, 418
Health maintenance organizations, 14-15
Health manpower shortage areas, 209
Health objectives
 for infants, children, and adolescents, 250
 for pregnant women, 220

Health practitioners, values for, 42
Health problems
    major, risk factors for, 16
    nutrition-related; see Nutrition-
        related health problems
    nutritional risk factors associated
        with, 307
Health promotion, 15-17
    community, 342
    objectives for, 17
    in workplace, 337, 386-387
Health Resources and Services
        Administration, 208, 209, 399
Health resources, local, 48-49
Health statistics resources, 48
Health status in community, indices
        of, 360
Health Systems Agencies, 393
Health trends, 12-13
"Healthy People in 1979," 17
Healthy People, the Surgeon General's
        Report on Health Promotion
        and Disease Prevention, 209,
        374
Heart to Heart: A Manual on
        Nutrition Counseling for the
        Reduction of Cardiovascular
        Disease Risk Factors, 385
Heart disease
    causes of, 360
    risk factors for, 16
Height
    for age, 182
        low, 252
    measurement of, 191-193, 281, 283
    reference data on, 182
    weight for, 182
Height velocity and puberty, 286-287,
        288
Helping strategies, 380
Hematocrit, 182-183
Hemoglobin, 182-183
HES; see Health Examination Survey
Hierarchy of objectives, 123
High blood pressure control, 322-323
History, 127, 185
    dietary, 186, 187
    in nutritional assessment of
        pregnant women, 232
    suggesting malnutrition, 190
HMOs; see Health maintenance
        organizations
HMSAs; see Health manpower
        shortage areas
Home Delivered Meals Program, 416
Home health services, 417
Hormones
    in adolescents, 288
    for lactation, 228
Hospital and Construction Act of
        1946, 391

Hospitals, changing nutrition services
        in, 342
Hot line, nutrition, 340
Household dietary studies, 186
Housing, 49-50
    congregate, 12
"How to Diagnose Nutritional
        Deficiencies in Daily Practice,"
        189
How to Prepare a Research Proposal,
        408
HSA; see Health Services
        Administration
Human milk, 257, 258
Human needs, Maslow's hierarchy of,
        95-96
Human Nutrition Information Service,
        336
Human Nutrition Research Center on
        Aging, 308
Human relations, 33
    vitamins of, 111
Human relations movement, 99
Human skill, 29-30
Humor, 108
"Hunger in America," 174
Hunger U.S.A., 9, 174
Hypertension
    in adults and elderly, 321-322
    in children, 284
Hypertension control, dietary changes
        for, 385
Hypertension Detection and Follow-
        Up Program, 385
Hypertensive diseases, costs associated
        with, 337
Hypothesis testing, 364

I
IDD; see Insulin-dependent diabetes
Imbalances, conditions related to,
        251-252
Immunological benefits of breast-
        feeding, 257
Impoverished leadership style, 102,
        103
Incidence versus prevalence, 357
Index of Nutritional Quality, 290-291
Individual dietary studies, 186
Indomethacin, 313
Industrial nutrition services, 342-343
Infants
    advisable intakes for, 255-256
    deficiencies and growth retardation
        in, 10
    digestion in, 253-254
    feeding practices for, 259, 295
    guidelines for feeding of, 274-277
    guidelines for patient management
        of, 260
    health objectives for, 250
    minimum requirements for, 255-256

Infants—cont'd
    mortality in, 13
    neuromuscular and psychosocial
        development in, 297-301
    nutrient requirements of, 255-259
    nutrient sources for, 256-259
    nutrition intervention and
        counseling for, 261, 274-277
    nutrition-related health problems
        of, 250, 251
    nutritional assessment of, 260-274
    at nutritional risk, 259-260
    physical growth of, 252-255
    physiology of nutrition in, 253-255
    psychosocial development of, 255
    quality assurance of health and
        nutrition care for, 278
    RDAs for, 255-256
    and referral for nutritional care,
        277-278
    supplements for, 274, 277
Inferential statistics
    classification matrix for, 367
    versus descriptive statistics, 363-364
Influence, 71
Information giving, 370
Information sources for community
        assessment profile, 46-47
Informational role of manager, 32-33
Innovation-decision process, 374-375
Inpatient care settings, quality
        assurance in, 148
Input, 351
INQ; see Index of Nutritional Quality
Instability of measurements, 127
Institution dietary studies, 186
Institutional nutrition, 9
Instrumentation, 127
Insulin-dependent diabetes, 323, 324
Insurance, 397
Integrated marketing organizations,
        84
Integrating models, 96-97
Integrative problem solving, 79-80
Interaction effects, 369
Internal environment, 84
Internal validity, 368
    threats to, 127-128
International agencies employing
        community dietitians/nutritionists, 8
Intervention/behavior change in
        nutrition counseling, 381-383
Intervention guidelines; see Nutrition
        intervention
Interviewing skills, 378, 379
Interviews, 49
Intestinal malabsorption and drugs,
        312-313
Iron deficiency, 177
    in human milk, 257
    in infants, 259

Iron deficiency—cont'd
  in pregnant and lactating women,
    10
Iron deficiency anemia
  in infants, 259
  during pregnancy, 222, 226
Iron intake, 179-180
  for adults and elderly, 311
Iron requirements
  for adolescents, 290-291
  for children, 279
Iron supplementation
  for infants, 274, 277
  during lactation, 231
  during pregnancy, 222, 226

J

JCAH; *see* Joint Commission on
    Accreditation of Hospitals
Job characteristics, 68-69, 70
Joint Commission on Accreditation of
    Hospitals, 134
Judiciary branch of government, 421

K

Kitchen facilities in community
    assessment, 49-50
Knowledge, 374
Knowles' adult learning concepts, 376

L

Labor-cost centers, 156-157
Laboratory assessment of nutritional
    status, 200-203
  of infants, 274, 275
  during pregnancy, 233
Laboratory studies, 185
Lactation
  and breast development, 228
  establishment and maintenance of,
    227
  hormones for, 228
  let-down reflex in, 228, 229
  management of, 228-229
  nutrition guidelines for, 243, 244
  nutritional demands of, 227,
    229-231
  RDAs for, 222
  stages of, 228
Laissez-faire leadership style, 100-101
Laxatives, 313
Leader behavior styles, 103, 104
Leader decision-making authority, 99
Leadership, 24, 98-104
  to achieve goals, 93-112
    communications, 104-111
    importance of motivation, 94
    motivation theories, 94-98
    vitamins of human relations, 111
  and guidelines for using
    management approaches, 102

Leadership—cont'd
  managerial grid in, 102-103
  and quality circles, 101-102
  styles of, 99-101
  tridimensional leader effectiveness
    model, 103-104
Learning, avoidance, 97
Learning process, 374
Learning theories, 374-376
Legislation, 421-422
  federal, supporting nutrition
    services, 415-416
Legislative branch of government, 421
Legislative issues related to nutrition,
    416-419
Legitimate power, 72
Length of infant, 260, 262-265
  measurement of, 191-193, 260, 270
  percentiles for, 266-269
Let-down reflex, 228, 229
Level of care model, 151-153
Licensure, 417
Life expectancy, 12-13, 305
  and health habits, 316
Life-style, 373, 375
Line of best fit, 370
Lipid requirements
  for adolescents, 289
  for children, 279
Lipids, measurement of, 233-236
Listening, 107, 378-379
Living situations and eating behavior,
    236
Loans, 397
Lobbying, 419-421
Local agencies employing community
    dietitians/nutritionists, 8-10
Local health resources, 48-49
Local-level nutrition strategies
  for adults and elderly, 337-343
  federal programs for, 209-210
  for infants, children, and
    adolescents, 295-296
  for pregnant women, 247
Local sources of nutrition
    information, 206-207
Long-range planning; see Strategic
    planning
Long-Range Planning, 41
Long-term care services, 336-337
  community-based, 314
Low-birth-weight infants, 220-221
Low-sodium products, 419

M

Macroenvironment, 85
Magnesium intake, 180
Main effects, 369
Mainframe, 350
Majority rule and dominance and
    suppression, 79

*Making Food Dollars Count—
    Nutritious Meals at Low Cost,*
    336
Malnutrition
  history suggesting, 190
  signs and symptoms of, 189-191,
    227
  in United States, 174-175
Management, 22-26
  and change, for twenty-first
    century, 33-34
  controlling, 24-25
  coordination as essence of, 25-26
  effective, 22-23
  leading in, 24
  and marketing skills, for community
    dietitian/nutrition services,
    18-19
  of nutrition services, control process
    in, 135
  by objectives, 97, 111
  organizing in, 24
  and participative leadership style,
    102
  planning in, 24
  span of, 68, 70
Management process, 23, 24, 33, 39,
    69, 95, 115
Management theory, 33
Managerial functions and
    coordination, 26-28
  time spent on, 31
Managerial grid, 102-103
Managerial performance, 28-29
Managerial skills and time allocation
  conceptual skill, 30-31
  human skill, 29-30
  technical skill, 29
Managers, roles of, 27-28, 32-33
Managing and managers in community
    nutrition, 22-26
  and evolution of management
    theory, 33
  external environment for, 34-35
  management and change for
    twenty-first century, 33-34
  managerial functions and
    coordination, 26-28
  performance in organization, 28-33
Managing organizational change,
    75-76
Managing professionals and conflict,
    78-79
Manipulation and co-option to
    overcome resistance to change,
    75, 76
Market data bases to assess nutritional
    status, 187-188
Market environment, 84
Market outlets or tools, 338

Market planning process, strategic, 84-85
Market survey, 338
Marketing
  and management skills, for community dietitian/nutrition services, 18-19
  in nutrition services, 82-87
    characteristics of effective marketing organization, 83-84
    marketing strategy, 85-86
    not-for-profit organization marketing, 83
    social marketing, 86-87
    strategic market planning process, 84-85
Marketing control system, 85, 86
Marketing information, 84
Marketing information system, 85
Marketing mix, 83, 85-86
Marketing organization, 83-84
Marketing plan, social, 87
Marketing planning system, 85, 86
Marketing strategy, 85-86
Maslow's hierarchy of human needs, 95-96
Massachusetts Maternal and Child Health Agency, 418-419
Massachusetts Nutrition Resource Center, 340
Matching procedures, 118-119
Maternal and Child Health Services, 209, 402, 403-404, 416
Maternal and Child Health Services Block Grant, 209, 418-419
Maternal nutrition
  guidelines for patient management, 231-237
  nutrition counseling for pregnant women, 222, 237-243
  nutrition guidelines for lactation, 229-231, 243, 244
  nutrition-related health problems of pregnant women, 220
  nutritional risk factors during pregnancy, 225-227
  physiological changes during pregnancy, 221-222
  and Pregnancy Nutrition Surveillance System, 220–221
  referral for services, 243–246
  support for, 243
  weight gain during pregnancy, 222-225
Maturation, 127
MBOs; see Management by objectives
McClelland, 96
MCH Services; see Maternal and Child Health Services
Mean, 364
Measurable indicators, 123

Measurement(s), 125; see also Anthropometric assessment
  common errors of, 195, 196
  in evaluation, 125
  and training for clinic personnel, 193
  validity of, 140
  of variables, in statistics, 368
Media attention to nutrition issues, 415
Mediators, managers as, 28
Medicaid, 9, 163, 418
Medical libraries, regional, 398
Medicare, 9, 163, 418
  home health services, 417
MEDLARS, 398
MEDLINE, 397
Megaloblastic anemia during pregnancy, 222, 226
Megavitamin diet during pregnancy, 225
Mental Retardation Planning Amendment, 416
MH; see Migrant Health
Microcomputer, 350
Middle-of-the-road leadership style, 103
Migrant Health, 402
Milk, 257-259
Mineral content of diet plans, 319
Mineral oil, 313
Mineral requirements
  of adolescents, 289-291
  of adults and elderly, 311
  of children, 279
  during pregnancy, 231
Minerals, measurement of, 233
Minicomputer, 350
Minnesota Heart Health Program, 341
Model criteria for quality assurance in ambulatory nutrition care, 285
  of adolescents, 293
  of children, 142, 143
  of infants, 142, 143, 278
  of pregnant women, 239-240
Model Workshop on Nutrition Counseling in Hyperlipidemia, 385
Monitoring in quality nutrition services, 214
Monitoring role of managers, 32
Monodisciplinary nutritional care audit, 151-153
Morbidity, 48
Morrill Act of 1862, 391
Mortality, 48; see also Death rates
  causes of, 15
  experimental, 127
  infant, 13
Motivation
  importance of, 94
  for quality assurance, 134

Motivation theories
  control theories, 94-96
  expectancy model, 97
  methods for behavior modification, 97-98
  process theories, 96-97
Multiple discriminant analysis, 371
Multiple-factor analysis of variance, 369
Multiple objectives, 83
Multiple publics, 83
Multiple time series, 118
Multivariate analysis, 370-371

N

National Academy of Sciences, 10, 415
National agencies employing community dietitians/ nutritionists, 8
National Cancer Institute, 392
  dietary recommendations of, 325-326
National Center for Health Statistics, 176
  growth grids, 260, 262-265
  percentiles for length, weight, and head circumference, 260, 266-269
  skinfold thickness, 271-274
National Conference on Quality Assurance in Ambulatory Nutrition Care, 143
National Health and Nutrition Examination Survey, 51, 176-179, 314, 318, 333
National health expenditures, 14
National Health Planning and Resources Development Act of 1974, 393
National Health Service Corps, 402
National Heart, Lung, and Blood Institute, 210, 316, 322, 384-385
National High Blood Pressure Education Program, 322, 323, 385
National Institute of Arthritis, Diabetes, and Digestive and Kidney Diseases, 316
National Institutes of Health, 210, 308, 392, 399
  Consensus Development Panel on Osteoporosis, 326
  Division of Research Grants, 393
  Nutrition Coordinating Committee, 356
  Office of Medical Applications of Research, 316
National Library of Medicine, 397, 398
National Nutrition Consortium, 414
National Nutritional Monitoring System, 176

National Research Council
  Food and Nutrition Board, 356
    Recommended Daily Dietary
      Allowances; *see* Recommended
      Daily Dietary Allowances
  protein requirement during
    lactation, 231
National School Lunch Act of 1946,
  294
National Science Foundation, 392
National sources of nutrition
  information, 207-209
National studies on nutritional status
  National Health and Nutrition
    Examination Survey, 51,
    176-179, 314, 318, 333
  Nationwide Food Consumption
    Survey, 179-180, 251, 336
  Preschool Nutrition Survey, 9, 176
  Ten-State Nutrition Survey, 9,
    175-176, 200, 314
Nationwide Food Consumption
  Survey, 179-180, 251, 336
Natural history of disease, 361
NCHS; *see* National Center for Health
  Statistics
NDB; *see* Nutrient Data Bank
Need, 122-123
Need/problem, 52-54
Needs assessment, 122-123
Negative evaluation results, 130
Negotiation and agreement to
  overcome resistance to change,
  75, 76
Negotiator role of manager, 32
"Net cost" studies, 158
NET program; *see* Nutrition
  Education and Training
  Program
Networks, 341
Neuromuscular and psychosocial
  development in infants,
  297-301
Neutrality-empathy, 109
New divorce–extended family, 12
New Federalism, 392
NFCS; *see* Nationwide Food
  Consumption Survey
NHANES; *see* National Health and
  Nutrition Examination Survey
NHBPEP; *see* National High Blood
  Pressure Education Program
NHLBI; *see* National Heart, Lung,
  and Blood Institute
NHSC; *see* National Health Service
  Corps
Niacin intake, 180
NIDD; *see* Non-insulin-dependent
  diabetes
NIH; *see* National Institutes of Health
Nominal group process, 80

Nominal variables, 364
Non-insulin-dependent diabetes,
  323-324
Nonequivalent control groups, 118,
  119
Nonexperimental designs, 119
Nonparametric tests, 369-370
North Carolina Public Health
  Nutrition Program, 295
North Karelia Project, 387
Not-for-profit organizations
  characteristics of, 39-41
  marketing for, 83
  strategic planning in, 39-41
Null hypothesis, 364
Numeric data bases, 350, 356
Numerical continuous variables, 364
Numerical discrete variables, 364
Nursing personnel, 8
Nutrient Data Bank Conference, 352
Nutrient levels, 180
Nutrient requirements
  of adolescents, 288-291
  of infants, 255-259
Nutrients
  blood-forming, measurement of,
    233
  calculation and evaluation of, using
    Quick Input Program, 352
  consumed by elderly, 329
  sources of, for infants, 256-259
Nutrition
  community; *see* Community
    nutrition
  computers and, 351-356
  consumer interest in, 4, 11
  current problems in, 10-11
  data bases for, 350
  good, food intake for, 282
  and health research studies, 332
  infant, physiology of, 253-255
  institutional, 9
  maternal, 219-248; *see also*
    Maternal nutrition
  and mortality and morbidity, 48
  public policy and legislative issues
    related to, 416-419
  relationship of cancer to, 324-325
*Nutrition and Your Health—Dietary
  Guidelines for Americans*, 16,
  415
*Nutrition Assessment: A Compre-
  hensive Guide for Planning
  Intervention*, 52
Nutrition Coordinating Committee,
  356
Nutrition counseling, 203
  algorithm for termination of, 383
  assessment in, 378
  for children, 284
  evaluation, 384

Nutrition counseling—cont'd
  goal of, 374, 376
  intervention/behavior change in,
    381-383
  model for, 376, 377
  for pregnant women, 237-243
    economic benefits of, 162
  treatment plan in, 380-381
Nutrition data retrieval system,
  computer in, 356
Nutrition education, 203-205
  for children, 284, 295, 296
  computer in, 354-356
  and decision to breast-feed, 247
  for pregnant women, 238
  in schools, 50
  and WIC, 246
Nutrition Education and Training
  Program, 10, 50, 419
Nutrition education plan, 206
Nutrition guidelines for lactation,
  243, 244
Nutrition hot line, 340
Nutrition information assistance,
  206-209
Nutrition intervention, 203-206
  for adults and elderly, 328-329,
    330-331, 337-343
  for children, 284
  for infants, 261, 274-277
  for pregnant women, 231, 245
Nutrition issues, coverage of, 415
Nutrition labeling, 419
Nutrition Monitoring Bill, 419
Nutrition policy, 414-415
Nutrition Program for Older
  Americans, 334
Nutrition program plan, 137, 138
Nutrition programs
  children's, 294-295
  financial assistance for, 396-397
  school, 50
Nutrition referral document, 206
Nutrition-related health problems
  of adults and elderly, 304-308
    guidelines for prevention of,
      316-327
  of infants, children, and
    adolescents, 250, 251, 280
  of pregnant women, 220
Nutrition research classification
  system, 355
Nutrition resources, 50
Nutrition science, analytical skills as
  tools of, 347-372
Nutrition services, 4
  action plans for, 67-91
  for adults and elderly, 334-343
  ambulatory; *see* Ambulatory
    nutrition care
  budget for, 390

Nutrition services—cont'd
  changing, in hospitals, 342
  controlling, for productivity
    categories of evaluation, 125-126
    characteristics of measures being
      evaluated, 126
    control process, 114, 115
    essential steps in program
      evaluations, 120-125
    evaluation, 114-117, 119-120
  controlling process in management
    of, 135
  evaluation design, 117-119
    threats to internal validity,
      127-128
    use of evaluation results, 128-130
  federal legislation supporting,
    415-416
  in health care delivery, 138-139
  implications of block grants for, 404
  industrial, 342-343
  for infants, children, and
    adolescents, 252-294
    nutrition-related health problems,
      250, 251
    Pediatric Nutrition Surveillance
      System, 250-252
    strategies at local level, 295-296
  marketing in, 82-87
  organizing for action in, 82-91
  quality; see Quality nutrition
    services
  referral system; see Referral
  regional, 339-340
  reimbursement for, 163-164
  related disciplines in, 348-349
  state, 340-342
Nutrition Services III, 211
Nutrition services delivery flowchart,
  205
Nutrition Services Payment System,
  163-164
Nutrition surveillance, 180-183
Nutrition Surveillance Program, 51-52
Nutrition surveillance system, 181-183
  Pediatric Nutrition Surveillance
    System, 250-252
  Pregnancy Nutrition Surveillance
    System, 220-221
  quality control in, 183
Nutrition surveys
  major, 327
  physical examination in, 191
  in United States, 174
  use of data from, 180-181
Nutritional Assessment in Health
  Programs, 191
Nutritional care
  ambulatory; see Ambulatory
    nutrition care
  of diabetic patients, 150-151

Nutritional care—cont'd
  local-level strategies for, 247
  referral for; see Referral
Nutritional care audits, 148, 149
  monodisciplinary, 151-153
Nutritional demands of lactation, 227
Nutritional Disorders of Children:
    Prevention, Screening, and
    Follow-Up, 260
Nutritional quackery, 11
Nutritional requirements, 308-310
  of adults and elderly, 308-311
  of children, 279
  during lactation, 229-231
  of pregnant women, 222
Nutritional risk, 176, 246
  associated with health problems and
    death, 307
  health consequences of infants at,
    259-260
  during pregnancy, 225-227
Nutritional screening and assessment
  process, 183-185
Nutritional status
  assessment of
    of adults and elderly, 327-333
    alternative approaches to
      consumption measurement
      methods, 187-189
    anthropometric, 191-199
    biochemical, 200-203
    of children, 281-284
    clinical, 189-191
    data collection in, 185
    dietary history methods for, 187
    dietary methodology for, 185-187
    of infants, 260-274, 275
    nutritional screening and,
      183-185
    of pregnant women, 231-237, 245
    and role of community dietitian/
      nutritionist, 203
  national studies on, 174-180
  and physiological changes of aging,
    309
Nutritional value of fast-food, 293
Nutritionist's guide to Washington,
  425-427
Nutritionists, public health, 5

O
Obesity, 10
  in adults and elderly, 316-318
  behavior modification for, 381-382,
    385-386
  and cardiovascular risk factors, 318
  in children, 280
  classification of, 316-317
  and diabetes, 323
  and hypertension, 322
  in infants, 259

Obesity—cont'd
  in pregnant women, 223-225
  in preschool children, 295
    case study of, 120-121
  statistics on, 316, 317
  treatment for, 316
Objective measuring criteria, 123
Objectives
  behavioral, 55
  in community assessment, 54-57
  excess number of, 57, 58
  hierarchy of, 123
  identifying and implementing, 123
  management by, 111
  multiple, 83
  setting, 123
Observational studies, 357
Occupational data, 51
Occupational therapists, 8
OEO; see Office of Economic
    Opportunity
Office of Disease Prevention and
    Health Promotion, 209-210
Office of Economic Opportunity, 392
Office of Management and Budget,
    316, 397, 422
Office of Prevention, Education, and
    Control, 210
Office of Technology Assessment, 158
Older Americans Act, 9, 314, 416
OMB; see Office of Management and
    Budget
Omnibus Budget Reconciliation Act of
    1981, 393, 403-404
Operational definition of variables in
    statistics, 368
Operational efficiency, 84
Operational planning versus strategic
    planning, 38-39, 40
Oral communication, 105
Ordinal scale variables, 364
Organization theory, 33
Organizational change, 34
  management of, 75-76
Organizational conflict and creativity,
    management of; see also
    Conflict; Creativity
  completing action plan, 87-91
  conflict, competition, and
    cooperation, 76-80
  organizational creativity, 80
Organizational design, 74-75, 85
Organizational purpose and mission,
    42-43
Organizations
  communications in, 109-111
  marketing, characteristics of, 83-84
  not-for-profit, 83
  performance in, 28-33
Organized sets of behavior, 31-33

Organizing, 24
  for action, in nutrition services,
      82-91
  basic elements of, 68-70
  for changing environments, 74-75
  division of work in, 68-70
  importance of, 68
Osteoporosis in adults and elderly, 326
OTA; see Office of Technology
      Assessment
Outcome criteria, 137
Outcomes, 123
  of care, for normal infant, 260
  for children, 281
  as measurement of quality, 138
Output, 351
Overabundance, dietary, 9

P

p-Value, 348
PAHO; see Pan American Health
      Organization
Pan American Health Organization, 8
Participation to overcome resistance
      to change, 75, 76
Participative leadership styles, 100,
      102
Partnership for Health Act, 175
Patient care audit, 144-148
Patient Care Audit, 134
Patient/client care criteria for
      nutrition services in health care
      delivery, 138-139
Patient management, guidelines for
  adolescents, 293
  children, 281
  infants, 260
Peace Corps, 392
Pearson product-moment correlation
      coefficient, 370
Pedagogy, 374
Pediatric Nutrition Surveillance
      System, 250-252
Pennsylvania Dietetic Association, 420
Performance
  measurement of, 114
  in organization
      managerial skills and time
          allocation, 29-31
      and roles of manager, 32-33
Performance budgeting, 156-157
Performance level for process and
      outcome criteria, 141
Persuasion, 374
Pert chart, 88, 89
Pharmacists, 8
Phenolphthalein, 313
Phosporus/calcium ratio, 326
Physical examination, 185
  in nutrition surveys, 191
  in nutritional assessment of
      pregnant women, 232

Physical goods versus services, 83
Physical growth of infants, 252-255
Physical therapists, 8
Physicians, 8
Physiological changes
  with aging, 309
  during pregnancy, 221-222
Physiological needs, 95
Physiology of infant nutrition, 253-255
Pickles and Ice Cream: The Complete
      Guide to Nutrition During
      Pregnancy, 339
Placebo program, 117
Planning, 24, 120
  coordination in early stages of, 26
  and decision making in community
      nutrition
      community assessment, 43-60
      decision making, 60-64
      strategic planning, 38-43
  operational, 38-39
  program, 39, 409
  quality assurance in, 137
  strategic, 38-43
Planning grant, 395
Planning process, 40, 41
  strategic market, 84-85
Policies, 137
Policy making, early stages of, 26
Political organizations, community, 49
Politicians, managers as, 28
Population
  distribution by age, 307
  elderly, 305-306
  of interest, in statistics, 368
  targeted in quality assurance
      criteria, 139-140
Population growth, zero, 12
Population study designs, 357
Positive reinforcement, 97
Poverty in adults and elderly, 314-315
Power, 71-72
PPOs; see Preferred payment
      organizations
PPS; see Prospective payment system
A Practical Guide to Values
      Clarification, 42
Precise measurements, 126
Preferred payment organizations, 14
Pregnancy
  anemia of, 226
  megavitamin and vegetarian diets
      during, 225-226
  nutritional counseling in, 162
  nutritional risk factors during,
      225-227
  physiological changes in, 221-222
  RDAs for, 222
  toxemia of, 226-227
  weight gain during, 222-225
Pregnancy Nutrition Surveillance
      System, 220-221

Pregnant women
  daily food guide for, 241, 243
  deficiencies in, 10
  federally supported food assistance
      programs for, 243-246
  health objectives for, 220
  intervention strategies and outcomes
      for, 231
  model criteria for quality assurance
      in ambulatory nutrition care
      for, 239-240
  nutrition counseling for, 237-243
  nutrition education for, 238
  nutrition-related health problems
      of, 220
  nutritional assessment of, 231-237
      anthropometric measurements,
          232-233
      biochemical determinations,
          233-237
      dietary assessment, 236-237
      history in, 232
      intervention guidelines for, 245
      physical examination in, 232
  nutritional needs of, 222
  obesity in, 223-225
Prepared formulas, infant, 257
Prepregnant weight as nutritional risk
      factor, 226
Preschool caregivers, nutrition
      education for, 295
Preschool children and obesity
  case study of, 120-121
  prevalence of, and feeding practices
      for infants, 295
Preschool Nutrition Survey, 9, 176
Prevalence versus incidence, 357
Primary prevention, 361
Priorities and role of managers, 28
Priority matrix, 57-60
Priority setting in community
      assessment, 57-60
Private foundation, 405
Private practice, 337-339
Proactive organization, 74
Problem identification in decision
      making, 61
Problem orientation, 108
Problem solving, integrative, 79-80
Procedures, 137
Proceedings of the Nutrition
      Behavioral Research
      Conference, 385
Process, 123
  as measurement of quality, 138
Process criteria, 137
Process guides, 384
Process theories, 96-97
Productivity
  controlling nutrition services for,
      113-131
  through people, 27

Professional-academic attention to nutrition issues, 415
Professional standards of practice, 137
Professional Standards Review Organizations, 134, 381
Professional Standards Review Procedure Manual, 134
Professionals, managing, as type of conflict, 78-79
Program, 351
Program of Projects, 209
Program administrators, implications of evaluation results for, 128-130
Program criteria for nutrition services in health care delivery, 138-139
Program evaluation; *see* Evaluation
Program planning, 39
  components of, 409
Program Planning and Proposal Writing, 408
Project grant, 395, 397
Project Head Start, 392
Promoting Health—Preventing Disease: Objectives for the Nation, 17, 209-210, 220, 304
Property and financial assistance, 397
Proposal Writing: A Manual and Workbook, 407
Proposals; *see* Grants
Prospective payment system, 418
Prospective studies, 357, 358
Protein intake, 179, 180
Protein requirements
  of adolescents, 289
  of adults and elderly, 310
  of children, 279
  during lactation, 229-231
Protocols, 206
Provider involvement in high blood pressure control, 322-323
PSROs; *see* Professional Standards Review Organizations
Psychological influences on adolescents, 291-293
Psychosocial and neuromuscular development in infants, 255, 297-301
Puberty and height velocity, 286-287, 288
Pubescence, 284
Public environment, 84
Public health nutrition personnel, 6
Public health nutritionists, 5, 6; *see also* Community dietitians/nutritionists
Public Health Service
  grant programs of, 399-402
  Groups Policy Statement, 394-395
  health promotion, health protection, and disease prevention, 209-210

Public Health Service—cont'd
  National Institutes of Health, 210
  Office of Disease Prevention and Health Promotion, 209-210
  regional offices, 401
  report on American health, 12-13
Public Health Service agencies, 399, 400
Public issue marketing, 86-87
Public policy, 414
  related to nutrition, 416-419
Public scrutiny, 83
Publics, multiple, 83
Published diet plans, 318, 319
Punishment, extinction and, 97-98

Q

QIP; *see* Quick Input Program
Quality assurance, 134, 135; *see also* Quality nutrition services
  in ambulatory nutrition care, 135-137
    for adolescents, 294
    for adults and elderly, 333-334
    characteristics of, 135
    for children, 142, 143, 284, 285
    for infants, 142, 143, 278
    measures for, 137-138
    for pregnant women, 239-240
  criteria for, 138-142
  dietetic audits, 148-153
  differentiated from evaluation, 135, 136
  implementing audit for, 144-148
  in inpatient or acute care settings, 148
  in program planning and evaluation, 137
  principles of, 134-135
  selecting population in, 139-140
Quality Assurance Committee of ADA, 134
Quality circles, 101-102
Quality control; *see also* Quality Assurance
  in anthropometric assessment, 195
  Nutrition Surveillance System, 183
Quality nutrition services
  assessment of nutritional status, 183-203
  coordination and referral system, 206-214
  delivering, 174-180
  elements of, 175, 183-214
  monitoring and evaluation in, 214
  national studies on nutritional status, 174-180
  nutrition intervention, 203-206
  nutrition surveillance in, 180-183
  nutrition surveys in United States, 174

Quasiexperimental studies, 118, 357
Questionnaires, food frequency, 186, 187
Quetelet index, 362
Quick Input Program, 352
"Quiet conflict," 78

R

r Coefficient, 370
Randomization, 117-119
Rank-order variables, 364
Ratifying criteria, 141-142
RD; *see* Dietetic registration
RDA; *see* Recommended Daily Dietary Allowances
Reactive organization, 74
Recall for data collection, 186, 187
  in elderly, 329
Reciprocal relationships for coordination, 26
Recommended Daily Dietary Allowances, 188-189
  for adolescents, 288, 289
  for adults and elderly, 310
  comparison of food consumption with, 187
  for infants, 255-256
  during lactation, 222, 229-231
  during pregnancy, 222
Record keeping in behavior modification, 382
Recording/documentation of care, 137
"Reference Collections Operated by the Foundation Center," 406
Reference power, 72
Referencing criteria, 141
Referral, 206, 207, 208
  coordination and, 206-214
    federal programs that support state and local nutrition services, 209-210
    Food Distribution Program, 214
    Food Stamp Program, 211-294
    nutrition information assistance, 206-209
  for food assistance programs, 210-214, 243-246
  for nutritional care
    for adolescents, 294
    for children, 284
    for infants, 277-278, 294-295
    for persons 60 years and older, 335
Referral data bases, 350, 356
Regional intervention strategies for adults and elderly, 337-343
Regional medical libraries, 398
Regional nutrition services, 339-340
Regression, 370
Regression artifacts, 127
Regression equation, 370

Reimbursement for nutrition services, 163-164
Reinforcement, positive, 97
Relationship analysis, 370
Relationship behavior, 103, 104
Relationship-building skills, 378-379
Reliability of measures, 126
  in statistics, 368
Report of Intended Expenditures, 404
Reporting system, statistical, 137
Reproductive performance as
      nutritional risk factor, 225
Research, health and nutrition, 332
Research classification system,
      nutrition, 355
Research grant, 395
Research hypothesis, 364
Research procedures, 363
Research support, biochemical, 394
Resistance by institution to evaluation
      results, 128
Resource allocation decisions, 158, 161
Resource analysis, 85
Resources
  in action plan, 88-90
  review of, in decision making, 63
Response rates of elderly in research
      studies, 332
Responsibility
  in action plan, 90
  of managers, 27
Retrospective studies, 357, 358
Reward power, 72
Riboflavin intake, 180
RIE; see Report of Intended
      Expenditures
Rogers-Shoemaker change process,
      374-375
Role perception, 94
RUMBA characteristics, 140
Rural Development Service, 397

S

Safety and security needs, 95
Sample, 364
Saturated fatty acid intake, program
      for decrease in, 320
Schedule in action plan, 88
School-age children, nutrition
      education for, 296
School Breakfast Program, 277, 294
School Lunch Program, 277, 294, 416
School nutrition programs, 50
Schools, nutrition education in, 50
Scientific management movement,
      98-99
Scientific method, 362-363
Secondary prevention, 361
Security and safety needs, 95
Select committee, 421
Selection for internal validity, 127

Self-disclosure, 379
Self-knowledge, 378
Self-realization needs, 95-96
Self-selection, 119
Service grant, 395
Service programs, evaluation in,
      119-120
Services versus physical goods, 83
Sheppard-Towner Act of 1921, 391
Shopping list, computer-planned, 354
Side effects of program, 126
Single-factor analysis of variance, 369
Single-parent families, 12
Skinfold measurements, 193-195
  of children, 284
  of infants, 271-274
Smoking
  and low birth weight, 220-221
  as nutritional risk factor, 226
Smoothing as manifestation of
      dominance and suppression, 79
Social activity and affection needs, 95
Social influences on food practices,
      243
Social marketing, 86-87
Social marketing plan, 87
Social Security Act, 9, 163, 209, 315,
      391-392
  Amendment of 1963, 416
  Amendment of 1983, 418
Social skills training, 382-383
Social welfare programs, 50-51
Social workers, 8
Societal trends and community
      nutrition programs, 11-15
Society for Nutrition Education, 419
Socioeconomic stratification, 47
Sociological concerns of adults and
      elderly, 314-315
Sodium in food groups, 178
Sodium-free products, 419
Sodium intake, 177, 178
  during pregnancy, 222, 227
Sodium levels, 10
Sodium requirements of adults and
      elderly, 311
Software, 351
Solid food and infants, 259
Special Food Service Program, 294
Special Projects of Regional and
      National Significance, 209
Special Supplemental Food Program
      for Women, Infants and
      Children, 9, 27, 48, 51, 243-
      246, 277-278, 416
  effect of, on birth weight, 247
  eligibility for, 246
  foods included in, 246
  nutrition education in, 246
Specialized services, provision of, 397
Spokesperson, manager as, 32

Spontaneity and communication,
      108-109
Standard deviation, 364
Standard error of estimate, 370
Standards, comparing performance
      against, 114
Stanford University Study, 386
State agencies employing community
      dietitians/nutritionists, 8-10
State Cooperative Extension Services,
      210
State intervention strategies for adults
      and elderly, 337-343
State nutrition services, 340-342
  and federal programs, 209-210
State program information, 165-167,
      168-169
State sources of nutrition information
      assistance, 206-207
State summary of expenditures and
      budget requests, 167, 168
Statistical regression, 127
Statistical reporting system, 137
Statistics
  basic concepts of, 363
  descriptive versus inferential, 363-
      364
  hypotheses in, 364
  population of interest in, 368
  procedures for, 368-370
  variables in, 364-368
Status and esteem needs, 95
Stewart's behavioral change plan, 376
Strategic market planning process,
      84-85
Strategic orientation, 84
Strategic planning
  in not-for-profit organizations,
      39-41
  process of, 41-43
  versus operational planning, 38-39,
      40
Strategy, 38
  in action plan, 88-90
  formulation of, 85
  marketing, 85-86
Strategy-spontaneity, 108-109
Structure as measure of quality, 138
Stuart-Meredith growth charts, 195
Students, nutrition education for, 296
Study and development grant, 395
Subscapular skinfold thickness, 273
Summer Food Service Program, 295
Superiority-equality, 109
Supplementation
  for adults and elderly, 311-312
  calcium, 326
  for infants, 259, 274, 277
  during lactation, 231
  during pregnancy, 222

Support and facilitation to overcome resistance to change, 75, 76
Supportive communication, 108-109
Suppression and dominance in conflict resolution, 79
Surveillance, 51-52
Surveys, 51-52
Swedish Diet and Exercise Program, 387
Sweeteners, artificial, 324
"System 4" organization structure, 74
Systems design, 85
Systems theory, 34

T

t Test, 369
Take Off Pounds Sensibly, 385
Task, 87
Task behavior, 103
Task force in action plan, 88, 90
Task Force on the Assessment of Infant Feeding Practices and Infant Health, 259
Task leadership style, 102, 103
Task planning sheet, 90
Team leadership style, 103
Technical information, dissemination of, 397
Technical skill, 29
Technological change, 33-34
Telephone interviewing in assessment of nutritional status, 187-188
Ten-State Nutrition Survey, 9, 175-176, 200, 314
Tennessee Department of Public Health growth chart guidelines, 199
Tertiary prevention, 361
Testing, 127
Tests, nonparametric, 369-370
Third-party reimbursement, 163-164, 416-417
    influence of, on health care services, 14
Thrifty Food Plan, 336
Time allocation
    to achieve process and outcome criteria, 141
    and managerial skills, 29-31
Time series, 118
Toxemia of pregnancy, 226-227
Training, 397
    for clinic personnel, in weighing and measuring, 193
Training grant, 395
Transportation, 51
Treatment plan in nutrition counseling, 380-381
Triceps skinfold measurement, 193-195, 271-274, 284
Tridimensional leader effectiveness model, 103-104

U

UNICEF; *see* United Nations Children's Emergency Fund
United Hospitals, Inc., 342
United Nations Children's Emergency Fund, 8
U.S. Census data, 44, 47
U.S. Commission on Inter-governmental Relations, 391
U.S. Department of Agriculture, 8, 50
    Daily Food Guide, 379
    Dietary Guidelines for Americans, 10
    Expanded Food and Nutrition Education Program, 210
    food assistance programs, 211
    Nationwide Food Consumption Surveys, 179-180
    Nutrient Data Bank, 351-352
    Thrifty Food Plan, 336
U.S. Department of Health and Human Services, 8, 208, 209
    Dietary Guidelines for Americans, 10
    Health Resources and Services Administration, 208, 209
    Nutrition and Your Health—Dietary Guidelines for Americans, 16
    nutrition problems affecting infants and children, 250
    Public Health Service; *see* Public Health Service
U.S. Senate Committee on Finance, 158
U.S. Senate Committee on Labor and Human Resources, 158
U.S. Senate Select Committee on Nutrition and Human Needs, 175, 356, 414, 415
Unsalted products, 419

V

Valence, 96
Validity
    internal, threats to, 127-128
    of measures, 126, 140
    in statistics, 368
Value drives, 27
Value formation, 42, 122, 125
Value shaping, 80
Values, 42
Variables in statistics, 364-368
Variance, analysis of, 369
Vegetarian diet during pregnancy, 225-226
Vegetarian food guide, 241
Verbal communication skills, 378-379
Verifying criteria, 141
VISTA, 392
Vitamin A intake, 177, 180
Vitamin B$_6$ intake, 180

Vitamin C intake, 177, 180
Vitamin content of diet plans, 319
Vitamin D
    in human milk, 257
    supplementation of, during lactation, 231
Vitamin requirements
    for adolescents, 289-291
    for adults and elderly, 311
    during pregnancy, 231
Vitamin supplements, 312
    for children, 259
Vitamins
    of human relations, 111
    measurement of, 233

W

War on Poverty programs, 392
Water requirements of adults and elderly, 311
Weighing
    of children, 283
    of infants, 260, 270
    training for clinic personnel in, 193
Weight
    for age, 182
    birth, 220
    of children, 281
    for height, 182
        high, 253
    of infants, 260, 262-265
        percentiles for, 266-269
    measurement of, 191
    during pregnancy, 221-222, 223-225, 227
    prepregnant, as nutritional risk factor, 226
    reference data on, 182
Weight control programs
    for adolescents, 296
    crash, 312
    published, 318, 319
Weight Watchers International, 316, 337, 382, 385-386
Weighted intake, 186
White House Conference on Aging, 326-327
White House Conference on Food, Nutrition, and Health, 9, 175, 414
WHO; *see* World Health Organization
WIC; *see* Special Supplemental Food Program for Women, Infants, and Children
Work, division of, 68-70
Workplace, health promotion and disease prevention in, 337, 386-387
World Health Organization, 8

World Health Organization—cont'd
   Expert Committee on Medical
      Assessment of Nutritional
      Status, 189, 190
Written audit system, 137
Written communication, 105-106

Z
ZBB; *see* Zero-based budgeting
Zero-based budgeting, 157
Zero population growth, 12

COMMON ABBREVIATIONS

ABNA	Achievable benefits not achieved
ADA	American Dietetic Association
AHA	American Hospital Association
APHA	American Public Health Association
ASTHO	Association of State and Territorial Health Officials
ASTPHND	Association of State and Territorial Public Health Nutrition Directors
BCHS	Bureau of Community Health Services
CBA	Cost-benefit analysis
CDC	Centers for Disease Control
CDP	Commodity Distribution Program
CEA	Cost-effectiveness analysis
CFDA	Catalog of Federal Domestic Assistance
DGA	Dietary Guidelines for Americans
DRG	Diagnosis-related groups
EFNEP	Expanded Food and Nutrition Education Program
EPSDT	Early and Periodic Screening, Diagnosis, and Treatment
FAO	Food and Agriculture Organization of United Nations
FCC	Federal Communications Commission
FDA	Food and Drug Administration
FSP	Food Stamp Program
FTC	Federal Trade Commission
HCFA	Health Care Financing Administration
HMO	Health Maintenance Organization
ICNND	Interdepartmental Committee on Nutrition for National Defense
IHS	Indian Health Service
IUNS	International Union of Nutritional Science
JCAH	Joint Commission on Accreditation of Hospitals
MCHS	Maternal and Child Health Services
NCI	National Cancer Institute
NET	Nutrition Education and Training Program